MW01593058

Pediatric Hematology/Oncology Series

BONE MARROW TRANSPLANTATION IN CHILDREN

Pediatric Hematology/Oncology Series

Bone Marrow Transplantation in Children
F. Leonard Johnson and Carl Pochedly, Editors; 530 pp., 1990

Developmental and Neonatal Hematology
James A. Stockman III and Carl Pochedly, Editors; 352 pp., 1988

Pediatric Hematology/Oncology Series

Bone Marrow Transplantation in Children

Editors

F. Leonard Johnson, M.D.

Chief, Section of Pediatric
Hematology/Oncology
University of Chicago Medical Center
Professor of Pediatrics
The University of Chicago
Chicago, Illinois

Carl Pochedly, M.D.

Section of Hematology/Oncology
University of Chicago Medical Center
Professor of Clinical Pediatrics
The University of Chicago
Chicago, Illinois

Raven Press 🐦 New York

Raven Press, 1185 Avenue of the Americas, New York, New York 10036

Made in the United States of America

Library of Congress Cataloging-in-Publication Data

Bone marrow transplantation in children / editors, F. Leonard Johnson, Carl Pochedly.
     p. cm. — (Pediatric hematology/oncology series)
    Includes bibliographical references.
    ISBN 0-88167-575-X
    1. Bone marrow—Transplantation. 2. Transportation of organs, tissues, etc. in children. I. Johnson, F. Leonard (Frank Leonard), 1945– . II. Pochedly, Carl. III. Series.
    [DNLM: 1. Bone Marrow—transplantation. 2. Bone Marrow Diseases—in infancy & childhood. 3. Bone Marrow Diseases—therapy. WH 380   B7126]
    RD123.5.B655 1990
    617.4'4—dc20
    DNLM/DLC
    for Library of Congress   89-10729
                                             CIP

9 8 7 6 5 4 3 2 1

*To the children and families whose
courage has taught and inspired us.*

Foreword

In 1949, Jacobson observed that mice could be protected from the otherwise lethal marrow aplasia induced by total body irradiation with the simple maneuver of shielding the spleen (a hematopoietic organ in the mouse). With this observation, he planted the seeds of an ever enlarging forest that has stimulated fundamental investigations into a more detailed understanding of the normal and malignant lymphohematopoietic system, and provided both pediatricians and patients with real hope for curative therapy of otherwise hopeless diseases. What was initiated by a few bold and courageous clinicians has in the past forty years developed into a world-wide subspecialty in clinical bone marrow transplantation.

Drs. Johnson and Pochedly have gathered together an impressive number of pediatric experts who describe for the reader the current status of bone marrow transplantation and the dramatic developments that have occurred in the past forty years.

Appropriately, the first two chapters regarding the history of bone marrow transplantation and the last chapter about the future of bone marrow transplantation are written by Dr. Robert A. Good, a pediatrician with enormous insight and curiosity who bridged the gap between clinical observations of the "experiments of nature," particularly in immunodeficiency diseases, and the further development in the laboratory of a better understanding of the immune system. Subsequent chapters deal in depth with the techniques, supportive care, the rationale and clinical results of marrow transplantation for diseases of marrow failure, genetic immunodeficiency diseases and lysomal storage diseases, and malignancy.

Furthermore, the clinical complications, including the pathological counterparts, are discussed in depth. Approaches to remaining problems are also elucidated.

In summary, this is an excellent book written primarily for the pediatrician with interests in immunology, hematology, and oncology, about the expanding field of bone marrow transplantation.

GEORGE W. SANTOS, M.D.
The Johns Hopkins Oncology Center
Baltimore, Maryland

Preface

"It is of use, from time to time, to take stock, so to speak, of our knowledge of a particular disease, to see exactly where we stand in regard to it, to enquire to what conclusions the accumulated facts seem to point, and to ascertain in what direction we may look for fruitful investigations in the future."

It is time to take stock, not as Osler did of a disease, but of a therapy—marrow transplantation in the treatment of childhood disease. It is 21 years since the first successful allogenic marrow transplant was performed in an infant with severe combined immunodeficiency at the University of Minnesota by a team led by Dr. Robert Good. Beginning as a desperate and experimental approach for patients with end-stage acute leukemia or for multiply transfused, often septic, patients with aplastic anemia, bone marrow transplantation has now become a curative therapy for many patients with a variety of life-threatening immunologic, hematologic, and oncologic pediatric diseases. It also has become clear over this period of time that marrow ablation followed by allogenic transplantation or autologous marrow rescue is often an expensive form of therapy with significant iatrogenic, immunologic, and infectious risks and a therapy that requires a dedicated medical team and an excellent supportive care system.

Where do we stand? When the marrow donor is a family member completely matched at the known loci of the major histocompatibility complex (MHC), allogenic marrow transplantation is the treatment of choice for several nonmalignant diseases, including severe combined or partial immunodeficiency syndromes and osteopetrosis in infants and severe aplastic anemia in children and adolescents. The results of marrow transplantation for thalassemia in Italy have been very encouraging, as have those in the very few patients transplanted for sickle cell anemia. Debate continues, however, about the optimal timing and ethics of marrow transplantation in the hemoglobinopathies. Using hemopoietic cells as a source of enzymes has also proved effective in reversing the enzyme deficiencies in selected patients with metabolic storage disorders, notably metachromatic leukodystrophy and Hurler's syndrome. Information from both human experience and animal models is conflicting, however, particularly in determining the effectiveness of marrow transplantation in preventing or reversing the neurological deterioration associated with these disorders.

In the treatment of malignant disease, few would argue that marrow trans-

Sir William Osler,
Gulstonian Lectures, 1885

plantation from an MHC-matched family member is the treatment of choice in acute lymphoblastic leukemia when a relapse has occurred in therapy, in acute nonlymphoblastic leukemia in first relapse, as well as in Philadelphia chromosome-negative chronic myelogenous leukemia and other myelodysplastic syndromes. As more effective chemotherapy regimens developed, however, optimal timing of marrow transplantation in other patients with leukemia is no longer so obvious. Current conventional wisdom in acute nonlymphoblastic leukemia (ANLL) is that marrow transplantation is indicated in all children with a MHC-matched sibling donor during the first remission. The few studies in children comparing marrow transplantation in first remission with maintenance chemotherapy have demonstrated that marrow transplantation results in a larger number of patients obtaining long-term hematologic remissions. The overall effectiveness of marrow transplantation, however, is blunted by attrition due to the consequences of chronic graft-vs.-host (GVH) disease. No studies have addressed this quality of life issue. As conventional chemotherapy for ANLL improves, the advantages of marrow transplantation (shorter duration of therapy) must be weighed against the potential problems of GVH disease. Perhaps more patients will be cured with less morbidity if marrow transplantation in ANLL is reserved until a first relapse occurs.

A similar situation exists in chronic myelogenous leukemia. This is a rare form of leukemia in children and most information comes from studies in adult patients. These studies demonstrate that the best results are obtained when transplantation is performed during the chronic phase of the disease when approximately 50 to 60 percent of patients obtain long-term continuing complete remissions. This compares to survival rates of 10 to 25% when transplantation is performed during "blast crisis" or in an advanced accelerated phase of the leukemia. What is not clear from these studies is the overall quality of life of these survivors, many of whom (up to 70% in some series) have developed chronic GVH disease. This compounds the ethical dilemma of undertaking a transplant with its substantial risks in a patient who may remain in the chronic phase for several years and whose life may be shortened by transplantation. Other approaches, now being tested, involve treating patients with conventional therapy or interferon and reserving transplantation until the very first sign of acceleration.

Should marrow transplantion be performed in patients with acute lymphoblastic leukemia (ALL) with poor prognostic features at diagnosis? Data from studies, with median follow-up periods of approximately 2 years, suggest that approximately 60% of patients with high-risk ALL, based on high initial white blood cell counts, remain disease-free if transplanted during a first remission. These results are similar to those being obtained with intensive chemotherapeutic approaches. Marrow transplantation in first remission, however, does appear to be indicated in children with leukemias of mixed phenotype or associated with certain chromosomal abnormalities, such as the Philadelphia chromosome-positive ALL, for whom effective chemotherapeutic approaches are still not available.

Relapse remains a continuing problem following transplants for leukemia and the most effective cytotoxic preparative regimens remain to be defined. Infants being treated by marrow transplantation for leukemia with regimens involving total body irradiation (TBI) face the additional problems of marked growth retardation and potentially serious neuropsychological sequelae. In this age group, we must meet the challenge of developing radiation-free conditioning regimens which, particularly in ALL, effectively prevent central nervous system relapse.

Infection still accounts for a considerable morbidity and mortality, especially in allogenic marrow transplantation. The use of prophylactic measures including laminar airflow insulation, intravenous gammaglobulin, acyclovir, and other prophylactic antibiotics remain unproved. However, a major advance over the past decade has been the demonstration that pneumonia due to cytomegalovirus (CMV), the major killer following marrow transplantation in the early 1970s, can be prevented in the setting of a patient who is CMV-negative, whose donor is CMV-negative, and when transfusion support is provided exclusively with CMV-negative blood products.

What options are available for the patient who does not have a MHC-matched family donor? The role of mismatched marrow transplantation, either from a partially matched family member or a MHC-matched unrelated individual, is still not established, as is illustrated by the sparse amount of information presented in the relevant chapters of this book. The success rate in these transplants has been disappointingly low, particularly in aplastic anemia, principally because of the increased morbidity and mortality from GVH disease and, less commonly, post-transplant lymphoproliferative syndromes. T cell depletion, although a logical approach to prevent GVH disease and to enable mismatched marrow transplantation, has been frustrated by an increased incidence of graft failure and relapse in transplants for leukemia.

The effectiveness of myeloablative cytotoxic therapy and autologous marrow rescue in the acute leukemias and selected malignant solid tumors is also being investigated as a means of circumventing the problem of lack of donors. To purge or not to purge? With what to purge? and What are the most effective cytotoxic preparative regimens? These are questions that still have not been answered. Interpreting the results following use of autologous marrow transplantation in the acute leukemias in studies done so far has been made difficult, if not impossible, by the different chemotherapy regimens used pre-transplant, the different preparative regimens, different durations between remission and transplant, various purging techniques (if purging is used at all) and the use of single or double transplants.

Finally, as we enter the third decade of pediatric marrow transplantation, we are now starting to see the extent of the problem of late effects following bone marrow transplantation. Fortunately, the majority of late effects appear to be transient in children who do not require radiation therapy as part of their preparative regimen. In contrast, children who require total body irradiation show a substantial incidence of endocrine problems.

Despite the unanswered questions and continuing challenges like those raised above or addressed in this book, progress in marrow transplantation over this relatively short period of 21 years has been remarkable. In 1966, D. E. Pegg concluded in the first monograph on marrow transplantation, "It is now abundantly clear that allogenic hemopoietic cell infusions are not yet established as a practical procedure in clinical medicine . . . the availability of hemopoietic stem cell infusions should not be used to justify extreme therapeutic measures which would otherwise certainly be fatal. A fatal outcome may not be averted, the tumor regression will certainly be disappointing, the patient's discomfort may be extreme and, finally, there is the danger of secondary disease to contend with." Two decades later, GVH disease with its attendant immunologic and infectious complications remains the major impediment to future success in allogeneic transplantation. There can be no doubt, however, that marrow transplantation is now a practical procedure in clinical medicine.

The literature on bone marrow transplantation is expanding rapidly and preparation of this book has required the combined efforts of many investigators, who represent many different areas of expertise. In a multiauthored book such as this one, then, divergent opinions are unavoidable and readers must be critical in formulating their own views.

We hope, that this book will serve as a practical guide for the present state of marrow transplantation in children and help determine the direction of fruitful investigations.

F. Leonard Johnson, M.D.
Carl Pochedly, M.C.
The University of Chicago
Chicago, Illinois

Acknowledgments

Publication of this book was supported in part by educational grants from **Cutter Biologicals** (Miles, Inc.), **Roche Laboratories,** and **Sandoz Pharmaceutical Corporation.**

We are grateful to Mable Pochedly, who provided vital assistance in corresponding with authors and the publisher, as well as in copyediting and proofreading of manuscripts. John Molyneux and Dorothea Dixon of Raven Press were most helpful and supportive throughout the planning and production of this book.

Contents

Contributors

Inga A. Aksamit, R.N., *Division of Bone Marrow Transplantation, Pacific Presbyterian Medical Center, Clay at Buchanan Street, San Francisco, California 94120*

Robert Ash, M.D., *Bone Marrow Transplantation Program, Milwaukee County Medical Center and Department of Medicine, Medical College of Wisconsin, Milwaukee Wisconsin 53201*

Kumar G. Belani, M.D., *Department of Anesthesiology, University of Minnesota Medical School, Minneapolis, Minnesota 55455*

Joel H. Berg, D.D.S., M.S., *Department of Pediatric Dentistry, University of Texas Dental Branch at Houston, Texas 77225*

Robert J. Berkowitz, D.D.S., *Department of Pediatric Dentistry, Children'sHospital National Medical Center, 111 Michigan Avenue, Washington, D.C. 20010*

William E. Beschorner, M.D., *Departments of Pathology and Oncology, The Johns Hopkins University School of Medicine, Baltimore, Maryland 21205*

Bruce Blazar, *University of Minnesota Medical School, Minneapolis, Minnesota 55455*

Nancy Bunin, M.D., *Division of Oncology, Children's Hospital of Philadelphia, and Department of Pediatrics, University of Pennsylvania, School of Medicine, Philadelphia, Pennsylvania*

Bruce Camitta, M.D., *Midwest Children's Cancer Center, Department of Pediatrics, Medical College of Wisconsin, Milwaukee, Wisconsin 53201*

James T. Casper, M.D., *Midwest Children's Cancer Center, Department of Pediatrics, Medical College of Wisconsin and Bone Marrow Transplantation Program, Children's Hospital of Wisconsin, 1700 W. Wisconsin, Milwaukee, Wisconsin 53201*

Pi-Nian Chang, Ph.D., *Department of Pediatrics, University of Minnesota Medical School, Minneapolis, Minnesota 55455*

Sandor Feldman, M.D., *Division of Infectious Diseases, Department of Pediatrics, University of Mississippi, 500 State Street, School of Medicine, Jackson, Mississippi 39216*

Gerald A. Ferretti, D.D.S., *School of Dentistry, University of Kentucky, Lexington, Kentucky 40506*

A. H. Filipovich, M.D., *Bone Marrow Transplantation Program, University of Minnesota Hospitals, 420 Delaware Street, S.E., and Division of Immunology, Department of Pediatrics, University of Minnesota Medical School, Minneapolis, Minnesota 55455*

John A. Fort, M.D., *Division of Hematology/Oncology, Children's Hospital National Medical Cancer Center, 111 Michigan Avenue, Washington, D.C. 20010*

Wayne L. Furman, M.D., *Department of Hematology/Oncology, St. Jude Children's Research Hospital, 332 North Lauderdale, Memphis, Tennessee 38101, and Department of Pediatrics, University of Tennessee College of Medicine, Memphis, Tennessee 38163*

Robert A. Good, M.D., Ph.D., *Department of Pediatrics, University of South Florida and All Children's Hospital, 801 Sixth Street, St. Petersburg, Florida 33701*

John Graham-Pole, M.D., *Division of Pediatric Hematology/Oncology, J. Hillis Miller Health Center, and Department of Pediatrics, College of Medicine, University of Florida, Gainesville, Florida 32610*

Richard Hong, M.D., *Departments of Pediatrics and Medical Microbiology, Center for Health Sciences, University of Wisconsin-Madison, Madison, Wisconsin 53792*

Willim Krivit, M.D., Ph.D., *Division of Pediatric Hematology/Oncology, University of Minnesota Variety Club Children's Hospital, and Department of Pediatrics, University of Minnesota Medical School, Minneapolis, Minnesota 55455*

Carl Lenarsky, M.D., *Division of Research Immunology and Bone Marrow Transplantation, Children's Hospital of Los Angeles, Los Angeles, California 90054-0700, and Department of Pediatrics, University of Southern California, School of Medicine, Los Angeles, California 90007*

David D. F. Ma, M.D., *Department of Hematology, Royal North Shore Hospital, St. Leonards, New South Wales, Australia 2065*

James S. Miser, M.D., *Division of Pediatric Hematology/Oncology, Mayo Clinic, Department of Pediatrics, Mayo Medical School, Rochester, Minnesota 55905*

Steven M. L. Neudorf, M.D., *Division of Hematology/Oncology, Children's Hospital Medical Center, Department of Pediatrics, College of Medicine, University of Cincinnati, Cincinnati, Ohio 45229*

Robertson Parkman, M.D., *Division of Research Immunology/Bone Marrow Transplantation, Children's Hospital of Los Angeles, Los Angeles, California 90027, and Departments of Pediatrics and Microbiology, University of Southern California, Los Angeles, California 90007*

Terry E. Pick, M.D., *Bone Marrow Transplant Services, Cook-Fort Worth Children's Hospital, 1212 W. Lancaster Avenue, Fort Worth, Texas 76102, and Department of Pediatrics, University of Texas Southwestern Medical Center at Sallas, 52-323 Harry Hines, Dallas, Texas 75235*

Daniel W. Pietryga, M.D., *Division of Hematology/Oncology, Children's Hospital Medical Center, and Department of Pediatrics, College of Medicine, University of Cincinnati, Cincinnati, Ohio 45229*

Norma K. C. Ramsay, M.D., *Pediatric Bone Marrow Transplantation Program, University of Minnesota Hospitals, and Department of Pediatrics, University of Minnesota Medical School, Minneapolis, Minnesota 55455*

Shahrokh Safarimaryaki, M.D., *Division of Pediatric Hematology/Oncology, The University of Texas Health Science Center, 7703 Floyd Curl Drive San Antonio, Texas 78284*

Jean E. Sanders, M.D., *Division of Oncology, Fred Hutchinson Cancer Research Center, Seattle, Washington, 98104, Children's Orthopedic Hospital and Medical Center, and Department of Pediatrics and Medicine, University of Washington, School of Medicine, Seattle, Washington 98104*

George Santos, M.D., *Bone Marrow Transplant Unit, The Johns Hopkins University School of Medicine, Baltimore, Maryland 21205*

Elsa Shapiro, Ph.D., *Department of Ophthalmology, University of Minnesota Medical School, Minneapolis, Minnesota 55455*

Dale Snover, M.D., *Department of Pathology, University of Minnesota Medical School, Minneapolis, Minnesota 55455*

Paul M. Sondel, M.D., Ph.D., *Departments of Pediatrics, Human Oncology, and Genetics, Center for Health Sciences, University of Wisconsin-Madison, Madison, Wisconsin 53792*

Jeffrey Sosman, M.D., *Department of Human Oncology, Center for Health Sciences, University of Wisconsin-Madison, Madison, Wisconsin, 53792*

Wayne E. Spruce, M.D., *Division of Hematology/Oncology, Bone Marrow Transplantation Program, Children's Hospital and Health Center, 8001 Frost Street, San Diego, California 92123; and Department of Basic and Clinical Research, Scripps Clinic and Research Foundation, La Jolla, California*

C. Gail Summers, M.D., *Department of Ophthalmology, University of Minnesota Medical School, Minneapolis, Minnesota 55455*

Michael E. Trigg, M.D., *Department of Pediatrics, University of Iowa, School of Medicine, and Pediatric Bone Marrow Transplantation Program, University of Iowa Hospitals and Clinics, Iowa City, Iowa 52242*

Robert Truitt, Ph.D., *Transplantation Immunology Laboratory, Midwest Children's Cancer Center, Children's Hospital of Wisconsin, Milwaukee, Wisconsin 53201*

Roger A. Vega, M.D., *Department of Pediatrics, Emory University School of Medicine and Bone Marrow Transplant Service, Henrietta Egleston Hospital for Children, 2040 Ridgewood Drive, N.E., Atlanta, Georgia 30322*

John E. Wagner, M.D., *Departments of Oncology and Pediatrics, The Johns Hopkins University, School of Medicine, Baltimore, Maryland 21205*

Kenneth I. Weinberg, M.D., *Division of Research Immunology/Bone Marrow Transplantation, Children's Hospital of Los Angeles, Los Angeles, California 90027 and Department of Pediatrics, University of Southern California School of Medicine, Los Angeles, California 90007*

Howard J. Weinstein, M.D., *Department of Pediatrics, Harvard Medical School, Pediatric Bone Marrow Transplant Unit, The Children's Hospital Medical Center, and the Dana-Farber Cancer Institute, Boston, Massachusetts 02115*

Chester B. Whitley, M.D., Ph.D., *Department of Pediatrics and Institute of Human Genetics, University of Minnesota Medical School, Minneapolis, Minnesota 55455*

Thomas E. Williams, M.D., *Division of Pediatric Hematology/Oncology, The University of Texas Health Science Center, 7703 Floyd Curl Drive, San Antonio, Texas 78284*

Gregory A. Yanik, M.D., *Department of Hematology/Oncology, Children's Hospital Medical Center, Cincinnati, Ohio 45229*

Andrew M. Yeager, M.D., *Department of Oncology and Pediatrics, The Johns Hopkins University, School of Medicine, Baltimore, Maryland 21205*

Axel R. Zander, M.D., *Division of Bone Marrow Transplantation, Pacific Presbyterian Medical Center, Clay at Buchanan Street, San Francisco, California 94120*

Bone Marrow Transplantation in Children, edited by F. Leonard Johnson and Carl Pochedly. Raven Press, Ltd., New York © 1990.

History. I. Early Studies in Transplantation Biology: Discovery of Two Separate Systems of Immunity

Robert A. Good

Department of Pediatrics, University of South Florida, St. Petersburg, Florida 33701

INTRODUCTION

Bone marrow transplantation has become a most useful approach to treatment of life-threatening human diseases. Indeed, it is now possible to cure more than 60 otherwise lethal diseases by treatments using bone marrow transplantation. As the methods and techniques used in bone marrow transplantation are refined and simplified, this powerful modality to therapy promises to become an even more important basis for treatment of an increasing number of human diseases.

To give perspective to the great progress that has been made, it seems important to reflect briefly on the events leading to the first successful allogeneic bone marrow transplantation carried out in Minnesota. This transplant resulted in the cure of an otherwise uniformly fatal disease, severe combined immunodeficiency disease (SCID) (1). Indeed, that very first patient and other patients in the vanguard who have been cured by bone marrow transplantation are now coming of age, that is, age 21, and their contributions to medical progress should be marked.

The Minnesota component of this story began in 1938 when Fred Kolouch accidentally discovered that anaphylactic shock in small rabbits could induce plasmacytosis in bone marrow and other lymphoid tissues (2). Kolouch had developed an interest in anaphylaxis as a medical student. In his study of hematology with Hal Downey at Minnesota, he observed plasmacytosis of blood and bone marrow in a patient who was suffering from serum sickness due to anti-tetanus antibody treatment (3). Kolouch's interest in a possible association of disease with plasma cells in the blood and tissues increased when he became aware of two Scandinavian investigators' interpretation of an experiment of nature represented by agranulocytosis (4,5). In this disorder, Bing and Plum had linked hyperglobulinemia and bone marrow plasmacytosis in several patients with aplastic anemia.

Kolouch successfully developed a model system for producing plasmacytosis in rabbits which were injected repeatedly with killed streptococcal vaccine. He presented a master's degree thesis that contained a description of his experiments and his extensive analysis of the literature dating back to 1895. He concluded that plasma cells were inextricably linked to immunization, infection, immunity and serum globulin formation (2,6,7). In his view, plasma cells that are derived from stem cells in the bone marrow (reticulum stem cells), from lymphocytes, or both, represented the cellular elements that produce antibody (2–4). Kolouch finished medical school and became a surgeon, but remained captivated by his earlier observations on lymphocytes and plasma cells and was seeking a way to pursue these pressing leads.

Thus, it was quite natural that Kolouch recognized that I, as a student training in virology and neurophysiology, might be able to explore further the cellular basis of immunity. My initiation as an experimental and clinical immunologist occurred when Kolouch told me about his analyses which suggested that plasma cells produce antibodies. He also raised his concerns as to whether it was the physiological events set in motion during anaphylaxis or the events that followed antigenic stimulation which led to production of antibodies that were responsible for the plasmacytosis he associated with anaphylactic shock (2–4).

To answer this question, I designed a simple experiment. Plasmacytosis was generated in marrow and lymphatic tissues during active anaphylaxis, following a second exposure to antigen. This plasmacytosis was compared to the bone marrow and lymphatic tissue changes that occurred following passive anaphylaxis, involving a single exposure to antigen. The results of this experiment were clear. Passive anaphylaxis did not lead to significant plasmacytosis, but active anaphylaxis did (8). A logical interpretation of these findings was that secondary exposure to an antigen generated much antibody and also produced impressive plasmacytosis, but primary exposure to antigen generated little antibody and induced only little plasmacytosis. In numerous subsequent experiments, I was able to link plasma cell formation to antigenic stimulation with a number of antigens in different species of animals and in many different tissues, including the brain (9–11). The number of bone marrow plasmacytes could be correlated with the slope of the curve of gamma-globulin accumulation in the serum following streptococcal infections, which led to occurrence of rheumatic fever (12). During this period of my studies, I became aware of the work which Merrill Chase had done at the Rockefeller Institute in collaboration with Landsteiner (13). He had shown that delayed hypersensitivity could be passively transferred by lymphoid cells from one guinea pig to another, but that this type of allergy was not passively transferable by serum or circulating antibody in such animals. Although Chase was not very receptive to Kolouch's and my concepts that plasma cells were the factories for antibody production, his experiments separated sharply delayed allergic reactions that were dependent on cells from circulating antibodies and linked the skin reactions in guinea pigs to the lymphocytes.

Multiple Myeloma and Hodgkin's Disease.

In the course of studying myeloma proteins obtained from patients with multiple myeloma, a plasma cell disease (14), and of studying C-reactive protein in patients with Hodgkin's disease (15), I recognized, rather accidentally at first and later showed in detailed experiments, that patients with different malignancies had very different immunodeficiencies. These immunodeficiencies led to different complicating infections. Thus, patients with myeloma, who had a profound antibody deficiency syndrome, suffered from repeated infections with pneumococci, *Hemophilus influenza,* streptococci and sometimes pseudomonas. All of these agents are potentially highly virulent encapsulated bacterial pathogens. By contrast, patients with Hodgkin's disease had different opportunistic infections that featured recurrent fungus infections, virus infections and often intracellular infections with bacteria of lower virulence (16,17).

We and others later showed that patients suffering from each of these two separate forms of cancer had very different immunological deficits (18). Those with myeloma could not make antibodies and had very low concentrations of normal immunoglobulins in their blood. They also had spikes of myeloma protein, which reflected the monoclonal gammopathy (14). By contrast, patients with Hodgkin's disease had normal or slightly raised levels of immunoglobulin and produced antibody well. But patients with Hodgkin's disease were anergic, had gross deficiencies of expression of delayed allergic reactions, and rejected homografts poorly (19–21). Their cell-mediated immunities were deficient. Myeloma was obviously a disease that involved plasma cells, while Hodgkin's disease was clearly a disease that involved lymphocytes. It was later recognized that Hodgkin's disease involved only certain lymphocyte subpopulations.

Agammaglobulinemia

In 1952, my reflections on these secondary immunodeficiency diseases were in the early stages of clarification. I tried to separate the immunological functions that are associated with antibodies and plasma cells on the one hand from the immunological functions that are associated with the cell-mediated immunities and lymphocytes, later attributed to T cells. Then we encountered another extraordinary challenge. Bruton (22) described for the first time a child with agammaglobulinemia. This 8-year-old boy suffered from repeated infections, could make no antibodies, and lacked gammaglobulin in his blood. As luck would have it, we had three such patients in our hospital at the time Bruton's paper was published. Each of these patients with X-linked agamma-globulinemia (1) lacked gammaglobulin in their blood, (2) could not make antibody at all after primary, secondary or tertiary stimulation with several of the most potent antigens available, (3) did not have plasma cells, and (4) could not develop plasma cells even in response to the most intensive anti-genic stimulation (23–26). In striking contrast, each patient had a normal capacity to develop delayed allergies to a variety of fungal antigens and bacte-rial antigens. Each also could be sensitized readily to 2–4 dinitrofluoroben-zine (25). These patients had normal numbers of lymphocytes. They not only lacked ability to produce plasma cells but also they did not have germinal centers in their lymph nodes (23,25,27). We later showed that they had a normal thymus (28).

Life for these patients consisted of one pneumococcal, hemophilus, strepto-coccal, meningococcal or pseudomonas infection after another. They always required antibiotics to cure their infections. By contrast, these patients showed normal resistance to certain viral infections, like measles and chicken pox, yet they had an unusual susceptibility to paralytic poliomyelitis (23,25,29,30). They seemed to have no problems with tuberculosis, fungal infections, atypical mycobacterial infections, or infections with lower-grade bacterial pathogens. Thus, like the patients with multiple myeloma, patients with X-linked agammaglobulinemia suffered from an antibody deficiency syn-drome but possessed intact cell-mediated immunity (25,29,30). We realized that these patients with X-linked agammaglobulinemia demonstrated that there are 2 major immunologic components of defense against microbes. On one hand, there were the high-grade encapsulated bacterial pathogens against which the defense was by antibodies, and on the other hand, there were the lower-grade, not so virulent bacterial pathogens, viruses and fungi against which the defense was lymphocytes (30).

These patients also helped us divide the lymphoid cell system into two separate compartments. Agammaglobulinemic patients had no plasma cells and could not develop plasma cells or germinal centers, but otherwise their lymphoid cell populations seemed to develop quite normally. We looked upon the agammaglobulinemic patients as well as the myeloma and Hodgkin's disease patients as representing extraordinary experiments of nature who were teaching us fundamental truths about the immune systems. Thus, with the help of these patients, we were able to speak of two microbial universes, two separate and distinct immunity systems and even two separate universes of viruses. These patients were susceptible to paralytic polio virus infection and hepatitis B infection and later were shown also to develop severe infections with echoviruses. However, they resisted and became immune to measles and chickenpox without being able to produce significant antibody responses to either. Although in one agammaglobulinemic patient, a skin graft was retained for a very long period (31), rejection of skin grafts, especially second-set skin grafts, proved to be quite vigorous in most agammaglobulinemic patients and was usually comparable to that of normal persons.

We thus began to speak quite confidently of there being two immunity systems; one subserving antibody production and the other subserving cell-mediated immunity, including delayed allergies. By their very nature, these patients, of course, at first had represented a potential major challenge to our concept that plasma cells produce antibodies. By then, this concept had been supported by the classical research of Fagraeus (32) with production of antibody in plasma cell-rich tissue cultures. The concept was also supported by the immunofluorescence microscopic studies of Coons and his colleagues (33–35). Agammaglobulinemic patients possessed no plasma cells at all and they lacked gammaglobulins, antibodies and antibody responses. Thus, these patients represented a powerful support to our concept (19,36) now espoused by several others, that plasma cells are the very cellular factories of antibody production (37,38).

Therefore, as an experiment of nature, the study of agammaglobulinemic patients made major contributions to understanding of the immune systems. These agammaglobulinemic patients showed that patients with primary immunodeficiency diseases are great teachers of immunology (19,23,25).

DISCOVERY OF THE BIOLOGIC FUNCTION OF THE THYMUS

The occurrence in the same patient of a thymoma and a broadly based immunodeficiency (23,25,39,41) also guided our thinking and our hands. In 1952, an unusual patient appeared in our clinic. Life for this patient over the prior 8 years had been a succession of severe lift-threatening infections. His microbial susceptibilities, however, like those of agammaglobulinemic children, were found to be associated with numerous episodes of infections that included several occurrences of pneumococcal pneumonia and also viral and fungal infections (39–41).

We found this patient to have a severe deficiency of allograft immunity. He failed to develop or express delayed allergies normally; his bone marrow and lymph nodes were virtually devoid of plasma cells and germinal centers. In addition to this increased susceptibility to infection, the patient had a huge thymoma, weighing 540 grams, located in the mediastinum. On biopsy, this enormous mass proved to be a benign stromal epithelial thymoma. Surgical removal of this thymoma did not correct the patient's immunodeficiency, but it caused us to rethink what the thymus was all about (38–40).

In this case, a distinct thymus abnormality occurred in a patient suffering from a broadly based life-threatening immunodeficiency, from which he ultimately died after he contracted hepatitis. This occurrence provoked us to begin extensive studies of the biological functions of the thymus. The experiments thus launched led us to discover a crucial function of the thymus in developmental immunobiology. To explore the relationship between the thymic tumor and the broadly based immunodeficiency in our patient, in 1955 we began to extirpate the thymus in baby rabbits 4–5 weeks old (41). We were disappointed that thymectomy did not produce any readily identifiable immunodeficiency in our rabbits. However, we still believed that our patient with the thymoma was somehow trying to teach us an important lesson in immunobiology (39,40).

Bursa of Fabricius

In 1957 I became aware, through discussions with Harold Wolfe of Wisconsin, of experiments carried out at Ohio State University. In 1955–1956, Glick, a graduate student was working with Knouff in the anatomy department at Ohio State. Knouff asked Glick to determine the function of the bursa described by Fabricius, the 16th century anatomist. Glick proceeded to carry out many studies to try to discover the function of the organ.

He had made little progress with this project when he was assigned to give a class demonstration of an antibody test. Glick had previously carried out this exercise, and so he asked a fellow graduate student, Chang, to immunize the chickens for the class demonstration. Chang, not fully receptive to Glick's emphasis on the importance of the bursa project, had taken for normal the very chickens which Glick had bursectomized while in the newly hatched period. When the class demonstration failed because bursectomized chickens that could not produce antibody had been used, Glick and Chang recognized the significance of their serendipitous discovery.

After several additional experiments had been carried out, they wrote a paper entitled, "The role of the bursa of Fabricius in development of antibody production in chickens." In this article, also published with Jaap, they showed that removal of the bursa of Fabricius in newly hatched chickens does indeed prevent development of ability to produce antibodies. When they submitted their paper describing these important experiments to *Science,* the paper was refused because "the results were of insufficient general interest." Eventually this seminal discovery defining the crucial role of the bursa of Fabricius, was published in a journal called *Poultry Science* (42). Of course, being published in this journal, the paper was missed by most immunologists.

Harold Wolfe's life work, or at least a large part of it, was embodied in 23 papers on "precipitin production in chickens." Thus, he had ready access to the paper of Glick and appreciated its importance. Using elegant methodologies, Wolfe and his students confirmed and extended the crucial contribution of Glick. When Wolfe learned that I was working on the genetics and origins of antibody production, he called me and shared his findings with me (43).

When Wolfe mentioned that the Ohio State researchers had discovered an important function of the bursa of Fabricius early in life, their finding rang a consonant note in Minneapolis. My teacher of hematology, Hal Downey, a comparative hematologist, had taught me that the bursa of Fabricius had a developmental history, histogenesis and morphology very suggestive of that of the thymus. Indeed, as early as 1911, Jolly (44,45) had done comparative studies on the development and involution of both the thymus and the bursa of Fabricius. He concluded that the bursa of Fabricius of birds was very similar to the thymus (44,45), and thus called the bursa the cloacal thymus.

These suggestions were enough to recommend to me that we resume our research on thymic function and extend it to removing the thymus as early in life as possible, even in the first hours of life. This we did, and by so doing showed that removal of the thymus in the immediate neonatal period in rabbits and mice dramatically inhibited development of both humoral antibody responses and all the so-called cell-mediated immunities (46).

Publication of these findings established the priority of my laboratory in the thymus discovery. Indeed, we had previously reported our suspicion that the thymus possessed important immunological functions from our encounter with the patient with the thymic tumor (41).

By the summer of 1961, we had done all the critical experiments in mice and rabbits to establish that neonatal thymectomy inhibits skin graft rejection, ability to initiate graft-vs.-host reaction, and ability to produce many antibody responses. We submitted our first completed reports for publication in 1962 (46–49). Thus, from our own research alone, we could be confident that the thymus exerts a crucial influence on development of all the cell-mediated immunities and also plays an important role in antibody production (49). We then launched numerous additional investigations of the crucial functions of the thymus and bursa in ontogenetic and phylogenetic perspective (50–54).

All of the studies mentioned above were either under way or had been completed by the time Miller reported the findings of his research. Miller approached the issue from an entirely different perspective, that is, from the research done by Jacob Furth on preventing leukemia by neonatal thymic extirpation in AKR mice. He presented experiments defining the biologic role of the thymus in developmental immunology (55,56), and thus had independently shown that neonatal extirpation of the thymus inhibits development of immunity in mice. He had been working on the role of thymic extirpation on the development of leukemia (57,58) and independently discovered that neonatal thymectomy in mice inhibits both graft rejection and antibody production. His article, published in *The Lancet* in 1961 (55), hit the scientific community like a bombshell and almost buried our parallel findings, even though we clearly had established priority and presented an equally clear definition of the consequences of neonatal thymic extirpation. In our phylogenetic studies we showed that the thymus first appeared in the lowest vertebrates, in conjunction with the first appearance of adaptive immunity. It was also clear that all vertebrates phylogenetically distal to the lowest vertebrates in which the thymus first appeared had a thymus. This finding established that thymic function comprised a critical survival advantage (59–61).

Soon thereafter, Parrott (62) and Waksman (63), the latter emphasizing especially the role of the thymus in development of cell-mediated immunities in rats, reported confirmatory experiments. A first golden era of the thymus was at hand (64).

Two Separate Lymphoid Systems

In 1962, a conference was held in Minneapolis which was designed to bring together all the competitors for credit for the discovery of thymic function. They were asked to describe their findings and to participate in an analysis of thymic function. The participants reviewed all of the crucial results in phylogeny, ontogeny and pathology which established the existence of separate central compartments, where immunity systems developed, and peripheral compartments, where lymphoid cells carried out their important functions (64).

In addition, two new directions were indicated. First, Warner and Szenberg (65) from Australia presented studies in chickens which suggested that the bursa controlled development of the antibody-producing cells. They showed that the thymus functioned primarily to develop cells involved in delayed allergic reactions (65). This conclusion electrified the conference. However, we saw a slightly different interpretation, since these studies had placed capacity to initiate graft-vs.-host reactions and capacity to exercise graft rejection in a category separate from that encompassing the cell-mediated immunities (66). Another important finding caused much less of a stir at the conference. Claman and others, in discussions, proposed that the cells of the thymus may be able to work together in cooperation with antibody-producing cells of bone marrow origin to produce truly vigorous antibody responses (67). Thus, it already could be suggested that "it takes two to tango" (68).

These two sets of findings convinced me that we should continue to pursue greater understanding of the influences of the thymus and of the bursa of Fabricius, until we could better define the cells and functions that developed in each of these central lymphoid organs. Which cell populations were trained in the thymus, and how did these populations function as immunological systems?

We wanted to look critically at these issues because the clinical case studies had provided us with a fairly clear concept of which major immunological processes were related to one another, and which were influenced together, and which of the immune cells and processes were dissociated from one another. I enlisted help from my colleagues and students in this line of research.

After some discussion, I turned to Max Cooper. Cooper paired with Ray Peterson and they were determined to learn approaches that could be used to address the central lymphoid organs: the bursa and thymus of the chicken. Cooper decided to use bursectomy, thymectomy or both to try to sort out the development of the cellular compartmentalization of the immunity systems.

Five years earlier, in studying the patients already described, I had already indicated my belief that two separate immunity systems exist: one responsible for antibody production and one that subserved cell-mediated immunities (19). In 1963, Cooper and Peterson, in my laboratory, carried out what proved to be truly definitive experimental studies in chickens to put this clinically derived insight on more solid experimental grounds. They studied chickens given near-lethal total body irradiation coupled with extirpation of the bursa of Fabricius, thymectomy, or both. These experiments were dramatically successful.

We found that when newly hatched chicks were subjected to thymectomy and near-lethal total body irradiation, a thymus-dependent lymphocyte population was depleted in the birds (69,70). This was shown to be located in the dense, nonfollicular lymphocyte population in the spleen. Therefore, another lymphoid system comprised of the germinal follicles and plasma cells throughout the body, was left essentially intact. Therefore, if the newly hatched chicks were given near-lethal total body irradiation, and if the bursa of Fabricius instead of the thymus had been extirpated at that time, all the plasma cells and all cells of the germinal centers were eliminated from development. However, the thymus and those thymus-dependent lymphoid accumulations developed quite normally.

Functionally, the irradiated-bursectomized chickens became agammaglobulinemic and could not make antibodies, but they reacted quite normally in cell-mediated immune functions. These chickens could reject allografts and could develop delayed allergies, and their spleen cells could initiate graft-vs.-host reactions. Chickens that had been irradiated and thymectomized accepted allografts, but did not develop delayed allergies, and they had lymphoid cells which did not initiate graft-vs.-host reactions. The irradiated, thymectomized chickens had immunoglobulins and could produce some antibodies. In studying such chickens, it became clear that there were two distinct and separate immunity systems, a thymus-*dependent* system and a thymus-*independent* system. These 2 systems subserved separate but interlocking immunological functions (69,70).

Van Alten, a professional embryologist collaborating with Cooper and Peterson in our laboratory, then showed that total body irradiation was not an absolutely essential component of the model that dissected the immunity systems into 2 separate compartments. Chicks were operated upon *in ovo* and, several days prior to hatching. Either the bursa, the thymus, or both of these central lymphoid organs were removed as completely as possible and the chicks were also given total body irradiation (71). By doing so it was shown that development of either one of the two separate lymphoid systems, or both together, could be thwarted. These experiments, taken together with the findings observed in the agammaglobulinemic children and in the patients with Hodgkin's disease or multiple myeloma, firmly established the existence of 2 separate and distinct lymphoid systems. Each of these systems was shown to have a separate and distinct central lymphoid organ. In chickens, the 2 systems have as their central lymphoid organ the thymus or the bursa of Fabricius, each with a dependent cell population.

In our laboratories, use of neonatal thymectomy alone, or irradiation and thymectomy, clarified this issue for mice, rats, hamsters and rabbits. Thus the same principles applied for all mammals. Later, Cooper and his associates working in London showed that the fetal liver can, at least in part, subserve the same function in humans as does the bursa in chickens (72).

Later, Paavo and Auli Toivanen confirmed that at a particular interval in development, nearly all the precursors of B lymphocytes are localized to the bursa, but this situation exists only for a brief time early in ontogeny (73–75). Later in ontogeny, the precursors of antibody-producing cells reside elsewhere, e.g., in the liver or the bone marrow (76–79).

Studies in Humans

When Cooper presented the results of his experiments with irradiation and either thymectomy or bursectomy, Angelo DiGeorge pointed out that a similar situation indeed does exist in man (80). He described athymic humans, who, like the irradiated athymic birds, lacked T-dependent cells and the T-dependent functions. But these athymic patients retained at least certain antibody responses and the ability to produce immunoglobulins. This experiment of nature, represented by the DiGeorge athymic children, could thus be interpreted in light of our experimental research, and could readily be defined in developmental cellular and functional immunological terms. The X-linked agammaglobulinemic patients, lacking plasma cells and germinal centers, represented the reverse side of the coin (81).

The earlier clear definition of the Swiss-type agammaglobulinemia, as a disease featured by immunological and lymphoid cellular abnormalities, appeared to be strikingly parallel to the model produced by using a combination of irradiation and both thymectomy and bursectomy (81). It had been shown earlier that the immunocompetent cells which developed in the thymus had indeed passed through the blood (82). Thus, we postulated that DiGeorge's athymic syndrome, like the immunodeficiency produced by neonatal thymectomy, should be correctable simply by a fetal thymic transplant. This postulate was first shown to be correct by Cleveland (83) and was confirmed by August (84), both of whom treated DiGeorge syndrome successfully by transplantation of an embryonic thymus. We also successfully carried out corrections of the DiGeorge syndrome by thymic transplantation, thereby launching cellular engineering in man (85,86). At this time we recognized that in patients with what I called the Swiss-type agammaglobulinemia, which was first described by Glanzmann and Riniker (87) and later studied clinically and immunologically by Hitzig and Willi (88) and pathologically by Tobler and Cottier (89), represented a disease in which putative lymphoid stem cell development had been thwarted and was thus a disease that might be corrected if treatment using normal stem cells could be provided.

SUMMARY

Our interest in the lymphoid cells and immunity evolved from studies in both humans and experimental animals. These studies indicated that plasma cell development was associated with antibody production. Critical experiments of nature represented by aplastic anemia and patients with serum sickness had pointed the way. Furthermore, the results from laboratory experiments with primary and secondary antigenic stimulation in rabbits were compatible with the view that plasma cell formation was the cellular event associated with antibody production. The very early *in vivo* studies in Minnesota were consonant with the latter view, and with the somewhat more definitive *in vitro* experiments of Scandinavian investigators. Along with the later studies of Coons and coworkers, all these studies served to link plasma cells to humoral immunities and antibody production.

The experiments of nature represented by X-linked agammaglobulinemia and, as counterpoints, by Hodgkin's disease and multiple myeloma, all challenged these ideas. They also contributed to the validity of distinguishing (1) a plasma cell-based immunity attributable to antibody production and (2) a separate and distinct cell-mediated immunity linked to lymphoid cells that could be separated from the plasma cell lineage. Thus, delayed allergy, allograft immunities and resistance to a different set of pathogens comprise the cellular immunities. It was clear that resistance to high-grade encapsulated bacterial pathogens could be attributed to plasma cells and antibody production. Likewise, resistance to certain viruses, fungi, intracellular bacterial and facultative intracellular bacterial pathogens was to be related to allograft immunities, delayed allergy and the majority of circulating lymphocytes.

From our very early studies, we considered there to be two separate and distinct cellular bases of immunity: lymphocytic vs. plasmacytic, or antibody-mediated vs. cell-mediated immunities, and thus, two distinct and separable bases of immune functions. These evolving concepts were consonant with experimental results of Merrill Chase, who had linked bacterial allergy and delayed allergy to lymphocytes and antibodies to "other" cells in guinea pigs.

All of these clinically based and laboratory based analyses reached fruition in experiments in which the thymus was removed in neonatal mice, rabbits, rats and hamsters, thus demonstrating interference with the development of cell-mediated immunities. Our experiments to remove the thymus in the neonatal period followed those of Glick, who, by inhibiting development of the bursa of Fabricius, had interrupted antibody production in birds. Experiments in our laboratory led by Cooper, Peterson and later Van Alten, using thymectomy, bursectomy or both, clarified the cellular bases of humoral and cell-mediated immunities. These analyses illuminated the two-separate-cellular-component concept of immunity. This concept in turn led to incisive new ways of viewing the immunological functions, and ultimately to successful approaches to correction or management of the different immunodeficiency diseases.

REFERENCES

1. Gatti RA, Meuwissen HJ, Allen HD, Hong R, Good RA: Immunological reconstitution of sex-linked lymphopenic immunological deficiency. *Lancet* 1968;2:1366–1369.
2. Kolouch F: A study of the bone marrow plasma cell of mammals with special reference to its origin in the rabbit under normal and experimental conditions. (Thesis.) University of Minnesota, 1938.
3. Kolouch F: Origin of bone marrow plasma cell associated with allergic and immune states in rabbits. *Proc Soc Exp Biol Med* 1938;39:147–148.
4. Kolouch F, Good RA, Campbell B: The reticulo-endothelial origin of the bone marrow plasma cells in hypersensitive states. *J Lab Clin Med* 1947; 32:749–755.
5. Bing J, Plum P: Serum proteins in leucopenia. (Contribution on question about place of formation of serum proteins.) *Acta Med Scandinav* 1937;92:415–428.
6. Cajal SR: *Manual de Anatomía Patológica General,* ed. 1, Barcelona, Spain, 1890.
7. Mas y Magro F: Morphologie, Genese und physiologie der zyanophilenzellen (plasmazellen) der hämatopoetischen organe. *Arch f Exper Zellforsch* 1929;8:415–431.
8. Good RA: Effect of passive sensitization and anaphylactic shock in rabbit bone marrow. *Proc Soc Exp Biol Med* 1948;67:203–205.
9. Good RA: The morphologic mechanisms of hyperergic inflammation in the brain; with special reference to the significance of local plasma cell formation. (PhD dissertation.) University of Minnesota, 1947.
10. Good RA: Experimental allergic brain inflammation, a morphological study. *J Neuropathol Exp Neurol* 1950; 9:78–92.
11. Campbell B, Good RA: Mechanisms of antigen-antibody reaction in neurotropic virus disease. In, *Congrès Neurologique International* IVe, 1949, vold.3: *Completes Rendus* (Proceedings). Paris, Masson Publisher, 1951, pp. 294–296.
12. Good RA, Campbell B: Relationship of bone marrow plasmacytosis to the changes in serum gamma globulin in rheumatic fever. *Am J Med* 1950;9:330–342.
13. Chase MW: The cellular transfer of cutaneous hypersensitivity to tuberculin. *Proc Soc Exp Biol NY* 1945;59:134.
14. Kunkel HG, Slater RJ, Good RA: Relation between certain myeloma proteins and normal gamma globulin. *Proc Soc Exp Biol Med* 1951;76:190–193.
15. Good RA: Acute-phase reactions in rheumatic fever. In, *Symposium on Rheumatic Fever.* Minneapolis, University of Minnesota Press, 1952, pp. 115–135.
16. Kelly WD, Good RA, Varco RL: Anergy and skin homograft survival in Hodgkin's disease. *Surg Gynecol Obstet 1958;107:565–570.*

17. Good RA, Kelly WD, Gabrielsen AE: Studies of the immunologic deficiency diseases: agammaglobulinemia, Hodgkin's disease, and sarcoidosis. In, Grabar P, Miescher P, (eds): *Mechanisms of Cell and Tissue Damage Produced by Immune Reactions.* Basel, Benno Schwabe Company, 1962, pp. 353–384.

18. Good RA, Martinez C, Gabrielsen AE: Progress toward transplantation of tissues in man. In, *Advances in Pediatrics,* Vol XIII. Yearbook Medical Publishers, Chicago, 1964, pp. 93–127.

19. Good RA: Morphological basis of the immune response and hypersensitivity. In, Felton HM, et al., (eds): *Host-Parasite Relationship in Living Cells.* Charles C. Thomas, Springfield, IL, 1957, p. 78.

20. Kelly WD, Lamb DL, Varco RL, Good RA: An investigation of Hodgkin's disease with respect to the problem of homotransplantation. *Ann New York Acad Sci* 1960;87:187–202.

21. Lamb D, Pilney F, Kelly WD, Good RA: A comparative study of the incidence of anergy in patients with carcinoma, leukemia, Hodgkin's disease and other lymphomas. *J Immunol* 1962;89:555–558.

22. Bruton OC: Agammaglobulinemia. *Pediatrics* 1953;9:722.

23. Good RA, Varco RL: A clinical and experimental study of agammaglobulinemia. *J Lancet* 1955;75:245–271.

24. Good RA: Absence of plasma cells from bone marrow and lymph nodes following antigenic stimulation in patients with agammaglobulinemia. *Revue d'Hematol.* 1954;9:502–503.

25. Good RA, Zak SJ: Disturbances in gamma globulin synthesis as "experiments of nature." *Pediatrics* 1956;18:109–149.

26. McQuarrie I, Good RA: The clinical significance of congenital deficiencies of specific plasma proteins. *Arch Rediatr Uruguay* 1955;26:192–210.

27. Good RA: Studies on agammaglobulinemia. II. Failure of plasma cell formation in the bone marrow and lymph nodes of patients with agammaglobulinemia. *J Lab Clin Med* 1955;46:167–181.

28. Good RA: General discussion. In, Good RA, Gabrielsen AE, (eds): *The Thymus in Immunobiology.* New York, Harper & Row, 1964, pp. 746–749.

29. Good RA, Kelly WD, Rotstein J, Varco RL: Immunologic deficiency diseases; agammaglobulinemia, hypogammaglobulinemia, Hodgkin's disease and sarcoidosis. *Progr Allergy* 1962;6:187–319.

30. Good RA, Finstad J, Gatti RA: Bulwarks of the bodily defense. In, Mudd S, (ed): *Infectious Agents and Host Reactions.* Philadelphia, W.B. Saunders Company, 1970, pp. 76–114.

31. Good RA, Varco RL: Successful homograft of skin in a child with agammaglobulinemia; studies on agammaglobulinemia. *JAMA* 1955;157:713–716.

32. Fagraeus A: Antibody production in relation to the development of plasma cells. *Acta Med Scandinav* (Suppl) 1948;130:7–122.

33. Leduc EH, Coons AH, Connolly JM: Studies on antibody production. II. The primary and secondary responses in the popliteal lymph node of the rabbit. *J Exp Med* 1955;102:61.

34. White RG, Coons AH, Connolly JM: Studies on antibody production. III. The alum granuloma. *J Exp Med* 1955;102–173.

35. White RG, Coons AH, Connolly JM: Studies on antibody production. IV. The role of the wax fraction of mycobacterium tuberculosis in adjuvant emulsions on the production of antibody to egg albumin. *J Exp Med* 1955;102:83.

36. Ehrich WE, Drabkin DL, Forman C: Nucleic acids and the production of antibody by plasma cells. *J Exp Med* 1949;90:157–168.

37. Barr D: The functions of the plasma cells. *Am J Med* 1952;9:722–727.

38. Good RA, Varco RL: A Clinical and experimental study of agammaglobulinemia. In, Good RA, Platou ES, (eds): *Essays on Pediatrics,* in honor of Irvine McQuarrie. Minneapolis, Lancet Publications, 1955, pp. 103–129.

39. MacLean LD, Zak SJ, Varco RL, Good RA: Thymic tumor and acquired agammaglobulinemia; a clinical and experimental study of the immune response. *Surgery* 1956;40:1010–1017.

40. Good RA, Mazzitello WF: Chest disease in patients with agammaglobulinemia. *Dis Chest* 1956;29:9–35.

41. MacLean LD, Zak SJ, Varco RL, Good RA: The role of the thymus in antibody production;

an experimental study of the immune response in thymectomized rabbits. *Transplant Bull* 1957;4:21–22.

42. Glick B, Chang TS, Jaap RG: The bursa of Fabricius and antibody production. *Poultry Sci* 1956;35:224.
43. Mueller AP, Wolfe HR, Meyer RK, Aspinall RL: Further studies on the role of the bursa of Fabricius in antibody production. *J Immunol* 1962;88:354.
44. Jolly J: Sur la function hematopoietique de la bourse de Fabricius. *Comp Rend Soc Biol* 1911;70:498.
45. Jolly J: La bourse de Fabricius et les organes lymphoepitheliaux. *Arch Anat Microbial* 1914;16:363.
46. Archer OK, Pierce JC: Role of the thymus in development of the immune response. *Fed Proc* 1961;20:26.
47. Martinez C, Kersey J, Papermaster BW, Good RA: Skin homograft survival in thymectomized mice. *Proc Soc Exp Biol Med* 1962;109:193.
48. Archer OK, Papermaster BW, Good RA: Thymectomy in rabbit and mouse; consideration of time of lymphoid peripheralization. In, *The Thymus in Immunobiology, op. cit.,* pp. 414–435. (See reference #28.)
49. Good RA, Dalmasso AP, Martinez C, et al.: The role of the thymus in the development of immunologic capacity in rabbits and mice. *J Exp Med* 1962;116:773.
50. Dalmasso AP, Martinez C, Good RA: Failure of spleen cells from thymectomized mice to induce graft-vs.-host reactions. *Proc Soc Exp Biol Med* 1962;110:205.
51. Dalmasso AP, Martinez C, Good RA: Studies of immunologic characteristics of lymphoid cells from thymectomized mice. In, *The Thymus in Immunobiology, op. cit.,* pp. 478–491. (See reference #28.)
52. Martinez C, Dalmasso AP, Good RA: Homotransplantation of normal and neoplastic tissue in thymectomized mice. In, *The Thymus in Immunobiology, op. cit.,* pp. 465–477. (See reference #28.)
53. Archer OK, Sutherland DER, Good RA: The developmental biology of lymphoid tissue in the rabbit; consideration of the role of thymus and appendix. *Lab Invest* 1964;13:259–271.
54. Sutherland DER, Archer OK, Peterson RDA, et al.: Development of "autoimmune processes" in rabbits after neonatal removal of central lymphoid tissue. *Lancet* 1965;1:130–133.
55. Miller JFAP: Immunological function of the thymus. *Lancet* 1961;2:748.
56. Miller JFAP: Effect of thymic ablation and replacement. In, *The Thymus in Immunobiology, op. cit.,* pp. 436–464. (See reference #28.)
57. Miller JFAP: Role of the thymus in murine leukæmia. *Nature* 1959;183:1069.
58. Miller JFAP: Studies on mouse leukæmia. The role of the thymus in leukæmogenesis by cell-free leukæmic filtrates. *Br J Cancer* 1960;14:93.
59. Papermaster BW, Condie RM, Finstad J, Good RA: Evolution of the immune response. I. The phylogenetic development of adaptive immunologic responsiveness in vertebrates. *J Exp Med* 1964;119:105–130.
60. Finstad J, Papermaster BW, Good RA: Evolution of the immune response. II. Morphologic studies on the origin of the thymus and organized lymphoid tissue. *Lab Invest* 1964;13:490–512.
61. Finstad J, Good RA: The evolution of the immune response. III. Immunologic responses in the lamprey. *J Exp Med* 1964;120:1151–1168.
62. Parrott DMV: Strain variation in mortality and runt disease in mice thymectomized at birth. *Transplant Bull* 1962;29:102.
63. Arnason BG, Jankovic BD, Waksman BH, Wennersten C: Role of the thymus in immune reactions in rats. II. Suppressive effect of thymectomy at birth on reactions of delayed (cellular) hypersensitivity and the circulating small lymphocyte. *J Exp Med* 1962;116:177.
64. Good RA, Gabrielsen AE, (eds): *The Thymus in Immunobiology. Structure, Function, and Role in Disease.* New York, Harper & Row, 1964. p. 778.
65. Warner NL, Szenberg A: Immunologic studies on hormonally bursectomized and surgically thymectomized chickens; dissociation of immunologic responsiveness. In, *The Thymus and Immunobiology, op. cit.,* pp. 395–413. (See reference #64.)
66. Good RA: General discussion. In, *The Thymus and Immunobiology, op. cit.,* pp. 395–413. (See reference #64.)

67. Claman MN, Chaperon EA, Triplett RF: Thymus marrow cell combination; synergism in antibody production. *Proc Soc Exp Biol Med* 1964;122:1167.
68. Azar H: General discussion. In, *The Thymus and Immunobiology, op. cit.*, p. 432. (See reference #64.)
69. Cooper MD, Peterson RDA, Good RA: Delineation of the thymic and bursal lymphoid systems in the chicken. *Nature* 1965;205:143–146.
70. Cooper MD, Peterson RDA, South MA, Good RA: The functions of the thymus system and the bursa system in the chicken. *J Exp Med* 1966;123:75–102.
71. Van Alten PJ, Cain WA, Good RA, Cooper MD: Gamma globulin production and antibody synthesis in chickens bursectomized as embryos. *Nature* 1968;217:358–360.
72. Owen JJT, Wright DE, Habu S, et al.: Studies on the generation of B lymphocytes in fetal liver and bone marrow. *J Immunol.* 1977;118:2067.
73. Toivanen P, Toivanen A, Good RA: Ontogeny of bursal function in chicken. I. Embryonic stem cell for humoral immunity. *J Immunol* 1972;109:1058–1070.
74. Toivanen P, Toivanen A, Linna TJ, Good RA: Ontogeny of bursal function in chicken. II. Postembryonic stem cell for humoral immunity. *J Immunol* 1972;109:1071–1080.
75. Toivanen P, Toivanen A, Good RA: Ontogeny of bursal function in chicken. III. Immunocompetent cell for humoral immunity. *J Exp Med* 1972;136:816–831.
76. Granfors K, Martin C, Lassila O, et al.: Immune capacity of the chicken bursectomized at 60 hr of incubation. Production of the immunoglobulins and specific antibodies. *Clin Immunol Immunopathol* 1982;23:459.
77. Jalkanen S, Granfors K, Jalkanen M, Toivanen P: Immune capacity of the chicken bursectomized at 60 hr of incubation: surface immunoglobulin and B-L (Ia-like) antigen bearing cells. *J Immunol* 1983;130:2038.
78. Jalkanen S, Korpela R, Granfors K, Toivanen P: Immune capacity of the chicken bursectomized at 60 hr of incubation. Cytoplasmic immunoglobulins and histological findings. *Clin Immunol Immunopathol* 1984;30:41.
79. Veromaa T, Jalkanen S, Granfors K, Toivanen P: Inability to transfer immune unresponsiveness of chickens bursectomized at 60 hours of incubation. *Transplantation* 1986;42:197–199.
80. DiGeorge AM: Congenital absence of the thymus and its immunologic consequences: Concurrence with congenital hypoparathyroidism. In, Good RA, Bergsma D, (eds): *Immunologic Deficiency Diseases in Man,* Birth defects original article series, vol. 4. New York, National Foundation Press, 1968. pp. 116–121.
81. Peterson RDA, Cooper MD, Good RA: The pathogenesis of immunologic deficiency diseases. *Am J Med* 1965;38:579–604.
82. Moore MAS, Owen JJT. Chromosome marker studies on the development of the hematopoietic system in the chick embryo. *Nature* 1965;208:956.
83. Cleveland WW, Fogel BJ, Brown WT, Kay HE: Fœtal thymic transplant in a case of DiGeorge's syndrome. *Lancet* 1968;2:1211.
84. August CS, Rosen FS, Filler RM, et al.: Implantation of a fœtal thymus restoring immunological competence in a patient with thymic aplasia (DiGeorge's syndrome). *Lancet* 1968;2:1210.
85. Biggar WD, Good RA, Park BH: Immunologic reconstitution of a patient with combined immunodeficiency disease. *J Pediatr* 1972;81:301–306.
86. Biggar WD, Park BH, Stutman O, et al.: Fetal thymus transplantation; experimental and clinical observations. In, Bergsma D, Good RA, Finstad J, (eds): *Immunodeficiency in Man and Animals.* Birth Defects: Original Article Series, Vol. XI. Sunderland, Mass., Sineauer Associates, 1975. pp. 361–366.
87. Glanzmann E, Riniker P: Essentielle lymphozytophthise. *Wien Med Wochschr* 1950;100:35.
88. Hitzig WH, Willi H: Hereditare lympho-plasmocytare Dysgenesie ("Alymphocytose mit Agammaglobulinamie") *Schweiz Med Wochschr* 1961;91:1625.
89. Tobler R, Cottier H: Familiare lymphopenie mit agammaglobulinamie und schwerer moniliasis. *Helvet Pardiatr Act* 1958;13:313.

Bone Marrow Transplantation in Children, edited by F. Leonard Johnson and Carl Pochedly. Raven Press, Ltd., New York © 1990.

History. II. The First Successful Treatment of Human Disease by Allogeneic Bone Marrow Transplantation

Robert A. Good

Department of Pediatrics, University of South Florida, St. Petersburg, Florida 33701

THE MHC AND HISTOCOMPATIBILITY TESTING IN MICE

Research which led to the next step that permitted successful bone marrow transplantation in humans was derived again from that incredible little teacher, the laboratory mouse. Gorer observed that inbred mice that were compatible and did not produce antibodies against their own red blood cells exhibited immune responses to immunizations with blood cells from a separate inbred strain (1). He and his associates, particularly George Snell, then showed that tumor transplantation and tissue grafting followed rules which would permit transplantation within the strain, but which predicted graft rejection when transplants were made between members of different inbred strains (2,3). In short, a major histocompatibility system, called H-2, could be readily defined. If a mismatch at H-2 existed between donor and recipient strains, grafts of tumor tissue would regularly be rejected, as would grafts of skin or other tissues. Tumor grafts between donor and recipient matched at this major histocompatibility complex (MHC), which Gorer called H-2, would regularly be accepted. Likewise, skin grafts would often be accepted without further manipulation if donor and recipient were matched at the MHC barrier.

BONE MARROW TRANSPLANTATION AFTER TOTAL BODY IRRADIATION

These findings with the mouse were supported by observations made by Jacobson. Jacobson discovered that if the entire spleen or a relatively small component of host marrow, such as marrow in one limb, was shielded while a rabbit was given total body irradiation, full recovery of hematopoiesis and recovery of all the lymphoid tissue would surely occur. However, if no such shielding were used, the hematopoietic and lymphoid systems would be irretrievably destroyed (4). Other studies then showed that lethal total body irradiation could be treated effectively and all hematopoiesis and lymphopoiesis restored if bone marrow cells from mice of the same inbred strain were given intravenously or intraperitoneally (5).

Thus, syngeneic bone marrow transplantation led to dramatic reconstruction of all hematopoietic elements, when the bone marrow cells were taken from a donor that was genetically identical to the irradiated recipient. This included reconstruction of thymic structure, as well as lymph nodes and spleen lymphoid components. Severe graft-vs.-host reactions or highly lethal so-called secondary disease were produced if the bone marrow transplantation was carried out in circumstances where donor and recipient were mismatched at the H-2 barriers. However, bone marrow transplants could be carried out without serious consequences, and generally without significant evidence of graft-vs.-host reactions or graft-vs.-host disease, if donor and recipient were matched at the H-2 barrier (6).

In our laboratory, as early as 1954, we had been trying to confirm the now classical experiments of Billingham, Brent, and Medawar (7). These workers had produced immunological tolerance to skin grafts by injecting cells from the prospective donor strain of mice into mice of the prospective recipient strain at birth. When this was done with mice of the appropriate strain combinations (initially C3H or CBA → A and A → C3H or CBA), tolerance that ultimately permitted indefinite skin graft survival after transplantation was achieved. We, however, attempted to reproduce these findings using transplantations with different inbred strains, e.g., A and C57BL/6 or C3H and C57BL/6, which are now known to be more disparate at both H-2 and non-H-2 determinants than are C3H or CBA and A. However, our experiments regularly failed. Tolerance as described by Billingham, Brent and Medawar could not be produced in our experiments.

After much frustration, we finally discovered what the problem was. The strains used by Billingham et al., shared determinants of the H-2 region, while the strains we were using were completely different at the H-2 locus and also were different at numerous non-H-2 histocompatibility determinants. With this insight, we changed our strategy and did many experiments using inbred strains of mice that were matched at the H-2 determinants and were disparate only at what we now call minor or multiminor histocompatibility barriers. Thus, we chose to use mice of the MHC-matched C3H and Ce strains or male—female disparaties at the Y histocompatibility determinants. When the mice were partly matched, it was easy to produce immunological tolerance by the technique of Billingham, Brent and Medawar. Furthermore, once this had been accomplished, it was possible to perform perfectly extraordinary feats of tissue and organ transplantation when such matching had been carried out.

Martinez, Mariani and I showed, for example, that production of lasting immunological tolerance, although easier to produce in neonates, could be produced throughout life if donor and recipient were matched at the MHC locus (8–12). We showed that parabiotic union established for a relatively brief period resulted in a long-lasting tolerant state in adult mice (13). In addition, with Aust we found that full immunologic tolerance would permit successful allogeneic pituitary, adrenal and even functioning ovarian transplants in the tolerant recipients (8,13,14). We even showed, as had Uphoff, that bone marrow transplants could readily be accomplished if donor and recipient were matched at the H-2 locus, and such marrow transplants produced a lasting tolerant state between MHC-matched strains.

THE HUMAN MAJOR HISTOCOMPATIBILITY COMPLEX (MHC)

Thus, we became convinced that functions of the major histocompatibility complex of humans were analogous to those of the MHC in laboratory mice. If so, matching between donor and recipient might be expected to permit feats involving long-lasting immunological tolerance, as were readily produced in mice. Our subsequent experiments were critical in developing this concept (15). We tried to reconstruct the lymphoid system following neonatal thymectomy. Such reconstruction was readily accomplished if the donated thymus was from a neonatal mouse of the same strain as the thymectomized recipient and the mouse was transplanted in the neonatal period (16–18). With H-2 matching, the reconstruction was prompt and complete. If the thymus had been taken from an MHC-mismatched donor, the graft often failed to reconstruct immunity functions completely. When reconstruction of immunity did occur it took place more slowly than when donor and recipient were matched at the major histocompatibility complex (19). Also, after mismatched thymus transplants, secondary disease sometimes occurred, and the neonatal mice were more susceptible to the ravages of secondary disease or graft-vs.-host reactions than were normal mice (20).

In another setting involving immunological reconstruction, the MHC proved to be crucial. Neonatally thymectomized mice could be quite fully reconstituted even though they had no thymus at all. This occurred if the mice had been given a sufficiently large number of fully mature peripheral lymphoid cells (either spleen cells alone or both spleen and lymph node cells) from donors matched with recipients at the H-2 determinants (15,21). If such matching had not been carried out, the recipient mice all had rapidly lethal graft-vs.-host reactions, the neonatally thymectomized mice being especially vulnerable to GVH disease as mentioned above.

FIRST BONE MARROW TRANSPLANTS

The first efforts to use marrow transplantation in man were all desperate attempts to treat patients who had experienced accidental exposure to total body irradiation or had exposure to excessive amounts of radionuclides (22–24). These attempts to treat hematopoietic failure or injury regularly failed. Indeed, some 200 efforts to achieve marrow transplants in this context were attempted, but none succeeded. In 1959, for example, Dr. William Krivit and I attempted to treat a patient with otherwise untreatable, highly lethal acute leukemia by using very large doses of total body irradiation followed by bone marrow transplantation from a paternal donor (25). The anti-leukemic therapy in our regimen was impressively effective, but a fatal acute graft-vs.-host reaction ensued.

Shortly thereafter, experiments with bone marrow transplants in dogs by E. Donnall Thomas showed occasional successes. Based on these studies, he treated patients with leukemia using high-dose total body irradiation from a twin-beam cobalt instrument and identical twins as donors. In these studies, a few relatively long-term remissions of leukemia and even apparent cures occurred. These trials showed that in man, as in mice, perfect matching at MHC barriers permitted bone marrow transplantation. These results were obtained after Thomas had achieved occasional impressive successes in bone marrow transplants with use of partially inbred beagle dogs as both donors and recipients (26). Although unpredictable, the occasional successes were sufficiently encouraging to cause increased interest in the possibility of treating human disease by bone marrow transplantation. Earlier, Uphoff had achieved successful marrow transplantation quite regularly in mice when donor and recipient were matched at H-2. Thus, when these mice were subjected to total body irradiation they showed long-term survival, without significant graft-vs.-host reactions or secondary diseases (6).

During the mid-1960s, knowledge of the MHC in man developed rapidly. Following Daussett's discovery of the antigen Mac in association with studies of autoimmune neutropenia, investigations of the major histocompatibility system located on chromosome 6 were investigated in earnest (27–29). It was clearly established that in man, as in mice, there existed a highly polymorphic histocompatibility system with multiple loci at which many alleles operate. This polymorphic histocompatibility system was found to be strung out along chromosome 6. The A and B loci were recognized first, followed by the C locus. Then important counterpart loci related to the class II antigens of the mouse were recognized, but these were located outside or distal to the loci responsible for the class I antigens of the A, C, and B loci. In this way, these MHC determining, serologically defined D loci (later designated DP, DQ, and DR) were identified.

It was soon clear that the MHC determinants of man were similar, although not identical, in distribution to those of the mouse. Then the possibility of treating human disease by MHC-matched bone marrow transplantation once again became attractive to us. Uphoff had shown in experimental systems that fetal liver transplants, in lieu of marrow transplants, were sometimes successful without MHC matching (30). We reasoned that fetal liver or bone marrow might provide a source of stem cells. We proposed that if such fetal liver cells were obtained prior to the fourteenth week of gestation, the time when immunocompetent lymphocytes appear in the liver, the fetal liver might be used as a source of stem cells to treat children suffering from severe combined immunodeficiency disease (SCID) (31).

TRANSPLANTATION FOR TREATMENT OF SCID

We were the first to try to use such a fetal liver transplant to treat SCID. We used liver tissue from a 13-to-14-week-old abortus. With that transplant we obtained prompt restoration of T and B cell function in the recipient with SCID (31). However, our patient developed anemia and, to correct the anemia, the patient was given a single blood transfusion. Whether the hazardous reactive lymphoid cells came from the fetal liver transplant or from the non-irradiated blood transfusion was not certain. In any case, we dramatically corrected the immunologic defect and thus apparently cured the severe combined immunodeficiency, but the patient developed a fulminant graft-vs.-host reaction and died (32).

In response to this devastating experience, I reasoned that the best way to correct SCID might be to employ an HLA- and mixed lymphocyte culture (MLC)-matched sibling donor, according to studies in mice. This setup should not produce graft-vs.-host reaction. Thus, we proposed treatment of SCID in infants by using marrow from a matched sibling (33), but we warned against the hazard of blood transfusion from MHC-mismatched donors. A golden opportunity to try our newly proposed treatment for SCID soon followed.

Our patient was the twelfth male child over three generations in a large family to suffer from SCID. The child was referred to us by a pediatrician, Dr. Herrieux, in Meriden, Connecticut, who was aware of our efforts to correct immunodeficiency disease by cellular engineering. The baby had four female siblings. The entire family came to Minneapolis for tissue typing, with the plan to correct SCID using an HLA-matched sibling as donor for a marrow transplant.

The tissue typing showed that one of the daughters was a fairly good match. But the prospective donor was mismatched at the A locus and was also a blood group ABO mismatch. The prospective donor was of blood group O and the intended recipient was of blood group A.

A bone marrow transplant was done by Richard Gatti, Richard Hong, Hugh Allen and I. We gave the cells for this first marrow transplant by the intraperitoneal route. The marrow transplant took and very promptly showed evidence of having corrected the immunological deficiency in our patient. Within three weeks, lymphocytes appeared in blood and marrow, plasma cells appeared for the first time in marrow, and immunoglobulins and antibodies attributable to the donor marrow appeared and were produced vigorously (1,34,35). However, after a few weeks, the child showed evidence of graft-vs.-host disease. The GVH disease took the form of skin rash, diarrhea, and liver function abnormalities, and the child also developed an iatrogenic, aregenerative aplastic anemia (36). Instead of trying to eliminate the offending graft, as many of our colleagues suggested, we performed a second transplant from the same sister donor to this child with SCID, who now had aplastic anemia.

This graft also took promptly and worked effectively to reconstruct the entire hematopoietic system. Thus, the marrow became responsible not only for a new immunity system but also for an entirely new hematopoietic system for the child with SCID. The patient's blood type switched promptly from his original type A to the sister's O. Also, levels of immunoglobulin became normal, and plasma cells and lymphocytes achieved normal numbers. All of the child's hematopoietic cells which could be made to divide were those that came from the female donor, and no cells of the male karyotype of the recipient were to be seen. The patient with SCID who had suffered from many recurrent infections became a healthy, vigorous, happy youngster capable of normal growth and development. Since the transplant of bone marrow from his MHC-matched sister was given, this child has remained in vigorous good health and is capable of all normal immunologic functions.

Thus, in our first case, we successfully treated by bone marrow transplantation both the inborn genetic disease X-linked SCID and also the complicating immunologically based aplastic anemia (34–36).

Soon thereafter, a matched sibling donor was used by Bach, Bortin and coworkers (37) with partial success to treat a 2-year-old boy who suffered from the complex immunohematologic entity, the Wiskott-Aldrich syndrome. Then with the guidance of Van Rood, Van Bekkum and Dicki, deKoning and Dooren in Holland, we successfully treated a child with the classical autosomal recessive form of SCID (38). These successful applications of bone marrow transplantation using matched sibling donors set the stage for further application of this form of cellular engineering to treat many otherwise lethal diseases.

SUMMARY

Our studies of patients with primary immunodeficiency diseases emerged from the experimentally based concept that there are two separate and distinct systems for humoral and cell-mediated immunity. This led to research which defined the cellular bases of immunity as being two distinct immunity systems, each with its own central lymphoid organ. We discovered that the thymus functions as the central developmental organ for one of these systems in mammals. We later showed, in extending Glick's work, that the bursa of Fabricius represents a central lymphoid organ for development of humoral immunity in all orders of birds and is the seat of plasma cell development. Concomitant experiments with transplantation immunity and study of the histocompatibility systems made it clear that matching of donor and recipient can foster tissue and organ transplantation, and can facilitate correction of immunodeficiency in neonatally thymectomized mice. These experimental investigations of our own were based on Gorer's monumental contributions which, along with the contributions of his coworker Snell, laid the groundwork for histocompatibility matching in mice.

Later, our investigations were affected in an important way by our inability at first to confirm the landmark contributions to tolerance development by Billingham, Brent and Medawar. Thus, for production of tolerance, we were forced to turn to donors and recipients who were matched according to the histocompatibility system. These investigations, together with our experimental analysis of the origins of the two immunity systems, led Peterson, Cooper and me to define the principal primary immunodeficiency diseases of man in a new context. We compared X-linked agammaglobulinemia to the immunodeficiency produced by bursectomy in chickens. We related the athymic DiGeorge syndrome to the consequences of neonatal thymectomy in rodents and chickens, and the Swiss type of severe combined immunodeficiency disease (SCID) was likened to the condition of chickens that were both thymectomized and bursectomized.

These concepts, the knowledge of how the immunity systems develop from stem cell precursors in bone marrow in birds and mammals, and our understanding of how these stem cells are distributed throughout the blood to the central lymphoid organs, led us to propose that bone marrow transplantation might cure SCID. When we tested this hypothesis, we were able to cure for the first time by bone marrow transplantation, a fatal human disease, severe combined immunodeficiency. This patient was cured of SCID and later, by a second marrow transplant, was cured of aplastic anemia that complicated the cellular reconstitution of his hematopoietic system. This event pointed the way for the application of bone marrow transplantation to the treatment of many human immunodeficiencies, aplastic anemias, hematopoietic disorders, leukemias, and cancers.

REFERENCES

1. Gorer PA: The detection of antigenic differences in mouse erythrocytes by the employment of immune sera. *Br J Exp Biol* 1936;17:42.
2. Gorer PA: The genetic and antigenic basis of tumor transplantation. *J Pathol Bacteriol* 1937;44:691.
3. Snell GD: Histocompatibility genes of the mouse. II. Production and analysis of isogenic resistant lines. *J Natl Cancer Inst* 1958;21:843.
4. Jacobsen LD, Simmons EL, Marks EK, Eldredge JH: Recovery from irradiation injury. A review. *Cancer Res* 1952;12:315.
5. Lorenz E. Uphoff D, Reid TR, Shelton E: Modification of irradiation injury in mice and guinea pigs by bone marrow injections. *J Natl Cancer Inst* 1951;12:197–201.
6. Uphoff DE: Genetic factors influencing irradiation protection by bone marrow. I. The F_1 hybrid effect. *J Natl Cancer Inst* 1957;19:123–130.
7. Billingham RE, Brent L, Medawar PB: "Actively acquired tolerance" of foreign cells. *Nature* 1953;172:603.
8. Shapiro F. Martinez C, Good RA: Homologous skin transplantation from F_1 hybrid mice to parent strains. *Proc Soc Exp Biol Med* 1959;101:94–97.
9. Shapiro F, Martinez C, Smith JM, Good RA: Tolerance of skin homografts induced in adult mice by multiple injections of homologous spleen cells. *Proc Soc Exp Biol Med* 1961;106:472–475.
10. Mariani T, Martinez C, Smith JM, Good RA: Induction of immunological tolerance to male skin isografts in female mice subsequent to the neonatal period. *Proc Soc Exp Biol Med* 1959;101:596–599.
11. Martinez C, Shapiro F, Kelman H, et al.: Tolerance of F_1 hybrid skin homografts in the parent strain induced by parabiosis. *Proc Soc Exp Biol Med* 1960;103:266.
12. Martinez C, Shapiro F, Good RA: Essential duration of parabiosis and development of tolerance to skin homografts in man. *Proc Soc Exp Biol Med* 1960;104:256–259.
13. Martinez C, Aust JB, Good RA: Acquired tolerance to ovarian homografts in castrated mice. *Transplant Bull* 1956;3:128.
14. Martinez C, Smith JM, Good RA: Acquired tolerance to homologous transplantation of endocrine glands in inbred strains of mice. *Br J Exp Pathol* 1958;39:574.
15. Yunis EJ, Hilgard HR, Martinez C, Good RA: Studies on immunologic reconstitution of thymectomized mice. *J Exp Med* 1965;121:607–632.
16. Yunis EJ, Martinez C, Good RA; Increased graft-vs.-host susceptibility of thymectomized recipients. *Proc Soc Exp Biol Med* 1967;124:418–421.
17. Dalmasso AP, Martinez C, Sjodin K, Good RA: Studies on the role of the thymus in immunobiology; reconstitution of immunologic capacity in mice thymectomized at birth. *J Exp Med* 1963;118:1089–1109.
18. Stutman O, Yunis EJ, Martinez C, Good RA: Reversal of post-thymectomy wasting disease in mice by multiple thymus grafts. *J Immunol* 1967;98:79–87.
19. Stutman O, Yunis EJ, Good RA: Thymus; an essential factor in lymphoid repopulation. *Transplant Proc* 1969;1:614–615.
20. Dalmasso AP, Martinez C, Good RA: Further studies of suppression of the homograft reaction by thymectomy in the mouse. *Proc Soc Exp Biol Med* 1962;111:143–146.
21. Yunis EJ, Fernandes G, Smith J, Good RA: Long survival and immunologic reconstitution following transplantation with syngeneic or allogeneic fetal liver and neonatal spleen cells. In, Dupont B, Good RA (eds): *Immunology of Bone Marrow Transplantation*, New York, Grune and Stratton, 1976, pp. 173–177.
22. Graw RG, Rogentine GN, Leventhal BG, et al.: Graft-vs.-host reaction complicating HLA-matched bone marrow transplantation. *Lancet* 1970;2:1053–1055.
23. Bortin MM: A compendium of reported human bone marrow transplants. *Transplantation* 1970;9:571–587.
24. Bortin MM: Allogeneic bone marrow transplantation in leukemia patients. In, Hickey RC, Clark BL (eds): *Current Problems in Cancer*, Chicago, Yearbook Medical Publishers, 1987.
25. Krivit W, Good RA: Unpublished observations.
26. Epstein RB, Storb R, Ragde H, Thomas ED: Cytotoxic typing antisera for marrow grafting in littermate dogs. *Transplantation* 1968;6:45–58.

27. van Rood JJ, van Leeuwen A: Major and minor histocompatibility systems in man and their importance in bone marrow transplantation. In: *Immunology of Bone Marrow Transplantation, op. cit.*, pp. 103–110. (See reference #21.)

28. Amos DB: The era of the immunogeneticist. *J Immunol* 1981;127:1727.

29. Klein J: *Immunology; the science of self-nonself discrimination.* New York, John Wiley & Sons, 1982.

30. Uphoff D: Mechanisms in graft-vs.-host reactions; an immunogenetic appraisal. In: *Immunology of Bone Marrow Transplantation, op. cit.*, pp. 167–171. (See reference #21.)

31. Cooper MD, Gabrielsen AE, Good RA: Central and peripheral lymphoid tissues in immunologic processes in human disease. In, Good RA, Bergsma D (eds): *Immunologic Deficiency Diseases in Man: Birth Defects Original Article Series* Vol. IV, No. 1. New York, National Foundation Press, 1968.

32. Hong R, Kay HEM, Cooper MD, et al.: Immunological restitution in lymphopenic immunologic deficiency syndrome. *Lancet* 1968;1:503–506.

33. Hong R, Gatti RA, Good RA: Hazards and potential benefits of blood transfusion in immunological deficiency. *Lancet* 1968;2:388–389.

34. Good RA: Immunologic reconstitution; the achievement and its meaning. *Hospital Practice* 1969;4:41–47.

35. Gatti RA, Meuwissen HJ, Allen HD, et al.: Immunological reconstitution of sex-linked lymphopenic immunological deficiency. *Lancet* 1968;2:1366–1369.

36. Meuwissen HJ, Gatti RA, Terasaki PI, et al.: Treatment of lymphopenic hypogammaglobulinemia and bone marrow aplasia by transplantation of allogeneic marrow; crucial role of histocompatibility matching. *N Engl J Med* 1969;281:691–696.

37. Bach FH, Albertini RJ, Joo P, et al.: Bone marrow transplantation in a patient with Wiskott-Aldrich syndrome. *Lancet* 1968;2:1364–1366.

38. deKoning J, Dooren LJ, van Bekkum DW, et al.: Transplantation of bone marrow cells and fetal thymus in an infant with lymphopenic immunological deficiency. *Lancet* 1969;1:1223–1227.

*Bone Marrow Transplantation in
Children*, edited by F. Leonard Johnson
and Carl Pochedly. Raven Press, Ltd.,
New York © 1990.

The Histocompatibility Barrier in Bone Marrow Transplantation

A. H. Filipovich

*Bone Marrow Transplant Program, University of Minnesota Hospitals, Division of
Immunology, Department of Pediatrics, University of Minnesota Medical School,
Minneapolis, Minnesota 55455*

INTRODUCTION: RECOGNITION OF THE HISTOCOMPATIBILITY BARRIER

The successful application of allogeneic bone marrow transplantation to an expanding spectrum of diseases in the 1970s and 1980s was preceded and propelled by progress in the definition of the allelic genes of the major histocompatibility complex (MHC) in man. The major histocompatibility complex is a major gene grouping which occupies an area of approximately 1/1000 of the human genome and is located on the short arm of chromosome 6 (6p) (1). The linked genes in this complex have largely retained their unique structure over millions of years, thus being highly conserved in evolution. This finding caused geneticists to speculate that the cell surface antigen products of the MHC have played a critical function in the survival of the human species in its present form.

Antigens from genes of the major histocompatibility complex, in particular products of the class I genes to be described later in this review, are present as integral membrane glycoproteins on virtually all nucleated cells. While little is known about the role of antigens of the major histocompatibility complex in the function of most body cells, it is now clear from cellular and molecular studies that MHC products are central to immune responsiveness.

Decades before the natural function of antigens of the major histocompatibility complex was elucidated, Gorer discovered an inherited mechanism which was implicated in experimental tissue graft rejection (2). This finding led to serologic analyses of the genetic system which came to be called the major histocompatibility complex (MHC) in the mouse. Confirmation of a homologous genetic region in human chromosomes quickly followed (3).

Before the recognition of a stringent histocompatibility barrier, codominantly inherited from both parents, early attempts at transfusion of bone marrow or blood from relatives into recipients with lethal immunodeficiencies inevitably met with failure. These early transplant attempts resulted in either (1) no effect, presumably due to non-engraftment, or (2) the development of lethal graft-vs.-host reactions (4). By the late 1960s, prototype methods had been developed to probe for histocompatibility among family members, and the first therapeutic successes with human marrow transplantation were recorded (5–7). In these cases, the donors were selected because they were identical or very similar to the recipients by serologic testing (8), because donor and recipient lymphocytes did not respond *in vitro* in mixed lymphocyte culture (MLC), or both studies indicated compatibility (9).

Since those pioneering treatments were done, thousands of allogeneic bone marrow transplants have been performed. More than 95% of the transplants have been carried out between donors and recipients who were siblings shown to be identical in the major histocompatibility complex. In the 1980s, there has been continued improvement in long-term disease-free survival following histocompatible bone marrow transplantation. As a result, there has been an upsurge of research interest in expanding the opportunities for transplantation to the estimated 60–65% of eligible patients who do not have genotypically histocompatible donors (10).

In the late 1970s, the Seattle bone marrow transplant team reported that the long-term outcome of marrow transplantation from closely matched relatives for the treatment of leukemias equaled the results following transplantation from genotypically matched siblings (11). More recently, the development of reliable methods of T cell depletion (12–15) has prompted investigation into the use of full haplotype mismatched related donors. Finally, computerized files of HLA types of voluntary blood donors in the United States and western Europe are now accessible to marrow transplantation centers in search of unrelated donors. These sources have been used to select closely matched unrelated donors for several hundred recipients, more than 100 of whom have already undergone the transplantation procedure.

Successful marrow transplantation between matched siblings requires the removal of two major immunologic barriers. The first barrier is immunologic resistance by the recipient against the foreign marrow graft. This barrier is influenced by incompatibility of major histocompatibility antigens, similar to the case with solid tissue allografts, as well as by differences between the host and donor at minor histocompatibility loci (16), differences of hematopoietic (or hybrid) histocompatibility genes or both (17). Failure of primary engraftment, or the occurrence of rejection, often results in prolonged pancytopenia and places the recipient at high risk for fatal opportunistic infections, for hemorrhage, or both. Attempts at retransplantation generally require additional immunosuppressive therapy which may further compromise the patient.

The second barrier, unique to hematopoietic cell transplants, is the potential for graft-vs.-host (GVH) reaction. This reaction is caused by immunocompetent cells which are contained in the marrow graft and are capable of injuring host ("foreign") tissues. It is generally accepted that T lymphocytes with cytotoxic potential are involved in the GVH reaction. Acute graft-vs.-host disease (GVHD) results in necrotizing lesions of the skin, gastrointestinal mucosa, and of the liver and biliary tract. Fever, maculopapular rash, watery (and often bloody) diarrhea, and jaundice can occur. Acute graft-vs.-host disease can be mild and self-limited. More often it does not resolve spontaneously but progresses, if not effectively treated, to a chronic condition persisting for months or years, as chronic graft-vs.-host disease. Severe acute GVH disease is often complicated by fatal opportunistic infections. Chronic GVH disease is marked by cutaneous manifestations of hyperkeratosis and hyperpigmentation, xerostomia, xerophthalmia, malabsorption or chronic liver disease, and profound immunodeficiency. (For reviews of graft-vs.-host disease see references 18 and 19.)

The strength of these two barriers, immunologic resistance by the recipient and graft-vs.-host immunoreactivity of the donor cells, is governed by genetic differences between host and donor. Thus, the risk of non-engraftment, severe GVH disease, or both, are magnified for the patient who receives a transplant from a donor who is mismatched at the major histocompatibility complex. Analysis of the available literature and our own experience at the University of Minnesota suggests that patients currently undergoing mismatched marrow transplantation require longer and more costly hospitalizations in order to achieve durable engraftment and to treat secondary complications.

An additional major challenge to successful transplantation across the histocompatibility barrier is the prolonged and sometimes incomplete process of post-transplant immunoreconstitution. Immune recovery in mismatched recipients is inferior when compared to results achieved with histocompatible donors. Failure of the recovery of functional cell-cell interactions has been implicated in the development of unusual and potentially lethal complications, such as alloimmune cytopenias and lymphoproliferative disorders.

This chapter reviews the progress which has been made in crossing the histocompatibility barrier and proposes some approaches to solving the remaining problems.

THE HUMAN MAJOR HISTOCOMPATIBILITY COMPLEX

The human immune system, which consists of T lymphocytes, B lymphocytes and macrophages, performs a number of helper and suppressor functions that are comprehensively integrated to protect the host from "foreign" antigens, including infectious agents. The genes of the major histocompatibility complex are critical to the regulation of the immune response(s). In concert with lymphocyte specific antigens, such as the T cell receptor, immunoglobulins and differentiation antigens (namely, CD_3 and CD_4) (20), the products of MHC genes control antigen recognition, production of antibodies, lymphocyte proliferation, cytotoxicity and suppression of the immune response. Incompatibility of antigens of the major histocompatibility complex among cooperating cell populations can disrupt the balance of opposing processes in the immune response.

The major histocompatibility complex, also referred to as the HLA (human leukocyte antigen) system, contains a set of tightly linked genes that are usually inherited as one group, or haplotype. A generic map of the HLA region on the short arm of human chromosome 6 appears in Figure 1. Each individual inherits a maternal and paternal copy of chromosome 6 and thus a maternal and paternal haplotype. Since HLA haplotypes assort independently into gametes, any two siblings have an overall chance of 25% to inherit the same set of maternal and paternal haplotypes; 50% of siblings inherit only one of the two haplotypes in common, and 25% inherit the genetically "opposite" maternal and paternal

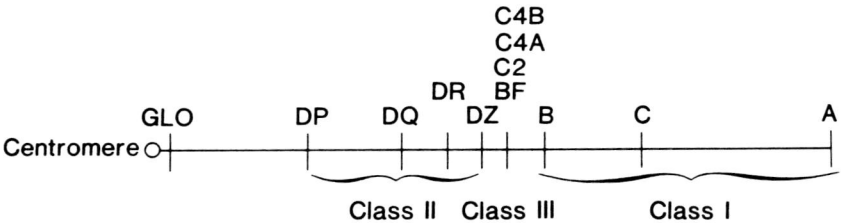

FIG. 1. A schematic representation of the major histocompatibility region located on the short arm of human chromosome 6(6p). GLO = glyoxylase, an enzyme mapped near the centromere (see text for description).

haplotypes. In sequence from the telomeric to the centromeric boundaries of the major histocompatibility complex, the HLA system consists of genes encoding so-called class I, class III and class II molecules.

Class I molecules include HLA-A, HLA-B and HLA-C loci. Their products are integral membrane glycoproteins found on nearly all nucleated cells. All class I molecules consist of a glycosylated heavy chain which anchors the molecule in the cell membrane. Class I heavy chain genes are highly polymorphic, that is, many different alleles (or structural variants) are encoded at the HLA-A, -B, and -C loci. Class I heavy chains are usually noncovalently bound to a smaller nonpolymorphic protein-beta-2 microglobulin, encoded on chromosome number 15. The heavy chains of class I molecules possess striking similarities to one another, and similarities to the constant region of the heavy chain of immunoglobulin G, in terms of amino acid composition and sequences.

Class II molecules are encoded by several loci within the HLA-D region, provisionally designated DZ, DR, DQ (or DC), and DP (formerly SB) in telomeric to centromeric order (21). Class II molecules are expressed on cells with immunologic function such as B lymphocytes, activated T lymphocytes and macrophages, as well as hematopoietic precursors. Class II molecules are dimeric, composed of two noncovalently-linked polypeptide chains (alpha and beta), both of which span the cell membrane. The beta, or heavy chains, and alpha, or light chains for each class II locus are encoded as separate genetic sequences and can combine in transposition. For example, alpha from the maternal haplotype can bond to beta from the paternal haplotype. Molecular studies indicate that class II light chains, in particular, are quite polymorphic; in other words, there are many alleles in a given population. Both alpha and beta chains of class II molecules resemble immunoglobulin heavy chains. (A complete listing of recognized HLA specificities for both class I and II antigens from the Ninth Histocompatibility Workshop is available [21]).

Class III molecules are polymorphic proteins belonging to the complement system; designated BF, C_2, C_4, and C_4B. Alleles of each complement component are easily distinguished by differences in electrophoretic mobility. Common class III gene combinations are designated as complotypes (22).

Two important genetic characteristics of the major histocompatibility complex affect the magnitude of histocompatibility within the human population, and define the probability of identifying a histocompatibility donor for any given patient. The first remarkable genetic feature of the major histocompatibility complex is the diversity of alleles which exist in the population for each of the major loci. Due to this enormous polymorphism, many parents will be heterozygous at both the class I and class II loci with classic Mendelian segregation of haplotypes in their children. Unfortunately, such heterogeneity in HLA types, along with the trend toward reduced family size in developed countries, results in the current situation where patients with full siblings have only a 30–40% chance of having a two-haplotype matched donor.

Another relevant genetic characteristic of the HLA system is the existence of linkage disequilibrium, which is the nonrandom association of alleles within haplotypes. The frequency of such a nonrandom association of alleles is defined as a statistically significant difference from the calculation which predicts the likelihood of specific genetic alleles at two or more loci coexisting as a haplotype. This calculation is predicated solely on the basis of the respective gene frequencies for those alleles in the population. An example of linkage disequilibrium is the greater than expected occurrence of the haplotype composed of the phenotypes HLA-A1, -B8, and -Dr3. The existence of linkage disequilibrium improves the chances of finding a phenotypically matched unrelated donor for patients who have inherited the more prevalent haplotypes. Since extended haplotypes have been identified in approximately 30% of all chromosomes in Caucasians, it has been predicted that about 50% of patients will possess one or two such haplotypes (23).

Non-MHC Histocompatibility Antigens

Two minor histocompatibility antigen systems have been identified in humans. Both were identified through the study of cytotoxic T lymphocytes obtained from marrow recipients after transplantation (16). Both are felt to be MHC-restricted in that cytotoxic cells will kill only target cells which share the same class I antigen *and* express the foreign minor antigen. The first minor histocompatibility antigen to be identified was H-Y, which is expressed only on male (or Y-bearing) cells. It has been speculated that H-Y may account for the higher incidence of graft-vs.-host disease which is observed when alloimmunized females (parous or transfused) serve as donors for histocompatibility brothers (24,25). The second minor histocompatibility antigen system, named HA, occurs in a high frequency, especially in HLA-A2 positive individuals. Its chromosomal localization has not yet been determined. In preliminary reports, incompatibility for HA is highly correlated with the occurrence of chronic graft-vs.-host disease following MHC-compatible transplantation (16).

Although there is abundant evidence for the existence of a hematopoietic histocompatibility (Hh) barrier in murine models of transplantation (17), the human counterpart has not yet been defined. The murine hematopoietic histocompatibility barrier controls the efficiency of marrow engraftment in irradiated recipients. Characteristics of the murine hematopoietic histocompatibility barrier include (1) the existence of multiple polymorphic genes, (2) the restricted expression of hematopoietic histocompatibility antigens on blood-forming (and leukemic) cells (27), (3) linkage with murine major histocompatibility complex in most cases (28), and (4) the necessity for coexistence of regulatory genes which control recognition or response to the hematopoietic histocompatibility gene products in order to express resistance to putative Hh incompatibility (29).

The role for serum factors in resistance to murine marrow engraftment is still controversial (30). The cells mediating hematopoietic histocompatibility (or hybrid incompatibility), i.e., resistance to engraftment, are radioresistant and share many characteristics with natural killer (NK) cells (31). Recently, preliminary information has been presented for a human assay of the *in vitro* regulation of hematopoiesis by so-called Mφ/NK cells, which may be able to predict failure of engraftment in mismatched transplantation (32).

TISSUE TYPING OF MAJOR HISTOCOMPATIBILITY COMPLEX FOR BONE MARROW TRANSPLANTATION

The HLA phenotype of an individual can be determined by a series of serologic and cellular techniques which identify the allelic specificity at the different major loci. The class I antigens HLA-A, HLA-B, and HLA-C, as well as the class II antigens HLA-DR, HLA-DC and HLA-DQ, are defined by their patterns of reactivity to a panel of typing antisera in the presence of xenogeneic complement. This technique is the microcytotoxicity assay (32). Human sera obtained from multiparous women, which have been carefully screened and characterized, have been widely used for tissue typing in the past. Monoclonal antibodies are now replacing these heterologous sera in tissue typing panels. In fact, monoclonal antibodies have already permitted more detailed definition of HLA types, including the so-called "splits." This results in more accurate assignment of genotypes in families where parents appear to share alleles at certain loci.

In practice, most laboratories can perform HLA typing for HLA-A and HLA-B loci of various family members within 24 hours. HLA-C typing is not as informative since there are still many "blank" or nontypable C specificities. Since the genes of the major histocompatibility complex are linked as a haplotype, the finding of HL-A and HL-B identity between full siblings conveys a 95% probability that they are, in fact, identical for all antigens of the major histocompatibility complex including HLA-D/DR. Persons with this degree of histocompatibility will be found to be nonreactive (or identical) in the mixed lymphocyte culture (MLC) test.

Compatibility in mixed lymphocyte culture, or HLA-D identity, provides, at present, the best indicator test for the successful outcome of allogeneic bone marrow transplantation in terms of engraftment and incidence of graft-vs.-host disease (16). Since the region of the major histocompatibility complex is a lengthy stretch of DNA, chromosomal breaks occur with significant frequency, being in an estimated 1–5% of offspring. These chromosomal breaks result in recombinations between the telomeric portion of the major histocompatibility complex, encoding HLA-A and/or HLA-B and the more centromeric regions encoding the HLA-D antigens, especially HLA-DP. Therefore, it is imperative that HLA-D identity be determined before final donor selection is made, especially if there are more than one HLA-A and HLA-B compatible donors available.

For many years, phenotypic identity for HLA-D has been based on the results of the mixed lymphocyte culture reactions in families. The mixed lymphocyte culture is a test of lymphocyte proliferation and requires 7 to 10 days to complete and interpret. Peripheral blood lymphocytes from the recipient and from potential donor(s) are cultured together in plastic microtitre wells. In order to assess the relative reactivity of the donor vs. recipient, and vice versa, so-called one-way mixed lymphocyte cultures are set up between fixed ratios of responding cells (e.g., donor = A) and irradiated stimulator cells (e.g., recipient = Bx). The irradiated cells (Bx) cannot proliferate, but serve to present the foreign histocompatibility antigens as stimuli to the responder cells.

After approximately 6 days of coculture, radiolabeled nucleotide (tritiated thymidine) is added for an additional 6 to 18 hours of culture before the experiment is terminated. Only untreated responder cells (A) can incorporate the isotope. Thus, the measure of radionucleotide in the cells at the end of the culture period [usually expressed as counts, or disintegrations, per minute, (cpm)] reflects the intensity of the responder vs. stimulator reaction (ABx). Siblings who are identical at the major histocompatibility complex will have very low mutual reactivity, being essentially indistinguishable from that of the responder stimulated by his or her own irradiated stimulator cells (thus, ABx = AAx). The experimental control for maximal responsiveness in the mixed lymphocyte culture is provided by a mixture of lymphocytes (pool = P) from unrelated individuals (APx). Results of crude data from the mixed lymphocyte culture are used to calculate a relative response (RR). This calculation can be used as a rough measure to compare the degree of HLA-D compatibility among responder-stimulator pairs in the same mixed lymphocyte culture experiment. The formula for percent relative response (22) is:

$$\%\mathrm{RR} = \frac{\mathrm{AB^x - AA^x}}{\mathrm{AP^x = AA^x}} \times 100$$

where AB^x, AA^x, and AP^x are expressed as radioactive counts per minute.

Each laboratory must establish its own standards for the percent relative response which represents a nonreactive or "negative" mixed lymphocyte culture response between HLA identical sibling pairs. For this reason the definition of "positive" responses in mixed lymphocyte culture varies from greater than 5% to greater than 18% relative response, depending on the reporting laboratory (22,33). With technical improvements and the availability of test systems to type for individual D region loci, such as DP, it is becoming apparent that some instances of "low reactivity" in mixed lymphocyte culture between seemingly HLA-identical siblings may reflect true antigenic differences. These differences may be due either to genetic recombination in centromeric regions of the major histocompatibility complex or phenotypic differences in the expression of class II antigens (described above).

Modifications of the mixed lymphocyte culture such as the use of (1) homozygous typing cells (HTC), which are homozygous for HLA-D specificities, and (2) prolonged culture with priming and restimulation, the primed lymphocyte test (PLT), can be performed in specialized laboratories. These technical modifications help to define the genetic bases of reactions in the primary mixed lymphocyte cultures between HLA identical donor-recipient pairs (22).

Complotypes are relatively easy to assign based on electrophoretic segregation (22). Complotypes are encoded between HLA-B and HLA-Dr, and thus they form part of the extended haplotypes (Figure 1). Complotypes are closely linked to HLA-D, since no recombinants between HLA-B and HLA-Dr have yet been identified where the complotype segregated with HLA-B. Thus, complotypes can be informative in establishing the chromosomal source of HLA-D material.

The usual approach used to identify a sibling who is identical at the major histocompatibility complex involves two steps: (1) serologic typing for HLA-A, -B and -DR of all family members, and (2) confirmation of identity between HLA-A, -B, and -DR identical siblings by observing mutual nonreactivity in mixed lymphocyte culture.

In contrast, protocols for selection of potential unrelated donors vary from one transplant center to another. It has not yet been established that phenotypic identity at non-HLA-D loci is of critical importance to the success of unrelated transplantation. For this reason, related or unrelated donors who are mismatched at one or more HLA-A or -B loci, but who are DR identical or unreactive in mixed lymphocyte culture have been employed as donors for marrow transplants if no donor candidates with complete phenotypic identity can be found.

The unrelated donor program established at the University of Minnesota, in conjunction with the St. Paul Red Cross Regional Blood Center, has accepted the following guidelines for donor selection:

1. A list of HLA-A and -B compatible or one HLA-A antigen mismatched subjects is abstracted from a roster of approximately 4000 regular donors of pheresis blood products, all of whom have been previously typed for HLA-A and -B.
2. Potential donors from this list, who are also matched with the recipient for both Dr alleles, are requested to provide blood samples for mixed lymphocyte culture testing with the recipient's cells.
3. A final selection is then made from among the MLC nonreactive donors, based largely on comparative percent relative response (% RR) as well as other practical considerations.

Reports from other centers suggest that the likelihood of two individuals who are identical by Dr or D typing to be nonreactive in mixed lymphocyte culture ranges from 10–30% (34–36). Additional information, such as DP typing, is also being collected prospectively in these cases. Where available, complotypes can be used to screen large donor lists for individuals who can be further typed for the major histocompatibility complex as potential unrelated donors (22).

Selection of a suitable matched sibling donor by the routine laboratory procedure for typing of the major histocompatibility complex can be complicated in cases where the recipients have severe combined immunodeficiency (SCID) or leukemia, particularly chronic myeloid leukemia (CML). HLA typing and MLC testing can be difficult in SCID for several reasons: (1) there may be extreme lymphopenia, (2) there may be aberrant expression of HLA antigens (as in the "bare lymphocyte syndrome") (37), and (3) there may be presence of silent maternal engraftment resulting in the finding of "too many" specificities by serologic HLA typing (39), and (4) there may be nonreactivity in mixed lymphocyte culture because of inherent defects of lymphocyte proliferation. Currently, tissue typing of infants with circulating maternal lymphocytes usually requires the physical separation of patient (generally non-T cells) from maternal (usually predominantly T) cells before typing of the major histocompatibility complex is performed.

Contamination of the peripheral blood mononuclear cell preparation with even small numbers of leukemic cells, as in chronic myeloid leukemia, can interfere with both serologic and cellular techniques of MHC typing. Leukemic cells can react anomalously to heterologous typing sera, confusing the interpretation of HLA-DR typing in particular. Leukemic cells generally incorporate radionucleotides at a higher rate than normal resting lymphocytes and, therefore, they can contribute to a high "autologous" background stimulation (AA^x) in mixed lymphocyte culture. Leukemic cells have also been shown to elicit reactivity by T cells of the HLA-identical sibling. As in the case of silent maternal engraftment, physical methods can be used to separate leukemic cells from the patient's normal lymphocytes which are then tested for compatibility at the major histocompatibility complex. In the future, many of these problems may be circumvented by the use of restriction fragment length polymorphisms (RFLP) for matching silbings in the 6p region (39).

Finally, it should be mentioned that blood-derived cells from siblings who are genetically identical at the major histocompatibility complex can, in fact, be different due to differential expression of class II molecules (16,35). Class II molecules are assembled from separate and allelic alpha and beta chains, and the chains of any given class II molecule may derive from either the father or mother or both. Thus, the theoretical possibility exists that one sibling's lymphocytes may express a predominance of class II molecules, e.g., HLA-Dr, composed of the maternal alpha chain and paternal beta chain, while the other sibling's cells express proportionally more class II molecules made up of the heterozygous paternal alpha chain and maternal beta chain. Conventional serologic techniques may not be sensitive enough to detect such relatively subtle differences, and the biologic importance of nonrandom alpha and beta chain assortment in the causation of graft rejection or graft-vs.-host disease is only speculative at this time. Murine experiments that were designed to reprobe the genetic basis of hematopoietic (hybrid) resistance, or hematopoietic histocompatibility (40), have demonstrated the preferential expression of "hybrid" class II molecules in transplant-resistant animals which may represent the putative (MHC-linked) hematopoietic histocompatibility antigens.

HUMAN MARROW TRANSPLANTATION ACROSS HISTOCOMPATIBILITY BARRIERS

Matched Transplantation

The large experience with transplantation among histocompatible siblings has served as the basis for developing protocols to achieve reliable multilineage engraftment for a variety of diseases. Today, graft rejection in matched transplantation for leukemias (both acute and chronic) has been virtually eliminated through the use of standardized protocols. These protocols employ chemotherapy in combination with high-dose single fraction or fractionated total body irradiation (41), whole donor marrow, and the use of either methotrexate or cyclosporine post-transplant to prevent graft-vs.-host disease (42,43). However, preliminary reports suggest that the substitution of *ex vivo* T cell depletion of donor marrow, in an attempt to further reduce the incidence of graft-vs.-host disease, increases the risk of nonengraftment in matched leukemic recipients who receive standard doses of pretransplant chemotherapy and radiotherapy (44–46).

For aplastic anemia the current widespread use of limited field (e.g., total lymphoid or thoracoabdominal) irradiation (47,48), or low dose radiation (49), in combination with cyclophosphamide has resulted in a rate of successful primary engraftment of about 95% for transfused patients. Post-transplant infusion of donor peripheral blood buffy coat cells partially overcomes the 30% rejection rate observed in transfused aplastic patients preconditioned with cyclophosphamide alone. However, this practice may carry an increased risk of chronic graft-vs.-host disease (50).

An estimated 90% of infants with severe combined immunodeficiency disease experience permanent engraftment of donor T lymphocytes without the need for any prior immunosuppressive cytoreductive therapy, provided they receive adequate numbers of marrow cells by the intravenous route (51).

A combination of chemotherapeutic agents, frequently consisting of busulfan and cyclophosphamide, is now commonly used to prepare patients with nonmalignant genetic conditions which may cause early death, such as partial immunodeficiencies, metabolic disorders and thalassemia major. This approach was designed to avoid adverse effects of high dose radiation and has also been successful in patients with leukemia (52). However, rejection remains a problem in an estimated 10–50% of matched recipients with metabolic diseases (53). These patients generally have not received prior chemotherapy, may be highly presensitized from chronic transfusions (as in children with thalassemia), or both.

Acute graft-vs.-host disease is a frequent complication of matched transplantation. Reported rates for series of patients who received *in vivo* immunosuppressive prophylaxis against graft-vs.-host disease range from 25% to over 70% (18,19). Chronic graft-vs.-host disease affects 30–40% of matched transplant recipients (54). The development of graft-vs.-host disease and the use of immunosuppressive drugs, principally steroids, for its treatment significantly delay immunologic recovery after transplant (55). The incidence of graft-vs.-host disease increases with age (48,57) and may be linked to the underlying diagnosis (25,56).

Since it has been shown that alleles encoded within the major histocompatibility complex predispose for or protect against the clinical expression of diseases (57), HLA associations with graft-vs.-host disease have also been investigated. Several HLA specificities appear to increase the risk of GVH disease. These include HLA B18 (58); HLA CW14, BW21, B49, and B50 (56). The risk of graft-vs.-host disease is decreased with HLA B8, B35 (58), HLA A19 and related specificities (56). These relationships still need to be substantiated in larger series of patients and corrected for the number of antigens tested. The mechanism or mechanisms by which HLA specificities or closely linked alleles influence the clinical expression of graft-vs.-host disease are not known. Possibilities include preferential interaction of certain HLA specificities with putative minor histocompatibility antigens (16), or presence of loci linked to the major histocompatibility complex which can modify the development of graft tolerance (59).

In our experience at the University of Minnesota, subtle differences in the relative response in mixed lymphocyte culture among histocompatibility siblings have also predicted a statistically significantly increased risk of acute graft-vs.-host disease. Only 38% of recipients who demonstrated truly negative mutual responses in mixed lymphocyte culture with donors (such as DR^x and $RD^x \leq 0\%$ of the autologous background DD^x or RR^x) experienced graft-vs.-host disease. In comparison, there was a 53% incidence of graft-vs.-host disease in recipients who showed slightly positive responses in mixed lymphocyte cultures (%RR or relative response = 1–5% in either direction): p = .001.

Figure 2 illustrates the effect of reactivity in mixed lymphocyte culture on the time to graft-vs.-host disease for histocompatible patients, separated according to their underlying diagnoses. These data were obtained as part of a larger analysis of several potential predictive factors. Along with donor age and sex matching, reactivity in mixed lymphocyte culture emerged as an independent predictive variable that could be used to select the "better" donor, in other words, the donor less likely to lead to graft-vs.-host disease, when more than one HLA identical donor was available within a family. The genetic bases

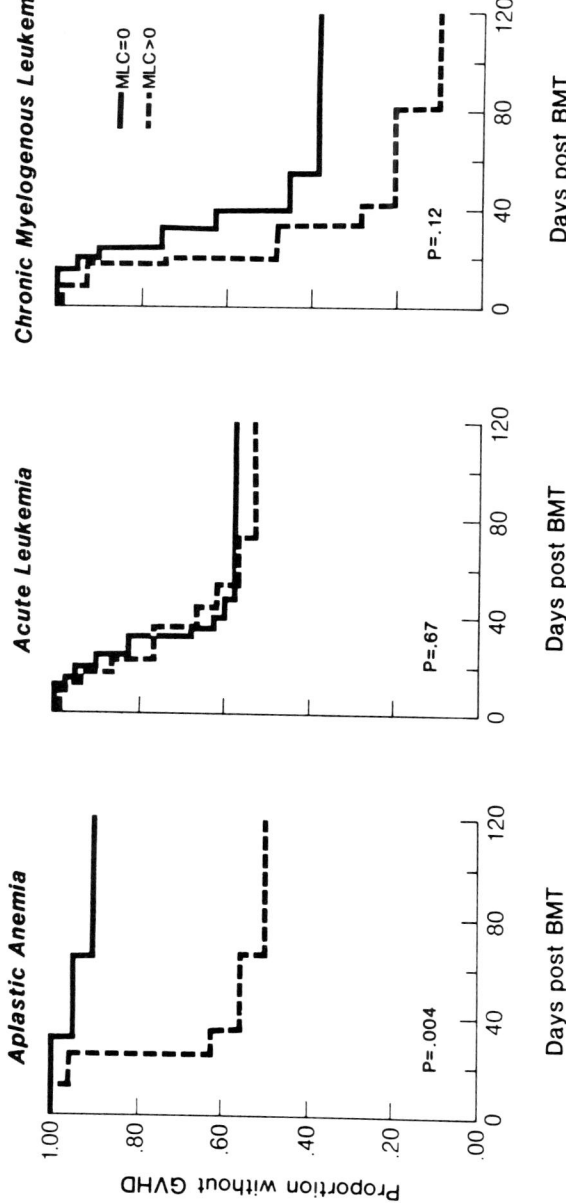

FIG. 2. Time to graft-vs.-host disease according to diagnosis and reactivity in the mixed lymphocyte culture (MLC) test. Overall p (all diagnoses) < .001. MLC = 0 refers to transplant recipients whose %RR in MLC in both directions: DR^x and RR^x was ≤ 0% of the autologous backgrounds, DD^x and RR^x; MLC > 0 refers to recipients with 1–5% RR in either or both one-way MLC tests with their HLA compatible sibling donor (see text for details).

of a positive mixed lymphocyte culture between HLA identical siblings have not been defined. However, possible explanations include: (1) the presence of a recombinant in the centromeric region of the major histocompatibility complex which would not be detected by conventional serologic HLA typing, (2) post-translational assortment or modification of class II molecule subunits resulting in subtle antigenic differences at class II loci between donor and recipient, and (3) differences in the inheritance of minor histocompatibility antigens, particularly if such loci are not on chromosome number 6. Assuming that these "slightly positive" responses in mixed lymphocyte culture are not simply the result of experimental error, additional study will be needed before biologic significance can be assigned to these observations.

In contrast to the well-recognized deleterious effects of graft-vs.-host disease, there also appears to be an advantage to allogeneic transplantation, and the occurrence of graft-vs.-host disease in particular, in reducing the incidence of post-transplant relapse of leukemia. It has been speculated that the occurrence of graft-vs.-host disease, the therapy given, or both, may be related to the lower relapse rate observed among recipients of allogeneic marrow compared with recipients of syngeneic (identical twin) marrow, since both groups received similar pretransplant antileukemic therapy (60). Among allogeneic recipients, the severity of graft-vs.-host disease has been inversely correlated with incidence of leukemic relapse (61).

Two analyses from our experience at the University of Minnesota also support the conclusion that graft-vs.-host disease can influence the rate of post-transplant relapse in patients with leukemias who are transplanted from histocompatible siblings. In these series, all patients were treated with a conditioning regimen that consisted of cyclophosphamide (60mg/kg/day for 2 days) and single dose (750 cGy), or fractionated total body irradiation (165 cGy for 8 doses). First, comparison of allogeneic and autologous (monoclonal-antibody treated) transplants in children and young adults revealed a similar rate of disease-free survival for recipients of either autologous grafts or allogeneic grafts in the absence of graft-vs.-host disease. The survival rate in either case was approximately 25%. An improved disease-free survival rate of approximately 40% at 2 years was seen among allogeneic recipients who had developed graft-vs.-host disease. This finding was significantly different by statistical analysis (62). In a separate analysis, time to relapse was examined according to the presence or absence of chronic GVH disease. Patients treated for acute lymphoblastic leukemia or chronic myeloid leukemia who developed chronic GVH disease had fewer relapses than patients who did not develop chronic GVH disease (63–64).

Partially Matched Related Transplantation Without T Cell Depletion

As one approach to expanding the number of potential donors, allografts of unmanipulated marrow from partially matched family members have been administered to selected patients who lacked histocompatible siblings. Until recently, such "mismatched related" transplants were restricted to donor-recipient pairs who were genotypically haplo-identical and were also phenotypically matched at one or more loci of the second haplotype.

In the treatment of aplastic anemia, unlike the current experience with use of histocompatible siblings, the results of transplantation from such closely matched relatives have been discouraging. Rejection of the primary graft has occurred in approximately half of patients in all published series, and long-term survival with adequate hematopoietic recovery has ranged from less than 10% to 28% (65–68).

In contrast, the use of partially matched related donors for treatment of hematologic malignancies while in remission, has resulted in a relapse-free survival rate that is comparable to that achieved with histocompatible transplantation (65,69,70). The rates of graft rejection, and related clinical problems such as delayed engraftment and prolonged granulocytopenia, were found to be statistically significantly greater in partially matched as compared to histocompatible recipients. However, overall engraftment failure in leukemia patients did not exceed 10% in any series. When compared to histocompatible donor-recipient transplants, the risk of graft-vs.-host disease is significantly increased by the use of partially matched donors, regardless of the form of post-transplant prophylaxis used. Thus, with use of methotrexate alone, the risk of GVH disease was 70% vs. 42% (for matched recipients) (69); with use of anti-thymocyte globulin, prednisone and methotrexate, the risk of GVH disease was 88% vs. 49% (65); and with use of cyclosporine A, the risk of GVH disease was 80% in mismatched recipients (70). The severity of graft-vs.-host disease was also increased in all series. The data shown in Table 1, comparing outcome of partially matched transplantation with the histocompatible "control" group from our Minnesota experience, is representative of the worldwide experience. Of note, patients undergoing mismatched transplantation experienced, on the average, longer and more costly hospitalizations due to the high rate of transplant-related complications.

TABLE 1. *Comparison of transplant outcome: Use of histocompatible sibling donors vs. partially matched related donors (total n).*

Outcome of Transplant	Aplastic anemia		Leukemia	
	Histocompatible (47)	Partially (7) Matched	Histocompatible (172)	Partially (9) Matched
Engraftment	> 96%	59%	> 99%	100%*
Graft-vs.-host disease	32%	50%	49%	88%
Disease-free survival	70%	28%	42%	44%

*3/9: mixed chimeras
Data from the University of Minnesota bone marrow transplantation experience, 1985.

A recent analysis of the relationship between HLA disparity and the risk of graft-vs.-host disease among 105 patients transplanted in Seattle failed to detect significant differences between patients who were mismatched at class I loci as compared with those mismatched at class II loci (69). However, the small group of patients who fared best were those who were phenotypically identical on HLA typing with their donors. More limited data from the Minnesota series is consistent with this finding, and also emphasizes the positive effect of donor-recipient mutual nonreactivity in the mixed lymphocyte culture (65).

A limited number of partially matched transplants have been performed for treatment of metabolic disorders (71). While mismatched transplants have produced metabolic correction in some patients, the barriers of graft rejection and severe graft-vs.-host disease still pose significant complications in this relatively young group of patients.

T Cell-depleted Haplo-identical Transplantation

The first reproducible successes with haplo-identical (usually parental) transplantation followed the development of an *ex vivo* technique for T cell elimination from human marrow, which was based on the principle of differential lectin-binding (72). This technique separated T cells, which produce graft-vs.-host disease, from normal marrow stem cells. The bone marrow was agglutinated with soybean lectin, followed by sheep red blood cell rosette formation and depletion (SBA/E/E^n). Although tedious, this procedure has been highly effective in removing T cells and preventing graft-vs.-host disease in marrow transplants performed across the major histocompatibility barrier.

Ex vivo SBA/E/E^n treatment with minor modifications has been used at many transplant centers in the United States, Europe, in the Middle East, and in Asia, particularly in the treatment of lethal congenital immunodeficiencies. Transplantation with use of T cell-depleted bone marrow from a parental donor for treatment of severe combined immunodeficiency (SCID) has proved to be attractive from both practical and scientific perspectives. Logistically, it has been estimated that less than 10% of SCID patients will have a histocompatible sibling (73). Furthermore, the barrier to engraftment is weak in patients with severe constitutional T cell deficiency; consequently, little or no immunosuppression is necessary for matched transplantation. Thus, SCID provides an ideal natural setting for the investigation of bone marrow transplantation using mismatched marrow, T cell-depleted marrow, or both.

The published reports of such transplants in SCID concur in their conclusions. Efficient T cell depletion has greatly decreased the very high anticipated rate of graft-vs.-host disease in haplo-identical transplantation (74,75). However, primary engraftment does not always occur without prior immunosuppression. As many as half of patients with severe combined immunodeficiency have required secondary T cell-depleted grafts, cytoreductive or immunosuppressive therapy, or both (76). Despite demonstrated chimerism, immunoreconstitution has not always been prompt or complete following such T cell-depleted transplants. B cell function in particular is not consistently corrected (75).

T cell depletion by mechanical methods as well as by immunologic methods, such as monoclonal antibody and complement lysis (77,78) or the use of immunotoxins (79), have also been applied to haplo-identical transplantation of leukemia and rare cases of genetic disorders. Although this area of clinical investigation is still in its formative stages, it is apparent that stable engraftment is rarely achieved when standard methods for pretransplant conditioning of histocompatible patients are used (78). To overcome this problem, several investigators have devised more intensive pretransplant immunosuppressive protocols to prepare haplo-identical recipients. Higher doses of total body irradiation and additional cytoreductive or immunosuppressive agents (78) have been tried with variable success. Significant morbidity from organ toxicity and opportunistic infections has developed despite an apparent improvement in engraftment.

Another major complication seemingly peculiar to T cell-depleted and mismatched transplantation, and particularly in patients with underlying immune deficiencies, is the appearance of fatal post-transplant B cell lymphoproliferative disorders. These tumors are frequently extranodal, they are rapidly progressive and resistant to both immunologic and cytotoxic therapy (80,81). Tumors have developed as late as 39 months following donor engraftment (82). The majority but not all of these B cell lymphoproliferative disorders have been associated with primary or reactivated Epstein-Barr virus infection. While it is tempting to attribute the emergence of lymphomas to ineffective immunoreconstitution, the predisposing factors have not yet been delineated.

Unrelated Transplantation

Successful cases of transplantation from phenotypically histocompatible, but unrelated, donors began to be published in the late 1970s (83,84). The systematic study of this approach as a therapeutic alternative for patients lacking histocompatible donors has been led by investigators at the University of Iowa. Their preliminary conclusion is that the use of partially matched unrelated donors is safe and feasible for the treatment of acute leukemias in remission and for chronic myeloid leukemia in chronic phase, (85) recently supported by data from the University of Minnesota (86).

The world's experience with unrelated transplantation (68 patients) was scrutinized at an international conference held at the National Institutes of Health in Bethesda, Maryland, USA, in May 1985. At that time the longest living survivor was 3.5 years post-transplant and the overall survival rate stood at 20% (87). Definition of the relative importance of matching for the different loci of the major histocompatibility complex, and possibly the importance of matching at minor histocompatibility loci, is a major goal of ongoing clinical trials of unrelated transplantation. If the therapeutic efficacy of transplantation of unrelated donor-recipient pairs is confirmed by ongoing studies, large-scale storage of cryopreserved cadaveric marrow may be used to supplement or supplant the use of living donors (87,88). Successful engraftment following infusion of cryopreserved cadaveric marrow has recently been reported (89).

LESSONS FROM EXPERIMENTAL ANIMAL STUDIES

Experimental animal models of bone marrow transplantation involving rodents, dogs and primates continue to play a critically important role by helping to define the necessary balance between factors determining acceptance (engraftment) and secondary complications of hematopoietic allografting (such as graft-vs.-host disease). Each of the animal models vary from one another in their inherent capacity to address different research questions relevant or parallel to human allogeneic transplantation. Rodent systems carry the advantage of extensive background information about immunogenetics, particularly in the mouse. Dogs and primates resemble humans more closely because of the composition of their hematopoietic and lymphoid organs, as well as in the practical aspects of medical treatment of larger, outbred species. However, each of these models has provided unique insights into the biology of allogeneic transplantation, as well as confirming general principles described in other species. Many of the methods which were used to overcome immunologic and/or genetic barriers to engraftment in lower animals have been successfully extrapolated to the human setting. Space does not permit a comprehensive review of animal studies pertaining to the histocompatibility barrier in marrow transplantation, but examples supporting current and future approaches will be mentioned here.

Studies in all major animal models have confirmed the importance of several factors affecting durable engraftment of marrow stem cells. These factors include: (1) the degree of histocompatibility (90,91), (2) the degree of matching for so-called non-MHC determinants, such as, allogeneic factors (92,93), (3) pretransplant conditioning of the recipient (94,95), (4) the dose (and route of administration) of transplanted cells (96), and (5) the composition of the hematopoietic graft (stem cells/"T" lymphocytes) (90,94).

Most animal models have employed single fraction, high-dose total body irradiation (referred to as "lethal" irradiation) to prepare recipients for grafting of hematopoietic tissues. In rat models of engraftment, chemotherapy alone (busulfan and cyclophosphamide) has been used (97). In these systems, genotypic identity at the major histocompatibility complex (mouse and monkey), DLA (dog) (91), and RT (rat) (97) confer an excellent prognosis for successful engraftment and the absence of serious graft-vs.-host disease. On the other hand, discrepancy in typing for only one of the major histocompatibility loci carries an increased risk of nonengraftment (91,97) under selective conditions (that is, less intensive pretransplant conditioning). Incompatibility at so-called "minor" as well as Hh (hematopoietic, or hybrid, histocompatibility) loci also imperils permanent engraftment (92,93). Animal studies have demonstrated that the cellular composition of the graft also influences the likelihood of sustained engraftment. These data indicate a significant impairment of engraftment of viable stem cells if other cells, such as T cells, NK cells, or both, have been removed from the transplant material (90).

Noteworthy advances have been made in the quest to overcome the barriers to hematopoietic transplantation posed by the histocompatibility of molecularly defined loci of the major histocompatibility complex and the functionally defined allogeneic resistance (hematopoietic histocompatibility) loci. Combinations of more intensive cytoreductive therapy, especially x-irradiation and more selective immunotherapy aimed at the elimination of residual host cells have been used. In the first instance, incompatibility at the major histocompatibility complex, depletion of post-thymic T cells (to prevent GVH disease, discussed below) combined with more intensive radiation and the use of other anti-T cell immunosuppressive agents have proved to be effective. Hematopoietic histocompatibility resistance, thought to be mediated primarily by NK-like cells, has been overcome with a variety of experimental approaches. These approaches include various schemes of "split dose" or larger fractions of radiation (each fraction being at least 300 cGy) (98), neutralization of host natural killer/macrophage function by infusion of anti-NK sera or other inactivating compounds such as anti-asialo GM1 (96, 108).

Animal models were instrumental in identifying T lymphocytes as the inciting factor or factors in the graft-vs.-host reaction. Several methods of T cell purging first shown to be efficacious in murine models have been applied to prevention of GVH disease in human transplantation. These methods are lectin-mediated separation of T cells from stem cells (72,101), monoclonal antibody and xenogenic or autologous complement lysis (102–105), and use of anti-T cell immunotoxins (79,106). Another approach to prevention of GVH disease and implicit T cell depletion is the physical separation and/or *ex vivo* propagation of hematopoietic stem cells prior to transplantation (96,107).

Furthermore, new genetic loci that regulate the expression of graft-vs.-host disease have been elucidated in mice (108,109). This knowledge has been used to explore alternate means of ameliorating the symptoms of graft-vs.-host disease by (1) pretransplant "conditioning" or sensitization of tolerizing cells in the donor via transfusions of recipient blood (110), or (2) the concurrent transplantation of allogeneic (mismatched T cell-depleted) marrow with autologous marrow (111).

Rodent transplant models have indicated that the graft-vs.-leukemia effect can often be distinguished from graft-vs.-host disease. Certain experiments have served to identify phenotypes of animals that are genetically resistant to hematologic malignancy irrespective of typing at the major histocompatibility complex (112), while others have demonstrated allogeneic "anti-tumor" effect without adverse clinical graft-vs.-host reactions (113).

Ongoing experiments with rodent models should also prove useful in directing the study of human post-transplant immunologic recovery. The limited examples available portend delayed expansion of a functional immunologic repertoire for histoincompatible (in other words, haplo-identical) recipients, compared with recipients of syngeneic cell transfer (114). Broad-ranging immunodeficiency has been observed secondary to subclinical chronic graft-vs.-host disease (115). The complexity and flexibility of immunologic development is based on current knowledge of the capacity for genetic rearrangement which leads to T and B cell diversity. These concepts support the belief that transplantation across histocompatibility barriers can result in functional immunoreconstitution.

FUTURE RESEARCH DIRECTIONS

Bone marrow transplantation has served medical science as a prototype of genetic engineering for the treatment of a number of systemic human diseases, both inherited and acquired. Investigators in the use of marrow transplantation have realized the potential of transferring near-perfect genetic information, regulated within the cellular package, to cure diseases which had previously proved fatal.

In the next century, we can anticipate that disease-specific therapies will replace the use of marrow transplantation for a number of conditions. In the treatment of leukemias, it is possible that minimal residual cancer will be eradicated by tumor-specific *in vivo* therapy, perhaps using a combination of targeted anti-tumor reagents (e.g., immunotoxins) and enhancement of natural anti-tumor effector mechanisms. It is likely that a number of inherited metabolic diseases will be treated by corrective gene insertion into autologous stem cells. For the remainder of the 20th century, however, whole cell marrow transplantation will thrive as a pivotal therapeutic and experimental modality for many human diseases. The judicious application of this approach will continue to supply the critical observer with biologic insights that will improve the treatment of premalignant, malignant, immunodeficient, and autoimmune diseases.

The need to improve the safety of marrow transplantation in the short term compels further exploration into the diversity of the human major histocompatibility complex. The continued development of MHC typing panels composed of monoclonal antibody specificities, and the use of DNA markers (such as restriction fragment length polymorphisms), will enhance the precision of genotypic matching between prospective marrow donors and recipients, thus improving our ability to select "best available" donors.

Modification in pretransplant conditioning may improve engraftment of T-depleted stem cells across histocompatibility barriers. Appropriate modifications might include the introduction of a significant delay (3 to 7 days) between total body irradiation and marrow infusion, the use of immunotherapies to neutralize residual sensitized T cells or augmented (interleukin-2-driven) natural killer cells, or a combination of both (116).

New approaches to prevention of graft-vs.-host disease should be tried under appropriate circumstances. Possible new approaches might be T cell subset depletion for MHC identical transplants, donor transfusion (with recipient cells), or combinations of allogeneic/syngeneic transplants in situations which do not place the donor at significant risk, and where autologous marrow is free of tumor.

Hopefully, post-transplant opportunistic infections, including Epstein-Barr virus associated lymphoproliferative disorders, will be resolved through the development of effective antiviral drugs.

Post-transplant immunoreconstitution after histocompatible grafting will continue to represent multifaceted, natural experiment. Study of this phenomenon will yield new information regarding the constraints, as well as the plasticity, of the human immunologic repertoire (117).

REFERENCES

1. Francke U, Pellegrino MA: Assignment of the major histocompatibility complex to a region of the short arm of chromosome 6. *Proc Nat'l Acad Sci (USA)* 1977; 74:1147–1151.
2. Gorer, PA, Lyman S, Snell GD: Studies on genetic and antigenic basis of tumour and transplantation: linkage between a histocompatibility gene and "fused" in mice. *Proc R Soc London* (B) 1948; 135:499–505.
3. Ceppellini R, Curtoni ES, Mattiuz PL, et al.: Genetics of leukocyte antigens. A family study of segregation and linkage. In: Curtoni ES, Mattiuz PL, Tossi RM, (eds); *Histocompatibility Testing 1967,* Copenhagen, Munksgaard 1967; p. 149–187.
4. Bortin MM, Rimm AA: Severe combined immunodeficiency disease: Characterization of the disease and results of transplantation. *JAMA* 1977; 238:591–600.
5. Meuwissen HJ, Gatti RA, Terasaki PI, et al.: Treatment of lymphopenic hypogammo-globulinemia and bone marrow aplasia by transplantation of allogeneic marrow. *N Engl J Med* 1969; 281:691–697.
6. Bach FH, Albertini RJ, Anderson JL, et al.: Bone marrow transplantation in patients with the Wiskott-Aldrich syndrome. *Lancet* 1968; ii:1364–1366.
7. DeKonig J, van Bekkum D, Dicke KA, et al.: Transplantation of bone marrow cells and fetal thymus in an infant with lymphopenic immunological deficiency. *Lancet* 1969; 1:1223–1227.
8. Duasset J, Colombani J, Legrand L, et al.: Genetics of the HLA system: deduction of 480 haplotypes. In: Terasaki PI, ed; *Histocompatibility Testing 1970,* Copenhagen, Munksgaard 1970, pp. 53–77.
9. Bach M, Bach F: Immunogenetic disparity and graft-vs.-host reactions. *Semin Hematol* 1974; 11:291–303.
10. O'Reilly, RJ: Allogeneic bone marrow transplantation: Current status and future directions. *Blood* 1983; 62:941–964.
11. Hansen JA, Clift RA, Thomas ED, et al.: Histocompatibility and marrow transplantation. *Transplant Proc* 1979; 11:1924–1929.
12. Reisner Y, Kapoor N, Kirkpatrick D, et al.: Transplantation for acute leukemia with HLA-A

and B nonidentical parental marrow cells fractionated with soybean agglutinin and sheep red blood cells. *Lancet* 1981; 2:327–331.

13. Blazar BR, Quinones RR, Heinitz KJ, et al.: Comparison of three techniques for the *ex vivo* elimination of T cells from human bone marrow. *Exp Hematol* 1985; 13:123–128.

14. Filipovich AH, Vallera DA, Youle RJ, et al.: Ex-vivo treatment of donor bone marrow with anti-T-cell immunotoxins for prevention of graft-vs.-host-disease. *Lancet* 1984; i(8375):469–472.

15. Slavin S, Waldmann H, Or R, et al: Prevention of graft-vs.-host disease in allogeneic bone marrow transplantation for leukemia by T cell depletion *in vitro* prior to transplantation. *Transplant Proc* 1985; 17:465–467.

16. Van Rood JJ, de Jongh B, Claas FHJ, et al. New facts on HLA genetics: Are they relevant in bone marrow transplantation? *Semin Hematol* 1984; 21:65–80.

17. Lotzova E: Involvement of MHC-linked hemopoietic-histocompatibility genes in allogeneic bone marrow transplantation in mice. *Tissue Antigens* 1977; 9:148–152.

18. Glucksberg H, Storb R, Fefer A, et al. Clinical manifestations of graft-vs.-host disease in human recipients of marrow from HL-A-matched sibling donors. *Transplantation* 1974; 18:295–304.

19. Neudorf S, Filipovich AH, Ramsay NKC et al. Prevention and treatment of acute graft-vs.-host disease. *Semin Hematol* 1984; 21:91–100.

20. Bernard A, Boumsell L, Dausset J, et al. Leucocyte typing. Human leucocyte differentiation antigens detected by monoclonal antibodies; Berlin, Springer-Verlag, 1984.

21. Bodmer J, Bodmer W: Histocompatibility 1984. *Immunol Today* 1984; 5:251–254.

22. Alper CA, Awdeh ZL, Rappeport J, et al. Complotypes in bone marrow transplantation. *Transplant Proc* 1985; 17:440–441.

23. Yunis EJ, Awdeh Z, Raum D, et al. The MHC in human bone marrow allotransplantation. *Clinics Haematol* 1983; 12:641–680.

24. Bortin MM, Gale RP, Rimm AA: Allogeneic bone marrow transplantation for 144 patients with severe aplastic anemia. *JAMA* 1981; 245:1132–1139.

25. Kersey JH, for the International Bone Marrow Transplant Registry. Personal communication to the author, 1986.

26. Gluckman E, Barrett AJ, Arcese W, et al.: Bone marrow transplantation in severe aplastic anemia. A survey of the European Group for Bone Marrow Transplantation. *Br J Haematol* 1981; 49:165–173.

27. Cudkowicz G, Hockman PS. Do natural killer cells engage in regulated reactions against self to ensure homeostasis? *Immunol Rev* 1979; 44:13–41.

28. Clark EA, Harmon RC: Genetic control of natural cytotoxicity and hybrid resistance. In: Klein F, Weinhouse S, eds.; *Advances in Cancer Research;* New York, Academic Press 1980; 31:226–285.

29. Warner JF, Dennert G. Bone marrow graft rejection as a function of antibody-directed natural killer cells. *J Exp Med* 1985; 161:563–576.

30. Kiessling R, Hochman PS, Haller O, et al.: Evidence for a similar or common mechanism for natural killer cell activity and resistance to hemopoietic grafts. *Eur J Immunol* 1977; 7:655–663.

31. Delmonte L: The MO/NK Cell: An inducer of HLA-independent graft-vs.-host disease? In: Cohen E, Singal DP, eds.; *Non-HLA Antigens in Health, Aging and Malignancy*, New York, Alan R. Liss, Inc.; 1983; 235–242.

31. Amos DB, Bashir H, Boyle W, et al.: A simple microcytotoxicity test. *Transplantation* 1969; 7:220.

32. Clift RA, Hansen JA, Thomas ED, et al.: Marrow transplantation from donors other than HLA identical siblings. *Transplantation* 1979; 28:235–242.

34. Dupont B, Hansen JA: Donor selection for bone marrow transplantation: The predictive value of HLA-D typing for MLR compatibility between unrelated individuals. *Transplant Proc* 1978; 10:53–56.

35. Van Rood JJ, Van Leeuwen A, Pahwa S, et al.: The importance of non-HLA systems and the feasibility of the use of unrelated donors in bone marrow transplantation. *Transplant Proc* 1978; 10:47–56.

36. Jeannet M, Speck B: Donor selection for bone marrow transplantation. Predictive value of

DR typing for mixed lymphocyte culture compatibility between unrelated individuals. *Transplant* 1978; 26:448–449.

37. Touraine JL, Betuel H, Souillet G, et al.: Combined immunodeficiency disease associated with absence of cell-surface HLA-A and -B antigens. *J Pediatr* 1978; 93:47–51.

38. Reinherz El, Acuto O, Fabbi M, et al.: Clonotypic surface structure on human T lymphocytes: functional and biochemical analysis of the antigen receptor complex. *Immunol Rev* 1984; 81:95–129.

39. Whitehead AS, Woods DE, Fleischnick E, et al.: DNA polymorphism of the C4 genes. A new marker for analysis of the major histocompatibility complex. *N Engl J Med* 1984; 310:88–91.

40. Drizlikh G, Schmidt-Sole J, Yankelevich B: Involvement of the K and I regions of the H-2 complex in resistance to hemopoietic allografts. *J Exp Med* 1984; 159:1070–1082.

41. Nesbit M, Woods W, Weisdorf D, et al.: Bone marrow transplantation for acute lymphocytic leukemia. In: Murphy S, ed: *Semin in Oncology,* New York, Grune and Stratton, 1985; 149–159.

42. Biggs JC, Atkinson K, Hayes J, et al.: After allogeneic bone marrow transplantation, cyclosporin A is associated with faster engraftment, less mucositis and three distinct syndromes of nephrotoxicity when compared to methotrexate. *Transplant Proc* 1983; 15:1487–1489.

43. Deeg HJ, Storb R, Buckner Cd, et al.: Acute nonlymphoblastic leukemia in first remission and chronic myelogenous leukemia in chronic phase treated by allogeneic marrow transplantation: A randomized study of methotrexate vs. incompatible host disease. *Blood* 1983; 62(5,suppl 1):A220.

44. Mitsuyasu RT, Champlin RE, Ho WG, et al.: Prospective randomized controlled trial of *ex vivo* treatment of donor bone marrow with monoclonal anti-T cell antibody and complement for prevention of graft-vs.-host disease: A preliminary report. *Transplant Proc* 1985; 17:482–485.

45. Martin PJ, Hansen JA, Storb R, et al.: A clinical trial of *in vitro* depletion of T cells in donor marrow for prevention of acute graft-vs.-host disease. *Transplant Proc* 1985; 17:486–487.

46. Filipovich AH, Vallera DA, Youle RJ, et al.: Graft-vs.-host disease prevention in allogeneic bone marrow transplantation from histocompatible siblings: A pilot study using immunotoxins for T cell depletion of donor bone marrow. *Transplant* 1987; 44:62–69.

47. Ramsay NK, Kim TH, McGlave P, et al.: Total lymphoid irradiation and cyclophosphamide conditioning prior to bone marrow transplantation for patients with severe aplastic anemia. *Blood* 1983; 62:622–626.

48. Gluckman E: Report of the workshop on anti-thymocyte globulin in severe aplastic anemia. In: Gale RP, ed; *Recent Advances in Bone Marrow Transplantation* New York, Alan R. Liss, Inc., 1983; 7:53–58.

49. Champlin R, Ho W, Winston DJ, et al.: Treatment of severe aplastic anemia. A comparison of antithymocyte globulin vs. allogeneic bone marrow transplantation. In: Gale RP, ed; *Recent Advances in Bone Marrow Transplantation* New York, Alan R. Liss, Inc. 1983; 7:29–38.

50. Storb R, Doney KC, Thomas ED, et al.: Marrow transplantation with or without donor buffy coat cells for 65 transfused aplastic anemia patients. *Blood* 1982; 59:236–246.

51. Good RA, Kapoor N, Pahwa RN, et al.: Current approaches to the primary immunodeficiencies. In: Fougereau M, Dausset J, eds: *Immunology 80;* New York, Academic Press, 1980; 906–929.

52. Santos GW, Tutschka PJ, Brookmeyer R, et al.: Marrow transplantation for acute nonlymphocytic leukemia after treatment with busulfan and cyclophosphamide. *N Engl J Med* 1983; 309:1347–1352.

53. Blazar BR, Ramsay NKC, Kersey JH, et al.: Pretransplant conditioning with busulfan (myleran) and cyclophosphamide for nonmalignant diseases: Failure of complete engraftment following histocompatible allogeneic bone marrow transplantation. *Transplantation* 1985; 39:597–603.

54. Sullivan KM, Shulman HM, Storb R: Chronic graft-vs.-host disease in 52 patients: Adverse natural course and successful treatment with combination immunosuppression. *Blood* 1981; 57:267–276.

55. Atkinson K, Farewell V, Storb R, et al.: Analysis of late infections after human bone marrow

transplantation: Role of genotypic nonidentity between marrow donor and recipient and of nonspecific suppressor cells in patients with chronic graft-vs.-host disease. *Blood* 1982; 60:714–720.

56. Bross DS, Tutschka PJ, Farmer ER, et al.: Predictive factors for acute graft-vs.-host disease in patients transplanted with HLA-identical bone marrow. *Blood* 1984; 63:1265–1270.

57. Tiwari JL, Terasaki PI: *HLA and Disease Associations,* New York, Springer-Verlag, 1985.

58. Storb R, Prentice RL, Hansen JA, et al.: Association between HLA-B antigens and acute graft-vs.-host disease in man. *Lancet* 1983; 2:816–819.

59. Tutschka PJ, Hess AD: Suppressor cells in transplantation tolerance. I. Suppressor cells in the mechanism of tolerance in radiation chimeras. *Transplantation* 1981; 32:203–209.

60. Weiden PL, Flournoy N, Thomas ED, et al.: Anti-leukemic effect of graft-vs.-host disease in human recipients of allogeneic marrow grafts. *N Engl J Med* 1979; 300:1068–1073.

61. Weiden PL, Sullivan KM, Flournoy N, et al.: The Seattle marrow transplantation unit: Antileukemic effect of chronic graft-vs.-host disease: Contribution to improved survival after allogeneic marrow transplantation. *N Engl J Med* 1981; 304:1529–1532.

62. Weisdorf D, Ramsay NKC: Personal communication to the author, 1986.

63. Henslee PG, Kersey JH: Personal communication to the author, 1986.

64. Henslee PJ, Ramsay NKC, Filipovich AH, et al.: Effect of chronic graft-vs.-host disease (CGVHD) on survival and relapse rate following bone marrow transplantation (Abstr). *Proceedings of the American Association for Cancer Research* 1985; 26:301.

65. Filipovich AH, Ramsay NKC, Arthur DC, et al.: Allogeneic bone marrow transplantation with related donors other than HLA MLC matched siblings, and the use of antithymocyte globulin, prednisone, and methotrexate for prophylaxis of graft-vs.-host disease. *Transplantation* 984; 39:282–285.

66. Dupont B, O'Reilly RJ, Pollack MS, et al.: Use of HLA genotypically different donors in bone marrow transplantation. *Transplant Proc* 1979; 11:219–224.

67. Hansen JA, Clift RA, Mickelson EM, et al.: Marrow transplantation from donors other than HLA identical siblings. *Hum Immunol* 1981; 1:31–40.

68. Stoch S, Gale RP, Champlin R, et al.: Partially mismatched marrow transplantation for acute leukemia and aplastic anemia. In: Gale RP, ed; *Recent Advances in Bone Marrow Transplantation,* New York, Alan R. Liss, Inc., 1983; 785–795.

69. Beatty PG, Clift RA, Mickelson EM, et al.: Marrow transplantation from related donors other than HLA-identical siblings. *N Eng J Med,* 1985; 313:765–771.

70. Powels R, Pedrazzini A, Crofts M, et al.: Mismatched family bone marrow transplantation. *Semin Hematol* 1984; 21:182–187.

71. Pearson ADJ: Survey of preparative regimens and complications of bone marrow transplantation in patients with lysosomal storage disease. In: Krivit W, and Paul, NW (eds); *Bone Marrow Transplantation for Treatment of Lysosomal Diseases,* New York, Alan R. Liss Inc., 1986; 153–164.

72. Reisner Y, Kapoor N, O'Reilly RJ, et al.: Allogeneic bone marrow transplantation using stem cells fractionated by lectins. VI. *In vitro* analysis of human and monkey bone marrow cells fractionated by sheep red blood and soybean agglutinin. *Lancet* 1980; 2(8208):1320–1323.

73. Levinsky RJ, Davies EG, Butler M. et al.: Problems of mismatched bone marrow transplantation for severe combined immunodeficiency using soybean lectin fractionation. *Exp Hematol* 1983; 11 (suppl. 113):89–90.

74. O'Reilly RJ, Kapoor N, Kirkpatrick D, et al.: Transplantation for severe combined immunodeficiency using histoincompatible parental marrow fractionated by soybean agglutinin and sheep red blood cells: Experience in six consecutive cases. *Transplant Proc* 1983; 15:1431–1435.

75. Friedrich W, Vetter U, Heymer B, et al.: Immunoreconstitution in severe combined immunodeficiency after transplantation of HLA-haploidentical, T-cell-depleted bone marrow. *Lancet* 1984; I(8380):761–764.

76. Filipovich AH: Progress in broadening the uses of marrow transplantation: availability of donors. *Vox Sang* 1986; 51 (supp 2) 95.

77. Spruce WE, McMillan R, Miller W, et al.: Transplantation of T-lymphocyte-depleted bone marrow between HLA-mismatched individuals. *Transplantation* 1983; 36:369–372.

78. Bozdech MJ, Sondel PM, Trigg ME, et al.: Transplantation of HLA-haploidentical T-cell

depleted marrow for leukemia: Addition of cytosine arabinoside to the pretransplant conditioning prevents rejection. *Exp Hematol* 1985; 13:1201–1210.

79. Filipovich AH, Vallera DA, Youle RJ, et al.: *Ex vivo* T depletion with immunotoxins in allogeneic bone marrow transplantation: The pilot clinical study for prevention of graft-vs.-host disease. *Transplant Proc* 1985; 17:442–444.

80. Shearer WT, Ritz J, Finegold MJ, et al.: Epstein-Barr virus-associated B-cell proliferations of diverse clonal origins after bone marrow transplantation in a 12-year-old patient with severe combined immunodeficiency. *N Engl J Med* 1985; 312:1151–1159.

81. McClain KL, Shapiro RS, Ramsay NKC, et al.: Virologic studies in four patients with posttransplant lymphomas following T-depleted mismatched bone marrow transplantation (BMT) (Abstr). *Blood* 1985; 66:242a.

82. Shapiro RS, Pietryga D, Blazar BR, et al.: B cell lymphoproliferative disorders following bone marrow transplantation. In: Gale RH, Champlin R, eds; *Recent Advances in Bone Marrow Transplantation* Vol 53, New York, Alan R. Liss, Inc. 1987; 647–657.

83. O'Reilly RJ, Dupont B, Pahwa S, et al.: Reconstitution in severe combined immunodeficiency by transplantation of marrow from an unrelated donor. *N Engl J Med* 1977; 297:1311–1318.

84. Horowitz SD, Bach FH, Groshong T, et al.: Treatment of severe combined immunodeficiency with bone-marrow from an unrelated mixed leukocyte-culture non-reactive donor. *Lancet* 1975; 2:431–433.

85. Gingrich RD, Howe CWS, Goeken NE, et al.: The use of partially matched, unrelated donors in clinical bone marrow transplantation. *Transplantation* 1985; 39:526–532.

86. McGlave P, Scott E, Ramsay N, et al.: Unrelated donor bone marrow transplantation therapy for chronic myelogenous leukemia. *Blood* 1987; 70(3): 877–881.

87. Kersey JH: Personal communication to the author, 1986.

88. Mugishima H, Terasaki P, Sueyoshi A. Bone marrow from cadaver donors for transplantation. *Blood* 1985; 65:392–396.

89. Blazar B, Lasky LC, Perentesis JP, et al.: Successful mononuclear and granulocytic engraftment in a recipient of bone marrow from a cadaveric donor. *Blood* 1986; 67: 1655–1660.

90. Wagemaker G, Vriesendorp HM, van Bekkum DW: Successful bone marrow transplantation across major histocompatibility barriers in rhesus monkeys. *Transplant Proc* 1981; 13:875–880.

91. Storb R, Thomas ED: Graft-vs.-host disease in dog and man: the Seattle experience. *Immunol Rev* 1985; 88:215–238.

92. Lotzova E, Savary CA: Natural resistance to foreign hemopoietic transplants: A possible model of leukemia surveillance. In: Mirand EA, Hutchinson WB, Enrick M, eds; *International Cancer Congress, Part C Biology of Cancer (2),* New York, Alan R. Liss, Inc., 1983; 125–135.

93. Korngold R, Sprent J: Lethal graft-vs.-host disease across minor histocompatibility barriers in mice. *Clin Haematol* 1983; 12:681–693.

94. Soderling CCB, Song CW, Blazar BR, et al.: A correlation between conditioning and engraftment in recipients of MHC mismatched T cell depleted murine bone marrow transplants. *J Immunol* 1985; 135:941–947.

95. Deeg HJ, Storb R, Shulman HM, et al.: Engraftment of DLA-nonidentical unrelated canine marrow after high-dose fractionated total body irradiation. *Transplantation* 1982; 33:443–446.

96. van Bekkum DW: The double barrier in bone marrow transplantation. *Semin Hematol* 1974; 11:325–340.

97. Oaks MK, Cramer DV: The genetics of bone marrow transplantation in the rat. *Transplantation* 1985; 39:69–76.

98. Miller SC: Genetically determined resistance to foreign bone marrow transplantation in mice: characterization of the effector cells. *J Immunol* 1983; 131:92–97.

99. Lotzova E, Savary CA, Pollack SB: Prevention of rejection of allogeneic bone marrow transplants by NK 1.1 antiserum. *Transplantation* 1983; 35:490–494.

100. Charley MR, Mikhael A, Bennett M, et al.: Prevention of lethal, minor-determinate graft-host disease in mice by the *in vivo* administration of anti-asialo GM_1. *J Immunol* 1983; 131:2101–2103.

101. Reisner Y, Biniaminov M, Rosenthal E, et al.: Interaction of peanut agglutinin with normal human lymphocytes and with leukemic cells. *Proc Natl Acad Sci (USA)* 1979; 76:447–451.
102. Vallera DA, Soderling CC, Carlson GJ, et al.: Bone marrow transplantation across major histocompatibility barriers in mice. Effect of elimination of T cells from donor grafts by treatment with monoclonal Thy-1.2 plus complement or antibody alone. *Transplantation* 1982; 33:243–248.
103. Prentice HG, Gilmore MJ, Price-Janes L, et al.: Depletion of T lymphocytes in donor marrow prevents significant graft-vs.-host disease in matched allogeneic leukæmic marrow transplant recipients. *Lancet* 1984; 1:472–476.
104. Thierfelder S, Cobbold S, Kummer U, et al.: Antilymphocytic antibodies and marrow transplantation. VII. Two of nine monoclonal anti-Thy-1 antibodies used for pretreatment of donor marrow suppressed graft-vs.-host reactions without added complement. *Exper Hematol* 1985; 13:948–955.
105. Goldman JM, Apperley JF, Jones L, et al.: Bone marrow transplantation for patients with chronic myeloid leukemia. *N Engl J Med* 1986; 314:202–207.
106. Vallera DA, Youle RJ, Neville DM Jr., et al.: Bone marrow transplantation across major histocompatibility barriers. V. Protection of mice from lethal graft-vs.-host disease pretreatment of donor cells with monoclonal anti-Thy1.2 coupled to the toxin ricin. *J Exp Med* 1982; 155:949–954.
107. Mauch P, Lipton JM, Hamilton B, et al.: Lethal graft-vs.-host disease: Modification with allogeneic cultured donor cells. *Blood* 1984; 63:1112–1119.
108. O'Toole MM, Bosma GC, Bosma MJ: Expression of Murine lm-1 locus. Lm-1 determinants on lymphocytes and macrophages, and effects of lm-1 incompatibility on bone marrow grafts. *J Exp Med* 1985; 162:607–624.
109. Click RE: Tolerance of histoincompatible marrow grafts. *Transplant Proc* 1979; 11:490–493.
110. Halle-Pannenko O, Pritchard LL, Bruley-Rosset M, et al.: Parameters involved in the induction and abrogation of the lethal graft-vs.-host reaction directed against non-H-2 antigens. *Immunol Rev* 1985; 88:59–85.
111. Ildstad ST, Sachs DH: Reconstitution with syngeneic plus allogeneic or xenogeneic bone marrow leads to specific acceptance of allografts or xenografts. *Nature* 1984; 307:168–170.
112. Singer DE, Hayner DR, William RM: Resistance to BM myelogenous leukemia in rat radiation chimeras. *Leuk Res* 1980; 4:337–342.
113. Truitt RL, Rose WC, Rimm AA, et al.: Graft-vs.-host leukemia. VIII. Selective reduction in anti-host reactivity without loss of antileukemia reactivity by treatment of donor mice with lipopolysaccharide. *Exp Hematol* 1978; 6:488–498.
114. Ildstad ST, Wren SM, Bluestone JA: Characterization of mixed allogeneic chimeras. Immunocompetence, *in vitro* reactivity and genetic specificity of tolerance. *J Exp Med* 1985; 162:231–244.
115. Shearer GM, Levy RB: Graft vs. host-associated immune suppression is activated by recognition of allogeneic murine I-A antigens. *J Exp Med* 1983; 157:936–946.
116. Filipovich AH, Malilay G, Condie RM, et al.: Preclinical studies directed at the prevention of allogeneic bone marrow rejection (Abstr) *Proc Am Soc Hematology, Blood* 1985; 66:66a.
117. Chu E, Umetsu D, Rosen F, et al.: Major histocompatibility restriction of antigen recognition by T cells in a recipient of haplotype mismatched human bone marrow transplantation. *J Clin Invest* 1983; 72:1124–1129.

Bone Marrow Transplantation in Children, edited by F. Leonard Johnson and Carl Pochedly. Raven Press, Ltd., New York © 1990.

Technique of Bone Marrow Transplantation

Carl Lenarsky

Division of Research Immunology and Bone Marrow Transplantation, Children's Hospital of Los Angeles, and Department of Pediatrics, University of Southern California School of Medicine, Los Angeles, California 90054-0700

A. Marrow harvesting technique
B. ABO incompatibility
C. Risks to the donor
D. Supportive services
    1. The transplant environment
    2. The transplant team
    3. Blood bank services
    4. Laboratory support
Summary

The number of medical centers performing bone marrow transplants has substantially increased over the past few years. As of 1987, the International Bone Marrow Transplantation Registry received data from 138 transplant teams worldwide in 31 countries (1). In addition, there are several transplant teams that do not report to the International Registry.

Although there are no strict guidelines and standards for the techniques of marrow transplantation, most transplant physicians utilize similar methods for the actual procurement and infusion of bone marrow. In contrast, differences exist in the supportive services provided for patients in various transplant centers. In this chapter, the basic procedures related to the transfer of bone marrow from donor to recipient will be reviewed. In addition, the supportive services needed for a successful pediatric bone marrow transplant program will be discussed.

MARROW HARVESTING TECHNIQUE

In 1970, Thomas and Storb reported a method for obtaining, preparing, and administering bone marrow which has not significantly changed in nearly 20 years (2). The marrow aspirations are carried out under sterile conditions in the operating room. General anesthesia is utilized most often, although it is possible to perform the procedure with spinal anesthesia (3). The donor is placed in the prone position and is slightly flexed at the waist. Bone marrow is aspirated from both posterior iliac crests (Figure 1). In most cases, not more than one or two skin punctures are necessary over each crest; the needle can be directed over the surface of the bone, and punctures made through the periosteum at multiple sites. In order to reduce contamination of marrow with peripheral blood, the needle and syringe should be gently rotated 360° during each aspiration, and the volume of each aspiration is limited to 5 to 10 ml.

The total volume of marrow obtained is dependent on the size of the recipient as well as the size of the donor. In general, one should attempt to collect 3×10^8 nucleated bone marrow cells per kilogram of recipient body weight. A volume of donor marrow of 10 to 15 ml. per kilogram of recipient body weight will usually contain an adequate number of marrow cells. How-

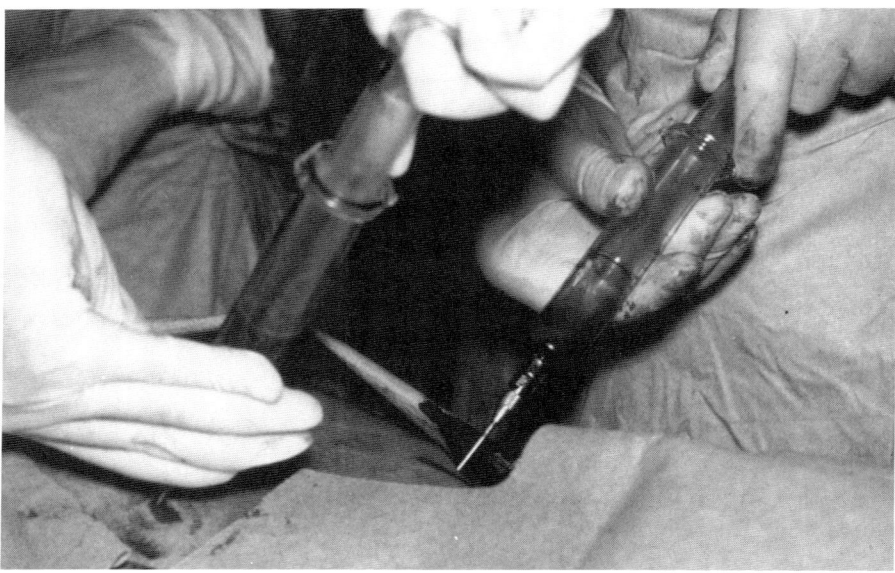

FIG. 1. Technique of bone marrow harvesting: bone marrow is aspirated from both posterior iliac crests by 2 operators.

ever, in many instances, with small donor and large recipient, this amount of marrow may be impossible to obtain. If necessary, additional marrow may be obtained from the anterior iliac crests, and very rarely, from the sternum or other long bones.

As the marrow is obtained, it is placed in a beaker containing a tissue culture medium and preservative-free heparin (Figure 2). After the marrow procurement procedure, the entire volume of bone marrow/medium and heparin is passed through 2 or 3 fine iron wire mesh filters to remove bone particles or clots (Figure 3). The filtered marrow is placed in a standard transfusion bag and eventually administered to the recipient intravenously (Figure 4).

The specific equipment and materials required for marrow procurement are all commercially available (Table 1, Figures 5 and 6). Alternatives for harvesting bone marrow have been utilized (4). A few investigators have reported utilizing circulating peripheral blood stem cells rather than marrow stem cells for autologous bone marrow transplantation (5). It remains to be determined whether sufficient numbers of stem cells can be isolated from peripheral blood to allow for allogeneic marrow engraftment.

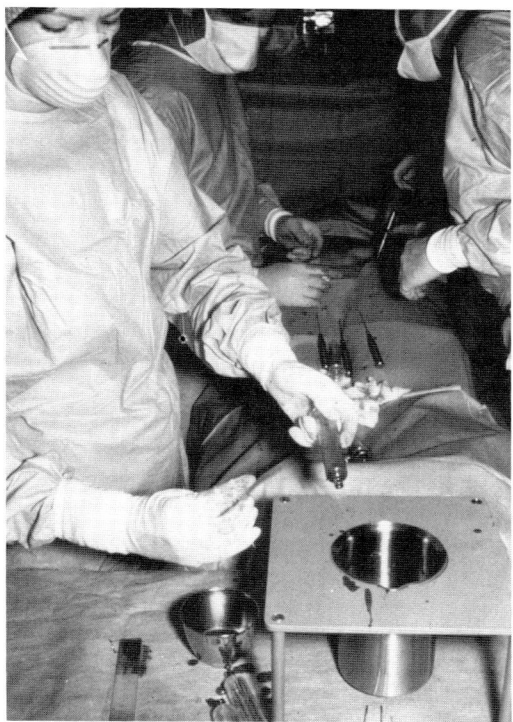

FIG. 2. An assistant places bone marrow into a sterile beaker containing physiologic medium and heparin.

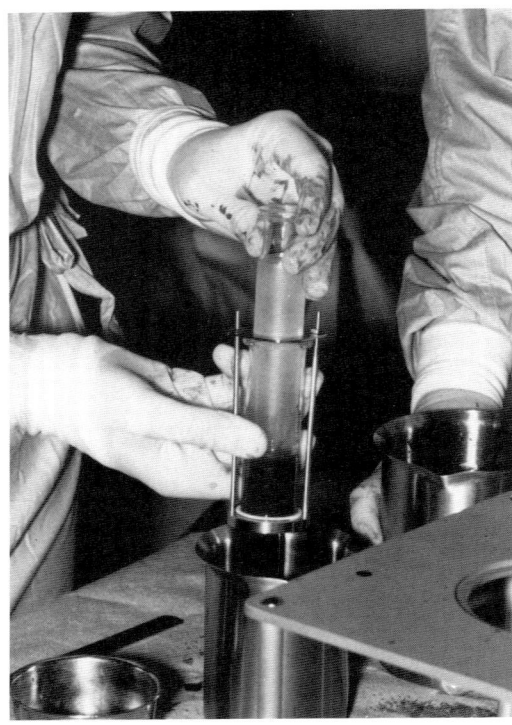

FIG. 3. Bone marrow is filtered to remove clots and bone particles.

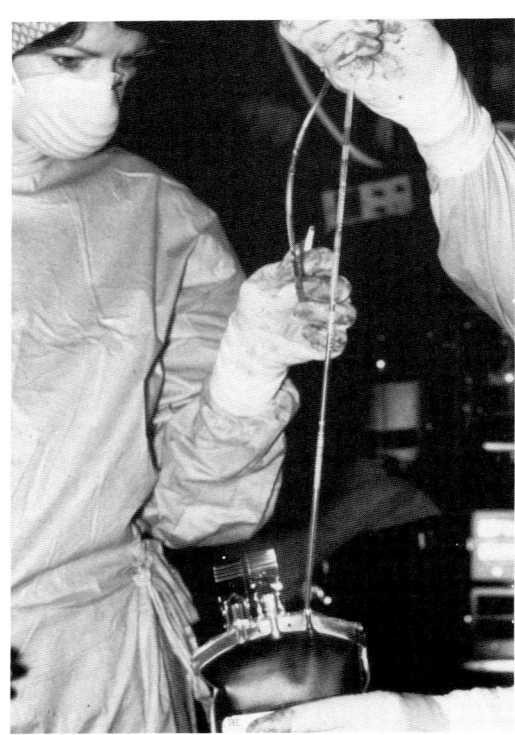

FIG. 4. Bone marrow is placed in transfusion bag and subsequently infused into recipient.

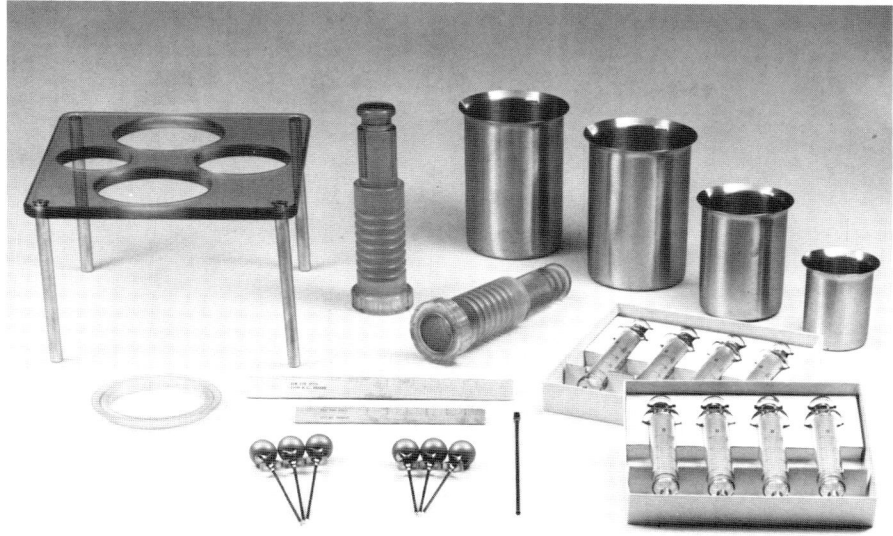

FIG. 5. Photograph of general apparatus needed for harvesting bone marrow.

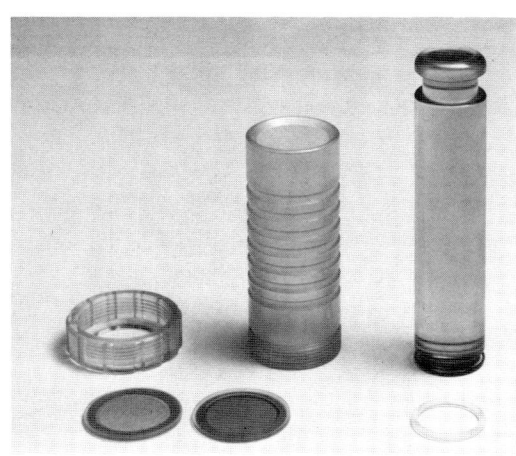

FIG. 6. Close-up of polycarbonate filter, which is commonly used to filter bone marrow in the operating room.

ABO INCOMPATIBILITY

Since the inheritance of the ABO blood group antigens is independent of inheritance of the HLA gene complex, transplants between ABO nonidentical individuals are frequently considered. Analysis of data from several centers indicate that ABO antigens are not clinically important targets of graft rejec-

TABLE 1. *Equipment and supplies needed for performing bone marrow transplantation*

Supplies and equipment	Number
Needles	
Ball top needle	3–5
Rosenthal needle	3–5
Thomas needle	5–10
Aspiration Syringes	
20 ml	10
30 ml	3–5
50 ml	3–5
Filtering Apparatus	
140 ml Polycarbonate filter	2–3
Fine screens	5–10
Coarse screens	5–10
Silicone gasket	5–10
Silicone O-ring	5–10
(Other filtering apparatus is available)	
Beaker Holder	
Polycarbonate	1–2
Beaker adapter	1–2
Stainless steel beakers	
1200 ml	2–4
250 ml	2–4
600 ml	2–4
Dipsticks (Used to measure and stir bone marrow in beaker)	
Dipstick for 1200 ml beaker	1–2
Dipstick for 600 ml beaker	1–2

The above list of equipment and supplies is a general recommendation. All equipment is available from University of Washington Scientific Instrument Division.

tion or graft-vs.-host disease. These studies also show that ABO incompatibility is not a significant barrier to successful bone marrow transplantation (6,7). Nevertheless, ABO incompatible transplants do present specific problems.

In the setting of bone marrow transplantation, a major ABO incompatibility is one in which the recipient possesses hemagglutinins capable of reacting with ABO antigens on the surface of the donor erythrocytes. Major incompatibility carries a high risk of hemolytic transfusion reactions, particularly if the hemagglutinin titer in the recipient is high. In the past, it was usually necessary to remove or to decrease the titer of recipient anti-donor ABO antibodies prior to infusion of the donor marrow cells to prevent a hemolytic transfusion reaction involving the erythrocytes contained in the marrow inoculum.

The technique commonly utilized for removing recipient ABO antibodies pretransplant is plasma exchange. An alternative approach is *in vitro* immunoadsorption, using synthetic ABO antigens linked to a crystalline silica matrix (8). However, these techniques involve large volume plasmapheresis or plasma exchange. They are time consuming, and they are not always safe and practical for use in small patients.

The simplest procedure to prevent reactions due to a major ABO incompatibility is to fractionate the donor bone marrow at the time of harvesting (9,10). Ho et al. have reported a simple technique to separate erythrocytes from bone marrow by sedimentation under gravity after addition of hydroxyethyl starch (Table 2) (11). This technique obviates the need for cumbersome and potentially hazardous large volume plasma exchange in the pediatric patient.

One delayed complication of marrow transplantation across major ABO incompatibilities is a persistent hemolysis post-transplantation. This occurs if the production of isohemagglutinins by the recipient is not sufficiently suppressed by the marrow ablative conditioning regimen. Hows et al., have reported that reticulocyte recovery in ABO incompatible transplants was significantly delayed and associated with prolonged red cell transfusion requirements, theoretically due to the immune destruction of erythrocytes after the late normoblast stage (12).

TABLE 2. *Procedure for gravity sedimentation of erythrocytes from bone marrow in major ABO incompatible transplants**

Materials and equipment
A 500 ml bottle of 6% HES (Hydroxyethyl starch—Volex or Hespan) Four 600 ml transfer pack units (with coupler) Three 300 ml transfer pack units (with coupler) Three sampling site couplers (injection site coupler) Three 60 ml sterile syringes with disposable needles Hemostats (or line clamps), tubes for cell count, hematocrit and other samples
Procedure

1. Record volume of unseparated marrow, then transfer aliquots of 300–350 ml into 600 ml transfer bags. Seal off the tail.
2. Insert injection site into one of the ports of each bag.
3. Add 6% HES (Hydroxyethyl starch—Volex or Hespan) to each bag via the injection site in a ratio of 1:8 (HES:marrow) by volume. Mix thoroughly by inverting several times.
4. Suspend each bag with the ports at the lower end and allow to stand for 30–45 minutes. Sedimentation of RBC occurs during this time.
5. Carefully attach a 300 ml transfer bag through the unused port of the bag containing the sedimented marrow and run off the RBC layer. Allow approximately 0.5 cm of RBCs to remain in the 600 ml bag in order to minimize loss of stem cells. (Use hemostat clamps to control the flow of RBC into the collecting bag.)
6. Pool the supernatant plasma, buffy coat layer and contaminating RBC into a single transfusion bag (generally another 600 ml bag). Mix well by agitating and remove appropriate samples for quality control (cell count, hematocrit, CFU-C and bacterial culture if necessary). Record volume of separated marrow and label the bag with the name of the donor.

*Adapted from Ho et al.[11]

A minor ABO incompatibility is one in which the donor possesses hemagglutinins capable of reacting with ABO antigens on the surface of the recipient erythrocytes. In order to prevent a minor hemolytic transfusion reaction at the time of marrow infusion, the marrow can be washed free of plasma prior to administration. This is rarely a significant problem in marrow transplantation in children, although occasionally donor derived erythrocyte antibodies and immune hemolysis have been observed after allogeneic marrow transplantation (13).

RISKS TO THE DONOR

The decision to perform a bone marrow transplant involves weighing the risks and benefits to the patient together with the risks to the donor (14). The occurrence of life-threatening complications in association with 3290 marrow donations were reviewed by the International Bone Marrow Transplant Registry. In that study, the incidence of such events was estimated at 0.27%; one fatality occurred in connection with a marrow donation (15).

Buckner et al. have reported the experience at a single institution in harvesting marrow for allogeneic transplantation on 1200 occasions from 1160 normal donors (16). Hospitalization time was 3 days or less for 99% of the procedures. Three donors developed cardiopulmonary problems during the donation, and one donor had a cerebrovascular accident after a second donation. Two donors developed life-threatening bacterial infections. Other potential risks to the donor included bleeding, infection at the operative site, and postoperative pain, although the complication rate was very low.

In general, young donors tolerate the procedure well. Sanders reported experience in harvesting marrow from 23 infant donors less than 2 years of age, with no major complications (17). The amount of pain experienced after the aspiration procedure was minimal and usually well controlled with acetaminophen. Interestingly, three of these infant donors were found to have significant medical problems during the pretransplant evaluation, including one with a stage I neuroblastoma. In a recent report, a patient with aplastic anemia was transplanted utilizing marrow from a 7-week-old sibling donor, without complications to the donor (18).

It should not be necessary to give a blood transfusion to a donor during or after the marrow procurement procedure. If the donor is substantially smaller than the recipient, then previously stored autologous blood can be transfused during the aspiration procedure to enable a larger volume of marrow to be obtained. Even in small donors, 10 to 15 ml/Kg of whole blood can be obtained and stored 7 to 10 days prior to the marrow aspiration. In the extremely rare event that nonautologous blood needs to be administered to the donor during the procurement of marrow, such blood must be irradiated to prevent the engraftment of non-HLA-identical immunocompetent cells in the recipient.

Special attention is required to support the emotional well-being of the donor. Adequate preoperative teaching and counseling to prepare the donor is required. Care must be taken to minimize the risks to the donor, and to insure that the donor is in good health before beginning the transplant process. Table 3 summarizes a suggested preoperative evaluation for bone marrow donors. Finally, if a patient does poorly following bone marrow transplantation, the donor may express feelings of responsibility for the unfavorable outcome. These issues must be addressed by the transplant team in preparing the family for the transplant.

SUPPORTIVE SERVICES

As the number of institutions performing bone marrow transplantation increases, questions naturally arise as to the basic facilities and supportive services required for a successful marrow transplant program. Although there are no universally accepted guidelines, most would agree that experience on the part of the medical and nursing staff in dealing with the transplant patient is of critical importance.

Furthermore, it is believed that bone marrow transplantation should be considered more than a clinical service for patients. The medical team should also be committed to the scientific investigation of the many existing barriers to successful transplantation, and to promptly report new developments which may arise from these investigations.

TABLE 3. *Laboratory studies needed for preoperative evaluation of bone marrow donors*

1. CBC, platelet count, reticulocyte count
2. SMA-12
3. Electrolytes
4. Hepatitis associated antibody
5. Hepatitis associated antigen
6. Herpes simplex antibody
7. Herpes zoster antibody
8. Epstein-Barr virus antibodies
9. Cytomegalovirus antibody
10. Human immunodeficiency virus antibody
11. RBC antigen typing
12. ABO typing
13. Isohemagglutinen titer
14. Peripheral chromosome karyotype analysis, with banding
15. Cellular immune function (options)
    a. mitogen blastogenesis
    b. antigen blastogenesis
16. Urinalysis
17. PT, PTT (optional)
18. Chest x-ray (optional)
19. EKG (adult donors)

The Transplant Environment

Many bone marrow transplant centers have separate nursing units designated for transplant recipients. Currently, bone marrow transplants are done in several different environments, according to the protocol of the institution in which they are performed. These choices include room isolation, reverse isolation, laminar airflow in a clean environment, or laminar airflow in a sterile environment. The patient care facility should have a proper air handling system, to prevent nosocomial infections due to microbial material disseminated from central heating or cooling systems (Figure 7).

Laminar airflow rooms in which strict sterile technique is used to maintain a germ-free environment are being used at many transplant centers (Figure 8). Transplant patients in this setting may be at less risk for infections, especially when there is acute graft-vs.-host disease, when compared to those patients transplanted under less stringent isolation (19–21). However, it has not

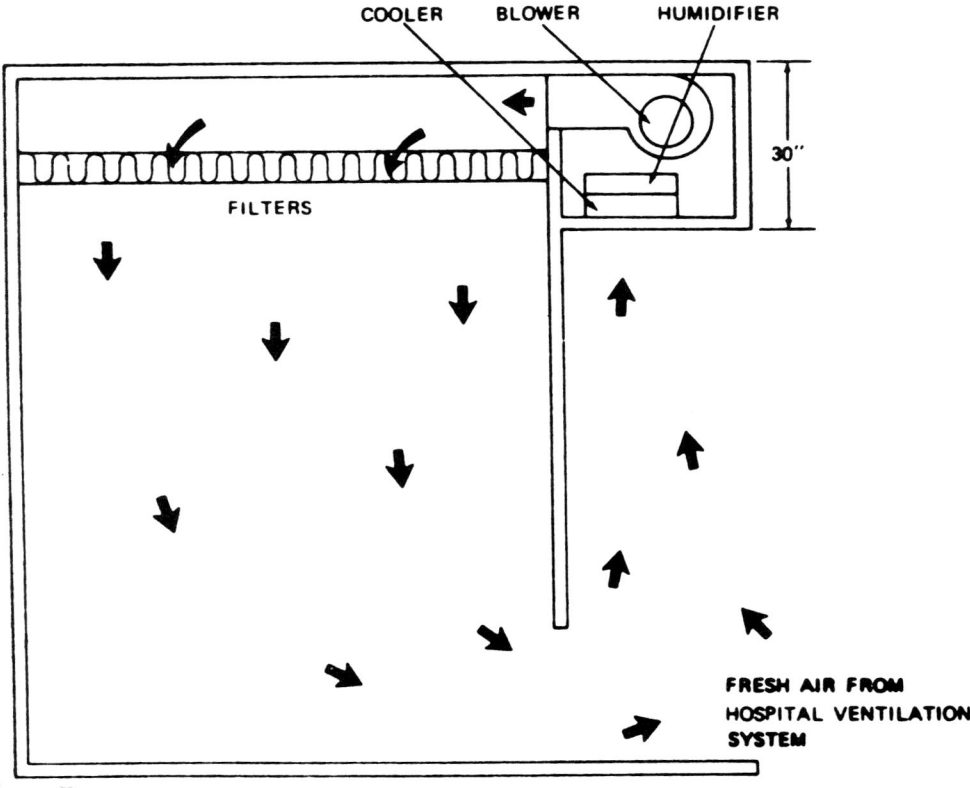

FIG. 7. Diagram of a laminar airflow room. The head of the patient's bed is adjacent to the filters, thus the flow of clean air is near the patient and flows away from him. This minimizes the likelihood of introducing airborne pathogens.

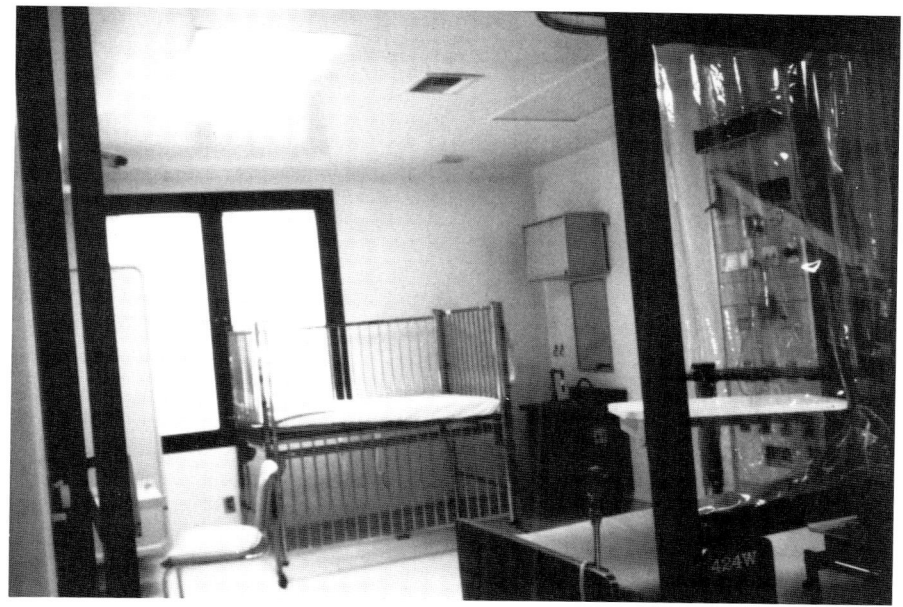

FIG. 8.   View of a laminar airflow room from outside.

been demonstrated that the extreme measures of patient isolation result in improved overall long-term survival.

The laminar airflow room is separated into two areas: the antechamber and the sterile patient area. A clear plastic curtain separates the sterile area from the antechamber (Figure 9). In the plastic curtain are several sets of plastic sleeves with access gloves that may be used by medical or nursing staff to examine the patient. An open portal is located at one end of the plastic curtain to allow individuals to enter the sterile area. Each staff member or visitor must scrub their hands, and don a sterile gown, mask, hood, booties, and two pairs of sterile gloves (Figure 10). Two pairs of gloves permit the replacement of a contaminated glove without introducing skin contaminants into the room.

In the sterile area, the patient will notice a constant low humming sound created by the fans in the wall behind the head of the bed. The fans pull air from the antechamber through filters, and then push the filtered air out into the sterile area. The filtered air flows down and out of the room.

Each room has a supply cart stocked daily with patient care items, linen, and miscellaneous medical supplies. Items are double wrapped and sterilized in the hospital central supply department, either with steam or ethylene oxide. All food entering the room is sterilized. The equipment, walls, and plastic curtains are cleaned several times every week. Table 4 lists many of

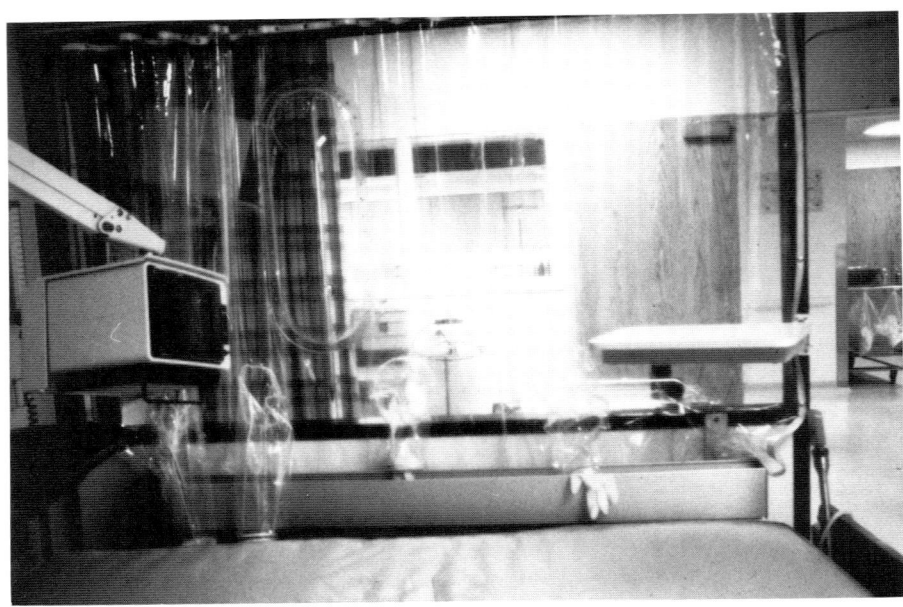

FIG. 9. View of outside from laminar airflow room, showing plastic curtain together with plastic sleeves and access gloves.

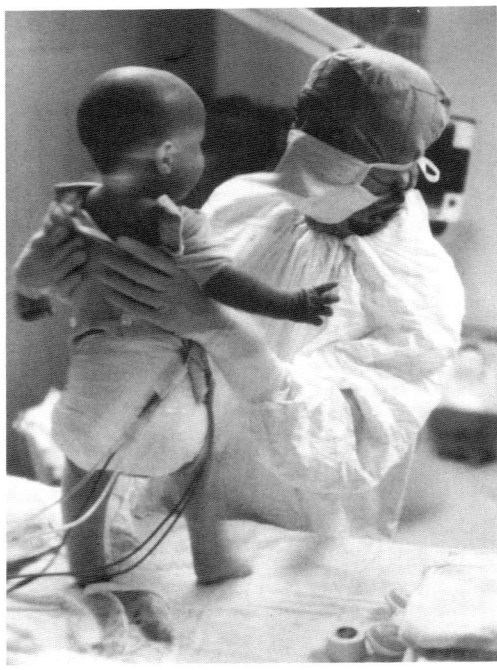

FIG. 10. Despite strict isolation procedures, close interaction with the patient is maintained.

TABLE 4. *Care and activities of patients being cared for in laminar airflow rooms*

1. Obtain weight, vital signs
2. Routine daily blood drawn from central catheter
3. IV line changes
4. Venous catheter dressing changes
5. Sterile sponge bath
6. Application of body creams and powders
7. Take oral nonabsorbable antibiotics
8. Take oral antifungal agents
9. Perform mouth care
10. Handwashing
11. Take body surveillance cultures
12. Exercise

the daily routine activities for the patient being cared for in a laminar airflow room.

The Transplant Team

The ability to support a patient through a bone marrow transplant is dependent upon the presence of competent and informed nurses. Communication between physicians and nurses is essential and can best be accomplished on a day-to-day basis by having nurses participate in daily patient rounds. The free flow of information between attending physicians, housestaff, and nurses will ultimately benefit the patient. Some transplant centers currently assign one nurse for one patient, although this 1:1 ratio may be increased or decreased as the level of care dictates.

A bone marrow transplant team is incomplete without the availability of a psychologist and social worker. Many patients and families will require the services of such professionals before, during, and after transplantation. The emotional stresses placed on the patient and family are enormous. Bone marrow transplantation is often the last option in an otherwise hopeless situation. Initially, the psychological stress is compounded by the fact that many patients are referred to bone marrow transplant centers that are far from home and familiar hospital personnel. In addition to concerns about the life of the patient and the welfare of the donor, the family is concerned about the high cost of the procedure and the loss of income that accompanies long vigils in the hospital.

In reality, a multidisciplinary team is required to support these patients and their families. The members of this complex team need to formally meet at least once every week to discuss and identify problems, and to work toward formulating solutions whenever possible.

Blood Bank Services

The ability to provide adequate blood product support is essential for the care of bone marrow transplant recipients. All recipients of allogeneic bone marrow grafts receive intensive immunosuppression with cytoreductive chemotherapy, radiotherapy, or both, before transplantation. This treatment results in severe pancytopenia lasting for several weeks. During this period, transfusions of red cells and platelets are necessary, and granulocyte transfusions are sometimes needed.

Care must be taken to minimize the risks of transfusion. Obviously, irradiated blood products must be available. The administration of cytomegalovirus (CMV) negative blood products will reduce the chances for transmission of infections due to this virus. Thus, use of CMV negative blood products results in development of fewer cases of serious CMV infections when patients who are CMV seronegative are transfused with blood products from donors who are CMV seronegative at the time of transplant (21). Blood banks should be committed to providing CMV negative blood products for such patients and, if necessary, should develop a pool of CMV negative volunteer donors. An on-site blood bank with the ability to perform apheresis is desirable for any marrow transplant center.

Laboratory Support

The full range of clinical laboratories is required for any successful transplant program. In addition, specialized laboratories in immunology, genetics and virology should be readily available.

SUMMARY

The technique of transferring bone marrow from one individual to another is simple. In contrast, the care of the transplant patient requires a major commitment on the part of the medical institution and personnel to provide the resources allowing for a successful bone marrow transplantation.

REFERENCES

1. International Bone Marrow Transplant Registry Newsletter, March 1987.
2. Thomas ED, Storb R: Technique for human marrow grafting. *Blood* 1970;36:507.
3. Filshie J: The anaesthetic management of bone marrow harvest for transplantation. *Anaesthesia* 1984;39:480.
4. Pflieger H, Wiesneth M. Schmeiser T, Kubanek B: A simple technique for processing of bone marrow for human marrow transplantation. *Blut* 1982;45:411.
5. Bell AJ, Hamblin TJ, Oscier DG: Circulating stem cell autografts. *Bone Marrow Transplantation* 1986;1:103.

6. Gale RP, Feig S, Ho W, et al.: ABO blood group system and bone marrow transplantation. *Blood* 1977;50:185.
7. Buckner CD, Clift RA, Sanders JE, et al.: ABO-incompatible marrow transplants. *Transplantation* 1978;26:233.
8. Bensinger WI, Baker DA, Buckner CD, et al.: Immunoadsorption for removal of A and B blood-group antibodies. *N Engl J Med* 1981;304:160.
9. Braine NG, Sesenbrenner LL, Wright, SK, et al.: Bone marrow transplantation with major ABO blood group incompatibility using erythrocyte depletion of marrow prior to infusion. *Blood* 1982;60:420.
10. Blacklock HA, Prentice HG, Evans JPM, et al.: ABO-incompatible bone marrow transplantation; removal of red blood cells from donor marrow avoiding recipient antibody depletion. *Lancet* 1982;1:1061.
11. Ho WG, Champlin RE, Feig SA, Gale RP: Transplantation of ABH-incompatible bone marrow: gravity sedimentation of donor marrow. *Br J Haematol* 1984;57:155.
12. Hows JM, Chipping PM, Palmer S, Gordon-Smith EC: Regeneration of peripheral blood cells following ABO incompatible allogeneic bone marrow transplantation for severe aplastic anemia. *BR J Haematol* 1983;53:145.
13. Hows J, Beddow K, Gordon-Smith E, et al.: Donor derived red blood cells antibodies and immune hemolysis after allogeneic bone marrow transplantation. *Blood* 1986;67:177.
14. Trigg ME: The decision in pediatrics to go ahead with bone marrow transplant for a pediatric malignancy. *Bone Marrow Transplantation* 1986;1:111.
15. Bortin MM, Buckner CD: Major complications of marrow harvesting for transplantation. *Exp Hematol* 1983;11:916.
16. Buckner CD, Clift RA, Sanders JE, et al.: Marrow harvesting from normal donors. *Blood* 1984;64:630.
17. Sanders J, Buckner CD, Bensinger WI, et al.: Experience with marrow harvesting from donors less than 2 years of age. *Bone Marrow Transplantation* 1987;2:45.
18. Valentino L, Lee K, Feig SA, Moss T: The use of a 7-week-old donor for bone marrow transplantation. *Clin Res* 1988;36:210A.
19. Buckner CD, Clift RA, Sanders JE, et al.: Protective environment for marrow transplant recipients; a prospective study. *Ann Int Med* 1978;89:893.
20. Storb R, Prentice RL, Buckner CD, et al.: Graft-vs.-host disease and survival in patients with aplastic anemia treated by marrow grafts from HLA-identical siblings. Beneficial effect of a protective environment. *N Engl J Med* 1983;308:302.
21. Sheretz R, Belani A, Kramer BS, et al.: Impact of air filtration on nosocomial Aspergillus infections. *Am J Med* 1987; 83:709.
22. Bowden RA, Sayers M, Flourney N, et al.: Cytomegalovirus immune globulin and seronegative blood products to prevent primary cytomegalovirus infection after marrow transplant. *N Engl J Med* 1986;314:1006.

Bone Marrow Transplantation in Children, edited by F. Leonard Johnson and Carl Pochedly. Raven Press, Ltd., New York © 1990.

Supportive Care in Bone Marrow Transplantation*

Wayne E. Spruce, M.D.*

Division of Hematology/Oncology, Bone Marrow Transplantation Program, Children's Hospital and Health Center, San Diego, California 92123, and Department of Basic and Clinical Research, Scripps Clinic and Research Foundation, La Jolla, California 92037

INTRODUCTION

The past two decades have seen significant improvements in the application of marrow transplantation to the treatment of a variety of malignant and

*Supported in part by grant #CA35048 from the National Cancer Institute, Bethesda, Maryland.

nonmalignant disorders (1–9). These advances have been made possible, in part, by parallel improvements in the ability to support patients through periods of prolonged bone marrow aplasia. Thus, improvements in blood banking and anti-microbial therapy have enabled patients to successfully undergo more aggressive cytoreductive therapy. Development of more effective anti-neoplastic agents and improved understanding of the actions of these drugs have also made therapy more effective. Improvements in the ability to provide nutritional support for patients both parenterally and orally have also contributed to the quality of the support offered to patients during prolonged periods of increased physiological stress.

The development of special care units in hospitals has also added to our ability to care for critically ill patients. These units are staffed with highly trained and motivated individuals who have special expertise in the care of these complex patients.

THE TRANSPLANT TEAM

The complex nature of marrow transplantation necessitates that many individuals with special skills be involved with the care of the patient. The patient's physician continues to have the ultimate responsibility but the transplant physician also requires that consultants be readily available from the entire spectrum of pediatric subspecialty areas in order to provide for the total care of the patient.

Skilled nursing care is critical to the success of any transplant unit, as transplant nurses are responsible for coordinating and carrying out details of the daily care of the patient. Their attention to detail and observations of the patient can often prevent problems or allow the problems to be dealt with before they become critical. In addition, they often become the patient's advocate with the physician, and they can provide insights into both the physical and emotional state of the patient which might not otherwise be evident.

The medical social worker provides essential support for the patient and family, tending to myriad details including housing, food, financial support, and transportation. Additionally, the social worker provides counseling for the patient and family and can be helpful in dealing with the emotional stresses associated with the transplant process. Frequently, the social worker can identify potential psychological problems and the need for intervention by a psychiatrist or psychologist. Most centers include psychiatric evaluation of the patient during the pre-transplant period and these specialists are an important part of the transplant team, providing support, not only for the patient and family, but also for the transplant team.

The clinical dietitian evaluates the nutritional status of the patient at the time of admission and helps to plan nutritional support for the patient both before and after the procedure. In patients who develop graft-vs.-host disease, the dietician can provide invaluable input into the care of the patient.

Several other disciplines are also important in the care of the transplant patient. The pharmacist provides important information about drug dosage, drug interactions and toxicity in transplant patients who invariably receive many medications. Recreational and occupational therapists can provide diversions for the patient and help to make isolation more bearable for the patient and family. A hospital-based school teacher can often provide the child with welcome diversion and help to give a degree of normalcy to the child's daily routine.

It is extremely important that the various members of the transplant team communicate on a regular basis. Regularly scheduled meetings of the team are helpful in providing for the ongoing care of the patient. This enables the entire team to provide input and, in our experience, adds immeasurably to the quality of care of the patient. These meetings also help to develop good working relationships among the team members.

PRE-TRANSPLANT EVALUATION

Before being admitted for transplantation, patients should be in as good clinical condition as possible. This ideal situation, however, is not always attained and there may not be time for infections or poor nutritional status to be corrected before beginning preparation for the transplant. This is especially true in patients with aplastic anemia, in patients with relapsed leukemia, and in children with immunodeficiency syndromes. However, in those patients where a short delay is possible, potentially complicating clinical conditions should be corrected.

All patients should have a thorough dental evaluation prior to coming to transplantation and, if the patient's condition allows, dental abnormalities should be corrected. Dental abscesses particularly are a source of infection and sepsis during the post-transplant period of profound neutropenia, and these should be treated before beginning the transplant process. Some centers use topical applications of fluoride and special mouth rinses after the transplant to counter the adverse effects of chemoradiotherapy on the oral cavity and the teeth (10–12).

Patients often come to the transplant center from another hospital. In this situation, it is essential to have a thorough review of the patient's medical and social history and to maintain direct and frequent contact between the referring institution and the transplant center.

The input from the medical social worker or psychologist from the referring center often provides the transplant team with helpful insights in dealing with the patient and his or her family. Many centers provide the family with a booklet describing the transplant center and giving details of the transplant procedure. Details about accommodations, the availability of financial support, and local transportation help the family before their arrival at the transplant center. If it is at all possible, the patient and the family should have the opportunity to meet the staff and tour the facility before the actual admission day.

Most centers schedule conferences between the family and the transplant staff during the initial evaluation period to provide information about the procedure and to enable the child and family to become acquainted with the staff. Many families will come to the transplant center with unrealistic expectations of what the procedure can offer and it is important that these subjects be discussed and that the family be given ample time to process the information and to discuss it with the staff.

NUTRITIONAL SUPPORT

Children undergoing marrow transplantation are unable to maintain adequate oral intake of food during cytoreductive chemotherapy and radiotherapy, and are given during the immediate post-transplant period. This inadequate intake is a result of the severe nausea, vomiting, oral mucositis, diarrhea, altered taste and decreased salivary secretion associated with the preparative regimens. The occurrence of fevers and sepsis also increase the patient's caloric needs. Patients who develop acute and chronic graft-vs.-host disease (GVHD) have a prolonged period of inadequate oral intake and various degrees of malabsorption.

Experience with surgical patients and children with chronic malabsorption in the 1960s demonstrated the effectiveness of parenteral nutrition in patients unable to eat for prolonged periods of time (13–17). Initial problems with venous access, sclerosis and sepsis, were overcome by the development of a silastic right atrial catheter by Broviac (18). This catheter has been modified by Hickman and now there are many different catheters available with single, double, and even triple lumens (19–21). In children, most atrial catheters are inserted in the operating room under general anesthesia. The type of catheter used depends on the size of the child. Double lumen catheters enable more nutrition to be delivered, since they do not require interruptions for injection of antibiotics or for infusion of blood products (22). However, in our experience, children under the age of 7 frequently do not have veins of sufficient diameter to accept the double lumen catheters. Some centers have inserted two single lumen catheters in this situation. These catheters are also used for routine blood sampling and for infusion of blood products and antibiotics. With proper care and attention by experienced nurses, problems with infection and catheter blockage are rare (21).

The patient's nutritional status should be reviewed by the physician and dietitian at the time the patient is evaluated for the transplant. Objective measures of nutritional status include the patient's current weight in relation to ideal body weight and usual weight. Anthropometric measurements of triceps, skin fold, midarm circumference, and muscle diameter are useful in assessing nutritional status. Nitrogen balance, creatinine height index and the measurements of visceral proteins (including albumin, transferrin, prealbumin and retinol binding protein) are also used to assess the patient's overall nutritional status (23–26). Static measurements are less valuable than serial ones. There is evidence from one center that the patient's nitrogen balance is one of the most important measurements in determining adequacy of parenteral nutrition (27).

Total daily caloric requirements can be determined from the recommended daily allowances for children of different ages or by using the Harris Benedict equations. In both systems, allowances must be made for increased requirements related to fever and sepsis. Both of these situations may increase baseline caloric requirements by as much as 50%. Total daily caloric requirements range from 70–90 calories/kg/day in a child 1 to 7 years old, and up to 50 calories/kg/day in adolescents. Protein requirements range from 2.5 g/kg/day in infants to 1.5 to 2 g/kg/day in older children (26). Crystalline amino acid solutions are used as the protein source and are available in 7%, 8.5% and 10% solutions (23).

Dextrose is the major source of nonprotein calories. It is usually begun at a concentration of 10% and increased to 20–25% over a period of three to four days. A ratio of nonprotein calories to grams of nitrogen of 150:1 has been shown to be optimal for protein synthesis (26). It has been the practice in our center to formulate the protein and dextrose concentrations in our hyperalimentation solutions to approximate this ratio as closely as possible. Excessive losses of protein in the stool in children with severe graft-vs.-host disease may make the delivery of optimal protein difficult. In addition to protein and dextrose, electrolytes, trace elements and multivitamins are added to the hyperalimentation solutions in appropriate concentrations to replace losses and to prevent deficiencies from developing.

Patients who are on prolonged parenteral nutrition can develop essential fatty acid deficiencies within a few weeks (28). This can be prevented by the use of lipid solutions using approximately 1–2 g/kg/day. In addition, these solutions are a good source of calories and can provide up to 50% of the patient's daily requirement. However, they should not exceed 60% of the total daily calories (26). Lipids are cleared slowly and it is necessary to evaluate the patient's serum turbidity 4–6 hours after the infusion. In occasional patients, clearance of lipids is so slow that the infusions can be given only two to three times a week.

While on hyperalimentation it is important to monitor the patient's electrolytes, serum glucose, creatinine, urine glucose, and liver function. Our practice has been to evaluate the electrolytes, glucose and creatinine daily and to assess liver function three times a week. If there are electrolyte disturbances or significant hyperglycemia, monitoring at more frequent intervals may be necessary. Fluid balance must also be followed closely to avoid fluid overload. For patients who develop hyperglycemia, it has been our practice to use continuous insulin infusions while hyperalimentation is being given. This allows adjustment of the rate of infusion without changing the entire hyperalimentation solution, which is necessary if the insulin is added directly to the hyperalimentation solution. Fortunately, it is only an occasional child who will require supplemental insulin while on hyperalimentation.

Except in patients who are significantly malnourished on admission to the transplant unit, we do not start hyperalimentation until the day after the transplant. This is done largely for practical reasons. Patients require high volumes of intravenous fluids during the cytoreductive therapy and simultaneous administration of these fluids makes the delivery of the parenteral nutrition more difficult. We do not routinely give lipid solutions to patients who are able to resume oral intake within the first three to four weeks after the transplant. However, in those who are unable to take oral nutrition within this time period, especially if there are severe gastrointestinal disturbances, lipids are added as outlined above.

The adequacy of the parenteral nutrition can be assessed by following the patient's daily weight, calculations of calories delivered, and nitrogen balance (23,24,26). In many instances, optimal amounts of parenteral nutrition cannot be delivered. Renal and hepatic abnormalities may prevent the administration of large volumes of fluid and limit the amounts of protein that can be safely administered (23,29). In patients with single intravenous lines, interruptions for administration of antibiotics and blood products can limit the time available for delivery of parenteral nutrition (22). Despite this, most patients can be adequately maintained on parenteral nutrition during the first three to four weeks after transplantation. A recent study from the University of Minnesota demonstrated that prophylactic total parenteral nutrition including lipids can improve overall survival and disease free survival in patients undergoing allogenic transplantation. While the mechanisms are not clear, they postulate an enhancement of the cytoreductive therapy by the amino acids and polyunsaturated fats. Total parenteral nutrition may also modify the acute catabolic effect of the cytoreductive regime on the host and enhance marrow recovery and immune function (30).

As patients gradually improve their oral intake, the volume of hyperalimentation can be reduced and slowly discontinued. In patients whose calorie intake is the limiting factor in determining the time of discharge from the hospital, home programs are now available to provide hyperalimentation for part of the day. In patients with severe gastrointestinal symptoms due to graft-vs-host disease, a home program may allow for earlier release from the hospital (29). Because of altered taste resulting from cytoreductive therapy, oral mucositis and graft-vs.-host disease, it is frequently a challenge to get children to eat. In some cases, oral supplements which are high in calories and protein may be necessary. Reward systems and positive reinforcement are frequently of value in encouraging the resumption of adequate oral intake. Except in the case of severe graft-vs.-host disease, most children will resume adequate oral intake after the fourth to fifth post-transplant week.

BLOOD COMPONENT THERAPY

Bone marrow transplantation is impossible without the availability of blood component therapy. Most patients with aplastic anemia and leukemia will require transfusion support before undergoing transplantation and for several weeks afterward.

SENSITIZATION AND GRAFT REJECTION

The deleterious effect of blood transfusion on engraftment was first shown in transplants between experimental animals mismatched for the major histocompatibility loci (31–33). Blood transfusions from the marrow donor given at variable times before the total body irradiation prevented engraftment (34). Loutit and Micklem showed in mice that the injection of spleen cells from histocompatible donor prior to irradiation also led to increased mortality (35). Storb and his co-workers demonstrated a high note of graft rejection in histocompatible dogs given pre-transplant transfusions from littermates. These studies also demonstrated that up to 30% of dogs given pre-transplant transfusions from unrelated animals become sensitized to marrow grafts from histocompatible littermates. These latter experiments clearly showed that presence of minor histocompatibility differences outside the HLA system were important in graft rejection (36,37).

Red cells that have been depleted of contaminating leukocytes by freezing, washing, or passage through nylon wool filters have been shown to decrease the likelihood of sensitization in both animals and humans (37,38). The degree of removal of leukocytes varies with the system. Studies in histocompatible dogs have shown that engraftment was not adversely affected by red cells, platelets, or mature granulocytes (38,39). Further studies have shown that the rejection rate using injections of mononuclear cells was similar to the rejection rate in patients receiving whole blood, thus implicating mononuclear cells in graft rejection. T lymphocytes have been excluded because infusions of T cells did not increase graft rejection. By exclusion, antigens present on the surface of monocytes and macrophages appear to play the major role in rejection (37,39,40).

Initially, graft rejection was a major problem in multitransfused patients with aplastic anemia, occurring in 30 to 60% of patients (40–45). In contrast, the rejection rate in patients transplanted for leukemia was less than 2% (47). This difference in rejection rate was thought to be due to the fact that the leukemic patient received the majority of his blood support while immuno-suppressed by chemotherapy, while the patient with aplastic anemia was trans-fused when still immunologically competent (40,48). In addition, the leuke-mic patient received more intense preparation for the transplant which might prevent him from responding immunologically to the donor marrow. The Seattle transplant team has clearly shown that patients who received no trans-fusions until immediately prior to beginning the conditioning for marrow transplantation have a significantly lower rejection rate than those who were transfused (49). The number of transfusions did not seem to correlate with rejection (46). This confirmed the earlier animal experience and indicated that the cause of the rejection was based on prior sensitization to non-HLA antigens. Under ideal circumstances, patients with aplastic anemia who are candidates for bone marrow transplantation should not receive blood prod-ucts unless it is absolutely necessary.

RECOMMENDATIONS FOR BLOOD PRODUCT SUPPORT PRIOR TO TRANSPLANTATION

Patients with acute leukemia who receive non-T cell depleted marrow trans-plants from histocompatibility matched sibling donors have a very low rejection rate regardless of their prior history of transfusions and no special precautions need be taken (47). It would seem prudent, however, to avoid transfusing the patient with blood from family members if at all possible, although this restric-tion is not mandatory (50). For example, in a life-threatening situation where the patient responds only to platelet transfusions from a family member, plate-lets from this donor should be used. Unnecessary platelet transfusions should be avoided in order to prevent or delay sensitization of the patient and the subsequent development of refractoriness to platelet transfusions (51–53).

In a patient with aplastic anemia, the primary physician should have HLA typing done on the patient and family. If the patient is found to have a compatible sibling, a transplant center should be contracted as soon as possi-ble. Transfusions of blood products should be given only if absolutely neces-sary. In the event that red cell transfusions are necessary, family members and especially the designated bone marrow donor should not be used as blood donors, for the reasons detailed above.

Frozen red cells, washed red cells, and cells that have been passed through nylon filters may be free of the offending mononuclear cells and have a lower risk of sensitizing the patient to non-HLA antigens (54–59).

Standard practice has been to give platelet transfusions to patients when the platelet count falls below 20,000/mm^3, (29,40), however, many patients will have no clinical bleeding with platelet counts below 10,000/mm^3. This is espe-cially true in patients who are free of infection. Slichter and Harker showed that the fecal loss of blood in patients with platelet counts between 5000 and

10,000/mm^3 was no greater than that in the general population (60). Therefore, in a stable infection-free patient it is probably not indicated to transfuse platelets at a particular level. In patients who are bleeding or are septic, platelet support is clearly necessary. Again, family members should be avoided as donors. The use of pooled platelets can usually provide adequate numbers of platelets to control bleeding, and sensitization is not generally a problem in the pre-transplant period (29,40). Mononuclear cell contamination can be reduced by centrifugation of pooled platelet concentrates at the risk of significant loss of platelets (61). Drugs such as semisynthetic penicillins and steroids can enhance stool blood loss in thrombocytopenic patients and, if possible, should be avoided (60).

While avoidance of transfusions in patients with aplastic anemia is clearly desirable, the majority of these patients coming to transplantation will have received some blood products. Several conditioning regimens have been successful in reducing the rejection rate (46,62–66).

BLOOD COMPONENT THERAPY AFTER MARROW TRANSPLANTATION

All patients undergoing transplantation for acute leukemia and aplastic anemia will require support for several weeks after the marrow graft. This is a result of the intense conditioning regimen and the time it takes the graft to function.

After the transplant, it is necessary to irradiate all blood products prior to transfusion. This prevents the replication of lymphocytes that contaminate packed red cells and platelet concentrates. Patients who are profoundly immunocompromised can develop graft-vs.-host disease from lymphocyte contamination of these products (67–72). It is now standard practice to irradiate all blood products with the exception of the donor marrow, or donor buffy coat in the case of patients with aplastic anemia. For irradiation of blood products most centers use 1500 to 3000 cGy from either a cessium source or a radiation therapy unit (29). Experiments have shown that irradiation effectively reduces thymidine incorporation into lymphocytes and that the functional qualities of the cells are not compromised (73,74).

It has recently been shown that patients who are cytomegalovirus (CMV) negative and whose donors are also CMV negative have a significantly lower rate of CMV infection when transfused with CMV negative blood products. This protection did not hold in patients who had CMV positive donors (75). Therefore, in the situation of a CMV negative patient and marrow donor blood support should be provided from donors who are CMV negative.

Red Cell Support

Most centers, including our own, maintain the patient's hematocrit in the range of 30%. The number of units of packed red cells that a child will require to maintain this level varies. Bleeding, infection, and the amount of blood removed for laboratory studies can all affect the quantity of packed red cells needed. In series of patients, including both adults and children, the number of units required post-transplant has been in the range of 8 to 15 (29,40) although in our center, most children undergoing transplantation for hematologic malignancies require 6 or 7 units of packed red cells. Many patients with severe graft-vs.-host disease or other complications may be transfusion-dependent for longer periods of time.

A mild to moderately severe hemolytic anemia occurs in some bone marrow recipients whose marrow donor was a minor blood group mismatch, such as when the donor is blood group O and the recipient group A or B (76). When these patients were transfused with donor specific red cells, they developed a Coombs' positive hemolytic anemia during the second post-transplant week. The cause of this reaction is not clear; however, the use of washed type O red cells alleviated the problem. Thus, it is now our routine practice to transfuse only type O red cells in patients whose marrow donor was a minor group mismatch. Experience in other centers has recently been reviewed (76a).

Platelet Support

Most centers attempt to keep the patient's platelet count in the range of $20,000/mm^3$. However, in some instances such as when there is severe oral or gastrointestinal bleeding, higher platelet levels may be required to provide adequate hemostasis. Similarly, in some patients levels lower than this may be safe. This is especially true in patients who have chronically low platelet counts associated with chronic graft-vs.-host disease. Most pediatric patients can be supported with random pooled platelets. One unit of platelets contains approximately 5.5×10^{10} platelets, and 50 to 60% of these platelets can be expected to be viable. One unit of platelets will raise the platelet count by $10,000/m^2$ of body surface area. If fluid volume becomes a problem, the blood bank can frequently reduce the quantity of plasma in the platelet concentrate (29). The use of blood group specific platelets is generally recommended; however, this is not mandatory and occasionally not possible.

Platelet requirements for individual patients vary and depend on many factors. These include the presence of severe oral mucositis, infections, graft-vs.-host disease, and alloimmunization. Patients are considered refractory when the one hour post-transfusion platelet count shows less than 5% of the predicted rise on two separate occasions (40). In some patients, refractoriness is temporary and is related to sepsis, severe bleeding, intravascular coagulatin or hepatosplenomegaly (29). It has been the author's experience that refractoriness to platelet transfusion is uncommon in pediatric patients and that the use of single donor platelets is seldom necessary.

In those patients who do become refractory, platelets obtained by single donor platelet pheresis, preferably obtained from the marrow donor or the patients parents, are given. If the marrow donor is of sufficient age and size, he or she would be the preferred donor. However this technique does not guarantee platelet survival and such platelet pheresis should only be continued if the single donor products provide superior results. As noted, factors other than alloimmunization may be responsible for poor platelet survival.

In patients whose family members are not available as platelet donors, the use of HLA match platelets may be helpful. Finding donors who are a complete HLA match (A match) may be difficult and requires a large potential donor panel. It has been shown that even partially matched donors and completely mismatched donors can provide adequate platelet support for some patients (77,78). This may be explained by the observation that HLA antigens are variably expressed on platelets and, therefore, the platelets can survive in patients in spite of the presence of corresponding antibodies (61,79).

Because of the variable clinical response to HLA matched platelets, several investigators have developed platelet cross-matching techniques in an attempt to predict successful response to platelet transfusions. These techniques attempt to demonstrate the presence of serum antibodies reactive with a panel of donor platelets (77,80–85). The predictive value of these tests is quite good and correlates with successful platelet transfusions. The tests, however, are available only in a few centers and this limits their usefulness.

In the rare instance where patients are refractory to all platelet products, high doses of corticosteroids have been used with variable success. In some instances platelets from both random donors and from single donor platelet pheresis given at frequent intervals, such as every 6 to 12 hours, may be helpful in sustaining a patient until the graft begins to function (40). This latter approach has been used by our group in several adult patients; these patients did not develop severe bleeding in spite of having platelet counts of less than 5000/mm^3 for up to two weeks. Patients may be refractory to platelets from a donor on one occasion but respond well on another; therefore, before the possible usefulness of a given donor is eliminated, a second try may be indicated (60).

Most patients with leukemia and aplastic anemia will begin to show platelet recovery during the third and fourth transplant week and will be transfusion-free by the end of the fourth or fifth week (40). Patients with severe infections and graft-vs.-host disease will often require support for much longer periods of time. Some patients will stabilize their platelet counts in the 25,000 to 50,000/mm^3 range, will have no bleeding problems and will not require regular transfusions.

Granulocyte Support

The role of granulocyte transfusions in neutropenic febrile patients remains unsettled. The majority of patients undergoing transplantation will become febrile and some septic during the immediate post-transplant period. Their clinical course is occasionally complicated and ultimate recovery depends on many factors, including age, general condition, infecting organism, site of infections, and the appropriateness of anti-microbial therapy. This makes the role of granulocyte transfusions difficult to evaluate (86).

There is little question that appropriate anti-microbial therapy is paramount in the management of these patients. The beneficial effects of therapeutic granulocyte transfusions in treating antibiotic resistant gram negative septicemia have been demonstrated in several experimental and clinical trials over the past 10 years (86–88). The role of granulocyte transfusions in treating nonsepticemic patients or those with nonbacterial infections is not so clear (90,91). Studies have used various methods of collecting white cells, and involved various matched patient populations. Some patients were treated with corticosteroids and some were not.

Prophylactic granulocyte transfusions in patients undergoing transplantation have generally shown a lower incidence of septicemia and local infections but no demonstrable effect on survival (92,93). This lack of benefit of granulocyte transfusions has also been shown in patients undergoing induction chemotherapy for leukemia (94,95). Therefore, prophylactic granulocyte transfusions are no longer routinely used in most transplant centers.

Therapeutic granulocytes are generally given to neutropenic patients with positive blood cultures who do not respond to appropriate antibiotics. In addition, patients who remain clinically septic while on broad spectrum antibiotics, even when the cultures are negative, may be candidates for granulocyte support (40). It has been our practice to also use granulocyte transfusions in patients with localized infections, such as perirectal abscesses. Most centers use the bone marrow donor and other family members as white cell donors. In pediatric patients, the donor is frequently too young to provide granulocytic support and parents or other family members are usually used. This provides a stable donor pool and reduces the patient's exposure to cytomegalovirus and hepatitis (29,40).

Patients continue to receive granulocytes until their neutrophil counts are greater than $200/mm^3$ (29,40). Volume limitations must be kept in mind and attention to the patient's fluid balance is important to avoid volume overload. Diuretics may occasionally be necessary in children who are also receiving large fluid volumes for administration of parenteral nutrition and antibiotics.

Patients have developed severe reactions characterized by fever, chills, hypertension or hypotension, tachycardia, and occasionally pulmonary infiltrates following granulocyte transfusions (86,89,90). These reactions can often be prevented by the use of antihistamines, acetaminophen, and corticosteroids.

They also may be the result of alloimmunization. If this occurs, it is probably wise to no longer use that particular donor.

Severe pulmonary reactions associated with the administration of granulocytes and amphotericin B have been reported (96–98). Some authors believe that bacteremia contributes to the pulmonary reactions in the absence of amphotericin B (98). However, other investigators have not found this association (99,100). It is probably prudent to be cautious in administering granulocytes in the presence of bacteremia when amphotericin therapy is being given. Separating the administration of amphotericin and the transfusion of granulocytes by as much time as possible may be useful.

Finally, granulocyte transfusions have also been associated with an increased risk of CMV infection (101). It has been our experience that therapeutic granulocyte transfusions are seldom necessary in the pediatric patient. However, it is essential that a marrow transplant program have the capability of providing such support.

SUMMARY

This chapter addressed the critical role of supportive care in the care of the child undergoing marrow transplantation. The complex nature of the procedure makes it necessary for a large number of individuals to be involved. Physicians, nurses, social workers, dietitians, pharmacists, and therapists in various disciplines all bring important skills to the care of the child. The team approach to the care of the patient is essential to the success of a transplant program.

Parenteral nutrition has become an integral part of the treatment and enables the child to better tolerate the physiologic stress of the procedure. The availability of improved venous access has facilitated the delivery of hyperalimentation, blood component and antibiotic therapy.

Guidelines for blood component therapy have also been summarized. Transfusions before transplantation for patients with aplastic anemia should be minimized to reduce the risk of rejection. After the transplant, the guidelines for all patients are similar. These guidelines are just that but the clinical condition of an individual patient may dictate a different approach.

The ability to provide intensive support to patients undergoing marrow transplantation has helped to reduce the mortality of this procedure.

REFERENCES

1. Thomas ED: The role of marrow transplantation in the eradication of malignant disease. *Cancer* 1982; 49:1963–1969.
2. Santos GW, Tutschka PJ, Brookmeyer R, et al.: Marrow transplantation for acute nonlymphocytic leukemia following treatment with busulfan and cyclophosphamide. *N Engl J Med* 1983; 309:1347–1353.

3. Powles RJ, Morgenstern G, Clink HM, et al.: The place of bone marrow transplantation in acute myelogenous leukemia. *Lancet* 1980; 1:1047–1050.
4. Storb R, Witherspoon RP, Sullivan KM, et al.: Allogeneic marrow transplants for treatment of severe aplastic anemia. In Gale RP (ed): *Recent Advances in Bone Marrow Transplantation* Alan R. Liss, New York, 1983, pp. 3–10.
5. Feig SA, Champlin R, Arenson E, et al.: Improved survival following bone marrow transplantation for aplastic anemia. *Br J Hematol* 1983; 54:509–517.
6. O'Reilly RJ, Kapoor N, Kirkpatrick D, et al.: Transplantation for severe combined immunodeficiency disease using histocompatible parenteral marrow fractionated by soybean agglutinin and sheep red blood cells; experience in six consecutive cases. *Transplant Proc* 1983; 15:1431–1435.
7. Speck B, Gratwhol A, Nissen C, et al.: Allogeneic marrow transplantation for chronic granulocytic leukemia. *Blut* 1982; 45:237–242.
8. Goldman JM, Baughan ASJ, McCarthy DM, et al.: Marrow transplantation for patients in the chronic phase of chronic granulocytic leukemia. *Lancet* 1982; 2:623–625.
9. Storb R, Thomas ED: Allogeneic bone marrow transplantation. *Immunol Rev* 1983; 71:77–102.
10. RaKocz M, Serota F, Nelson L, et al.: Dental management of the child undergoing bone marrow transplantation. *JADA* 1982; 104:455–488.
11. Berkowitz RJ, Crock J, Strickland R, Gordon EM: Oral complications associated with bone marrow transplantation. *Am J Pediatr Hematol/Oncol* 1983; 5:53–57.
12. Shannon I, Trodahl J. Starcke E: Remineralization of enamel by a saliva substitute designed for use by irradiated patients. *Cancer* 1978; 41:1746–1750.
13. Wilmore DW, Dudrick SJ: Growth and development of an infant receiving all nutrients exclusively by vein. *JAMA* 1968; 203:860–864.
14. Dudrick SJ, Wilmore DW, Vars HM, Rhoads JE: Long-term parenteral nutrition with growth and development and positive nitrogen balance. *Surgery* 1968; 64:134–142.
15. Dudrick SJ, Wilmore DW, Vars HM: Long-term parenteral nutrition with growth in puppies and positive nitrogen balance in patients. *Surg Forum* 1967; 18:356–357.
16. Jeejeebhoy KN, Langer B, Tsallas G, et al.: Total parenteral nutrition at home; studies in patients surviving four months to five years. *Gastroenterology* 1976; 71:943–953.
17. Heizer WD, Orringer EP: Parenteral nutrition at home for five years via arterio-venous fistulae. *Gastroenterology* 1977; 72:527,532.
18. Broviac JW, Cole JJ, Scribner BH; A silicone rubber atrial catheter for prolonged parenteral alimentation. *Surg Gynecol Obstet* 1973; 136:602–606.
19. Hickman RO, Buckner CD, Clift RA, et al.: A modified right atrial catheter for access to the venous system in marrow transplant recipients. *Surg Gynecol Obstet* 1979; 148:871–875.
20. Blacklock HA, Hill RS, Clarke AG, et al.: Use of modified subcutaneous right atrial catheter for venous access in leukemia patients. *Lancet* 1980; 1:993–994.
21. Raaf JH: Results from use of 826 vascular access devices in cancer patients. *Cancer* 1985; 55:1312–1321.
22. Aker SN, Cheney CL, Sanders JE, et al.: Nutritional support in marrow graft recipients with single vs. double lumen right atrial catheters. *Exp Hematol* 1982; 10:732–737.
23. Cunningham BA, Lenssen P, Aker SN, et al.: Nutritional considerations during marrow transplantation. *Nursing Clin N Am* 1983; 18:585–596.
24. Grant JP: *Handbook of Total Parenteral Nutrition.* W.F. Saunders, Philadelphia, 1980.
25. Barale K, Cheney C, Lenssen P, et al.: Anthropometric measurement in a protective environment. *Perspectives in Practice* 1981; 78:359–361.
26. Kerner JA: *Manual of Pediatric Parenteral Nutrition.* John Wiley & Sons, New York, 1983.
27. Schmidt GM, Blume KG, Bross KJ, et al.: Parenteral nutrition in bone marrow transplant recipients. *Exp Hematol* 1980; 8:506–511.
28. Riella MC, Broviac JW, Wells M, Schribner BH: Essential fatty acid deficiency in human adults during total parenteral nutrition. *Ann Intern Med* 1975; 83:786–789.
29. Petz LD, Scott EP: Supportive care. In, Blume KG, Petz LD, (eds): *Clinical Bone Marrow Transplantation.* Churchill Livingstone, New York, 1983; pp. 199–205.
30. Weisdorf SA, Lysne J, Wind D, et al.: Positive effect of prophylactic total parenteral nutrition on long-term outcome of bone marrow transplantation. *Transplantation* 1987; 43:833–838.

31. Barnes D, Loutit JF: What is the recovery factor in the spleen? *Nucleonics* 1954; 12:68–71.
32. Van Putten LM, Van Beckkum DW, de Vries MJ, Balner H: The effect of preceding blood transfusions on the fate of homologous bone marrow grafts in lethally irradiated monkeys. *Blood* 1967; 30:749–757.
33. Storb R, Floersheim GL, Kolb JH, et al.: Effect of prior blood transfusions on marrow grafts; abrogation of sensitization by procarbazine and antithymocyte serum. *J Immunol* 1974; 112:1508–1516.
34. Weiden PL, Storb R, Kolb JH, et al.: Effect of time on sensitization to hematopoietic grafts by preceding blood transfusion. *Transfusion* 1975; 19:240–244.
35. Loutit JF, Micklem HS: Active and passive immunity to transplantation of foreign bone marrow in lethally irradiated mice. *Br J Exp Pathol* 1961; 42:577–586.
36. Storb R, Epstein RB, Rudolph RH, Thomas ED: The effect of prior transfusion on marrow grafts between histocompatible canine siblings. *J Immunology* 1970; 105:627–633.
37. Storb R, Weiden PL, Deeg HS, et al.: Rejection of marrow from DLA identical littermates given transfusions before grafting antigens are expressed on leukocytes and skin epithelial cells but not on platelets and red cells. *Blood* 1979; 54:477–484.
38. Miller WV, Schmidt R, Luke RG, Craywood BE: Effect of cytotoxicity antibodies in potential transplant recipients of leukocyte poor transfusions. *Lancet* 1975; 1:893–895.
39. Deeg HJ, Torok-Storb B, Storb R, et al.: Rejection of DLA-identical canine littermate marrow after transfusion induced sensitization antigens involved are expressed on cotton wool adherent but not nonadherent mononuclear cells, granulocytes, or thoracic duct lymphocytes. In, Baun SI, Ledney GD, Kahn A, (eds): *Experimental Hematology Today.* S. Karger, Basel, 1981.
40. Storb, R., Weiden P: Transfusion problems associated with transplantation. *Semin Hematol* 1981; 18:163–177
41. Storb R, Thomas ED, Buckner CD, et al.: Allogeneic marrow grafting for treatment of aplastic anemia. *Blood* 1974; 43:157–180.
42. Bone Marrow Transplant Registry: Bone marrow transplantation from histocompatible allogeneic donors for aplastic anemia. *JAMA* 1976; 236:1131–1135.
43. Effenbein GJ, Anderson PN, Humphrey RL, et al.: Immune system reconstruction following allogeneic bone marrow transplantation in man; a multiparameter analysis. *Transplant Proc* 1976; 8:641–646.
44. Effenbein GJ, Anderson PN, Klein DL, et al.: Difficulties in predicting bone marrow graft rejection in patients with aplastic anemia. *Transplant Proc* 1978; 10:441–445.
45. Gluckman E, Devergie A, Morty N, et al.: Allogeneic bone marrow transplantation in aplastic anemia; report of 25 cases. *Transplant Proc* 1978; 10:141–145.
46. Storb R, Doney KC, Thomas ED, et al.: Marrow transplantation with or without buffy coat for 65 transfused aplastic anemia patients. *Blood* 1982; 59:236–246.
47. Thomas ED, Storb R, Cleft RA, et al.: Bone marrow transplantation. *N Eng J Med* 1979; 292:832–843 and 895–902.
48. Holohan TV, Terasaki PI, Deisseroth AB: Suppression of transfusion related alloimmunization in intensity treated cancer patients. *Blood* 1981; 58:122–128.
49. Storb R, Thomas ED, Buckner CD, et al.: Marrow transplantation in 30 "untransfused" patients with severe aplastic anemia. *Ann Intern Med* 1980; 92:30–36.
50. Ho WG, Champlin RE, Winston D, et al.: Bone marrow transplantation in patients with leukæmia previously transfused with blood products from family members. *Brit J Hem* 1987; 67:67–70.
51. Van Eys J, Thomas D, Olivos B: Platelet use in pediatric oncology; a review of 393 transfusions. *Transfusion* 1978; 18:169–173.
52. Tejada R, Bias WB, Santos GW, et al.: Immunologic response of patients with acute leukemia to platelet transfusions. *Blood* 1973; 42:405–412.
53. Dutcher JP, Schiffer CA, Aisner J, et al.: Long-term follow-up of patients with leukemia receiving platelet transfusions; identification of a large group of patients who do not become alloimmunized. *Blood* 1981; 58:1007–1011.
54. Michinton RM, Waters AH, Baker LR, et al.: Platelet, granulocyte and HLA antibodies in renal dialysis patients transfused with frozen blood. *Br Med J* 1980; 12:218:113–114.
55. Polesky HF: Leukocyte-poor blood; a study in the evolution of component therapy. In,

Myhre B (ed): *A Seminar on Blood Components* Washington D.C. American Association of Blood Banks, 1977; p. 53.

56. Polesky HF, McCullough J, Helgeson MA, et al.: Evaluation of methods for interpretation of HLA-antigen poor blood. *Transfusion* 1973; 13:383–387.

57. Sirchia G, Parravicine A, Rebulla P. et al.: Evaluation for three procedures for the preparation of leukocyte-poor and leukocyte-free blood cells for transfusion. *Vox Sang* 1980; 38:197–204.

58. Sirchia G, Parravicine A, Rebulla P, et al.: Effectiveness of red blood cells filtered through cotton wool to prevent anti-leukocytic antibody production in multitransfused patients. *Vox Sang* 1982; 42:190–197.

59. Myrovic V, Brozovic B, Hughes ASB, et al: Leukocyte depleted blood; a comparison of filtration techniques. *Transfusion* 1983;30–32.

61. Slichter SJ, Harker LA: Thrombocytopenia; mechanisms and management of defects in platelet production. *Clin Haemotol* 1978; 7:523–539.

61. Brand A, Claas FH, Falkenburg JF, et al.: Blood component therapy in bone marrow transplantation. *Semin Hemat* 1984; 21:141–155.

62. Storb R, Thomas ED, Buckner CD, et al.: Marrow transplantation for aplastic anemia. *Semin Hematol* 1984; 21:27–36.

63. Ramsay NKC, Kim TH, McClave P, et al.: Total lymphoid irradiation and cyclophosphamide conditioning prior to bone marrow transplantation for patients with severe aplastic anemia. *Blood* 1983; 62:622–626.

64. Gale RP, Ho W, Feig S, et al.: Prevention of graft rejection following bone marrow transplantation. *Blood* 1981; 57:9–12.

65. Devergie A, Gluckman E: Bone marrow transplantation in severe aplastic anemia following cytoxan and thoraco-abdominal irradiation. *Exp Hematol* 1982; 10 (Suppl 10) 17–18.

66. Hows JM, Palmer S, Gordon-Smith EC: Use of cyclosporin A in allogeneic bone marrow transplantation for severe aplastic anemia. *Transplantation* 1982; 33:382–386.

67. Parkman R, Mosier D, Umansky I, et al.: Graft-vs.-host disease after intrauterine and exchange transfusions for hemolytic disease of the newborn. *N Eng J Med* 1974; 290:359–363.

68. Rosen RC, Huestis DW, Cerrison JJ: Acute leukemia and granulocyte transfusion; fetal graft-vs.-host reaction following transfusion of cells obtained from normal donors. *J Pediatr* 1978; 92:268–270.

69. Seemoyer TA, Bolanche RP: Thymic involution mimicking thymic dysplasia; a consequence of transfusion-induced graft-vs.-host disease in a premature infant. *Arch Pathol Lab Med* 1980; 104:141–144.

70. Weiden PL, Zuckerman N, Hansen JA, et al.: Fatal graft-vs.-host disease in a patient with lymphoblastic leukemia following normal granulocytic transfusion. *Blood* 1981; 57:328–332.

71. Von Fliedner V, Higby DJ, Kim U: Graft-vs.-host reaction following blood product transfusion. *Am J Med* 1982; 72:951–961.

72. Siimes MA, Koskimies S: Chronic graft-vs.-host disease after blood transfusions confirmed by incompatible HLA antigens in bone marrow. *Lancet* 1982; 1:42–43.

73. Holley TR, Van Epps DE, Harvey RL, et al.: Effect of high dose of radiation on human neutrophil chemotaxis, phagocytosis, and morphology. *Am J Pathol* 1974; 75:61–72.

74. Button LN, De Wolf WC, Newburger PE, et al.: The effects of irradiation on blood components. *Transfusions* 1981; 21:419–426.

75. Bowden RA, Sayers M,, Flournoy N, et al.: Cytomegalovirus immune globulin and seronegative blood products to prevent cytomegalovirus infection after marrow transplantation. *N Engl J Med* 1986; 314:1006–1010.

76. Hows J, Beddow K, Gordon-Smith E, Branch D, et al.: Donor derived RBC antibodies and immuno-hemolysis after allogeneic bone marrow transplantation. *Blood* 1986; 67:177–181.

76a. Lasky LC, Warkentin PI, Kersey JH, et al.: Hemotherapy in patients undergoing blood group incompatible bone marrow transplantation. *Transfusion* 1988; 23:277–281.

77. Duquesnoy RJ, Filip DJ, Rodey GE, et al.: Transfusion of platelets matched and selectively mismatched for HLA antigens to alloimmunized thrombocytopenic patients. *Am J Hematol* 1977; 2:219–226.

78. Tomasulo PA: Management of the alloimmunized patient with HLA matched platelets. In,

Schiffer CA (ed): *Platelet Physiology and Transfusion.* American Association of Blood Banks, Washington, D.C., 1978, p. 69.

79. Aster RH, Szatkowski N, Liebert M, et al.: Expression of HLA-B12, HLA-B8, W2 and W6 platelets. *Transplant Proc* 1977; 9:1695–1696.

80. Brand AV. Leeuwen A, Eernisse JG, et al.: Platelet transfusion therapy; optimal donor selection with a combination of the lymphocytoxicity and platelet immunofluorescense test. *Blood* 1978; 51:781–788.

81. Tosato G, Applebaum FR, Deisseroth AB: HLA matched platelet transfusion therapy for severe aplastic anemia. *Blood* 1978; 52:846–855.

82. Tosato G, Applebaum FR, Trapani RJ: Use of *in vitro* assay in selection of compatible platelet donors. *Transfusion* 1980; 20:47–54.

83. Slichter SJ: Selection of compatible platelet donors. In, Schiffer CA (ed): *Platelet Physiology and Transfusion.* American Association of Blood Banks, Washington D.C., 1978, p. 83.

84. Kickler TS, Braine HG, Ness PM, et al.: A radiological antiglobulin test for cross-matching platelet transfusions. *Blood* 1983; 61:238–242.

85. Myers TJ, Kim BK, Steiner M, Baldini MG: Selection of donor platelets for alloimmunized patients using a platelet associated IgG assay. *Blood* 1981; 58:444–450.

86. Schiffer, GA, Aisner J: Platelet and granulocyte transfusion therapy for patients with cancer. In, Petz LD, Swisher SK (eds): *Clinical Practice of Blood Transfusion.* Churchill Livingstone, New York, 1981. p. 551.

87. Graw RG, Herzig G, Perry S, Henderson ES: Normal granulocyte transfusion therapy; treatment of septicemia due to gram negative bacteria. *N Engl J Med* 1972; 287:367–375.

88. Vogler WR, Winton EF: The efficacy of granulocyte transfusions in neutropenic patients. *Am J Med* 1977; 63:548–555.

89. Herzig R, Herzig G, Graw RG, et al.: Efficacy of granulocyte transfusion therapy for gram negative sepsis; a prospective randomized controlled study. *N Engl J Med* 1977; 296:701–705.

90. Huestis DW: Adverse effects of granulocyte donation. *Prog Clin Biol Res* 1982; 88:101–104.

91. Higby DJ, Burnett D: Granulocyte transfusion; current status. *Blood* 1980; 55:2–8.

92. Clift RA, Sanders JE, Thomas Ed, et al.: Granulocyte transfusions for the prevention of infection in patients receiving bone marrow transplants. *N Engl J Med* 1978; 298:1052–1057.

93. Winston DJ, Ho WG, Young LS, Gale RP: Therapeutic granulocyte transfusions during human bone marrow transplantation. *Am J Med* 1980; 68:893–905.

94. Strauss RG, Cossett JE, Gale RP, et al.: A controlled trial of prophylactic granulocyte transfusions during initial induction chemotherapy for acute myelogenous leukemia. *N Engl J Med* 1981; 305:507–602.

95. Ford JM, Cullen MH, Roberts MM, et al.: Prophylactic granulocyte transfusions; results of a randomized controlled trial in patients with acute myelogenous leukemia. *Transfusions* 1982; 22:311–316.

96. Wright DG, Robichaud KJ, Pizzo PA, Deisseroth AB: Lethal pulmonary reactions associated with the combined use of amphotericin B and leukocyte transfusion. *N Engl J Med* 1981; 304:1185.

97. Wright DG, Robichaud K, Pizzo PA, Deisseroth AB: Pulmonary reactions associated with amphotericin B and leukocyte transfusions (Letter). *N Engl J Med* 1981; 305:585.

98. De Gregorio MW, Lee WMF, Ries CA: Pulmonary reactions associated with amphotericin B and leukocyte transfusions (Letter). *N Engl J Med* 1981; 305:585.

99. Foman SJ, Robinson GV, Wolf JA, et al.: Pulmonary reactions associated with amphotericin B and leukocyte transfusions (Letter). *N Engl J Med* 1981; 305:584.

100. Dana BW, Durie BGM, White RF, Huestis DW: Concomitant administration of granulocyte transfusions and amphotericin B in neutropenic patients; absence of significant pulmonary toxicity. *Blood* 1981; 57:90–94.

101. Winston DJ, Ho WG, Young, LS, et al.: Prophylactic granulocyte transfusions during human bone marrow transplantation. *Am J Med* 1980; 68:893–896.

Bone Marrow Transplantation in Children, edited by F. Leonard Johnson and Carl Pochedly. Raven Press, Ltd., New York © 1990.

Immune Recovery Following Bone Marrow Transplantation

Axel R. Zander and Inga A. Aksamit

Division of Bone Marrow Transplantation, Pacific Presbyterian Medical Center, San Francisco, California 94120

Introduction
A. The mucous membrane defense system
B. Phagocytes and killer cells
C. T cell mediated immunity
D. B cell mediated immunity
E. Effect of cytomegalovirus infection on recovery of immunity
F. Influence of the conditioning regimen on immune recovery
G. Immune recovery after autologous transplantation
H. Techniques used to enhance reconstitution of immune functions follow-
      ing marrow transplant
Summary

INTRODUCTION

The technique of marrow transplant consists of intravenous infusion of a bone marrow cell suspension into the specially prepared recipient. Preparation for the transplant is directed against the underlying disease. But at the same time this preliminary treatment creates space for engraftment and produces immunosuppression in the recipient to permit the infused stem cells to engraft and to establish a new immunohematopoietic system. From the time of the conditioning to when there is full development of hematopoietic and immunologic functions, the recipient is at risk for the development of potentially life-threatening bacterial, fungal, viral and protozoal infections.(1–4) (Figure 1).

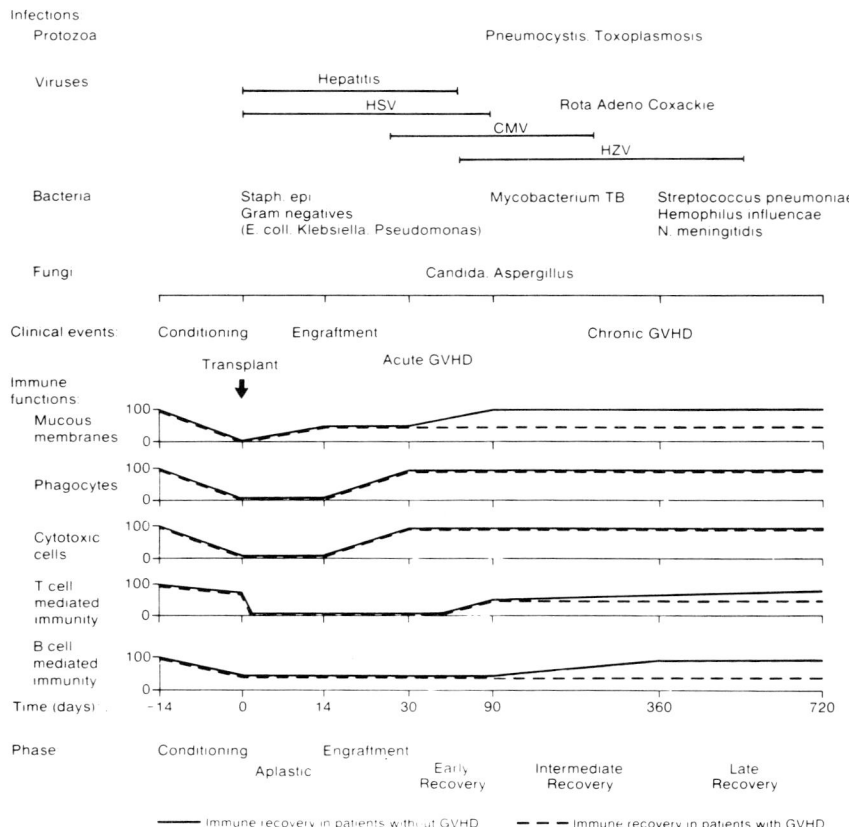

FIG. 1. Graph showing sequence of events and timetable for recovery of various immunologic functions, as well as times of increased risk of various infections following bone marrow transplant.

Rapidity of recovery and occurrence of clinical complications depend on the source of the hematopoietic stem cells used for transplantation. Patients who undergo syngeneic or autologous transplantation generally experience fewer life-threatening infections than patients given allogeneic transplants. Great emphasis needs to be placed on the prevention of serious infections in recipients of allogeneic bone marrow transplants, even beyond one year post-bone-marrow transplantation. On the other hand, the preventive measures needed for recipients of autologous and syngeneic marrow are somewhat less stringent.

The time periods or landmarks before and following a bone marrow transplant can, for the sake of the discussion, be divided into 6 phases (Table 1). First is the conditioning phase of between 2 days and 2 weeks duration. During this time the patient receives chemotherapy or combined chemoradio-

TABLE 1. *Time table or landmarks for assessment of events that occur before and following bone marrow transplantation*

1. The conditioning phase (pre-transplant)
2. The day of bone marrow infusion
3. Time to establish granulopoiesis (pre-engraftment phase)
4. Time when engraftment is complete
5. Early recovery phase
6. Intermediate recovery phase
7. Late recovery phase

therapy. Second is the day of bone marrow infusion, which is generally termed day 0. The third period is from the day of infusion until recovery of a granulocyte count of more than $200/mm^3$, which usually takes 1 to 4 weeks. This time period is called the pre-engraftment or aplastic phase. The engraftment phase is completed by 3 to 6 weeks post-transplant when the granulocyte count exceeds $1000/mm^3$, thus permitting the patient to be discharged from the transplant unit.

During the early recovery phase, from day 30 to day 90, the patient is closely followed as an outpatient. The final event is the intermediate recovery phase which extends from day 90 to day 360. The length of this phase can be most variable. Patients who receive an infusion of syngeneic or autologous bone marrow will be at only minimal or moderate risk for serious clinical complications. However, recipients of allogeneic bone marrow transplants will be at higher risk for intercurrent infections, particularly if they are suffering from chronic graft-vs.-host disease.

We will discuss the major compartments of the host defense system, the kinetics of their recovery, and clinical correlates. The host defense system consists of the first line defense of the mucous membranes, the phagocytic cytotoxic system, as well as T cell and B cell mediated immunity.

Mononuclear cells of the immune system in blood, bone marrow and other organs have been shown to be of donor origin by several techniques. These include chromosomal analysis in cases of sex mismatched transplants, immunoglobulin allotyping, and the use of DNA probes to distinguish donor and recipient by the means of restriction fragment length polymorphism (RFLP) (5–9). Besides the peripheral blood lymphocytes and monocytes, the sessile alveolar and hepatic macrophages are also of donor origin. The complete replacement of the lung and liver tissue macrophages might take several months post-transplant (9).

THE MUCOUS MEMBRANE DEFENSE SYSTEM

The mucous membranes of the body cover a vast surface area. They separate the host from the external environment in the gastrointestinal, respira-

tory and urogenital tracts. The musocal defense system consists of nonim-
munological defenses, such as the intact epithelial lining, the mucous coat, the
native microbial flora, immunologic components with secretory immunoglobulins, as well as cell mediated immunity of intra-epithelial lymphocytes
and lymphoid aggregates.

The mucosal defense system is impaired by the conditioning regimen given
prior to transplant (10). Most regimens will impair the intact epithelial lining of
the gastrointestinal tract, and thereby allow invasion of gut-associated flora. A
second factor which may lead to the development of mucositis is the type of
drugs given post-transplant for prevention of graft-vs.-host disease in allogeneic transplantation (11–12). Methotrexate, even if given in small doses, will
aggravate the existing injury of the mucous membranes caused by the conditioning regimen. This can lead to prolonged severe mucositis and secondary septice-
mias. Severe mucositis is seen less often with the use of cyclosporine.

Acute graft-vs.-host disease can affect the gut and might lead to significant
epithelial denudation allowing entry of bacteria and fungi. Chronic graft-vs.-
host disease may lead to debilitation and weight loss due to mucositis,
esophageal stenosis, anorexia from liver disease, and rarely, primary malabsorption (13). The sicca syndrome of chronic graft-vs.-host disease is characterized by insufficient tear production, dry mouth, and frequently by mucosal
abnormalities of the genital tract and respiratory tract as well (14). Secretory
immunoglobulin IgA levels, such as in saliva and tears, are decreased in
patients with chronic graft-vs.-host disease and, therefore, microbial invasion
may occur (15). Additional suppression of the mucosal defense system is
caused by treatment given for chronic graft-vs.-host disease. These defects of
the mucosal defense system can last for several years beyond the intermediate
recovery phase.

PHAGOCYTES AND KILLER CELLS

Granulocytes recover within 3 to 4 weeks post-bone-marrow transplantation, with recovery of the absolute neutrophil count to levels which are protective against most bacterial infections. The mechanism of action of granulocytes
in host defense consists of phagocytosis of microorganisms. The engulfed organisms are coated by antibodies and complement components in preparation for
subsequent intracellular killing. The overall impairment of granulocyte function in the early post-transplant period appears to be of only moderate degree
(18). There is some dispute as to what degree chemotaxis is deficient (16–18).
One study reported normal neutrophil chemotaxis and random migration,
whereas other workers found some degree of impairment of chemotaxis.
(17,18).

Intracellular killing of *Candida albicans* or *Staphylococcus aureus* and neutrophil iodinization capacity reflect the capacity to phagocytize and kill in-

tracellularly. Those functions are both normal (18). Opsonization capacity, as measured by the use of granulocytes from healthy donors and serum from the patient, can be deficient (17,18). It appears, therefore, that phagocytic defects in neutrophils do not contribute significantly to depression of host immune defenses, once the numbers of neutrophils have reached close to normal levels. Monocyte functions, as measured by chemotaxis, phagocytosis, adherence and cytotoxicity, recover early following transplant (19). Tissue macrophages change from being of host origin to donor origin. Complete replacement of lung and liver tissue macrophages can take several months. The "changing of the guard" of the lung tissue macrophages might be a contributing factor to the development of interstitial pneumonia, occurring 2 to 3 months post-transplant (9).

A specific defect is present in monocyte-associated fibronectin (20). Fibronectin on monocytes participates in opsonization primarily of gram positive bacteria. A defect in fibronectin binding was seen shortly after bone marrow transplant and in long-term survivors with chronic graft-vs.-host disease. It is proposed that this deficiency might contribute to the impaired resistance of recipients after marrow transplantation (20). Accessory functions of monocytes during early and late post-transplant phases are essentially normal. Monocytes are capable of presenting bacterial antigens in a T cell proliferation assay (20). They also provide accessory cell function in immunoglobulin production which is T cell dependent and stimulated by pokeweed mitogen (22). Monocytes secrete normal amounts of interleukin-1 in the early post-transplant period, as well as in patients with chronic graft-vs.-host disease, when T lymphocytes are defective in secretion of interleukin-2 (23).

Studies of natural killer (NK) cells in allogeneic bone marrow transplantation have shown contradictory findings (24–38). NK cells are implicated in a number of immunologic responses. NK cells of host origin can mediate resistance against allogeneic marrow grafts (32–34). In one study, high activity of natural killer cells early after transplant was associated with the occurrence of acute graft-vs.-host disease (26). Another study did not show a significant association between cytotoxic activity and such complications as infections, graft-vs.-host disease and recurrence of leukemia (24). As many as 20% of otherwise healthy long-term survivors have persistent defects in NK cell activity (24). These conflicting results may be due to the heterogeneity of the NK cell population (35).

Cytotoxicity of natural killer cells is mediated by several subsets of effector cells. Cloned cell lines derived from circulating lymphocytes are able to demonstrate subtle anti-leukemic effects which are obscured when effector cells from whole blood are tested (30).

Other studies have shown that NK cell responses and cytotoxic T lymphocyte responses to cytomegalovirus after grafting predict the outcome of cytomegalovirus infections (25). A correlation between pre-transplant natural killer cell activity and the occurrence of graft-vs.-host disease after bone marrow transplantation has been reported (27). Patients with normal natural killer cell activity against fibroblasts infected by herpes simplex virus (HSV) type I have a high likelihood to develop graft-vs.-host disease. On the other hand, patients with low NK activity do not show this tendency to develop graft-vs.-host disease. These findings were confirmed by a combined evaluation of two centers (39). Natural killer cell activity against fibroblasts infected by Herpes simplex virus, but not against K562, was of predictive value for acute graft-vs.-host disease (39).

It is generally believed that the more primitive phagocytic and cytotoxic functions of the immune system recover earlier and that the more specialized functions requiring cell-cell interaction and fine regulation recover later. Thus, this sequence of events in immunologic recovery repeats the ontogeny of the immune functions (40). However, there is recent evidence that the population of large granular lymphocytes, which comprise NK cells, produces lymphokines which can influence B lymphocytes as well (41–45). NK cells can inhibit B cell growth and differentiation (36,46,47). However, when large granular lymphocytes are activated, they can secrete at least 4 lymphokines: interleukin-1, interleukin-2, B cell growth factor (BCGF), and B cell differentiation factor (BCDF). All of these lymphokines can augment B cell growth and differentiation (41,42,44,45). Besides secreting stimulatory factors, these lymphokines can induce B lymphocytes to be responsive to the various factors.

T CELL MEDIATED IMMUNITY

Recovery of T cell mediated function after bone marrow transplantation has been evaluated by several techniques. These include determination of T lymphocyte surface markers, measurement of delayed-type hypersensitivity and *in vitro* assays to determine lymphoblastic responses to mitogens, helper cell activity for the synthesis of immunoglobulin T cell mediated cytotoxicity, and T cell colony formation. Repopulation of T and B lymphocytes of donor origin in the peripheral blood occur in the first 3 months post-transplant (48–55). Expression of lymphocyte surface markers is influenced by a variety of clinical events, such as acute and chronic graft-vs.-host disease, cytomegalovirus infections, T cell depletion of the donor graft, and type of immunosuppression used to prevent graft-vs.-host disease (48–55).

This variety of influences that affects lymphocyte surface markers accounts for the discrepant findings seen in many studies. Most studies agree that helper-inducer (CD4) cells are reduced both in relative proportion and in absolute numbers in the early post-transplant phase. It is also agreed that the number and proportion of suppressor cytotoxic (CD8) cells are higher than normal in the early and late recovery phases (48–56). However, in one study lymphocyte surface markers were determined in the very early aplastic and engraftment phase, starting on day 4 following allogeneic transplant. In this study, it was noted that the very first cell population returning was CD4 cells, followed 4 to 7 days later by CD8 cells (73). Most patients in the early post-transplant course had a positive helper-suppressor (CD4/CD8) ratio which became reversed 3 weeks post-transplant. This reversal of the helper-suppressor ratio was noted in patients undergoing either autologous or allogeneic transplants. In the subset of allogeneic transplant recipients, early reversal of the CD4/CD8 ratio correlated with the occurrence of acute graft-vs.-host disease.

Other studies of immune follow-up measure lymphocyte surface markers at a later time post-transplant (48,52,54,56). The helper and suppressor cell types are determined by Fc-Igm and Fc-IgG receptors on T cells. Use of this technique has confirmed the presence of an increase in suppressor cells and a decrease in helper cells for more than a year post-transplant (57). Some studies report normalization of helper-suppressor cell ratios in healthy bone marrow recipients after one year (52–53). Patients with chronic graft-vs.-host disease will maintain a reversed helper-suppressor cell ratio for years (48,55,58). Several studies found a correlation between the presence of a low helper-suppressor cell ratio and the occurrence of cytomegalovirus infections (51,59,61).

Various studies have noted that from less than 3% to more than 25% of cells in the peripheral blood are positive for class II antigens (62–68). A correlation of this finding with acute graft-vs.-host disease has been claimed (67). Class II antigens like HLA-DR and HLA-DQ are normally not expressed on peripheral blood T lymphocytes (63). However, between 30 and 80% of freshly isolated T lymphocytes from recently transplanted patients express HLA-DR but less than 8% express HLA-DQ (50,51,54,58,62). HLA-DR and HLA-DQ are expressed by *in vitro* activated T cells (69).

Recovery of cellular immunity *in vivo* is measured by delayed-type hypersensitivity (DTH) skin testing. Cellular immunity shows abnormally low responses, particularly in patients with acute and chronic graft-vs.-host disease. Responses to recall antigens can be suppressed for as long as 3 to 4 years after bone marrow transplant, particularly in patients with chronic graft-vs.-host disease (70).

Proliferative responses to mitogens and alloantigens remain depressed for 6 months. In patients with chronic graft-vs.-host disease, these responses are depressed for longer than one year (56,70,75).

Helper and suppressor cell functions of T lymphocytes have been explored to explain the immunologic deficiencies seen after transplant. Various *in vitro* systems have been used to determine the influence of T lymphocytes on immunoglobulin production (76–83). One such culture system for production of immunoglobulins employs pokeweed mitogen together with autologous or allogeneic T lymphocytes and a B cell enriched population (76–79). T lymphocytes from most marrow transplant recipients did not express helper cell function, but in most cases showed significant suppressor cell function (78). When T lymphocytes were fractionated into subpopulations of helper cells and suppressor cells, it was shown that CD4 cells could exert help as well as suppression (81). T cell defects were less frequent in patients who did not suffer from chronic graft-vs.-host disease (81).

T lymphocyte colony formation was studied after bone marrow transplantation (84–86). Under normal conditions, a T cell colony forming cell is a mature T cell of helper phenotype (87–89). T cell depleted cell populations can be driven toward T cell colony production in the presence of exogenous interleukin-2 (101). One study found defective T cell colony formation more than one year post-transplant, while others noted recovery of T cell colony formation to near normal by one year (84–86). Exogenous interleukin-2 caused a modest increase in colony formation, but it could not increase colony formation to near normal levels (84,86).

The effect of depletion of T lymphocytes from donor marrow on immune recovery is still controversial. Drugs to prevent graft-vs.-host disease generally given by themselves to a recipient of unmanipulated bone marrow, have immunosuppressive effects. A similar recovery of the numbers of B cells and T cells and recovery of T cell function by day 28 was observed in patients who received T cell depleted bone marrow, when compared with a historical control group. The control group received prophylaxis against graft-vs.-host disease in the form of methotrexate alone or as a combination of methotrexate and prednisone plus antithymocyte globulin or the OKT3 antibody (92). Helper cytotoxic and proliferating T lymphocyte precursors may be enumerated by using the method of limiting dilutions. By use of this technique, T lymphocyte functions were found to be more severely impaired for the first 180 days after transplantation in patients given T cell depleted bone marrow than in recipients of untreated marrow. After the first 6 months, recipients of T cell depleted marrow had blood T cell counts comparable to those observed in patients given untreated marrow (92).

B CELL MEDIATED IMMUNITY

The repopulation of B cells to normal numbers in the peripheral blood of a recipient of allogeneic or syngeneic bone marrow transplantation occurs within 2 to 3 months following the transplant (72,73,75). Early in the post-transplant course, immature B cells bearing the CD5 T cell antigen are present in the circulation (93).

Levels of IgG and IgM immunoglobulins in the serum return to normal 3 months post-transplant, but IgA levels may be suppressed for years (73–75). IgE levels have been reported to be increased with acute graft-vs.-host disease, and in the presence of infections due to viruses and other microbial pathogens (94–96).

Recipients of allogeneic and syngeneic marrow transplants have severely depressed responses to immunization with neoantigens, including keyhold-limpet hemocyanin, pneumococcal polysaccharide type 3 antigen, and bacterophage OX (163). These depressed responses are seen in the first 6 months post-transplant and recover by one year in healthy recipients, but the responses to immunizing antigens remain suppressed in patients who suffer from chronic graft-vs.-host disease (107,108). Patients with chronic graft-vs.-host disease show impaired primary response to the bacteriophage, and a deficit in converting from IgM to IgG in secondary response (107).

Besides presence of chronic graft-vs.-host disease, administration of anti-thymocyte globulin was a determinant factor in causing delay of antibody production to neoantigens (107). Antibody responses to recall antigens like tetanus toxoid, diphtheria toxoid, and measles virus can be detected in the early phase post-bone-marrow transplant (99–101). The study of recall antigens in healthy long-term recipients of bone marrow transplants shows positive IgG titers in two-thirds of the recipients tested for antibodies against tetanus toxoid, diphtheria toxoid, and the measle virus (101). In recipients with chronic graft-vs.-host disease, positive antibody titers are seen in only one-third of cases (101). The derivation of the antibodies to recall antigens in the early post-transplant period has not been fully clarified. It is conceivable that the immunity is either transferred from mature donor cells or is derived from residual host cells. Host-derived antibody can be measured by following isohemagglutinin titers in ABO incompatible marrow graft recipients. In 80% of cases no measurable titers can be detected following day 80, and no cases have measurable titers by day 120 post-transplant (107). However, we recently observed a persistent elevation in isohemagglutinin titer in a patient who experienced mixed chimerism until day 150 (102).

Support for the hypothesis that immunity to recall antigen is derived from donor cells comes from two sources. Lum et al., reported that B cells immune to recall antigens can be transferred in T cell depleted marrow grafts (103). All 9 short-term recipients had antitetanus toxoid titers while 3 out of 7 had antibodies against diphtheria toxoid. In long-term recipients, 5 out of 6 had antitetanus titers and 3 out of 5 had antidiphtheria titers. Among historical controls consisting of short-term recipients who received unmanipulated marrow, 221 out of 235 had antibody titers against tetanus toxoid and 176 out of 232 had antidiphtheria titers. The persistence of antibody synthesis in long-term recipients shows that immunity can be transferred in T cell depleted marrows. A similar transfer of immunity from donor-derived T cell depleted marrow is enhanced by immunization of the recipient and the donor prior to transplantation (104).

Despite normalization of serum immunoglobulin IgG levels, IgG subclasses, particularly IgG-2 and IgG-4, may be suppressed for years in patients with chronic graft-vs.-host disease. These IgG subclasses contain antibodies to bacterial polysaccharides (105). Antibodies to *Hemophilus influenzae* type B capsular polysaccharide were suppressed for more than 2 years after transplantation in patients with chronic graft-vs.-host disease. *Hemophilus influenzae* and *Streptococcus pneumoniae* are responsible for the high incidence of fatal gram-positive infections in long-term survivors after allogeneic bone marrow transplants. The above mentioned study showed that most patients who developed *Hemophilus influenzae* type B pneumonia showed virtually no immuno-globulin antibody response to the antigen (105).

Tests of B cell function *in vitro* have been carried out to further assess the B cell defects seen after allogeneic bone marrow transplantation. B cell anti-body secretion by lymphocytes was studied by use of an indirect hemolysis assay. This study revealed a statistically significant increase of IgG plaque forming cells in patients who had acute graft-vs.-host disease, whereas pa-tients with chronic graft-vs.-host disease had deficient IgM production (76–78). T cell and T cell subset functions are more frequently altered in patients with chronic graft-vs.-host disease than in long-term healthy recipients (106,107). Patients with chronic graft-vs.-host disease have pan-T cells, CD4, and CD8 cells that significantly suppress immunoglobulin synthesis by normal T cells and B cells (107).

B cells from the same marrow recipients respond differently when activated by pokeweed mitogen, Epstein-Barr virus, Herpes simplex type I virus, and tetanus toxoid to induce immunoglobulin production (107). These studies show defective B cell function, lack of pan-T cell or CD4 helper cell activity, and increased pan-T, CD4 or CD8 cell suppressor activity after stimulation with various activators. From these studies it appears likely that there are different functional groups of cells within each subset. However, in these studies no correlations were found between serum titers and *in vitro* immune responses to the various polyclonal activators. The discrepancies seen be-tween the *in vivo* and *in vitro* functions indicate a need for development of newer and more specific *in vitro* assays for assessing B cell functions.

A more recent evaluation of an antitetanus toxoid system shows significant correlations between seropositivity and *in vitro* IgG production of IgG anti-bodies against tetanus toxoid (108,109). Recipient B cells failed to produce antibody in the presence of donor T cells, whereas T cells from long-term survivors provided helper activity to immune donor B cells in most cases. The presence of specific helper T cell activity against tetanus toxoid in most seropositive long-term recipients suggests that a specific immunity can be transferred from the bone marrow donor to the bone marrow recipient.

Further studies with this *in vitro* system suggests that the defect responsible for B cell deficiencies in long-term marrow recipients is multifaceted. This defect is due in part to a low antigen specific precursor frequency and in part due to deficient B cell functions. The deficiency is manifested by decreased proliferative and differentiative responses, as well as by decreased ability to synthesize immunoglobulin after appropriate stimulation (108,110).

EFFECT OF CYTOMEGALOVIRUS INFECTION ON RECOVERY OF IMMUNITY

Cytomegalovirus (CMV) infections have been identified as one of the major causes of morbidity and mortality following bone marrow transplantation. *De novo* CMV infection or reactivation of cytomegalovirus occurs in 50 to 70% of recipients of allogeneic bone marrow transplants. Cytomegalovirus is the most common pathogen associated with interstitial pneumonia, which carries a fatality rate as high as 80% (111,113). Patients who are CMV positive or have CMV positive bone marrow donors have a higher risk of developing CMV infection. CMV viremia may be silent or may have such clinical manifestations as late central or peripheral thrombocytopenia, neutropenia, fever, hepatitis, interstitial pneumonia and colitis. Cytomegalovirus infection can be documented on routine culturing in about 50% of recipients of allogeneic transplants, with a peak frequency between the 7th and 9th week post-transplant (114).

CMV infections have a profound effect on the immune system of otherwise healthy persons (115). Lymphocyte proliferative responses to mitogens and Herpes virus antigens are diminished during cytomegalovirus mononucleosis. Acute CMV infection is associated with the reversal in the normal ratio of helper and suppressor T lymphocytes. There are relative and absolute decreases in T helper cells and corresponding increases in T suppressor cells. Concomitantly diminished lymphocyte responses to mitogen and concanavalin A are noted. During convalescence, helper T lymphocytes increase, helper-suppressor cell ratios normalize, and lymphoblastic responses return to normal (115). Cytomegalovirus infections have a profound impact on *in vitro* immune parameters following autologous and allogeneic transplants (116–119). Patients who are CMV titer positive have a more protracted inversion of helper-suppressor cell ratios than patients who are CMV negative (116–119).

HLA-restricted cytotoxic T lymphocytes have been found active in the immune response to human CMV infections (120). Low cytotoxic response in the presence of CMV infection predicts poor outcome (114,120,121). CMV-specific cytotoxic lymphocytes either are absent or are present in very low numbers in blood from patients who developed fatal cytomegalovirus infections.

Vilmer et al., studied the relationship between immune status, graft-vs.-host disease, and CMV viremia (114). A seroconversion to CMV occurs after a mean of 10 weeks, with a range of 3 to 20 weeks. Lymphocyte proliferative responses to CMV antigen are noted after a mean of 15 weeks (range 3–20), and stay suppressed in patients who had developed graft-vs.-host disease or who soon developed this complication. When the patients develop a CMV lymphocyte response after transplant, CMV can no longer be recovered by culture of blood. (114). By use of modification of the lymphocyte proliferation test specific for CMV antigen and the *in vitro* CMV IgG synthesis test, CMV infection could be detected much earlier. By this technique, CMV infection was detected at a mean of 45 days after bone marrow transplant, which is about 30 days earlier than CMV growth was detected in culture (122). The sensitivity and early reactivity of the lymphocyte proliferation test and the *in vitro* IgG production assay may lead to early detection of CMV infection after bone marrow transplantation.

Graft-vs.-host disease has been associated with a significant increase in the incidence of CMV pneumonia. But it is not associated with an increased frequency of idiopathic pneumonitis and *Pneumocystis carinii* pneumonia (113). A study was done comparing the incidence of various types of interstitial pneumonia in 100 recipients of syngeneic bone marrow as compared with 351 allogeneic bone marrow recipients. In this study, no cases of CMV pneumonia were seen in the twin (syngeneic) transplants compared with an incidence of CMV pneumonia of 19% in the recipients of allogeneic transplants (134). The seroconversion from CMV negative to CMV positive was comparable in both groups. The explanation for the correlation between graft-vs.-host disease and CMV could be that graft-vs.-host disease may reactivate latent CMV infections. The explanation could also be that CMV infection may alter surface antigens on host cells leading to a more aggressive immune response. The incidence of graft-vs.-host disease was significantly higher in patients with viremia than in patients who had no viremia or who were seronegative (114).

A strong association between CMV infection and acute graft-vs.-host disease was noted (124). Acute graft-vs.-host disease preceeded CMV infection by more than a month. Patients who developed CMV infection had received larger amounts of cellular blood products post-transplant. These findings suggest that CMV infection may occur through reactivation of a latent virus in seropositive patients or through exposure to the virus by transfusion. It is of interest that a significant correlation was also found between CMV immunity of the donor and chronic, not acute, graft-vs.-host disease in the bone marrow recipient (125). The 2-year cumulative probability of developing chronic graft-vs.-host disease was 55% when the donor was immune to CMV and only 16.5% when the donor was nonimmune to CMV. No correlation between recipient pre-transplant CMV immunity and chronic graft-vs.-host disease was observed. Other studies found a correlation between cytomegalovirus seroconversion and the incidence of chronic graft-vs.-host disease, but there was no correlation between CMV infection and acute graft-vs.-host disease (126). Cytomegalovirus infection always appeared before chronic graft-vs.-host disease. In another series, recipients of marrow from CMV seropositive donors had an increased risk for severe graft-vs.-host disease (127,128). The interaction between immunosuppression, graft-vs.-host disease, and CMV infection might be mutual, with important contributions from all 3 components in the process of pathogenesis (Figure 2).

A correlation between CD8-positive, HNK-1-positive T cells and cytomegalovirus infection was seen in recipients of allogeneic marrow who had reactivated CMV infection. However, the association between DMV seropositivity and graft-vs.-host disease could not be explained by an increase of CD8-positive, HNK-1-positive T cells in CMV seropositive donors. It is possible that the association between CMV seropositivity of the donor and the occurrence of active CMV infection post-bone marrow transplantation might be explained by transmission of virus with the graft. It appears that a clear

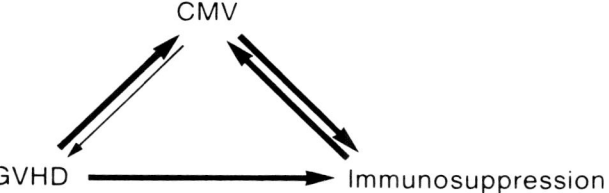

FIG. 2. Schema showing dynamic interaction of cytomegalovirus infection, graft-vs.-host disease, and immunosuppression in the patient following bone marrow transplantation.

definition of the relationship between cytomegalovirus infection and graft-vs.-host disease has to wait for completion of larger studies.

Prevention of cytomegalovirus infection in CMV-negative recipients of CMV-negative bone marrow has been most effective if strict transfusion policies were adhered to in cases where CMV-negative platelets and red cells were administered (129). The effectiveness of CMV hyperimmune plasma to prevent CMV infection in CMV negative or positive recipients is controversial (130–138).

INFLUENCE OF THE CONDITIONING REGIMEN ON IMMUNE RECOVERY

Gamma irradiation in conjunction with chemotherapy is widely used as a bone marrow ablative (conditioning) regimen to prepare patients for bone marrow transplantation. It had been generally assumed that the immune system of the host is completely ablated by the conditioning regimen, and that recovery of the immune system post-transplant is due to the function of the infused marrow cells. Recent studies have shown that even after supralethal conditioning treatment, fractions of host cells can still be found in blood and bone marrow (139–143). But mixed chimerism in most cases is only a transient phenomenon. To what degree surviving host cells participate in the regeneration of the immune system in man is not known.

Experimental studies in the mouse model suggest that the type of conditioning regimen given may influence immune recovery post-transplantation. In mice receiving syngeneic bone marrow transplants, persistent hypoplastic peripheral lymph nodes are found for many months following successful transplantation (144). Since the irradiated animals had been infused with syngeneic hematopoietic and lymphoid tissue, these findings indicate an impairment of receptiveness of host peripheral blood lymph nodes for circulating and donor-derived lymphocytes. The ability of normal blood-borne lymphocytes to enter peripheral nodes was markedly decreased in mice which had been exposed to 750 cGy (rad) of gamma irradiation. The irradiation-induced effect lasted longer than 6 months following syngeneic transplants and was caused by persistent anatomic changes in the lymphocyte receptive areas of the endothelium. Electromicroscopic studies showed significant intracellular edema, with occlusion of many microvascular lumina by edematous endothelial cells. Similar ultrastructural changes have been found in lymph nodes from human bone marrow transplant recipients (144).

The relative effect of gamma irradiation and busulfan on tissue specific localization of lymphocytes and recovery of immune function was tested in the same model. This study showed that busulfan had little effect on lymphocyte recirculation and the structures of the peripheral lymph nodes. Comparison of the effects of the two preparative regimens on recovery of contact hypersensitivity showed faster regeneration in busulfan-treated animals than in those given irradiation (145).

Conditioning regimens consisting of combination chemotherapy alone have challenged the more traditional preparative regimens which included total body irradiation (146). Results obtained with conditioning regimens consisting of combination chemotherapy alone are very encouraging. This includes studies in recipients of allogeneic transplants among patients with acute myeloid leukemia and chronic myelogenous leukemia, as well as recipients of autologous transplants in patients with Hodgkin's disease and non-Hodgkin's lymphoma (146,146(a)).

Recipients of an allogeneic bone marrow transplant who are conditioned with busulfan and cyclophosphamide retain host-type lymphocytes for up to 1 year. These lymphocytes retain their capacity of delivering interleukin-2 during the early recovery phase (146,147). The immune recovery of 21 patients conditioned with total body irradiation and 9 patients conditioned with high-dose chemotherapy (consisting of cyclophosphamide, BCNU, and etoposide) were compared during the early post-transplant phase in an earlier study. The natural killer (NK) response to K562 and the lymphoblastic responses to phytohemagglutinin were significantly lower in the group conditioned by chemotherapy. No significant differences were seen in the surface marker studies or other functional assays (56). Prospective comparisons of immune functions in patients conditioned with chemotherapy alone and the combination of chemotherapy and total body irradiation have not yet been carried out.

IMMUNE RECOVERY AFTER AUTOLOGOUS TRANSPLANTATION

Early recovery of immune functions after autologous transplantation is similar to the findings observed following allogeneic and syngeneic transplantation (71,74). Autologous bone marrow transplantation can serve as a model for immune recovery after ablative treatment since there are no histocompatibility differences and no immunosuppressive treatments which retard recovery. The incidence of late death related to transplantation is less after autografting. However, late death due to infection does occur even in patients who have recovered normal numbers of granulocytes and lymphocytes (146(a),148).

Usually, T cells recover as fast after autologous transplant as after allogeneic marrow transplantation and, like allogeneic bone marrow transplantation, an inverted helper-suppressor cell ratio is noted (55,149,153). In most studies this inverted T helper-suppressor cell ratio remained below 1.0 during the period of observation (55,62). Immature lymphocytes expressing Ia and CD8 surface antigens are seen for the first 6 months after transplant, similar to findings from allogeneic transplant studies (62,86). Proliferative capacity of T lymphocytes, as measured in T cell colony assays, is suppressed for more than 2 years after transplant (84–86). This T cell colony forming capacity can be partially reconstituted by adding human recombinant interleukin-2 to the culture (84–86). These observations give hope that interleukin-2 administration will be useful for immunologic reconstitution after autologous bone marrow transplantation.

Autologous transplantation can be performed with hematopoietic stem cells derived from the peripheral blood. This method is used for treatment of patients with hematologic malignancies and solid tumors and has recently attracted increasing interest (151–158). Evidence in mice, dogs, and nonhuman primates indicate that hematopoietic progenitor cells capable of repopulating ablated bone marrow circulate in peripheral blood (159,160). The hematopoietic recovery in most cases is faster than that observed following infusion of bone marrow stem cells, when grafts containing adequate numbers of stem cells are given (156–158,161).

Data on immune recovery following infusion of blood-derived stem cells are scarce. In one case of Burkitt's lymphoma, which was treated with myeloablative conditioning consisting of total body irradiation and cyclophosphamide, the number of peripheral blood T lymphocytes was within the normal range by day 8 post-transplant (161). The number of circulating B cells reached normal values by day 34 post-transplant. In another report, 8 patients underwent bone marrow transplantation with circulating stem cells for treatment of leukemia. In these patients, a lymphocyte count of $500/mm^3$ was reached by day 14 post-transplant, and the lymphocyte count reached $1500/mm^3$ by day 24 (162). The number of CD8-positive cells returned to normal in 3 patients by the end of 4 weeks. The number of CD4-positive cells also returned to normal by 4 weeks in one of 3 patients tested. Two patients studied at 3 and 7 months post-transplant had normal numbers of CD4-positive cells. These preliminary data suggest that autografting with blood-derived stem cells might lead to faster immune recovery than autografting with bone marrow stem cells.

TECHNIQUES USED TO ENHANCE RECONSTITUTION OF IMMUNE FUNCTIONS FOLLOWING MARROW TRANSPLANT

Thymus transplantation after allogeneic bone marrow grafting and treatment with thymosin fraction 5 have been undertaken in an effort to enhance reconstitution of immune functions and to prevent chronic graft-vs.-host disease. Neither thymus transplantation nor thymosin fraction 5 altered the incidence of chronic graft-vs.-host disease, infection, or leukemic relapse. Nor did use of these modalities accelerate immunologic reconstitution (163,164). One of the major problems encountered in doing thymus transplantation was rejection of the mismatched thymus graft. Modification of the technique which allows administration of cultured thymic epithelial monolayer cells might decrease the problem of graft rejection (163).

Thymosine alpha-1, thymopoietin and serum thymic factor are other thymic hormones being considered for use in reconstitution of T cell immunity (165). Recombinant growth factors like interleukin-2, interleukin-3, interleukin-4 and B cell differentiating factor will soon be available for testing in transplant recipients. Because of the problems associated with the disparity of transplantation antigens and graft-vs.-host disease in allogeneic transplants, the primary focus of investigation of the use of thymic hormones and hematopoietic growth factors might be in the reconstitution of recipients of autologous bone marrow grafts. The multitude of *in vivo* actions of growth factors needs to be further explored in preclinical models (166–169).

The question of whether bone marrow recipients should be immunized is controversial (Table 2). It has been proposed that patients who do not develop antibody titers in the early post-transplantation phase to clinically relevant antigens should be immunized (40).

No live vaccines should be used. Diphtheria toxoid, tetanus toxoid, and inactivated polio vaccines have been used without undue toxicity. Patients who do not develop graft-vs.-host disease can be successfully immunized (170–172). In patients who have developed chronic graft-vs.-host disease, immunization will be successful only after this disorder has been resolved.

For future studies, immunization of the donor and the recipient with rele-

TABLE 2. *Factors influencing immune recovery following bone marrow transplantation*

1. Source of stem cells
   a. Syngeneic or autologous donor
   b. Allogeneic matched donor
   c. Allogeneic mismatched donor
2. Composition of the graft
   a. T cell-depleted
   b. Peripheral blood mononuclear cells
   c. Bone marrow and mononuclear cells from peripheral blood
3. Conditioning regimen
   a. Chemotherapy only
   b. Chemotherapy and total body irradiation
4. Clinical events
   a. Intercurrent virus infections, particularly cytomegalovirus
   b. Drugs given to prevent or treat graft-vs.-host disease
   c. Presence and absence of graft-vs.-host disease

vant antigens appears most promising. It has been documented that memory cells are retained after T cell depletion, and presence of these cells allows for secondary antibody responses after booster injections (171).

SUMMARY

Rapidity of immune recovery and occurrence of clinical complications depend on the source of the hematopoietic stem cells used for transplantation. Patients who undergo syngeneic or autologous transplantation generally experience fewer life-threatening infections than patients given allogeneic transplants. Phagocytes and cytotoxic cells recover faster; T cell mediated and B cell mediated immunity recover in a delayed fashion. Cytomegalovirus infection delays immune recovery in recipients of allogeneic and autologous marrow transplants. Conditioning regimens consisting of chemotherapy alone without total body irradiation lead to persistence of host-type lymphocytes and their capacity of delivering interleukin-2 during the early recovery phase. The investigation into enhancement of immune recovery by lymphokines and monokines focuses on recipients of autologous bone marrow grafts because of the problems associated with the disparity of transplantation antigens and graft-vs.-host disease in allogeneic transplant recipients. Precautions for recipients of allogeneic and autologous bone marrow transplant need to be carefully tailored to their immune status.

REFERENCES

1. Young LS: An overview of infection in bone marrow transplant recipients. In, Prentice HG (ed): "Infections in Hæmatology" issue of *Clinics in Hæmatology,* 13(3):661–678, W.B. Saunders Company, London, 1984.
2. Meyers JC, Thomas ED: Infection complicating bone marrow transplantation. In, Rubin RH, Young LS (eds): *Clinical Approach to Infection in the Compromised Host.* Plenum Publishing Corporation, New York, 1981.
3. Appelbaum FR, Meyers JD, Fefer A, et al.: Nonbacterial nonfungal pneumonia following marrow transplantation in 100 identical twins. *Transplantation* 1982;33:265.
4. Atkinson K, Storb R, Prentice RL, et al.: Analysis of late infections in 89 long-term survivors of bone marrow transplantation. *Blood* 1979;53:720.
5. Storb R, Thomas ED, Buckner CD, et al.: Allogeneic marrow grafting for treatment of aplastic anemia. *Blood* 1974;43:157–180.
6. Gale RP, Sparkes RS, Golde DW: Bone marrow origin of hepatic macrophages (Kupffer cells) in humans. *Science* 1978;201:937–938.
7. Thomas ED, Ramberg RE, Sale GE, et al.: Direct evidence for a bone marrow origin of the alveolar macrophage in man. *Science* 1976;192:1016–1018.
8. Witherspoon RP, Schanfield MS, Storb R, et al.: Immunoglobulin production of donor origin after marrow transplantation for acute leukemia or aplastic anemia. *Transplantation* 1978;26:407–408.
9. Winston DJ, Territo MC, Ho WG, et al.: Alveolar macrophage dysfunction in human bone marrow transplant recipients. *Am J Med* 1982;73:859–866.
10. Beschorner W, Yardley J, Tutschka P, Santos G: Deficiency of intestinal immunity with graft-vs.-host disease in humans. *J Infect Dis* 1981;114:38–46.

11. Storb R, Deeg JH, Thomas ED, et al.: Marrrow transplantation for chronic myelocytic leukemia; a controlled trial of cyclosporine vs. methotrexate for prophylaxis of graft-vs.-host disease. *Blood* 1985;66:698.
12. Storb R, Deeg HJ, Whitehead J, et al.: Marrow transplantation for leukemia; methotrexate and cyclosporine compared with cyclosporine alone for prophylaxis of acute graft-vs.-host disease after marrow transplantation for leukemia. *N Engl J Med* 1986;314:729.
13. Sullivan KM: Graft-vs.-host disease. In, Blume KG, Petz LD (eds): *Clinical Bone Marrow Transplantation*, Churchill Livingstone, New York, 1983, pp. 109–129.
14. Sullivan KM, Shulman HM, Weiden PL, et al.: The spectrum of chronic graft-vs.-host disease in man. In, Gale RP, Fox CF (eds): *Biology of Bone Marrow Transplantation*. Academic Press, New York, 1980, p. 69.
15. Izutsu KT, Sullivan KM, Schubert MM, et al.: Disordered salivary immunoglobulin secretion and sodium transport in human chronic graft-vs.-host disease. *Transplantation* 1983;35:441.
16. Clark RA, Johnson FL, Klebanoff SJ, Thomas ED: Defective neutrophil chemotaxis in bone marrow transplant patients. *J Clin Invest* 1976;58:22.
17. Territo MC, Gale RP, Cline MJ, and the UCLA Bone Marrow Transplantation Team: Neutrophil function in bone marrow transplant recipients. *Br J Haematol* 1977;35:245.
18. Sosa R, Weiden PL, Storb R, et al.: Granulocyte function in human allogeneic marrow graft recipients. *Exp Hematol* 1980;8:1183.
19. Winston DJ, Territo MC, Ho WG, et al.: Alveolar macrophage dysfunction in human bone marrow transplant recipients. *Am J Med* 1982;73:859.
20. Klingemann HG, Maunder RJ, Storb R: Reduced monocyte-associated fibronectin in patients after allogeneic marrow transplantation. *Transplantation* 1987;43(3):454–456.
21. Tsoi M-S, Dobbs S, Brkic S, et al.: Cellular interactions in marrow-grafted patients. II. Normal monocyte antigen-presenting and defective T-cell proliferative functions early after grafting and during chronic graft-vs.-host disease. *Transplantation* 1984;37:557.
22. Shiobara S, Witherspoon RP, Lum LG, Storb R: Immunoglobulin synthesis after HLA-identical marrow grafting. V. The role of peripheral blood monocytes in the regulation of *in vitro* immunoglobulin secretion stimulated by pokeweed mitogen. *J Immunol* 1984;132:2850.
23. Brkic S, Tsoi M-S, Mori T, et al.: Cellular interactions in marrow-grafted patients. III. Normal interleukin-1 and defective interleukin-2 production in short-term patients and in those with chronic graft-vs.-host disease. *Transplantation* 1985;39:30.
24. Livnat S, Seigneuret M, Storb R, Prentice R; Analysis of cytotoxic effector cell function in patients with leukemia or aplastic anemia before and after marrow transplantation. *J Immunol* 1980;124:481.
25. Quinnan GV Jr, Kirmani N, Esber E, *et al.:* HLA-restricted cytotoxic T lymphocyte and nonthymic cytotoxic lymphocyte responses to cytomegalovirus infection of bone marrow transplant recipients. *J Immunol* 1981;126:2036.
26. Gluckman E, Tursz T: Natural killer cell activity in human bone marrow recipients; early reappearance of peripheral natural killer activity in graft-vs.-host disease. *Transplantation* 1981;31:61.
27. Lopez C, Sorell M, Kirkpatrick D, O'Reilly RJ and Ching C: Association between pre-transplant natural killer and graft-vs.-host disease after stem-cell transplantation. *Lancet* 1979;4:1103–1106.
28. Brenner MK, Reittie JE, Grob J-P, et al.: The contribution of large granular lymphocytes to B cell activation and differentiation after T cell depleted allogeneic bone marrow transplantation. *Transplantation* 1986;42:257–261.
29. Rooney CM, Wimperis JZ, Brenner MK, et al.: Natural killer activity following T cell depleted allogeneic bone marrow transplantation. *Br J Haematol* 1986;62:413.
30. Delmon L. Ythier A, Moingeon P, et al.: Characterization of anti-leukemia cells' cytotoxic effector function; implications for monitoring natural killer responses following allogeneic bone marrow transplantation. *Transplantation* 1986;42(3):252–256.
31. Warner JF, Dennert G: Effects of a cloned cell line with NK activity on bone marrow transplants, tumor development and metastasis *in vivo*. *Nature* 1982;300:31.
32. Harrison DE, Carlson GA: Effects of the beige mutation and irradiation on natural resistance to marrow grafts. *J Immunol* 1983;130:484.
33. Tolstad B, Benestad HB: The "natural resistance" to bone marrow allografts in normal and athymic nude rats. Rapid cytotoxic reactions both *in vivo* and *in vitro*. *Eur J Immunol* 1984;14:793.

34. Borland A, Mowat A, Parrott DMV: Augmentation of intestinal and peripheral natural killer cell activity during the graft-vs.-host reaction in mice. *Transplantation* 1983;36:513.
35. Ortaldo JR, Herberman R: Heterogeneity of natural killer cells. *Ann Rev Immunol* 1984;2:359.
36. Pattengale PK, Gidlund M, Milssow K, et al.: Lysis of fresh human B lymphocyte derived leukemia by interferon activated natural killer (NK) cells. *Int J Cancer* 1982;1:7.
37. Pattengale PK, Sundstrom C, Yu A, Levine A: Lysis of fresh leukemia blasts by interferon activated human natural killer cells. *National Conference on Immune Cells and Growth Regulators.* 1984;3:165.
38. Beran M, Hansson M, Kiessling R: Human natural killer (NK) cells can inhibit clonogenic growth of fresh leukemic cells. *Blood* 1983;61:596.
39. Lopez C, Kirkpatrick D, Livnat S, Storb R: Natural killer cells in bone marrow transplantation. *Lancet* 1980;3:1025.
40. Lum LG: The kinetics of immune reconstitution after human marrow transplantation. *Blood* 1987;69:369–380.
41. Kasahara T, Djeu JY, Dougherty SF, Oppenheim JJ: Interleukin mediated immune interferon (IFN-gamma) production by human T cells and T cell subsets. *J Immunol* 1983;130:1784.
42. Scala G, Allavena P, Djeu YU, et al.: Human large granular lymphocytes are potent producers of interleukin-1. *Nature* 1984;309:56.
43. Djeu YU, Stocks N, Zoon K, et al.: Positive self-regulation of cytotoxicity in human natural killer cells by production of interferon upon exposure to influenza and herpes viruses. *J Exp Med* 1982;156:1222.
44. Vyakarnam A, Brenner MK, Reittie JE, Lachmann PJ: Human cell clones with NK function activate B cells and secrete B cell differentiation factor. *Eur J Immunol* 1985;15:606.
45. Pistoia V, Cozzolino F, Tarcia M, et al.: Production of B cell growth factor by a Leu-OKM1 non-T cell with the features of large granular lymphocytes. *J Immunol* 1985;134:3179.
46. Brenner MK, Munro AJ: T cell help in human *in vitro* antibody producing systems; role of inhibitory T cells in masking allogeneic help. *Cell Immunol* 1981;57:280.
47. Arai S, Yamamoto H, Itah K, Kumagai K: Suppressive effect of human natural killer cells on pokeweed mitogen-induced B cell differentiation. *J Immunol* 1983;131:651.
48. deBruin HG, Astaldi A, Leupers T, et al.: T lymphocyte characteristics in bone marrow transplanted patients. II. Analysis with monoclonal antibodies. *J Immunol* 1981;127:244.
49. Atkinson K, Hansen JA, Storb R, et al.: T cell subpopulations identified by monoclonal antibodies after human marrow transplantation. I. Helper-inducer and cytotoxic-suppressor subsets. *Blood* 1982;59:1292.
50. Forman SJ, Nocker P, Gallagher M, et al.: Pattern of T cell reconstitution following allogeneic bone marrow transplantation for acute hematological malignancy. *Transplantation* 1982;34:96.
51. Schroff RW, Gale RP, Fahey JL: Regeneration of T cell subpopulations after bone marrow transplantation; cytomegalovirus infection and lymphoid subset imbalance. *J Immunol* 1982;129:1926.
52. Friedrich W, O'Reilly RJ, Koziner B, et al.: T-lymphocyte reconstitution in recipients of bone marrow transplants with and without graft-vs.-host disease; imbalances of T cell subpopulations having unique regulatory and cognitive functions. *Blood* 1982;59:696.
53. Gratama JW, Naipal A, Iljans P, et al.: T lymphocyte repopulation and differentiation after bone marrow transplantation. Early shifts in the ratio between T4+ and T8+ T lymphocytes correlate with the occurrence of acute graft-vs.-host disease. *Blood* 1984;63:1416.
54. Favrot M, Janossy G, Tidman N, et al.: T cell regeneration after allogeneic bone marrow transplantation. *Clin Exp Immunol* 1983;54:59.
55. Verdonck LF, de Gast GC: Is cytomegalovirus infection a major cause of T cell alterations after (autologous) bone marrow transplantation? *Lancet* 1984;1:932.
56. Zander AR, Reuben JM, Johnston D, et al.: Immune recovery following allogeneic bone marrow transplantation. *Transplantation* 1985;40(2):177–183.
57. Bacigalupo A, Mingari MC, Moretta L, et al.: T cell subpopulations after allogeneic bone marrow transplantation. In, Thierfelder S, Rodt H, Kolb HJ (eds): *Immunobiology of Bone Marrow Transplantation.* Berlin, Springer-Verlag, 1980, p. 135.
58. Saxon A, McIntyre RE, Stevens RH, Gale RP: Lymphocyte dysfunction in chronic graft-vs.-host disease. *Blood* 1981;58:746–751.
59. Persson U, Myrenfors P, Ringden O, et al.: T lymphocyte subpopulations in bone marrow

transplanted patients in relation to graft-vs.-host disease and cytomegalovirus-induced infection. *Transplantation* 1987;43(5):663–668.

60. Verdonck LF, de Gast GC: Is cytomegalovirus infection a major cause of T cell alterations after (autologous) bone-marrow transplantation? *Lancet* 1984;1:932.

61. Lonnquist B, Ringden O, Wahren B, et al.: Cytomegalovirus infection associated with and preceding chronic graft-vs.-host disease. *Transplantation* 1984;38:465.

62. Gebel HM, Kaizer H, Landay AL: Characterization of circulating suppressor T lymphocytes in bone marrow transplant recipients. *Transplantation* 1987;43(2):258–262.

63. Fu SM, Chiorazzi N, Wang CY, et al.: Ia bearing T lymphocytes in man; their identification and role in the generation of allogeneic helper activity. *J Exp Med* 1978;148:1423.

64. Fox R, McMillan R, Spruce E, et al.: Analysis of T lymphocytes after bone marrow transplantation using monoclonal antibodies. *Blood* 1982;60:578.

65. Hansen JA, Atkinson K, Martin PJ, et al.: Human T lymphocyte phenotypes after bone marrow transplantation T cells expressing Ia-like antigens. *Transplantation* 1983;36:277.

66. Uchiyama T, Nelson DL, Fleisher TA, Waldmann TA: A monoclonal antibody (anti-TAC) reactive with activated and functionally mature human T cells. II. Expression of TAC antigen on activated cytotoxic killer T cells, suppressor cells, and on one of two types of helper T cells. *J Immunol* 1981;126:1398.

67. Anderson MJ, Rappeport JM, Ault KA, et al.: Clinical correlates of unusual circulating lymphocytes appearing post-marrow transplantation (BMT). *Proc Am Soc Hematol* (Abstract). 1985;66:257a.

68. Uchiyama T, Broder S, Waldmann T: A monoclonal antibody (anti-TAC) reactive with activated and functionally mature human T cells. I. Production of anti-TAC monoclonal antibody and distribution of TAC(+) cells. *J Immunol* 1981;126:1393.

69. Chen Y-X, Evans RL, Pollack MS, et al.: Characterization and expression of the HLA-DC antigens defined by antileu 10. *Hum Immunol* 1984;10:221.

70. Witherspoon RP, Matthews D, Storb R, et al.: Recovery of *in vivo* cellular immunity after human marrow grafting. *Transplantation* 1984;37:145.

71. Witherspoon RP, Lum LG, Storb R: Immunologic reconstitution after human marrow grafting. *Semin Hematol* 1984;21:2.

72. Noel DR, Witherspoon RP, Weiden PL, Thomas ED: Does graft-vs.-host disease influence the tempo of immunologic recovery after allogeneic human marrow transplantation? An observation on 56 long-term survivors. *Blood* 1978;51:1087.

73. Gale RP, Opelz G, Mickey MR, et al.: For the UCLA Bone Marrow Transplant Team. Immunodeficiency following allogeneic bone marrow transplantation. *Transplant Proc* 1978;10:223.

74. Fass L, Ochs HD, Thomas Ed, et al.: Studies of immunological reactivity following syngeneic or allogeneic marrow grafts in man. *Transplantation* 1973;16:630.

75. Elfenbein GJ, Anderson PN, Humphrey RL, et al.: Immune system reconstitution following allogeneic bone marrow transplantation in man; a multiparameter analysis. *Transplant Proc* 1976;8:641.

76. Ringden O, Witherspoon R, Storb R, et al.: B cell function in human marrow transplant recipients assessed by direct and indirect hemolysis-in-gel assays. *J Immunol* 1979;123:2729.

77. Ringden O, Witherspoon RP, Storb R, et al.: Increased *in vitro* B cell IgG secretion during acute graft-vs.-host disease and infection; observations in 50 human marrow transplant recipients. *Blood* 1980;55:179.

78. Witherspoon RP, Lum LG, Storb R, Thomas ED: *In vitro* regulation of immunoglobulin synthesis after human marrow transplantation. II. Deficient T and non-T lymphocyte function within 3–4 months of allogeneic, syngeneic, or autologous marrow grafting for hematologic malignancy. *Blood* 1982;59:844.

79. Pahwa SG, Pahwa RN, Friedrich W, et al.: Abnormal humoral immune responses in peripheral blood lymphocyte cultures of bone marrow transplant recipients. *Proc Natl Acad Sci USA* 1982;79:2663.

80. Korsmeyer SJ, Elfenbein GJ, Goldman CK, et al.: B cell, helper T cell, and suppressor T cell abnormalities contribute to disordered immunoglobulin synthesis in patients following bone marrow transplantation. *Transplantation* 1982;33:184.

81. Witherspoon RP, Goehle S, Kretschmer M, Storb R: Regulation of immunoglobulin production after human marrow grafting; the role of helper and suppressor T cells in acute graft-vs.-host disease. *Transplantation* 1986;41:328.

82. Dosch H-M, Gelfand EW: Failure of T and B cell cooperation during graft-vs.-host disease. *Transplantation* 1981;31:48.
83. Okos AJ, Lum LG, Storb R: Epstein-Barr virus (EBV)-induced immunoglobulin (Ig) production and suppression by EBV immune T cells in bone marrow transplant recipients. (Abstract). *Proc Am Soc Hematol* 1983;62;227a.
84. Luckhurst E, Chapman G, Atkinson K, et al.: Abnormal T lymphocyte colony formation following human allogeneic bone marrow transplantation. *Transplant Proc* 1985;17(2):1717–1720.
85. Donnenberg AD, Elfenbein GJ, Santos GW: Cell-cell cooperation in lymphocyte colony formation; studies in human allogeneic marrow transplantation. *J Immunol* 1982;129:1080.
86. Mitsuyasu RT, Li S, Champlin RE, Gale RP: Abnormal T-lymphocyte colonies (CFU-TL) following bone marrow transplantation. *Exp Hematol* 1986;14:1049–1055.
87. Rozenszayn LA, Goldman I, Kalechman I, et al.: T lymphocyte colony growth *in vitro;* factors modulating clonal expansion. *Immunol Rev* 1981;54:157.
88. Gelfand EW, Lee JWW, Dosch H, Price GB: Human T cell colony formation in microculture; analysis of growth requirements and functional activities. *J Immunol* 1981;126:1134.
89. Rey A, Klein B, Illnicki C, et al.: The role of interleukin-2 in T-colony formation by human pre-T cells (pTCFC). *Clin Exp Immunol* 1987;58:154.
90. Mitsuyasu RT, Champlin RE, Ho WG, et al.: Prospective randomized controlled trial of *ex vivo* treatment of donor bone marrow with monoclonal anti-T cell antibody and complement for the prevention of graft-vs.-host disease; a preliminary report. *Transplant Proc* 1985;17:482.
91. Filipovich AH, Vallera DA, Youle RJ, et al.: Graft-vs.-host disease prevention in allogeneic bone marrow transplantation from histocompatible siblings. A pilot study using immunotoxins for T cell depletion of donor bone marrow. *Transplantation* 1987;44(1):62–69.
92. Daley JP, Rozans MK, Smith BR, et al.: Retarded recovery of functional T cell frequencies in T cell-depleted bone marrow transplant recipients. *Blood* 1987;70(4):960–964.
93. Antin JH, Ault KA, Rappeport JM, Smith BR: B cell reconstitution after marrow transplant (BMT). (Abstract). *Proc Am Soc Hematol* 1985;66:257a.
94. Walker SA, Rogers TR, Perry D, et al.: Increased serum IgE concentrations during infection and graft-vs.-host disease after bone marrow transplantation. *J Clin Pathol* 1984;37:460.
95. Ringden O, Persson U, Johansson SGO, et al.: Markedly elevated serum IgE levels following allogeneic and syngeneic bone marrow transplantation. *Blood* 1983;61:1190.
96. Saryan JA, Rappeport J, Leung DY, et al.: Regulation of human immunoglobulin E synthesis in acute graft-vs.-host disease. *J Clin Invest* 1983;71:556.
97. Witherspoon RP, Storb R, Ochs HD, et al.: Recovery of antibody production in human allogeneic marrow graft recipients; influence of time post-transplantation, the presence or absence of chronic graft-vs.-host disease, and antithymocyte globulin treatment. *Blood* 1981;58:360.
98. Witherspoon RP, Kopecky K, Storb R, et al.: Immunological recovery in 48 patients following syngeneic marrow transplantation for hematological malignancy. *Transplantation* 1982;33:143.
99. Lum LG, Shiobara S, Culbertson NJ, Storb R: T and B cell collaboration for tetanus toxoid induction of *in vitro* IgG antitetanus toxoid synthesis after human marrow grafting. (Abstract). *Exp Hematol* 1984;12:390
100. Donnenberg AD, Hess AD, Saral R, Santos GW: Adoptive transfer of immunity after allogeneic bone marrow transplantation in man; role of immunization immediately after marrow infusion. (Abstract). *Exp Hematol* 1984;12:390.
101. Lum LG, Munn NA, Schanfield MS, Storb R: The detection of specific antibody formation to recall antigens after human bone marrow transplantation. *Blood* 1986;67:582.
102. Cockerill KJ, Zander AR: Red cell aplasia due to host-type isohemagglutinins with exuberant red cell pregenitor production of donor-type in an ABO mismatched allogeneic bone marrow transplant recipient. *Blood* (Abstract). (Suppl 1), 1987;70(5):304a.
103. Lum LG, Noges JN, Culbertson NJ, et al.: Transfer of specific immunity in recipients who received T cell depleted marrows. (Abstract #212). *Exp Hematol* 1986;14:447.
104. Wimperis JZ, Brenner MK, Prentice HG, et al.: Transfer of a functioning humoral immune system in transplantation of T lymphocyte-depleted bone marrow. *Lancet* 1986;1:339.
105. Aucouturier P, Barra A, Intrator L, et al.: Long lasting IgG subclass and antibacterial

polysaccharide antibody deficiency after allogeneic bone marrow transplantation. *Blood* 1987;70(3):779–785.

106. Lum LG, Seigneuret MC, Orcutt-Thordarson N, et al.: Immunoglobulin production after marrow transplantation. III. The functional heterogeneity of FC-IgG receptor positive and negative T cell subpopulations. *Clin Exp Immunol* 1982;48:675–684.

107. Lum LG, Seigneuret MC, Orcutt-Thordarson N, et al.: The regulation of immunoglobulin synthesis after HLA-identical bone marrow transplantation. VI. Differential rates of maturation of distinct functional groups within lymphoid subpopulations in patients after human marrow grafting. *Blood* 1985;65(6):1422–1433.

108. Shiobara S, Lum LG, Witherspoon RP, Storb R: Antigen-specific antibody response of lymphocytes to tetanus toxoid after human marrow transplantation. *Transplantation* 1986;41(5):587–592.

109. Lum LG, Seigneuret MC, Storb R: The transfer of antigen-specific humoral immunity from marrow donors to marrow recipients. *J Clin Immunol* 1986;6(5):389–396.

110. Jin N-R, Lum LG: IgG antitetanus toxoid antibody production induced by Epstein-Barr virus from B cells of human marrow transplant recipients. *Cellular Immunol* 1986;101:266–273.

111. Meyers JD, Flournoy N, Thomas ED: Cytomegalovirus infection and specific cell-mediated immunity after marrow transplant. *J Infect Dis* 1980;142:816.

112. Lonnqvist B. Ringden O, Wahren B, et al.: CMV infection associated with and precedes chronic graft-vs.-host disease. *Transplantation* 1984;38:465.

113. Neiman PE, Reeves W, Ray G, et al.: A prospective analysis of interstitial pneumonia and opportunistic viral infection among recipients of allogeneic bone marrow grafts. *J Infect Dis* 1977;136:754.

114. Vilmer E, Mazeron MC, Rabian C, et al.: Clinical significance of cytomegalovirus viremia in bone marrow transplantation. *Transplantation* 1985;40(1):30–35.

115. Carney WP, Rubin RH, Hoffman RA, et al.: Analysis of lymphocyte subsets in cytomegalovirus mononucleosis. *J Immunol* 1981;126:2114.

116. Paulin T, Ringden O, Lonnqvist B: Faster immunological recovery after bone marrow transplantation in patients without cytomegalovirus infection. *Transplantation* 1985;39(4):377–384.

117. Gratama JW, Middeldorp JM, van der Meer JWM, et al.: Immune reactivity in relation to cytomegalovirus infection after allogeneic bone marrow transplantation. *Transplant Proc* 1985;17(1):488–492.

118. Wursch AM, Gratama JW, Middeldorp JM, et al.: The effect of cytomegalovirus infection on T lymphocytes after allogeneic bone marrow transplantation. *Clin Exp Immunol* 1985;62:278–287.

119. Persson U, Myrenfors P, Ringden O, et al.: T lymphocyte subpopulations in bone marrow transplanted patients in relation to graft-vs.-host disease and cytomegalovirus-induced infection. *Transplantation* 1987;43(5):663–668.

120. Quinnan GV Jr, Kirmani N, Esber E, et al.: HLA-restricted cytotoxic T lymphocyte and nonthymic cytotoxic lymphocyte responses to cytomegalovirus infection of bone marrow transplant recipients. *J Immunol* 1981;126(5):2036–2041.

121. Quinnan GV, Kirmani N, Rook AH, et al.: Cytotoxic T cells in cytomegalovirus infection. *N Engl J Med* 1982;107:7.

122. Ljungman P, Lonnqvist B, Gahrton G, et al.: Cytomegalovirus-specific lymphocyte proliferation and *in vitro* cytomegalovirus IgG synthesis for diagnosis of cytomegalovirus infections after bone marrow transplantation. *Blood* 1986;68(1):108–112.

123. Meyers JD, Flournoy N, Wade JC, et al.: Biology of interstitial pneumonia after marrow transplantation. In, Gale RP (ed): *Recent Advances in Bone Marrow Transplantation.* Alan R. Liss, Inc., New York, 1983, pp. 405–423.

124. Miller W, Flynn P, McCullough J, et al.: Cytomegalovirus infection after bone marrow transplantation; an association with acute graft-vs.-host disease. *Blood 1986;67(4):1162–1167.*

125. Jacobsen N, Andersen HK, Skinhoj P, et al.: Correlation between donor cytomegalovirus immunity and chronic graft-vs.-host disease after allogeneic bone marrow transplantation. *Scand J Hæmatol* 1986;36:449–506.

126. Lonnqvist B, Ringden O, Wahren B, et al.: Cytomegalovirus infection associated with and preceding chronic graft-vs.-host disease. *Transplantation* 1984;38(5):465–468.

127. Gratama JW, de Groot-Swings G, Slats J, et al.: Correlation between the fraction size of the peripheral-blood T8+ T lymphocyte subset of marrow donors and the development of acute graft-vs.-host disease. *Exp Hematol* 1984;12(Suppl 12):51–52.

128. Gratama JW, Fibbe WE, Naipal AMIH, et al.: Cytomegalovirus immunity and T lymphocytes in bone marrow donors and acute graft-vs.-host disease. *Bone Marrow Transplantation* 1986;1:141–146.

129. Bowden RA, Sayers M, Flournoy N, et al.: Cytomegalovirus immune globulin and seronegative blood products to prevent primary cytomegalovirus infection after transplantation. *N Engl J Med* 1986;314:1006–1010.

130. Ringden O, Pihlstedt P, Volin L, et al.: Failure to prevent cytomegalovirus infection by cytomegalovirus hyperimmune plasma; a randomized trial by the Nordic Bone Marrow Transplantation Group. *Bone Marrow Transplantation*. 1987;2:299–305.

131. Condie RM, O'Reilly RJ: Prophylaxis of CMV infection in bone marrow transplant recipients by hyperimmune CMV gamma globulin. In, *Developments in Biological Standardization*. Vol. 52. S Karger, Basel, 1982, pp. 501–513.

132. Winston DJ, Pollard RB, Ho WG, et al.: Cytomegalovirus immune plasma in bone marrow transplant recipients. *Ann Intern Med* 1982;97:11–18.

133. Meyers JD, Leszczynski J, Zaia JA, et al.: Prevention of cytomegalovirus infection by cytomegalovirus immune globulin after marrow transplantation. *Ann Intern Med* 1983;98:442–446.

134. Condie RM, O'Reilly RJ: Prevention of cytomegalovirus infection by prophylaxis with an intravenous, hyperimmune, native, unmodified cytomegalovirus globulin. *Am J Med* 1984;76(3A):134–141.

135. Winston DJ, Ho WG, Lin C-H, et al.: Intravenous immunoglobulin for modification of cytomegalovirus infections associated with bone marrow transplantation: preliminary results of a controlled trial. *Am J Med* 1984;76(3A):128–133.

136. Kubanek B, Ernst P, Ostedorf P, et al.: Preliminary data of a controlled trial of intravenous hyperimmune globulin in the prevention of cytomegalovirus infection in bone marrow transplant recipients. *Transplant Proc* 1985;17:468–469.

137. Winston DJ, Ho WG, Lin C-H, et al.: Intravenous immune globulin for prevention of cytomegalovirus infection and interstitial pneumonia after bone marrow transplantation. *Ann Int Med* 1987;106:12–18.

138. Ringden O, Paulin T, Pihlstedt P, et al.: Cytomegalovirus antibody screening of blood donors from immunocompromised seronegative patients. *Lancet* 1984;2:1044.

139. Branch DR, Gallagher MT, Forman SJ, et al.: Endogenous stem cell repopulation resulting in mixed hematopoietic chimerism following total body irradiation and marrow transplantation for acute leukemia. *Transplantation* 1982;34(4):226–228.

140. Knowlton RG, Brown VA, Braman JC, et al.: Use of highly polymorphic DNA probed for genotypic analysis following bone marrow transplantation. *Blood* 1986;68(2):378–385.

141. Ginsburg D, Antin JH, Smith BR, et al.: Origin of cell populations after bone marrow transplantation. Analysis using DNA sequence polymorphisms. *J Clin Invest* 1985;75:569–603.

142. Petz LD, Yam PY, Wallace RB, et al.: Mixed hematopoietic chimerism following bone marrow transplantation for hematologic malignancies. *Blood* 1987;70(5):1331–1337.

143. Yam PY, Petz LD, Knowlton RG, et al.: Use of DNA restriction fragment length polymorphisms to document marrow engraftment and mixed hematopoietic chimerism following bone marrow transplantation. *Transplantation* 1987;43(3):399–407.

144. Samlowski WE, Johnson HM, Hammond EH, et al.: Marrow ablative doses of gamma-irradiation and protracted changes in peripheral lymph node microvasculature of murine and human bone marrow transplant recipients. *Lab Invest* 1987;56(1):85–95.

145. Samlowski WE, Crump CL: Recovery of contact hypersensitivity response following murine bone marrow transplantation; comparison of gamma-irradiation and busulfan as preparative marrow-ablative agents. *Blood* 1987;70(6):1910–1920.

146. Tutschka PJ, Copelan EA, Klein JP: Bone marrow transplantation for leukemia following a new busulfan and cyclophosphamide regimen. *Blood* 1987;70(5):1382–1388.

146(a). Jagannath S, Dicke KA, Armitage JO, et al.: High-dose cyclophosphamide, carmustine, and etoposide and autologous bone marrow transplantation for relapsed Hodgkin's disease. *Ann Int Med* 1986;104:163–168.

147. Tutschka PJ: Personal communication to the author, 1987.

148. Armitage J: Personal communication to the author, 1987.
149. Singer CRJ, Tansey PJ, Burnett AK: T lymphocyte reconstitution following autologous bone marrow transplantation. *Clin Exp Immunol* 1983;51:455–460.
150. Linch DC, Knott LJ, Thomas RM, et al.: T cell regeneration after allogeneic and autologous bone marrow transplantation. *Br J Haematol* 1983;53:451–458.
151. Bosly AE, Staquet PJ, Doyen CM, et al.: Recombinant human interleukin-2 restores *in vitro* T cell colony formation by peripheral blood mononuclear cells after autologous bone marrow transplantation. *Exp Hematol* 1987;15:1048–1054.
152. Ueda M, Harada M, Shiobara S, et al.: T lymphocyte reconstitution in long-term survivors after allogeneic and autologous marrow transplantation. *Transplantation* 1984;37(6):552–556.
153. de Gast GC, Verdonck LF, Middeldorp JM, et al.: Recovery of T cell subsets after autologous bone marrow transplantation is mainly due to proliferation of mature T cells in the graft. *Blood* 1985;66(2):428–431.
154. Zander AR, Cockerill KJ: Autologous transplantation with circulating hemopoietic stem cells. *J Clin Apheresis* 1987;3:191–201.
155. Kessinger A, Armitage JO, Landmark JD, et al.: Is there a correlation between the number of autologous peripheral mononuclear cells and peripheral stem cells infused and rate of marrow recovery? *Exp Hematol 1986;14:541.*
156. Körbling M, Martin H, Ho AD, et al.: Autologous blood stem cell transplantation (ABSCT): a new therapeutic concept. (Abstract #92). *Exp Hematol* 1987;15(5):471.
157. Juttner CA, To LB, Kimber RJ: Autografting using peripheral blood stem cells (PBSC) collected during very early remission of acute non-lymphoblastic leukæmia (ANLL). (Abstract #250). *Exp Hematol* 1987;15(5):540.
158. Marit G, Bernard P, David B, et al.: Autologous blood stem cells transplantation in leukemic patients; a report of 11 cases. (Abstract #369). *Exp Hematol* 1987;15(5):592.
159. Goodman JW, Hodgson GS: Evidence for stem cells in the peripheral blood of mice. *Blood* 1962;19:702.
160. Cavins JA, Kasakura S, Thomas ED, Ferrebee JW: The recovery of lethally irradiated dogs given infusions of autologous leukocytes preserved at −80 degrees C. *Blood* 1964;23:38–42.
161. Körbling M, Dorken B, Ho AD, et al.: Autologous transplantation of blood-derived hemopoietic stem cells after myelo-ablative therapy in a patient with Burkitt's lymphoma. *Blood* 1986;67(2):529–532.
162. To LB, Juttner CA, Stomski F, et al.: Immune reconstitution following peripheral blood stem cell autografting. *Bone Marrow Transplantation* 1987;2(1):111.
163. Witherspoon RP, Hersman J, Storb R, et al.: Thymosin fraction 5 does not accelerate reconstitution of immunologic reactivity after human grafting. *Br J Hæmatol* 1983;55:595.
164. Atkinson K, Storb R, Ochs HD, et al.: Thymus transplantation after allogeneic bone marrow graft to prevent chronic graft-vs.-host disease in humans. *Transplantation* 1982;33(2):168–173.
165. Goldstein AL, Low TLK, Thurman GB, et al.: Current status of thymosin and other hormones of the thymus gland. *Recent Prog Horm Res* 1981;37:369.
166. Metcalf D, Begley CG, Williamson J, et al.: Hemopoietic effect in mice of recombinant CSFs. (Abstract #2). *Exp Hematol* 1987;15(5):429.
167. Kulkarni SS, Pizzini RP, Dicke KA: Augmentation of mitogen response and natural killer cell activity by *in vivo* administration of murine interleukin-3 in mice. (Abstract #297). *Exp Hematol* 1987;15(5):562.
168. Slavin S, Ekerstein A, Weiss L, et al.: New therapeutic strategies for autologous and allogeneic bone marrow transplantation. (Abstract #374). *Exp Hematol* 1987;15(5):595.
169. Yatsiv I, Weiss L, Ekerstein A, Slavin S: Potential role of *in vivo* recombinant Il-2 in allogeneic bone marrow transplantation. (Abstract #375). *Exp Hematol* 1987;15(5):595.
170. Franceschini F, Gale RP: Immune reconstitution following bone marrow transplantation in man. In, Gale RP, Champlin R (eds): *Progress in Bone Marrow Transplantation*. Alan R. Liss, Inc., New York, 1987, pp. 607–622.
171. Kodo H, Gale RP, Saxon A: Antibody synthesis by booster tetanus toxoid immunization in humans. *J Clin Invest* 1984;73:1377.
172. Witherspoon RP, Matthews D, Storb R, et al.: Recovery of *in vivo* cellular immunity after human marrow grafting. *Transplantation* 1984;37:145.

Bone Marrow Transplantation in Children, edited by F. Leonard Johnson and Carl Pochedly. Raven Press, Ltd., New York © 1990.

Hematopoietic Reconstitution Following Bone Marrow Transplantation*

David D. F. Ma

Department of Hematology, Royal North Shore Hospital, St. Leonards, New South Wales, Australia 2065

Introduction
A. Normal hematopoiesis
   1. *In vitro* assessment of hematopoietic progenitor cells
   2. The hematopoietic microenvironment
   3. Hematopoietic growth regulators
B. Hematopoietic reconstitution after bone marrow transplantation
   1. Kinetics of peripheral blood regeneration
   2. Hematopoietic stem cell reconstitution
   3. Significance of progenitor cell assays in clinical marrow transplantation
   4. Hematopoietic stroma following marrow transplantation
   5. Factors affecting hematopoietic reconstitution
   6. Hematopoietic chimerism
C. Conclusions and future prospects
Summary

INTRODUCTION

Intensive ablative chemotherapy and radiotherapy given prior to bone marrow infusion destroys the existing lymphohematopoietic tissues. During the

*This work was supported by grants from the Australian National Health and Medical Research Council, New South Wales State Cancer Council, and Leo and Jenny Leukemia Foundation.

period of aplasia, before marrow reconstitution occurs, bone marrow transplant patients require support with blood products and they are extremely vulnerable to serious infections and hemorrhage.

This chapter focuses on the nonlymphoid component of hematopoietic events that occur after bone marrow grafting, the application of *in vitro* cell cultures in understanding the kinetics of hematopoietic reconstitution, and the factors that influence the development of mature functioning blood cells following the infusion of donor bone marrow. Bone marrow transplantation provides a unique opportunity to study the control of hematopoiesis in man. Increased understanding of the processes that affect hematopoietic reconstitution will improve the outcome of human bone marrow transplantation.

NORMAL HEMATOPOIESIS

Hematopoiesis is a process by which circulating and functioning blood cells are produced (Figure 1). The hematopoietic system has been arbitrarily divided into two major components, the myeloid system and the lymphoid system. The myeloid system includes all blood cells except lymphocytes. The lymphoid system includes bone marrow derived (B) lymphocytes and thymic derived (T) lymphocytes. Rapid progress has occurred in our understanding of the functions of both the myeloid and lymphoid systems, but this discussion will concentrate on the development of the myeloid system.

In the embryo, hematopoiesis begins in the yolk sac and subsequently switches to the liver, spleen, thymus, bone marrow and other lymphoid tissues. During infancy, active hematopoiesis (myelopoiesis) occurs in the marrow of nearly all bones of the body, but in adults, hematopoiesis is seen largely in the ends of long bones and the axial skeleton. Lymphopoiesis also occurs in the thymus and other lymphoid tissues. In humans, soon after birth, all circulating erythrocytes, neutrophils and platelets are produced in the bone marrow. Each day the bone marrow of a normal adult produces over one hundred thousand million (100,000,000,000 or 1×10^{11}) neutrophils and twice that number of erythrocytes.

The production of large numbers of functioning endstage cells in the circulation is achieved by proliferation and differentiation of a small population of stem cells which possess the capacity for self-regeneration. These pluripotent stem cells produce committed progenitor cells which proliferate to form morphologically recognizable immature hematopoietic cells in the bone marrow. These, in turn, form the mature circulating blood cells. Hematopoiesis is a dynamic process which can respond rapidly to certain stimuli, such as hemorrhage and infection. This process is controlled by a precise and complex regulatory system. Hematopoiesis is influenced by humoral factors as well as by cellular and extracellular elements within the hematopoietic tissues (1,2).

Most bone marrow cells represent morphologically recognizable stages in the

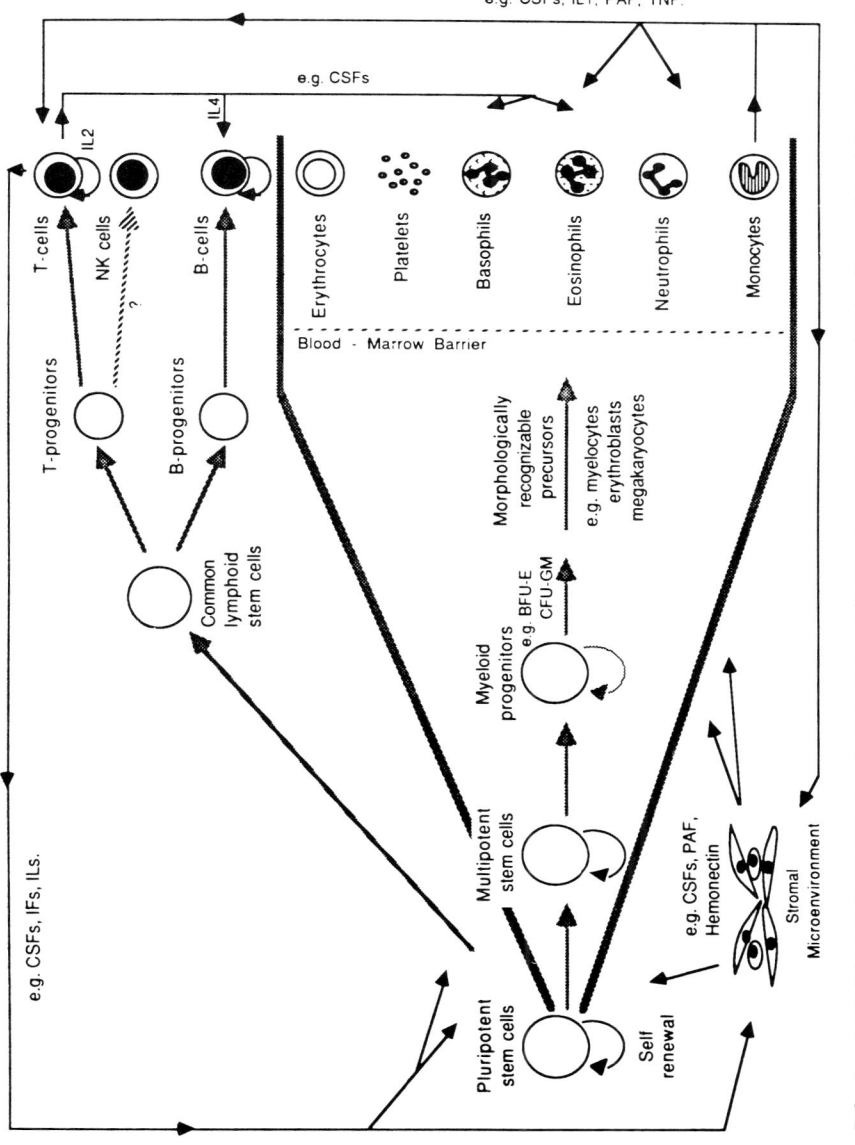

FIG. 1. A simplified model of hematopoiesis in adults, including some of its regulators. CSF = Colony Stimulating Factors, IFs = Interferons, ILs = Interleukins, PAF = Platelet Activating Factor, TNFs = Tumor Necrotizing Factors, ⟶ = stimulation or inhibition.

maturation of pluripotent stem cells. Although stem cells and early committed progenitors cannot be identified by morphology, they can be detected by an *in vivo* method, by *in vitro* cultures, and more recently by detection of cell surface antigens (3). Hematopoietic stem cells can form colonies on the surface of the spleen (CFU-S) in lethally irradiated mice which have been injected with normal mouse bone marrow cells (4). Splenic colonies are heterogeneous and not all CFU-S colonies contain cells of all hematopoietic lineages. Some of these colonies are derived from committed progenitors, and others are derived from the pluripotent stem cells. The pluripotent CFU-S colonies appear relatively late and are resistant to suppression by 5-fluorouracil (5). There is convincing evidence that lymphoid and myeloid cells originate from a common base of hematopoietic stem cells (1,2).

It has not been possible to demonstrate stem cells by the spleen colony forming assay in other animals and in humans, but splenic colonies containing hematopoietic cells have been found in patients who died within the first year following bone marrow transplantation (6). Evidence for existence of pluripotent stem cells has been obtained indirectly by karyotypic and isoenzymatic analysis of cells in chronic myeloid leukemia (CML). The philadelphia (Ph[1]) chromosome is present in erythroid, granulocytic and megakaryocytic cells in these patients (7). Furthermore, both lymphoid and myeloid blastic transformation can occur in chronic myeloid leukemia. Studies in patients with CML, who are also glucose-6-phosphate dehydrogenase (G-6-PD) heterozygotes, indicate that lymphoid and myeloid cells share a common stem cell (8).

In Vitro Assessment of Hematopoietic Progenitor Cells

The committed progenitor cells can be detected in semisolid cultures, and are called the colony forming cells (CFC) or unit (CFU) (Figure 2). In this *in vitro* system, the marrow derived cells are immobilized in a semisolid medium, such as agar, methylcellulose or a plasma clot. Colony growth depends on the addition of a hematopoietic growth supplement containing colony stimulating factors (CSF). The colonies of the granulocyte-macrophage series are named, depending on the type(s) of cells present in the colonies, CFU-GM (granulocyte-macrophages), CFU-G (granulocytes), or CFU-M (macrophages). Myeloid colonies were first identified in mice in the late 1960s (9,10) and in man in 1970 (11). Colonies of human eosinophils, erythroid cells, megakaryocytes, basophils and lymphocytes can all be grown in culture. Recently, human multipotent progenitor cells can be detected *in vitro*. These multipotent cells are called CFU-GEMM (granulocyte-erythrocyte-macrophage-megakaryocyte) or simply CFU-Mix (12). These cells have some capacity for self-renewal and have the ability to produce cells of myeloid, erythroid, megakaryocytic, and even lymphoid lineages, at least of the T cell type (13).

In 1982, Ogawa and colleagues (14) described an assay which supports the

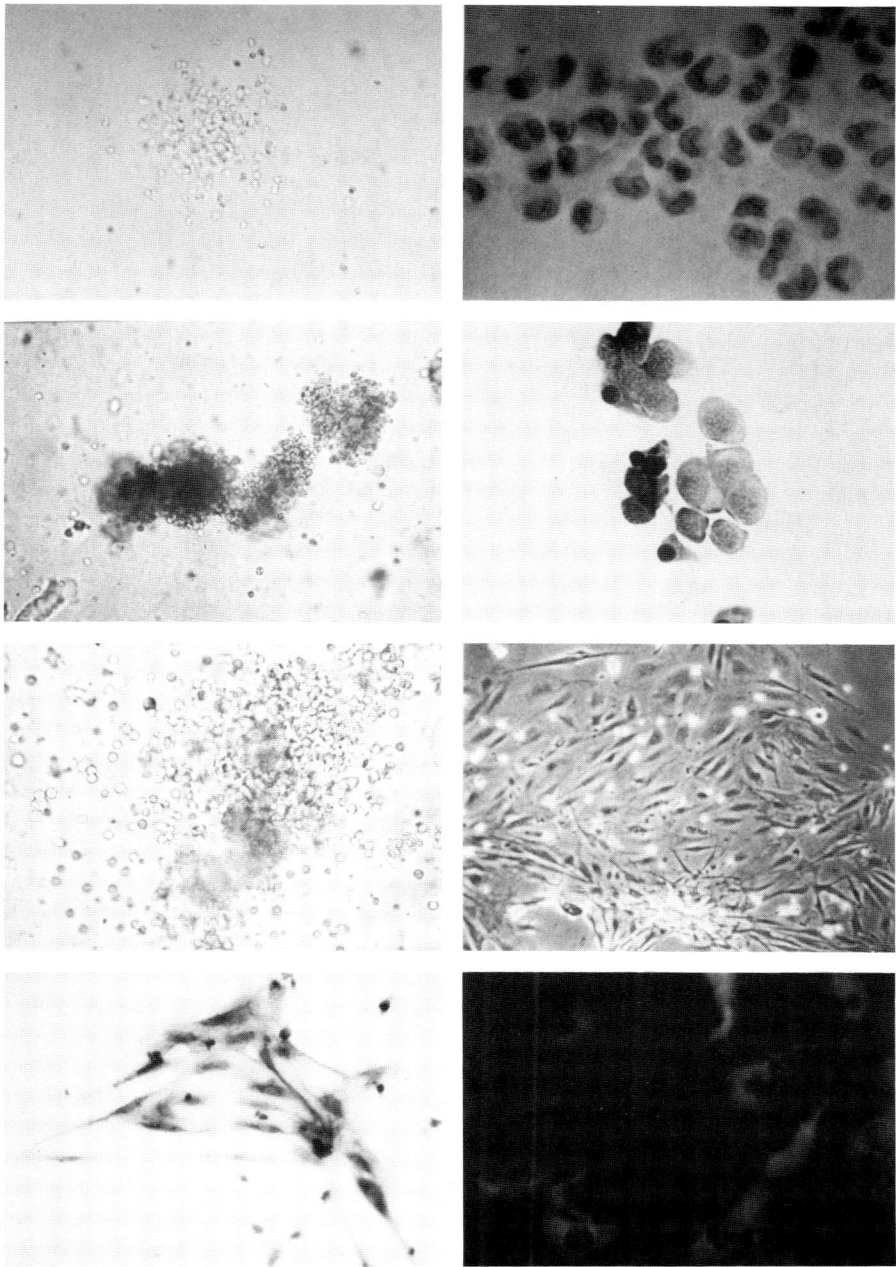

FIG. 2. Microphotographs of some hematopoietic colonies grown *in vitro* from human bone marrow cells. Top left, a CFU-G colony; top right, cells from such a colony. Second row, a BFU-E colony; and nucleated red cells from such a colony. Third row, a CFU-Mixed colony; and a bone marrow endothelial cell colony containing cells of cobblestoned appearance, typical of endothelial cells. Immunoperoxidase Factor VIII antigen (bottom right); and immunofluorescent Ulex lectin stainings of a small endothelial cell colony (bottom left).

growth of blast cell colonies from human umbilical cord blood. These colonies can self-replicate *in vitro*. Similar types of colonies have been reported in human bone marrow (15). These colony forming cells may represent a progenitor even more primitive than the CFU-GEMM, and possibly more primitive than the pluripotent hematopoietic stem cells.

The Hematopoietic Microenvironment

As mentioned, hematopoiesis is normally restricted to specific sites in the body, although stem cells and their progenitors circulate in the blood. The microenvironment of the bone marrow must differ from that in other tissues. The role of tissue stroma in creating the hematopoietic microenvironment is most obvious for the lymphoid tissues, particularly the thymus. There is ample evidence that T cell differentiation is regulated by the stromal cells within the thymus.

The growth regulating influence of stromal cells is less obvious for the bone marrow. The bone marrow stroma contains both cellular and noncellular elements. The stromal cells include fibroblasts, macrophages, fat cells, vascular endothelial cells, lymphocytes and neural cells. Collagen, glycosaminoglycans, and fibrin are some of the noncellular elements found in the stromal matrix (16,17). *In vivo* evidence for the regulatory role of marrow stroma has come from experimental work on CFU-S colony formation (spleen colony forming assay) in irradiated mice and in marrow transplantation in mice with hypoplastic anemia. These studies are discussed below.

Recently, an *in vitro* culture for adherent stromal cells has been developed (18,19). Bone marrow adherent cells are grown in liquid medium containing hydrocortisone and fetal calf and horse sera over a period of weeks. The culture contains fibroblastoid cells, macrophages, fat cells, some lymphocytes and endothelial-like cells. Clonogenic assays, such as the CFU-F (fibroblasts) and endothelial cell colonies (20,138), are possible for some of these cells. Extracellular matrix is also formed in the culture. This long-term culture (LTC) of bone marrow stroma can support the proliferation and differentiation of hematopoietic progenitors, including CFU-GEMM, for an extended period. Thus, long-term bone marrow culture provides an *in vitro* system to study the role of bone marrow stroma in bone marrow transplantation.

Hematopoietic Growth Regulators

A number of soluble factors including prostaglandins, lactoferrin and transferrin have been shown to affect hematopoiesis *in vitro* (2). However, major efforts in hematopoiesis research have been concentrated on the isolation of a family of glycoproteins, known as colony stimulating factors (CSF) or hematopoietic growth factors (21). These factors are specific for hematopoietic cells.

Most of them are produced by a wide variety of tissues and cells, including vascular endothelium and lectin stimulated T lymphocytes.

These growth factors include colony stimulating factors for granulocyte and macrophage lineages (designated GM-CSF, M-CSF, and G-CSF), erythropoietin, and interleukin-3 (IL-3) or multi-CSF, as well as growth factors that affect lymphoid differentiation, such as IL-2 and IL-4. Most of these factors are shown to play a role at different stages of hematopoietic stem cell development. For example, GM-CSF is required for the survival of the myeloid progenitor cell since it induces the progenitor cell to proliferate and differentiate. GM-CSF is also essential for the function of mature neutrophils (22). A number of these hematopoietic growth factors have been genetically isolated and are available in pure recombinant forms. These purified hematopoietic growth factors may be effective as therapeutic agents to promote hematopoietic reconstitution in patients following bone marrow transplantation.

HEMATOPOIETIC RECONSTITUTION AFTER BONE MARROW TRANSPLANTATION*

The regeneration of hematopoiesis after bone marrow transplant is influenced by clinical factors which, unlike studies done in experimental animals, are often beyond the control of clinical and laboratory investigators. The patient population is heterogeneous in age, sex, race, physical condition, and disease status. Patients with aplastic anemia are usually given immunosuppressive therapy prior to receiving the marrow transplant, but patients with leukemia or malignant solid tumors require intensive chemotherapy with or without irradiation to totally ablate the cancer cells. These latter patients have already received significant anticancer therapy. This prior therapy with drugs, irradiation, or both, might have caused substantial damage to the bone marrow stem cells, to the stromal cells, and to other organs. On the other hand, most patients with severe combined immunodeficiencies can be successfully given bone marrow transplants without significant preceding cytoreductive therapy.

The cellular composition of the bone marrow infusion depends on the type of marrow transplanted. In allogeneic marrow transplantation, the harvested bone marrow may be treated to remove T cells to prevent graft-vs.-host (GVH) disease (23), or to deplete the content of red blood cells in preparation for ABO incompatible marrow transplants (24). In autologous marrow transplants, the bone marrow may be treated to remove residual tumor cells, or the infused bone marrow may have been cryopreserved (25,26). In the postgrafting period, events such as infection, transfusion, drug therapy, leuke-

---

*For this chapter, allogeneic bone marrow transplant implies HLA compatible sibling bone marrow transplant, unless stated otherwise.

mic relapse and GVH disease also contribute to the rate of recovery of the hematopoietic system. In spite of the large number of possible clinical and procedural problems, successful engraftment occurs in most patients unless they succumb to the transplant-related complications.

After preconditioning and bone marrow infusion, there is a period of pancytopenia. Evidence of bone marrow regeneration is usually present at 10 to 14 days postinfusion. At that time the marrow is hypocellular and contains aggregates of immature but morphologically distinguishable myeloid and erythroid precursors. This growth of precursor cells coincides with a gradual rise of the peripheral blood counts. Initially, the leukocytes in the peripheral blood are mainly mononuclear cells and atypical lymphocytes, and later granulocytes appear. This pattern of reappearance of leukocytes is similar for both allografts and autografts.

Careful examination of the blood usually reveals circulating erythroblasts and myelocytes during the first 2 weeks following transplant. The numbers of these cells reach a peak between 3 and 6 weeks (27). Bone marrow cellularity increases gradually unless marrow rejection occurs. Most patients develop a normocellular bone marrow 9 to 12 months postgrafting. Autopsies on some patients who died following transplantation of bone marrow show the presence of extramedullary hematopoiesis in the liver during the first 3 weeks and in the spleen up to 1 year post-transplant (6,28). Medullary hematopoiesis is also noted in the femoral shafts. These findings indicate that tissues which provide a suitable hematopoietic microenvironment during fetal development can be reutilized after marrow transplantation.

Kinetics of Peripheral Blood Regeneration (Figure 3)

A rise in the reticulocyte count is detected at about 2 weeks after grafting (29). In our studies (30), the percentage of reticulocytes, corrected for anemia, rises above 0.5% by 4 weeks. Maximal reticulocytosis occurs about 4 to 6 weeks post-transplant and is usually accompanied by a significant increase in the platelet count. Red cell regeneration is also characterized by the appearance of certain features of fetal erythrocytes, namely, macrocytosis, increased fetal hemoglobin and surface "i" antigen (31,32). Studies by Macklis et al. (33), suggest that these findings result from differentiation of erythroid progenitors in which fetal genes are reactivated.

In uncomplicated allogeneic bone marrow transplantation, the neutrophils rise above 500/mm^3 within 2 to 3 weeks and above 1000/mm^3 in 3 to 4 weeks (29,30). The neutrophil count in most patients increases rapidly, but it does not reach normal levels until 3–6 months postgrafting. The recovery of neutrophils is more variable following transplantation of autologous bone marrow, and this recovery is often delayed in patients with leukemia (34–36). Studies of neutrophil function have shown that neutrophil chemotaxis is impaired as

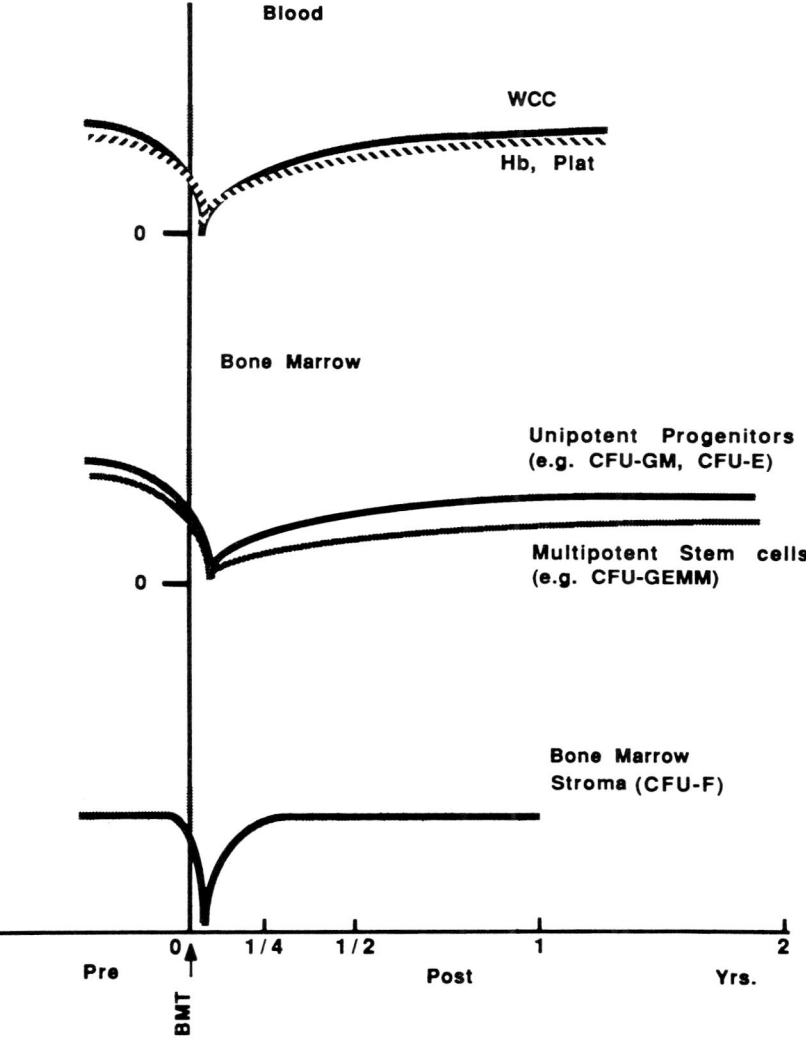

FIG. 3. Time course of the peripheral blood and bone marrow changes after bone marrow transplantation. Shaded areas represent normal ranges. Note functional defects may exist in some cell lineages despite normalization of their numbers.

long as 4 months after allogeneic marrow transplants (37–39), but phagocytic oxidation remains normal (37,40). The increase in bacterial and fungal infections during the early post-transplant period may be due to impaired neutrophil function. In contrast, monocyte function appears to recover more rapidly. Production of interleukin-1 and the cytotoxic and antigen presenting functions of monocytes are normal by 6 to 8 weeks postgrafting (41–43).

Increase of lymphocytes may precede the increase of the neutrophils and monocytes by several days. Some of these early appearing lymphocytes are of monocytoid appearance. They are CD3+, CD8+ and some also express HLA-DR antigens (34). Although the number of lymphocytes in the peripheral blood attains normal values by 3 to 4 months, the CD4/CD8 (helper-suppressor) ratio is reversed. CD8+ (T8) lymphocytes are the first to recover to higher than normal levels; CD4+ (T4) lymphocytes recover more slowly. This CD4/CD8 ratio returns to normal by 1 year except in patients with chronic graft-vs.-host disease. Increased numbers of CD38+ (OKT10+) T cells may also be found during the first year postgrafting. Levels of serum IgG and IgM return to normal after 3 to 4 months, but IgA may remain low for years postgrafting. In general, the immune system appears to be normal by one year after bone marrow transplantation except in patients with chronic GVH disease. The kinetics of lymphocyte reconstitution after marrow transplant is beyond the scope of this review, and readers are referred to Chapter 6 of this monograph and to excellent recent review articles on this topic (44–46).

Platelet production is the last component in the blood to recover. Assessing recovery of platelet production is complicated by such factors as giving platelet transfusions during the early post-transplant period and development of immune thrombocytopenia. Usually, the mean platelet count reaches 50,000/mm³ within 3 to 5 weeks, but this level of platelet count may not occur until as late as 6 to 7 weeks following allogeneic marrow transplant (29,30). The platelet count usually reaches the normal value by 6 months postgrafting. In autologous transplants, platelet regeneration may be slower than that following allogeneic bone marrow transplants, particularly in patients who were given a second autologous transplant (47,48,77). It is important to note that most autologous marrow transplant patients have had significant prior cytotoxic therapy.

Hematopoietic Stem Cell Reconstitution

The kinetics of hematopoietic progenitor cell regeneration (see Figure 3) postgrafting can be followed by the clonogenic assays described above. During the interval after intensive preconditioning and prior to bone marrow infusion, no CFU-GM, BFU-E, CFU-E and CFU-Mix are detected in the recipient's bone marrow or blood (49,138). Following bone marrow transplantation, myeloid and erythroid progenitors appear in the blood within the first 3 days post-transplant, they disappear, then they reappear 30 to 40 days later (49). In contrast, CFU-GM and BFU-E of the bone marrow are undetectable until 1 to 4 weeks after marrow transplant (49–51). The persistence of circulating progenitor cells immediately after transplant suggests trapping of stem cells and progenitor cells in extramedullary sites, such as in the liver, spleen, and lungs. Subsequently there is differentiation of the stem cells with release of their progenitors from these extramedullary sites. The early persistence of progenitor cells may also represent damage to the blood-bone marrow barrier (52) by the conditioning regimen, since interstitial edema may be seen in bone marrow biopsies during the first week postgrafting (27).

Myeloid progenitors have been found to reach normal numbers within the first 2 months following transplantation in most patients (50,51,53). However, results of large studies (27,54–57) show that growth of marrow CFU-GM is significantly below normal during the first 6 months. In some cases, the number of myeloid progenitor cells is below normal for several years after bone marrow transplantation. Peripheral blood CFU-GM and BFU-E are also reduced, but peripheral blood levels of neutrophils, platelets, and hemoglobin are normal at 4 to 6 months after successful transplant. The cause for the discrepancy between the decrease of hematopoietic progenitors and normal blood cell values is unclear. Studies in transplantation of mice and dogs (58,59) are consistent with this clinical observation. Depletion of pluripotent stem cells (CFU-S) has been observed following marrow transplantation in mice (58,60). Mice treated with busulphan have near normal blood counts and bone marrow cellularity despite markedly reduced numbers of CFU-GM and CFU-S (61).

How can this paradox be explained? One possibility is that in order to maintain adequate circulating mature cells, an increased demand for differentiation is placed on a limited number of stem cells, and this does not allow complete regeneration of the stem cell pool. This assumes that stem cells can regenerate to the normal levels. Results of studies in humans support such an hypothesis. A severe and sustained decrease in multipotent progenitor cells (CFU-Mix) is seen in recipients even several years postgrafting (56,57). An increased number of CFU-Mix cells in cell cycle (57) postgrafting also reflects an attempted compensation for a decreased stem cell reserve, as part of the effort to produce blood cells. Proliferative abnormalities in CFU-GM have also been noted by others (54,56).

The situation of a reduced stem cell reserve in the presence of normal blood counts is not unique to bone marrow transplant patients. Reduced numbers of CFU-GM are seen in 3 other clinical settings: in patients with severe aplastic anemia whose blood cell counts have recovered to normal or near normal (62), in patients with acute lymphoblastic leukemia who have been off long-term maintenance therapy and in remission for several years (63), and in patients with acute myeloid leukemia in long-term remission (64).

The impaired recovery of hematopoietic progenitor cells after bone marrow transplantation may result from abnormal interaction between hematopoietic progenitors and regulatory cells. Mature T cells and monocytes may enhance or inhibit myelopoiesis and erythropoiesis *in vitro* (62,65,66). T cell functions are defective for a prolonged period postgrafting (44,45); therefore, impaired stem cell function after marrow transplant may result from defective T cells. This notion is supported by the observation that E rosette forming T cells cause suppression of myeloid progenitor cell growth (55).

After marrow grafting, *in vitro* myeloid progenitor cell growth is enhanced by cyclosporin (an anti-T cell agent) and by antibodies to gamma interferon (67). In contrast, CD4+ lymphocytes obtained early in the period following transplantation of allogeneic bone marrow enhance erythroid progenitor growth *in vitro*. No enhancing effect is observed in CD4+ lymphocytes obtained in the later post-transplant period (68). Thus, the effect of regulatory cells on hematopoiesis is complex and dependent on various factors. These variables include time postgrafting, as well as the amount and the type of stimuli and cells involved in the interaction with the hematopoietic stem cells.

Regardless of cause, decreased stem cell numbers post-transplant suggests a reduced hematopoietic reserve and may thus have clinical implications. Reduced hematopoietic reserve could partly explain the increase in serious and often rapidly fatal infections, the increased susceptibility to the myelosuppressive effect of drugs such as trimethoprimsulfamethoxizole, and the increased incidence of infection-associated thrombocytopenia that occurs in patients more than 6 months post-transplant (69).

The presence of reduced stem cell numbers despite normal bone marrow cellularity suggests certain clinical problems. Perhaps one cannot rely on the recommended number of infused nucleated bone marrow cells as being adequate for bone marrow engraftment in certain situations, such as in autologous marrow grafting in acute leukemias. In fact, marrow CFU-GM content in patients with acute myeloid leukemia in remission is approximately 50% that of the normal despite the presence of normocellular marrow (70). Patients who have received a second transplant of autologous marrow show a prolonged delay in recovery of neutrophil and platelet counts as compared to the rate of recovery following their first autograft (47,48). Recently, use of stem cells obtained from peripheral blood for transplantation have been advocated. Thus, a more reliable assay of stem cells other than nucleated cell count is required to assess the transplantability of cells harvested from bone marrow or peripheral blood.

Significance of Progenitor Cell Assays in Clinical Marrow Transplantation

Culture of myeloid progenitor cells is the most widely used method to evaluate engraftment in bone marrow transplantation. Since neutrophils are derived from CFU-GM, there is a strong correlation between the dose of CFU-GM units infused and the time for neutrophil recovery in patients undergoing transplantation of autologous marrow (71–76). The number of marrow CFU-GM units infused also directly affects the rate of recovery of reticulocytes and platelets in patients transplanted with purged autologous bone marrow (76). In allogeneic marrow transplants, engraftment is further complicated by genetic disparity, by immunosuppression given both pre-transplant and post-transplant for prevention of graft rejection and prevention of GVH disease, as well as by donor-recipient mismatches as to sex and ABO blood groups. Despite these complicating factors, the dose of donor marrow CFU-GM is closely correlated with the speed of neutrophil reconstitution (27,32,53,77,78). The CFU-GM content in the infused marrow also correlates with the time required for reticulocytes (27) and platelets (83) to regenerate in the recipients of transplanted bone marrow.

Certain studies suggest that the number of erythroid progenitors (BFU-E) transplanted directly affects the time required for recovery of granulocytes and reticulocytes (27,74), but this finding is inconsistent (53,77). There are few reported studies on the association between CFU-Mix and engraftment (57,74,77). It is emphasized in all these studies that the correlation between peripheral blood reconstitution postgrafting and the progenitor cell dose is nonlinear. In contrast to these studies, the dose of marrow CFU-GM does not correlate with engraftment in either allogeneic (57,79,80) or autologous bone marrow transplantation (81,82). Conflicting results have also been reported on the correlation between hematopoietic engraftment and BFU-E and CFU-Mix contents of the infused marrow.

The discrepancies in the literature concerning the predictive value of number of progenitor cells infused require analysis. The *in vitro* methods used to determine the colony forming cells vary considerably. Many variables are not standardized. These variables include semisolid media (agar vs. methylcellulose), the source of colony stimulating factors, the bone marrow cell separation methods (sedimentation vs. density gradient centrifugation), the incubation time (ranging from 7 to 16 days), carbon dioxide concentration, and humidity content. Thus, the cloning efficiency may vary making it difficult to compare the reported results. This is particularly true for erythroid progenitors which show a large variation even in normal controls. Standardization of these *in vitro* assays could be achieved by the use of identical reagents and culture conditions, and the use of purified recombinant colony stimulating factors.

The criteria used to express colony assay results and to define peripheral blood reconstitution also differ. Time to engraftment of individual cell lineage is used for analysis in some studies (75,77,78) but not by others (57,79,81). The accuracy of colony scoring (e.g., CFU-Mix colonies) and peripheral blood counting (e.g., the inaccuracy of manual reticulocyte measurement) (77), undoubtedly affects the analysis. The influence of platelet, red cell and neutrophil transfusions on the increase in blood counts has been clearly defined in the analysis by some (27,72,76,77) but not by others (57,79,81).

In spite of the above discrepancies, evidence in humans and in animals (83) indicates that progenitor cell content, especially CFU-GM of the infused marrow, predicts the rate of hematological engraftment in patients following bone marrow transplantation. This correlation is mostly nonlinear (see above). This nonlinear correlation implies that there is a threshold above which a further increase in progenitor cells infused will not shorten the time taken for hematopoietic reconstitution. On the other hand, there is also a lower threshold of detection with use of the current progenitor culture method. Failure to grow progenitor colonies implies that the period of aplasia may be prolonged but reconstitution may still occur. This finding is in agreement with some *ex vivo* marrow purging studies, where marked reduction or absence of myeloid or multipotent progenitor growth by purging does not appear to affect autologous marrow reconstitution in some patients (82).

Measurements of CFU-GM or even CFU-Mix provide an indirect measurement of the repopulating potential of the pluripotent stem cells. Recent studies indicate that CFU-GM assay is equivalent to CFU-Mix in predicting hematopoietic recovery in bone marrow recipients (77,84). In general, faster hematological recovery is expected in patients given allogeneic bone marrow, with a dose of more than 3×10^4 CFU-GM/Kg of bodyweight (77). Likewise hematological recovery is faster in autologous marrow transplant patients who receive more than 1×10^3 marrow CFU-GM/Kg bodyweight (75), or over 30×10^4 blood CFU-GM/Kg bodyweight (84). It is not surprising that the amount of CFU-GM required for engraftment in allogeneic marrow transplants is higher than that needed for autografting because of the genetic disparity which complicates allogeneic transplants.

Alternative methods to assess transplantability of stem cells, such as long-term marrow culture and immunophenotyping, have been attempted. Long-term culture provides a workable alternative but this assay is difficult to quantify. At present, the *in vitro* progenitor cell assay represents the most convenient and quantitative method to assess the transplantability of hematopoietic pluripotent stem cells. It allows clinicians to assess the amount of myelotoxicity due to procedures such as cryopreservation (26), cell separation (85), and *in vitro* purging (76) and, therefore, this technique is valuable in patient management. Total nucleated cell counts will not identify stem cells that may be damaged as the result of the cryopreservation, cell separation and *in vitro* purging. The development of specific monoclonal antibodies against stem cells would allow rapid quantitation of the stem cell content in the marrow.

Hematopoietic Stroma Following Marrow Transplantation

Compared to the large number of studies on hematopoietic progenitor cells performed in conjunction with clinical bone marrow transplantation, less effort has been given to study of the hematopoietic microenvironment (see Figure 3). Damage to the microenvironment may explain the impairment or failure of hematopoiesis following marrow transplantation. Transplantation of stem cells from mice with congenital hypoplastic anemia (S1/S^d) to normal mice following high-dose radiation can protect the transplanted mice from the lethal effects of irradiation. Transplantation of stem cells from normal mice does not cure the anemia of S1/S^d mice, but heterotopic transplantation of splenic tissue, which presumably provides an appropriate stroma, does correct the anemia (86). Sublethal radiation (87), curettage of the bone marrow (88), or ectopic bone marrow grafting (89) result in temporary marrow damage, and hematopoietic recovery is invariably preceded by regeneration of the stroma.

In humans, the reported failure of syngeneic marrow transplantation in treatment of aplastic anemia may be due to defects in the bone marrow stroma (90). *In vitro* evidence suggests that damage to the stroma by irradiation or cytotoxic agents, used under similar conditions to that of clinical marrow transplantation, affects the ability of the stroma to support hematopoiesis (91,92). It has also been shown that host megakaryocytic progenitor (CFU-Mk) growth prior to transplant correlates with the rate of hematopoietic engraftment by the donor cells (57). CFU-Mk may reflect the growth requirements of hematopoietic stem cells and, thus, this assay may indicate the functional ability of the host stroma to support growth of the transplanted stem cells.

In one of our studies (20), stromal fibroblastic colony growth (CFU-F) was suppressed and the number of CFU-F cells in proliferative state was increased during the first month after transplant of allogeneic marrow. These changes were brief and returned to normal within 6 weeks postgrafting. As mentioned earlier, hematopoietic progenitors do not increase to near normal until 6 months postgrafting (56). Thus, stromal reconstitution, at least of the CFU-F cells, precedes hematopoietic recovery in marrow transplantation. This pattern of marrow regeneration is similar to that seen following mechanical or radiation damage (87,88). Phenotypically, post-transplant stromal CFU-F cells resemble normal CFU-F cells, but the functional characteristics of CFU-F cells post-transplant have not been fully elucidated.

Endothelial cells are recognized components of the marrow stroma both *in vitro* and *in vivo*. Cultures of vascular endothelium support the growth of human CFU-Mix, CFU-GM, and BFU-E (93). Messenger RNAs of several colony stimulating factors (e.g., GM-CSF, G-CSF, and M-CSF) are detected in cultured endothelial cells following stimulation with inflammatory mediators, such as IL-1 and tumor necrosing factor (94,95). However, most of these studies were performed using cultured umbilical vein endothelial cells or endothelial cell lines. Pure bone marrow endothelial cells were not used. It is known that endothelial cells of different tissues possess distinct features (95). Bone marrow endothelial cell colonies have been grown from enzyme digested bone marrow fragments (138). These colonies are morphologically distinct from CFU-F colonies and, they are positive for factor VIII antigen and *Ulex europeus* lectin (Figure 2). Studies on the reconstitution of marrow stromal endothelial cells following marrow transplantation are needed.

Several investigators have identified some of the noncellular components of the stroma which may have a role in hematopoietic regulation. Extracellular matrix derived from human LTC can modulate myeloid leukemia cell growth *in vitro* (97). Glycosaminoglycans obtained from bone marrow stroma but not from other tissues have been found to bind GM-CSF *in vitro* (98), thus, selective binding of hematopoietic growth factors could explain why these factors are not detectable in stromal culture supernatant. A new hematopoietic regulator called hemonectin has recently been isolated and characterized from stroma matrix (99). Altered non-cellular components of the stroma may also be important in the regeneration of hematopoiesis after bone marrow transplantation.

Factors Affecting Hematopoietic Reconstitution

Inheritance of the ABO blood group system is independent of the HLA antigens. Thus, ABO mismatch is not a contraindication for marrow transplant provided hemolytic transfusion reaction due to ABO mismatch is controlled. A number of methods are being used to circumvent this problem (24). ABO mismatch does not appear to influence the success of marrow engraftment, the rate of rejection, or the development of graft-vs.-host disease (100,101). Reports differ on the effects of ABO mismatch on the rate of recovery of peripheral blood cells post-transplant. There may be delay in reconstitution of erythrocytes, leukocytes, and platelets, leading to an increased requirement for transfusions of red cells and platelets (29,102). The basis for this delay may be related to the presence of ABH antigens on marrow progenitors, namely, CFU-GM, BFU-E and CFU-E (103). But other studies did not show a delay in hematopoietic reconstitution (104,105). This discrepancy may be due to the concentration of the antibodies and their avidity for the antigens involved. High titers of ABO blood group antibodies are sometimes associated with delayed reconstitution of reticulocytes (106) and neutrophils (102).

Isolated thrombocytopenia and neutropenia have been recorded in recipients of allogeneic and autologous bone marrow who have engrafted (107–109). Both transient and chronic thrombocytopenia and neutropenia have been observed in patients for up to several years postgrafting (107,110). Platelet and neutrophil autoantibodies have been detected, but their presence does not indicate future development of a cytopenia (109). Coomb's positive hemolytic anemia (138) in addition to other forms of immune dysfunction have been observed post-transplant. Autoimmunity is a likely mechanism for development of isolated cytopenias in some patients.

A major cause of morbidity and mortality following allogeneic marrow transplant is graft-vs.-host disease. Impaired progenitor cell growth and delay in peripheral blood recovery is seen in patients with this complication (57,77,111). The T cell appears to play a central role in development of GVH disease. T cell abnormalities in patients with this condition (112) may be the reason for the suppression of progenitor cell growth. It is interesting that removal of donor T cells for preventing GVH disease also causes delay in hematopoietic recovery. These different influences of T cell on hematopoiesis indicates the complexity of T cell involvement in the regulation of hematopoiesis.

Several other clinical parameters are known to influence hematopoietic recovery. Methotrexate therapy causes a greater delay of peripheral blood reconstitution than cyclosporine (113). Viral infections in nontransplanted patients, such as infections due to cytomegalovirus and Epstein-Barr virus may be associated with thrombocytopenia, neutropenia, or both. Also, virus infections may have a direct toxic effect on hematopoietic progenitors, such as occurs with parvovirus (114). Cytomegalovirus infection delays platelet recovery in autologous marrow transplantation (115), and herpes simplex infection delays neutrophil recovery in allogeneic transplants (80). But these findings are not universally observed.

Hematopoietic Chimerism

In allogeneic marrow transplantation, complete chimerism implies the total replacement of hematopoietic cells in the recipient by the engrafted donor cells. Stable or transient mixed chimerism, that is a mixture of host and donor cells, or a mixture of normal and leukemic cells, can occur. Return of peripheral blood cells after marrow regeneration could also be the result of autologous marrow recovery. Different methods have been used to study engraftment. These include cytogenetics, isoenzyme analysis, red cell phenotyping, HLA typing, immunoglobulin allotyping, and DNA restriction fragment polymorphism. Studies of chimerism have provided useful information regarding hematopoiesis following transplantation of bone marrow.

The use of sex chromosomes as markers of cellular origin in sex mismatch transplants is a convenient method to study chimerism. For example, 45 leukemic patients who were transplanted with allogeneic marrow were studied (116). Successful engraftment was characterized by the presence of donor cells in the marrow within 2 weeks and in the blood by 3 weeks postgrafting. Mixed chimerism was seen in 3 patients who had no leukemic relapse. Eight cases of leukemic relapse occurred, but in none was leukemia found in the donor cells. Leukemia occurrence in donor cells has been observed using cytogenetic analysis, but such cases are rare (117–119). In a study of 96 patients with severe aplastic anemia who had sex mismatch transplants (120), transient mixed chimerism occurred in 58% of the patients up to 13 months postgrafting. The rejection rate is higher and the incidence of graft-vs.-host disease is lower in the mixed chimeric group. None of these patients remained as mixed chimeras as determined by cytogenetic techniques. Most patients convert to the donor phenotype and the rest reject their grafts. Thus, long term stable mixed chimerism appears to be uncommon after marrow transplantation for treatment of aplastic anemia.

Autosomal polymorphism has also been used to document chimerism. Hematopoietic engraftment was detected in 14 out of 39 cases by autosomal polymorphism. Using this method, a high incidence of mixed chimerism and graft failure following infusion of T cell depleted marrow was observed (121). There seems to be a high sensitivity of detection of chimerism by this cytogenetic method. However, there are problems associated with cytogenetic analysis. The method depends on the proliferative rate of the cells and it is often difficult to obtain sufficient metaphases for study in the period soon after marrow transplantation. Proliferative differences may exist between host and donor cells. For example, peripheral blood cells of one patient, when stimulated with phytohemagglutinin, were found to be entirely of donor origin. But when these blood cells were stimulated with pokeweed mitogen they were found to be of mixed host and donor origin (116).

Red cell phenotyping is easy to perform, and it is also a sensitive method for determining the cellular origin. However, transfusion of red cells affects the assay. Immunoglobulin allotyping has been used to detect B cell origin following marrow transplant, and has been found to be extremely sensitive (122). This assay is not readily available and interpretation is also affected by recent transfusions. Other genetic characteristics, such as hereditary spherocytosis and thalassemia trait (32), have been used to confirm donor marrow engraftment. But these methods are not applicable to most patients.

Recently, DNA restriction fragment length polymorphisms (RFLPs) have been applied to the study of bone marrow transplantation. After restriction endonuclease digestion, variation in DNA sequences among individuals produces DNA fragments of different lengths. These fragments are called restriction fragment length polymorphisms. RFLPs are codominantly inherited and can be detected by the Southern blotting method. Thus, RFLPs can be used to detect donor and host cells in allogeneic marrow transplantation. The current method can detect a minor population of DNA (as little as 1–2%) in a mixture of 2 cell populations. The sensitivity of this technique may be further increased using methods such as the polymerase chain reaction (123). Unlike the above methods, RFLP analysis is not affected by red cell transfusions and it is independent of the mitotic rate of the cells. Both DNA or whole cells can be stored easily. In some cases, RFLP analysis can still be informative even though the pre-transplant host marrow sample is not available (122). The efficiency of this method depends on the restriction enzymes, and the number and type of RFLP probes used. The probability of detecting a difference in restriction fragment pattern between two siblings has been determined to be 99.7% by using 5 highly polymorphic probes (124). The hypervariable minisatellite probes may detect a difference in almost all donor-recipient pairs with one single analysis (125).

By applying analysis with restriction fragment length polymorphism to separated hematopoietic cell populations, a higher percentage of mixed chimerism has been demonstrated than was previously reported (122,126,127). In one series, specific RFLP markers were detected in all 27 patients studied (122). Transient mixed chimerism was not uncommon, but the occurrence of a progressive increase in the percentage of host cells indicates the likelihood of leukemic relapse. Thus, the studies of chimerism by DNA RFLPs have yielded clinically useful information regarding hematopoietic reconstitution following bone marrow transplantation.

The origin of stromal cells is a subject of debate. In one study, stromal cells derived from patients following marrow transplantation and grown in long term culture were shown to be of donor origin by use of sex chromosome analysis (128). This finding suggests a common stem cell for both the hematopoietic marrow and its stroma. This view is supported by enzyme marker studies in patients with clonal myeloproliferative disorders (129). But the concept is challenged by a recent study (13) which shows, by *in situ* hybridization, that the stromal cells in long term culture are of recipient origin. The adherent cells in long term culture were phenotypically diverse, and the origin of individual stromal cells could not be assessed easily. Clonogenic assays of individual cell types will unequivocally determine the origins of these cells. A number of other studies have shown conclusively that stromal fibroblasts are of recipient origin in patients transplanted with sex mismatched bone marrow. These stromal fibroblasts are highly resistant to chemotherapy and radiotherapy; they can repopulate the bone marrow within weeks postgrafting in patients with either aplastic anemia or leukemia (20,131).

CONCLUSIONS AND FUTURE PROSPECTS

Reconstitution of hematopoietic stem cells following bone marrow transplantation is a complex phenomenon affected by a variety of factors (Figure 4). Regeneration of the peripheral blood and bone marrow are evident in the second to third weeks postgrafting, but the blood cell counts and their functions do not return to normal until several months later, even in uncomplicated cases. Prolonged suppression of multipotent and unipotent progenitor cells has been observed following transplantation. This delay in hematopoietic reconstitution is influenced by many factors, such as ABO blood group, graft-vs.-host disease, immunosuppressive agents and certain infections (such as those due to cytomegalovirus). The basis for the finding of a reduced marrow reserve in association with normal cell counts in the peripheral blood during the late post-transplant period is unknown. Reduced stem cell reserve may be an explanation for increased susceptibility to severe infection and thrombocytopenia in some of these patients after marrow transplant.

In vitro progenitor cell assays allow quantitative assessment of hematopoietic progenitor cells. Studies using these assays have improved our understanding of the recovery of hematopoiesis following bone marrow transplantation. The

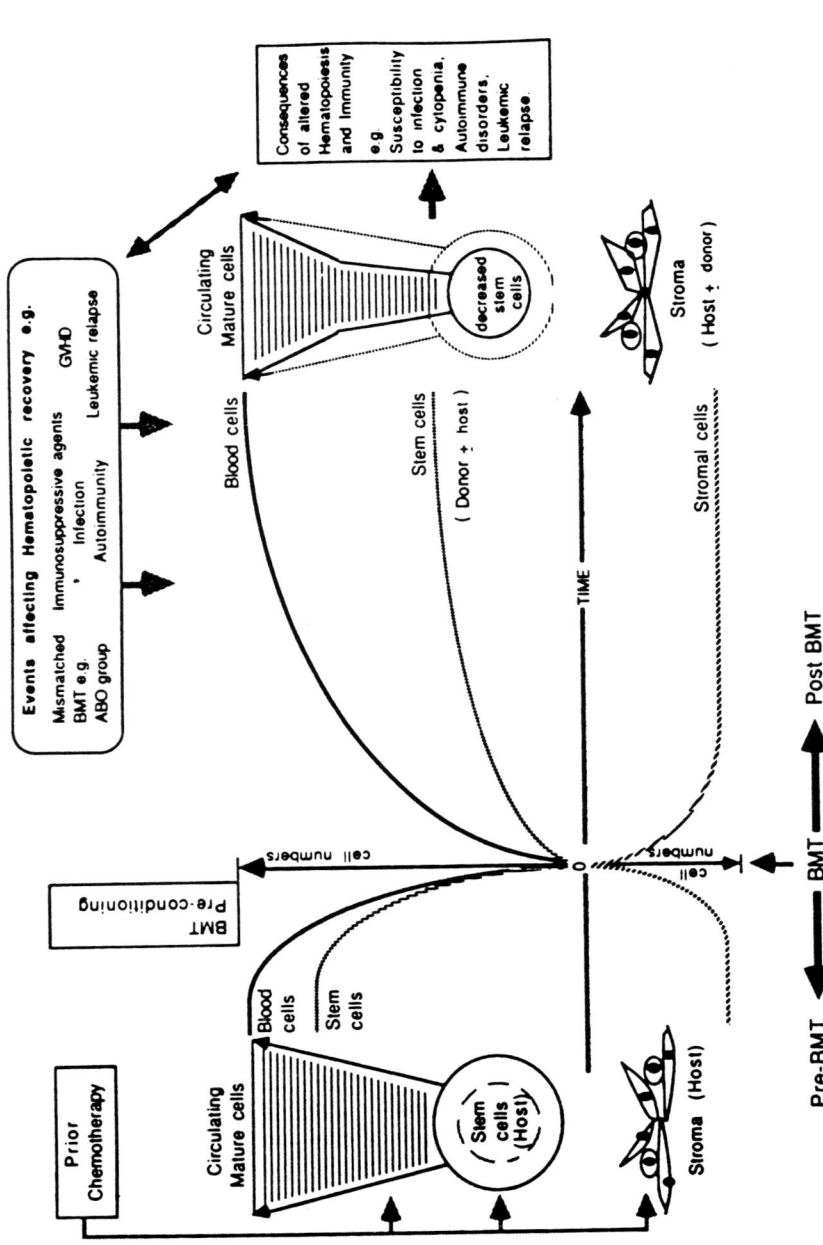

FIG. 4. An overview of the kinetics of hematopoietic reconstitution following bone marrow transplantation in humans.

number of colony forming cells, especially CFU-GM, of the infused bone marrow, correlate with the rate of recovery of the cells of the peripheral blood. Within limitations, CFU-GM assay assesses indirectly the transplantability of pluripotent stem cells. This assay is particularly useful in autologous bone marrow transplantation involving cryopreservation and *ex vivo* purging, or following a second autologous marrow transplant. The assay is useful in these situations because total nucleated cell counts cannot assess stem cell damage. Further development of methods of assessing pluripotent stem cells and marrow stromal elements will increase the usefulness of *in vitro* assay of stem cells in the management of bone marrow transplant patients.

Changes in the stromal microenvironment following marrow transplant is less clearly known. Radiation and some cytotoxic agents used to prepare patients for bone marrow transplantation have been shown to affect the ability of stromal cells produced in long term culture to support hematopoiesis. Evidence from successful marrow transplants shows that in contrast to hematopoietic stem cell regeneration, which is derived from the infused donor marrow, bone marrow stromal cells result from autologous regeneration. DNA-RFLP analysis of bone marrow of patients transplanted with allogeneic marrow has shown that transient or stable mixed chimeras are not uncommon. This technique provides a sensitive and convenient way to monitor hematopoietic engraftment and disease relapse in patients following allogeneic and autologous marrow transplantation. Use of this technique will help to improve our knowledge of hematopoietic events following transplant of bone marrow.

The changes in hematopoietic growth factors (HGFs) and their effects on marrow reconstitution require further attention. For example, megakaryocytic colony stimulating activities in patients' sera change rapidly during the early post-transplant period (132). Sera of mice with graft-vs.-host disease have increased erythroid colony stimulating activity (133). An increasing number of hematopoietic growth factors are being identified and many have been cloned. Measurement of these factors in patients undergoing bone marrow transplantation will help in our understanding of their role in bone marrow reconstitution. *In vivo* infusion of some of these agents, such as GM-CSF (134,135), has been shown to enhance hematopoietic reconstitution following high-dose chemotherapy in animals. These HGFs are currently being tested as therapeutic agents in clinical marrow transplantation.

Recombinant human GM-CSF have been shown to accelerate hematopoietic recovery following allogeneic and autologous BMT in a small number of patients (136,137). The immediate toxicity is minimal but long-term effects of HGFs on normal and malignant stem cells are unknown. Better understanding of the effects of hematopoietic growth factors on normal and malignant cells, and changes in these growth factors during bone marrow transplantation will permit rational use of these agents. It is possible that hematopoietic growth factors could be used to maintain and to increase the harvested stem cells *in vitro* before infusion. One could also explore the possible selectivity of these growth factors and other agents (such as monoclonal antibodies, 4-hydroperoxy-cyclophosphamide, and synthetic oligopeptides) to purge leukemic cells both *in vitro* and *in vivo*. Research in hematopoiesis continues to improve our understanding of the kinetics of hematopoietic reconstitution in bone marrow transplantation, and offers promise for improving the management of these patients.

SUMMARY

Hematopoietic reconstitution after bone marrow transplantation provides a unique opportunity to study the regulation of hematopoiesis in man. Evidence of hematopoietic recovery, as shown by an increase in the number of peripheral blood cells and increase in bone marrow cellularity, occurs at about 2 weeks post-transplant. However, peripheral blood neutrophils, lymphocytes, platelets and red cells remain below normal for at least 3 to 6 months. The hematopoietic multipotent and unipotent progenitor cells remain suppressed even several years after the transplant.

This pattern of hematopoietic regeneration with features resembling fetal hematopoietic development, is similar for both allogeneic and autologous marrow transplants. The process of hematological reconstitution is affected by factors such as graft-vs.-host disease and *ex vivo* manipulation of the harvested bone marrow. Possible causes of the reduced progenitor cell growth post-transplant include decreased stem cell reserve, and altered hematopoietic regulation by accessory cells, such as lymphocytes, monocytes and marrow stroma. Prolonged impairment of the marrow reserve and the presence of a defective immune system contribute to the morbidity and mortality following bone marrow transplantation.

Changes in the hematopoietic microenvironment and hematopoietic growth regulators post-transplant are poorly understood. In hematopoietic regeneration following physical injuries (such as marrow curettage) or ectopic marrow grafting, stromal regeneration precedes hematopoietic stem cell reconstitution in the bone marrow. Hematologic reconstitution following marrow transplantation appears to follow the same sequence of events. A defective microenvironment may be a significant factor delaying hematopoietic recovery.

A number of hematopoietic growth factors have been identified and are available in pure recombinant forms. Some of these factors are currently being studied in clinical trials of bone marrow transplantation. Changes in hematopoietic growth factors during bone marrow transplantation are poorly understood. Further studies in this area are needed and these will provide a rational basis for the use of these growth factors in bone marrow transplantation. The application of molecular biology, immunophenotyping and *in vitro* culture assays in bone marrow transplantation contribute to our knowledge of the complexity of hematopoiesis in this procedure. Increased understanding of hematopoiesis provides a rational basis for the management of patients undergoing bone marrow transplants.

REFERENCES

1. Metcalf D: The basic biology of hemopoiesis. In, Metcalf D (ed): *Hematopoietic Colony Stimulating Factors.* Amsterdam: Elsevier Science Publishing. New York, 1984, pp. 1–26.
2. Gordon M, Barrett AJ: Normal hematopoiesis. In, Gordon MY, Barrett AJ (eds): *Bone Marrow Disorders; The Biological Basis of Clinical Problems.* Oxford, Blackwell Scientific Publications, 1985, pp. 1–138.
3. Bodger MP, Izaguirre CA, Blacklock HA, Hoffbrand AV: Surface antigenic determinants on human pluripotent and unipotent hematopoietic progenitor cells. *Blood* 1983;61:1006–1010.
4. Till JE, McCulloch EA: A direct measurement of the radiation sensitivity of normal mouse bone marrow cells. *Radiat Res* 1961;14:213–222.
5. Hodgeson GS, Bradley TR: Properties of hematopoietic stem cells surviving 5-fluorouracil treatment; evidence of a pre-CFU-S cell? *Nature* 1979;281:381–382.
6. Antin JH, Weinberg DS, Rappeport JM: Evidence that pluripotential stem cells form splenic colonies in humans after marrow transplantation. *Transplantation* 1985;39:102–105.
7. Whang T, Free E III, Tjio JH, et al.: The distribution of the Philadelphia chromosome in patients with chronic myelogenous leukemia. *Blood* 1963;2:664–667.
8. Fialkow PJ: Cell lineages in hematopoietic neoplasia studied with glucose to phosphate dehydrogenase markers. *J Cell Physiol* 1982;(Suppl)1:37–43.
9. Ichikawa Y, Pluznik DH, Sachs L: *In vitro* control of the development of macrophage and granulocyte colonies. *Proc Natl Acad Sci USA* 1966;56:495–499.
10. Bradley TR, Metcalf D: The growth of mouse bone marrow cells *in vitro. Aust J Exp Biol Med Sci* 1966;44:297–300.
11. Pike BL, Robinson WA: Human bone marrow colony growth in agar gel. *J Cell Physiol* 1976;76:77–84.
12. Fauser AA, Messner HA: Granuloerythropoietic colonies in human bone marrow, peripheral blood and cord blood. *Blood* 1978;52:1243–1248.
13. Messner HA, Izaguirre CA, Jamal N: Identification of T lymphocytes in human mixed hemopoietic colonies. *Blood* 1981;58:402–405.
14. Nakahata T, Ogawa M: Hemopoietic colony forming cells in umbilical cord blood with extensive capability to generate mono-multipotential hemopoietic progenitors. *J Clin Invest* 1982;70:324–328.
15. Gordon MY, Hibbin JA, Kearney LU, et al.: Colony formation by primitive hemopoietic progenitors in co-cultures of bone marrow cells and stromal cells. *Br J Hæmatol* 1985;60:129–138.
16. Travassoli M, Friedenstein A: Hemopoietic stromal microenvironment. *Am J Hematol* 1983;15:185–203.
17. Bentley SA: Bone marrow connective tissue and the hemopoietic microenvironment. *Br J Hæmatol* 1982;50:1–6.
18. Dexter TM, Allen TD, Laythan LG: Conditions controlling the proliferation of hemopoietic cells *in vitro. J Cell Physiol* 1977;91:335–344.
19. Gartner S, Kaplan HS: Long-term culture of human bone marrow cells. *Proc Natl Acad Sci USA* 1980;77:4756–4758.
20. Da WM, Ma DDF, Biggs JC: Studies of hematopoietic stromal fibroblastic colonies in patients undergoing bone marrow transplantation. *Exp Hematol* 1986;14:266–270.
21. Stanley GR, Jubinsky PT: Factors affecting the growth and differentiation of hemopoietic cells in culture. *Clin Hematol* 1984;13:329–348.
22. Metcalf D: Actions of colony stimulating factors on hemopoietic cells. In, Metcalf D: *The Hemopoietic Colony Stimulating Factors.* Amsterdam, Elsevier, 1984, pp. 229–276.
23. Prentice HG, Blacklock HA, Janossy G, et al.: Depletion of T lymphocytes in donor marrow prevents significant GVHD in matched allogeneic leukemic marrow transplant recipients. *Lancet* 1985;1:472–475.

24. Dodds AJ, Ma DDF: Apheresis in bone marrow transplantation. In, *Therapeutic Hemapheresis.* 1986;163–170.
25. Santos GW, Colvin OM: Pharmacological purging of bone marrow with reference to autografting. *Clin Hematol* 1986;15:67–84.
26. Ma DDF, Johnson LA, Chan PM, Biggs JC: Factors affecting myeloid stem cell survival after cryopreservation of human marrow and chronic granulocytic leukæmia cells. *Cryobiology* 1982;19:1–9.
27. Arnold R, Schmeiser T, Wolfgang H, et al.: Hemopoietic reconstitution after bone marrow transplantation. *Exp Hematol* 1986;14:271–277.
28. Arnold R, Calvo W, Heymer B, et al.: Extramedullary hemopoiesis after bone marrow transplantation. *Scand J Hematol* 1985;34:9–12.
29. Hows JM, Chipping PM, Palmer S, et al.: Regeneration of peripheral blood cells following ABO incompatible allogeneic bone marrow transplantation for severe aplastic anemia. *Br J Hæmatol* 1983;53:145–151.
30. Ma DDF, Varga DE, Biggs JC: Donor marrow progenitors (CFU-Mix, BFU-G, CFU-GM) and hemopoietic engraftment following HLA-matched sibling bone marrow transplantation. *Leuk Res* 1987;11:141–147.
31. Alter BP, Rappeport JM, Heissman TH, Schroeder WA: Fetal erythropoiesis following bone marrow transplantation. *Blood* 1976;48:843–853.
32. Biggs JC, Ma DDF, and the St. Vincent's Hospital Marrow Transplant Team: Bone marrow transplantation; a preliminary study in aplasia and leukemia. *Med J Aust* 1980;2:603–608.
33. Macklis RM, Javid T, Lipton N, et al.: Synthesis of hemoglobin F in adult simian erythroid progenitor derived colonies. *J Clin Invest* 1982;70:752–761.
34. Martin PJ, Anderson CC, Jones HM, et al.: A rise in the percentage of large unstained cells in peripheral blood determined by the Hemalog D90 automated differential counter is a feature of impending myeloid engraftment following bone marrow transplantation. *Clin Lab Hematol* 1986;8:1–8.
35. Anderson KC, Ritz J, Takvorian T, et al.: Hematologic engraftment and immune reconstitution post-transplantation with Anti-B1 purged autologous bone marrow. *Blood* 1987;69:597–804.
36. Kersey JH, Weisdorf D, Nesbit ME, et al.: Comparison of autologous and allogeneic bone marrow transplantation for treatment of high risk refractory acute lymphoblastic leukemia. *N Engl J Med* 1987;317:461–467.
37. Sosa R, Weiden PL, Storb R, et al.: Granulocyte function in human allogeneic marrow graft recipients. *Exp Hematol* 1980;8:1183–1188.
38. Territo MC, Gale RP, Cline. MJ, and the UCLA Bone Marrow Transplantation Team: Neutrophil function in bone marrow transplant recipients. *Br J Hæmatol* 1977;35:245–251.
39. Clark RA, Johnson FL, Klebanoff SJ, Thomas ED: Defective neutrophil chemotaxis in bone marrow transplant patients. *J Clin Invest* 1976;58:22–27.
40. Rappeport JM, Newburger PE, Goldblum RM, et al.: Allogeneic bone marrow transplantation of chronic granulomatous disease. *J Pediatr* 1982;101:952–955.
41. Winston DJ, Territo MC, Ho WG, et al.: Alveolar macrophage dysfunction in human bone marrow transplant recipients. *Am J Med* 1982;73:859–864.
42. Shiobara S, Witherspoon RP, Lum LG, Storb R: Immunoglobulin synthesis after HLA-identical marrow grafting. V. The role of peripheral blood monocytes in the regulation of *in vitro* immunoglobulin secretion stimulated by pokeweed mitogen. *J Immunol* 1984;132:2850–2853.
43. Tsio MS, Dobbs S, Bokic S, et al.: Cellular interactions in marrow grafted patients. II. Normal monocyte antigen-presenting and defective T cell proliferative functions early after grafting and during chronic graft-vs.-host disease. *Transplantation* 1984;35:557–562.
44. Burakoff SJ, Lipton JM, Nathan DG: Recapitulation of immune response and hematopoietic system in bone marrow transplantation. *Clin Hematol* 1983;12:695–720.
45. Witherspoon RP, Lum LG, Storb R: Immunologic reconstitution after human marrow grafting. *Sem Hematol* 1984;21:2–10.
46. Lum LG: The kinetics of immune reconstitution after human marrow transplantation. *Blood* 1987;69:369–380.
47. Kingston JE, Malpas JS, Stiller CA, et al.: Autologous bone marrow transplantation contributes to hemopoietic recovery in children with solid tumors treated with high-dose melphalan. *Br J Hæmatol* 1984;58:589–595.

48. Linch DC, Burnett AJ: Clinical studies of ABMT in acute myeloid leukemia. *Clin Hematol* 1986;15:167–186.
49. Naganuma K, Ishii E, Ihiguro A, et al.: Hemopoietic progenitors before and after bone marrow transplantation. *Acta Hematol Jpn* 1986;49:852–861.
50. Moore MAS, Hansen JA, Everson LK, et al.: Hematological analysis of clinical bone marrow grafting evaluated by *in vitro* cultures. *Transplant Proc* 1976;8:647–654.
51. Gordon MY: Relevance of colony forming assays to bone marrow transplantation with particular reference to grafting for aplastic anemia. *Br J Hæmatol* 1971;42:61–71.
52. Tavassoli M: The marrow blood barrier. Br J Hæmatol 1979;41:297–302.
53. Faille A, Maraninchi D, Gluckman E, et al.: Granulocyte progenitor compartments after allogeneic bone marrow grafts. *Scand J Hematol* 1981;26:202–214.
54. Barrett AJ, Adams T: A proliferative defect of human bone marrow after transplantation. *Br J Hæmatol* 1981;49:159–164.
55. Li S, Champlin R, Fitchen JH, Gale RP: Abnormalities of myeloid progenitor cells after successful bone marrow transplantation. *J Clin Invest* 1985;75:234–241.
56. Ma DDF, Varga DE, Biggs JC: Hemopoietic reconstitution after allogeneic bone marrow transplantation in man; recovery of hemopoietic progenitors (CFU-Mix, BFU-E and CFU-GM). *Br J Hæmatol* 1987;65:5–10.
57. Messner HA, Curtis JE, Minden MD, et al.: Clonogenic hematopoietic precursors in bone marrow transplantation. *Blood* 1987;70:1425–1432.
58. Siminovitch L, Till JE, McCulloch EA: Decline in colony-forming ability of marrow cells subjected to serial transplantation into irradiated mice. *J Cell Comp Physiol* 1964;64:23–31.
59. Ragnavachar A, Prummer O, Fliedner TM, Steinback KH: Functional studies on myeloid progenitor cell reconstitution after autologous stem cell transplantation. *Exp Hematol* 1983;11 (Suppl 14):71.
60. Wolf NS, Priestly GV, Avercill LE; Depletion of reserve in the hemopoietic system. III. Factors affecting the serial transplantation of bone marrow. *Exp Hematol* 1983;11:762–771.
61. Morley A. Trainor K, Blake J: A primary stem cell lesion experimental chronic hypoplastic marrow failure. *Blood* 1975;45:681–688.
62. Bacigalupo A, Podesta M, Mingari L, et al.: Immune suppression of hematopoiesis in aplastic anemia; activity of T gamma lymphocytes. *J Immunol* 1980;125:1449–1453.
63. Layward L, LeVinsky RJ, Butler M: Long-term abnormalities in T and B lymphocyte function following treatment for acute lymphoblastic leukemia. *Br J Hematol* 1981;49:251–258.
64. Peschel C, Konwinka D, Geissler B, et al.: Studies of myelopoiesis *in vitro* on blood and bone marrow cells of patients with acute leukemia in long-term remission. *Leuk Res* 1983;7:397–406.
65. Nathan DG, Chess L, Hillman DG, et al.: Human erythroid burst forming unit; T cell requirement for proliferation *in vitro*. *J Exp Med* 1978;147:324–339.
66. Bagby GC, McCall E, Layman DC: Regulation of CSA production; interactions of fibroblasts, mononuclear phagocytes and lactoferrin. *J Clin Invest* 1983;71;340–344.
67. Raghavacher A, Frickhofen N, Arnold R, et al.: Hematopoietic colony formation after allogeneic bone marrow transplantation; enhancement by cyclosporin A and anti-immune interferon antiserum *in vitro*. *Exp Hematol* 1986;14:621–625.
68. Nakao S, Harada M, Ueda M, et al.: Enhancement of *in vitro* erythropoiesis by peripheral blood mononuclear cells from allogeneic marrow recipients in the early post-transplant period. *Scand J Hematol* 1986;36:180–185.
69. Winston DJ, Gale RP, Meyer DV, Young LS, and the UCLA Marrow Transplant Group: Infectious complications of human bone marrow transplantation. *Medicine* 1979;58:1–31.
70. Dickie KA, Jagannath S, Spitzer G, et al.: The role of autologous bone marrow transplantation in various malignancies. *Sem Hematol* 1984;21:101–122.
71. Spitzer G, Verma DS, Fisher R, et al.: The myeloid progenitor cell; its value in predicting hematopoietic recovery after autologous bone marrow transplantation. *Blood* 1980;55:317–323.
72. Abrams R, Polacek L, Hansen R, et al.: Variable precryopreservation recovery of CFU-GM following ficoll-hypaque processing of autologous bone marrow collections. *Blood* 1983;62 (suppl 1):216.
73. Harada M, Yoshida T, Ishino C, et al.: Hematologic recovery following autologous and allogeneic bone marrow transplantation. *Exp Hematol* 1983;11:841–848.

74. Vellekoop L, Spitzer G, Tucker SL, et al.: Predictive value of progenitor assays for time of hemopoietic recovery after autologous bone marrow transplantation. In, Dickie K, et al. (eds): *Proceedings of the First International Symposium on Autologous Bone Marrow Transplantation.* Houston, University of Texas M.D. Anderson Hospital, 1984, pp. 477–480.
75. Douay L, Gorin N-C, Mary J-Y, et al.: Recovery of CFU-GM from cryopreserved marrow and *in vivo* evaluation after autologous bone marrow transplantation are predictive of engraftment. *Exp Hematol* 1986;14:358–365.
76. Rowley SD, Zuehlsdorf M, Braine HG, et al.: CFU-GM content of bone marrow graft correlates with time to hematologic reconstitution following autologous bone marrow transplantation with 4-hydroperoxy-cyclophosphamide-purged bone marrow. *Blood* 1987;70:271–275.
77. Ma DDF, Varga DE, Biggs JC: Donor marrow progenitor (CFU-Mix, BFU-E and CFU-GM) and hemopoietic engraftment following HLA-matched sibling bone marrow transplantation. *Leuk Res* 1987;11:141–147.
78. Jansen T, Goselink HM, Veenhif WFJ, et al.: The impact of the composition of the bone marrow graft on engraftment and graft-vs.-host disease. *Exp Hematol* 1983;11:967–971.
79. Atkinson K, Norrie S, Chan P, et al.: Lack of correlation between nucleated bone marrow cell dose, marrow CFU-GM dose or marrow CFU-E dose and the rate of HLA-identical sibling marrow engraftment. *Br J Hæmatol* 1985;60:245–251.
80. Torres A, Alonso MC, Gomez-Villagran JL, et al.: No influence of number of donor CFU-GM on granulocyte recovery in bone marrow transplantation for acute leukemia. *Blood* 1985;50:94–98.
81. Beaujean F, Hartman O, LeForestier C, et al.: Successful infusion of 40 cryopreserved autologous bone marrows; *in vitro* studies of the freezing procedure. Biomed Pharmacol 1984;38:348–352.
82. Kaizer H, Stuart RK, Brookmeyer R, et al.: Autologous bone marrow transplantation in acute leukemia; a phase 1 study of *in vitro* treatment with 4-hydroperoxy-cyclophosphamide to purge tumor cells. *Blood* 1985;65:1504–1509.
83. Jones RJ, Sharkis SJ, Celano P, et al.: Progenitor cell assays predict hematopoietic reconstitution after syngeneic transplantation in mice. *Blood,* 1987;70:1186–1192.
84. To LB, Dyson PG, Branford AL, et al.: CFU-Mix are no better than CFU-GM in predicting hemopoietic reconstitutive capacity of peripheral blood stem cells collected in the very early remission phase of acute nonlymphoblastic leukemia. *Exp Hematol* 1987;15:351–354.
85. Ma DDF, Biggs JC: Comparison of two methods for concentrating stem cells for cryopreservation and transplantation. *Transfusion* 1982;22:217–219.
86. Bernstein SE: Tissue transplantation as an analytical and therapeutic tool in hereditary anemias. *Am J Surg* 1970;119:448–451.
87. Knospe WH, Blom T, Crosby WH: Regeneration of local irradiated bone marrow. I. Dose dependent long-term changes in the rat with particular emphasis upon vascular and stromal reaction. *Blood* 1966;28:398–415.
88. Patt HM, Maloney MA: Reconstitution of bone marrow in a depleted medullary cavity. In, Stohlman F (ed): *Hemopoietic Cellular Proliferation,* Grune & Stratton, New York, 1970; pp. 56–66.
89. Tavassoli M, Crosby WH: Transplantation of marrow to extramedullary sites. *Science* 1968;161:54–58.
90. Appelbaum FR, Fefer A, Cheever MA, et al.: Treatment of aplastic anemia by bone marrow transplantation in identical twins. *Blood* 1980;55:1033–1039.
91. Gualtieri RJ, Shadduck RK, Baker DG, Quesenberry P: Hematopoietic regulatory factors produced in long-term murine bone marrow cultures and the effect of *in vitro* irradiation. *Blood* 1984;64:516–525.
92. Greenberger TS, Palaszynsky EW, Pildci JH, et al.: Biological effects of prolonged L-phenylalanine mustard treatment of murine long-term bone marrow cultures and IL3 dependent hematopoietic progenitor cell lines. *J Natl Cancer Inst* 1985;74:247–262.
93. Ascensao JL, Vercelbotti GM, Jacob HS, Zanjani ED: Role of endothelial cells in human hematopoiesis; modulation of mixed colony growth *in vitro. Blood* 1985;63:553–558.
94. Sieff CA, Tsai S, Faller DV: Interleukin induced cultured human endothelial cell production of granulocyte-macrophage colony stimulating factor. *J Clin Invest* 1987;79:48–51.

95. Seelentag WK, Mermod JJ, Montesano R, Vassali P: Additive effects of interleukin-1 and tumor necrosis factor on the accumulation of the three granulocyte and macrophage colony stimulating factor m RNAs in human endothelial cells. *EMBO* 1987;6:2261–2265.

96. Zetter BR: The endothelial cells of large and small blood vessels. *Diabetes* 1981,30 (Suppl 2):24–28.

97. Luikart, SD, Sackrison JL, Maniglia CA: Bone marrow matrix modulation of HL-60 phenotype. *Blood* 1987;70:1119–1123.

98. Gordon MY, Riley GP, Watt SM, Greaves MF: Compartmentalization of hematopoietic growth factors (GM-CSF) by glycosaminoglycans in the bone marrow microenvironment. *Nature* 1987;326:403–405.

99. Campbell AD, Long MW, Wicha MS: Hæmonectin, a bone marrow adhesion protein specific for cells of granulocyte lineage. *Nature* 1987;329:744–746.

100. Storb R, Thomas ED, Weiden PL, et al.: Aplastic anemia treated by allogeneic bone marrow transplantation; a report on 49 new cases from Seattle. *Blood* 1976;48:817–841.

101. Gale RP, Feig S, Ho W, et al.: ABO blood group system and bone marrow transplantation. *Blood* 1977;50:185–194.

102. Blacklock HA, Gilmore M, Prentice HG, et al.: ABO incompatible bone marrow transplantation; removal of red blood cells from donor marrow avoiding recipient antibody depletion. *Lancet* 1982;ii:1061–1064.

103. Sieff C, Bicknell D, Caine G, et al.: Changes in cell surface antigen expression during hemopoietic differentiation. *Blood* 1982;60:703–713.

104. Storb R, Weiden PL: Transfusion problems associated with transplantation. *Semin Hematol* 1981;18:163–176.

105. Ho WG, Champlin RE, Feig SA, Gale RP: Transplantation of ABH incompatible bone marrow; gravity sedimentation of donor marrow. *Br J Hæmatol* 1984;57:155–162.

106. Falkenburg JHF, Schaafsma MR, Jansen T, et al.: Recovery of hematopoiesis after blood group incompatible bone marrow transplantation with red blood cell depleted grafts. *Transplantation* 1984;39:514–520.

107. Minchinton RM, Waters AH: Autoimmune thrombocytopenia and neutropenia after bone marrow transplantation. *Blood* 1985;66:752–755.

108. First LR, Smith BR, Lipton J, et al.: Isolated thrombocytopenia after allogeneic bone marrow transplantation; existence of transient and chronic thrombocytopenia syndrome. *Blood* 1985;65:368–371.

109. Minchinton RM, Waters AH, Malpas JS, et al.: Selective thrombocytopenia and neutropenia occurring after bone marrow transplantation; evidence of an autoimmune basis. *Clin Lab Hematol* 1984;6:157–164.

110. Spruce W, Forman S, McMillan R, et al.: Idiopathic thrombocytopenic purpura following bone marrow transplantation. *Acta Hematol* 1983;69:47–52.

111. Atkinson K, Norrie S, Chan P, et al.: Hemopoietic progenitor cell function after HLA-identical sibling bone marrow transplantation. Influence of chronic graft-vs.-host disease. *Int J Cell Cloning* 1986;4:203–220.

112. Noel DR, Witherspoon RP, Storb R, et al.: Does graft-vs.-host disease influence the tempo of immunologic recovery after allogeneic human marrow transplantation? An observation of 56 long-term survivors. *Blood* 1978;51:1087–1105.

113. Hows TM, Haffaf S, Palmer S, et al.: Regeneration of peripheral blood cells following allogeneic bone marrow transplantation for severe aplastic anemia. *Br J Hematol* 1982;52:551–557.

114. Young NS, Mortimer PP, Moore JG, Humphries RK: Characterization of a virus that causes transient aplastic crisis. *J Clin Invest* 1984;73:224–230.

115. Verdonck, LF, Van Heugten H, de Gast GC: Delay in platelet recovery after bone marrow transplantation. Impact of cytomegalovirus infection. *Blood* 1985;66:921–925.

116. Lawler SD, Baker MC, Harris H, Morgenstern GR: Cytogenetic studies on recipient of allogeneic bone marrow using sex chromosomes as markers of cellular origin. *Br J Hæmatol* 1984;56:431–443.

117. Failkow PJ, Bryant JI, Thomas ED, Neiman PE: Leukemic transformation of engrafted human marrow cells *in vivo. Lancet* 1971;1:251–255.

118. Goh K, Klemperer I: *In vivo* leukemic transformation; cytogenetic evidence of *in vivo* leukemic transformation of engrafted marrow cells. *Am J Hematol* 1977;2:283–290.

119. Newburger PE, Latt SA, Pesando JM, et al.: Leukemic relapse in donor cells after allogeneic bone marrow transplantation. *N Engl J Med* 1981;304:712–714.
120. Hill RS, Petersen FB, Storb R, et al.: Mixed hematologic chimerism after allogeneic marrow transplantation for severe aplastic anemia is associated with a higher risk of graft rejection and a lessened incidence of acute graft-vs.-host disease. *Blood* 1986;67:811–816.
121. Bertheas MF, Mascret B, Maraninchi D, et al.: Cytogenetic evidence of partial chimerism after T cell-depleted allogeneic bone marrow transplantation in leukemic HLA-matched patients. *Transplant Proc* 1987;19:2738–2740.
122. Lee MS, Chang KS, Cabanillas F, et al.: Detection of minimal residual cells carrying the t(14;18) by DNA sequence amplification. *Science* 1987;237:175–178.
123. Yam PY, Petz LD, Knowlton RG, et al.: Use of DNA restriction fragment length polymorphisms to document marrow engraftment and mixed hematopoietic chimerism following bone marrow transplantation. *Transplantation* 1987;43:399–407.
124. Knowlton RG, Brown VA, Braman JC, et al.: Use of highly polymorphic DNA probes for genotypic analysis following bone marrow transplantation. *Blood* 1986;68:378–383.
125. Jeffreys AJ, Wilson V, Thein SL: Hypervariable minisatellite regions in human DNA. *Nature* 1985;314:67–70.
126. Ginsberg D, Antin JH, Smith BR, et al.: Origin of cell populations after bone marrow transplantation; analysis using DNA sequence polymorphism. *J Clin Invest* 1985;75:596–602.
127. Blazar BR, Orr HT, Arthur DC, et al.: Restriction fragment length polymorphisms as markers of engraftment in allogeneic marrow transplantation. *Blood* 1985;66:1436–1441.
128. Keating A, Singer JW, Killen PD, et al.: Donor origin of the *in vitro* hematopoietic microenvironment after marrow transplantation in man. *Nature* 1982;298:280–283.
129. Singer JW, Keating A, Cuttner T, et al.: Evidence for a stem cell common to hematopoiesis and its *in vitro* microenvironment; studies of patients with clonal hematopoietic neoplasia. *Leuk Res* 1984;8:535–545.
130. Simmons PJ, Przepioska D, Thomas GD, Torok-Storb B: Host origin of marrow stromal cells following allogeneic bone marrow transplantation. *Nature* 1987;328:429–432.
131. Ma DDF, Da WM, Purvis-Smith S, Biggs JC: Chromosomal analysis of bone marrow stromal fibroblasts in allogeneic HLA-compatible sibling bone marrow transplantations. *Leuk Res* 1987;11:661–663.
132. deAlarcon PA, Schmieder TA: Megakaryocyte colony stimulating activity in serum from patients undergoing bone marrow transplantation. *Progr Clin Biol Res* 1986;215:335–340.
133. Kanamaru A, Okamoto T, Matsuda K, et al.: Elevation of erythroid colony stimulating activity in the serum of mice with graft-vs.-host disease. *Exp Hematol* 1984;12:763–767.
134. Metcalf D, Begley CG, Johnson GR: Hemopoietic effects of purified bacterially synthesized multi-CSF in normal and marrow transplanted mice. *Immunobiology* 1986;172:158–167.
135. Donahue RE, Wang EA, Stone DK, et al.: Stimulation of hematopoiesis in primates by continuous infusion of recombinant human GM-CSF. *Nature* 1986;321:872–875.
136. Brandt SJ, Kurtzberg J, Atwater SK, et al.: Effect of recombinant human granulocyte-macrophage colony stimulating factor (rHuGM-CSF) on hematopoietic reconstitution following high-dose chemotherapy and autologous bone marrow transplantation (ABMT). *Blood* 1987; 70 (suppl 1);378 (abstr).
137. Link H, Freund M, et al.: Recombinant human granulocyte-macrophage colony stimulating factor (rhGM-CSF): preliminary results in patients following bone marrow transplantation. *Blood* 1987;70 (Suppl 1):1094 (Abstr).
138. Ma DDF: Unpublished observations, 1987.

List of Abbreviations

BMT   bone marrow transplantation
HLA   histocompatible leukocyte antigen
CFU-S   colony forming unit—spleen
CFU-GM   granulocytes-macrophages colony forming unit (myeloid progenitor cells)

CFU-Mix	or CFU-GEMM, granulocytes-erythrocytes-macrophages-megakaryocytes colony forming unit (multipotent progenitor cells)
BFU-E	Burst forming unit—erythrocytes (early erythroid progenitor cells)
CFU-E	colony forming unit—erythrocytes (late erythroid progenitor cells)
CFU-Mk	colony forming unit—megakaryocytes
CSFs	colony stimulating factors
CFU-F	colony forming unit—fibroblasts
LTC	Dexter long-term bone marrow culture
Ils	interleukins
HGFs	hematopoietic growth factors
GVHD	graft-vs.-host disease
CD3	cluster of differentiation antigen number 3
RFLP	restriction fragment length polymorphism

Bone Marrow Transplantation in
Children, edited by F. Leonard Johnson
and Carl Pochedly. Raven Press, Ltd.,
New York © 1990.

Pathology of Bone Marrow Transplantation

*John E. Wagner, *Andrew M. Yeager, and
**William E. Beschorner

*Departments of Oncology and Pediatrics and **Pathology and Oncology, The Johns
Hopkins University School of Medicine, Baltimore, Maryland 21205

Since the first human bone marrow transplants were performed in the late 1950s, mainly in patients with end-stage leukemia, much clinical and scientific knowledge has been acquired. There are organ toxicities related to the various preparative regimens. Other complications, such as post-transplant infections, interstitial pneumonitis, and acute and chronic graft-vs.-host disease (GVHD), have been documented and studied (1–4). The major advances that have occurred since the inception of clinical trials on the use of this modality are, in part, due to a better understanding of the pathology of bone marrow transplantation (BMT).

Numerous complications related to bone marrow transplantation occur after a variable period of time following the preparative therapy and marrow infusion (5,6). Although the complications are frequently interrelated and occur simultaneously, each complication will be discussed in the order in which it usually occurs. In this chapter, we will focus on both the gross and microscopic tissue changes associated with the various disease processes.

TOXICITIES OF THE PRE-TRANSPLANT PREPARATIVE REGIMENS

High-dose chemotherapy and total body irradiation (TBI) are administered to the bone marrow transplant recipient before marrow infusion. This is done for 3 reasons: (1) to suppress the host immune system sufficiently to allow engraftment, (2) to make "space" for the new graft, and (3) in the case of cancer, to eradicate the primary disease. Most preparative regimens for marrow transplantation employ high-dose cyclophosphamide (7). This drug is given either alone or in combination with TBI or another chemotherapeutic agent, such as busulfan. Such intensive therapy is both immunosuppressive and myelosuppressive. In addition, each of the agents and/or modalities employed has well-known toxicities and pathological effects on extramedullary tissues.

Cyclophosphamide

At high doses (over 200 mg/kg), cyclophosphamide has been associated with hemorrhagic myocardial necrosis, which is the dose-limiting toxicity of this alkylating agent (8–10). With the doses of cyclophosphamide now being used in bone marrow transplantation, the frequency of myocardial necrosis is low. Hemorrhagic cystitis, however, is noted frequently but with variable severity (11). This complication is apparently due to the direct irritation of the mucosal cells by cyclophosphamide metabolites, such as acrolein. Toxicity to the bladder may be minimized by forced diuresis or by the administration of sulfhydryl-containing compounds, such as acetylcysteine or MESNA (12,13).

Ulceration of the bladder mucosa with presence of overlying fibrin and blood clots, as well as thickening and trabeculation of the bladder wall, have all been observed (Figure 1). Moreover, hemorrhages and edema have been noted on histologic examination of the lamina propria and muscularis mucosa of the bladder after giving high doses of cyclophosphamide. In the absence of gross hemorrhage, microscopic alterations, such as telangiectasias, atypia of mesenchymal cells in the lamina propria, and desquamation and atypia of bladder epithelial cells are frequently observed. Cytological examination of the urine sediment may reveal enlargement of the nuclei and nucleoli, as well as presence of multinucleate cells, karyorrhexia and vacuolization of the cytoplasm in the exfoliated urothelial cells.

Hemorrhagic cystitis in the post-marrow-transplant period, however, is not exclusively caused by cyclophosphamide. Similar cytopathological changes are seen after irradiation of the bladder. Furthermore, viral agents, such as adenovirus and papovavirus (14–16), have been implicated in cases of hemor-

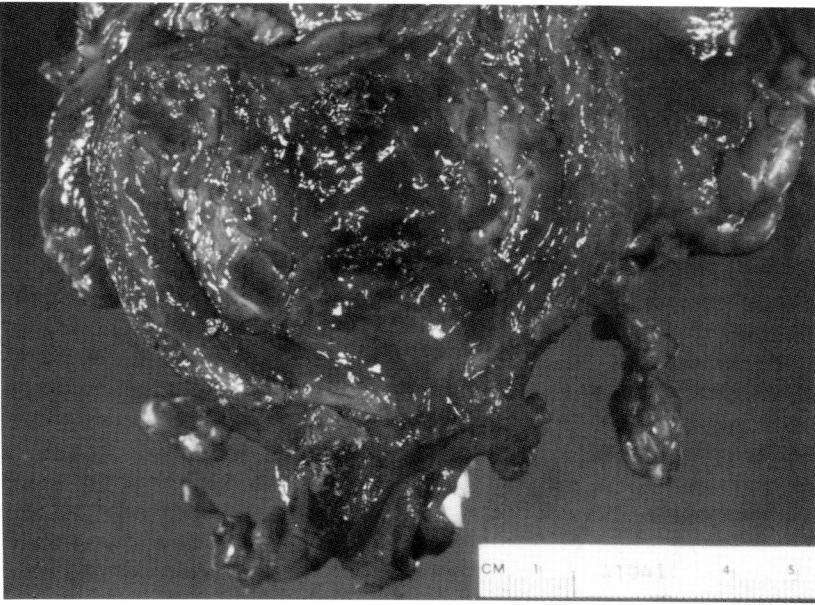

FIG. 1. Hemorrhagic cystitis related to high-dose cyclophosphamide. Urethral opening in the lower section. Note the extensive submucosal hemorrhage in the bladder.

rhagic cystitis; however, this occurs later in the post-transplant period. Viral cultures of the urine and viral detection methods such as enzyme-linked immunosorbent assays (ELISAs) may therefore be useful in delineating the etiology of this condition.

High-dose cyclophosphamide has been associated with a noninflammatory toxic vasculitis characterized by destruction of the muscularis with "moth-eaten" changes, fibrinoid necrosis, and telangiectases of venules and capillaries. This generalized vasculitis usually occurs within 3 weeks of cyclophosphamide administration. A toxic vasculitis may be responsible for the syndrome of fluid retention, pulmonary edema without cardiac failure, prerenal azotemia, and respiratory distress: the so-called capillary leak syndrome. This syndrome has been observed in patients receiving cyclophosphamide as part of the preparative regimen prior to bone marrow transplant (10,17).

Cyclophosphamide is also highly toxic to the gonadal tissues or gonads (18,19). After the administration of high-dose cyclophosphamide to males, there is significant depletion of germ cells of the testes, with a relative sparing of the seminiferous tubules, Leydig cells, and Sertoli cells. Similarly, cyclophosphamide given to postpubertal, premenopausal females results in a loss of primordial and mature ovarian follicles (20). Whether prepubertal gonads demonstrate similar sensitivity to cyclophosphamide is not known at this time.

Total body irradiation

Total body irradiation (TBI) is probably the single most effective immuno-suppressive conditioning regimen currently available (21), but there are numerous toxicities associated with its administration. These toxic effects are dependent on both the total dose of TBI administered and the rate of delivery of irradiation. Moreover, analysis of pathological alterations after TBI in bone marrow transplant recipients is complicated by several additional factors. Factors that complicate analysis of toxicity of TBI include inter-institutional variability in the doses and dose rates, as well as use of other chemotherapeutic modalities, such as cyclophosphamide, cytosine arabinoside, and etoposide, used in the preparative regimens.

The immediate side effects of total body irradiation include nausea, vomiting, diarrhea and hypotension. Like cyclophosphamide, the short-term effects of TBI include a generalized capillary leak syndrome, the adult respiratory distress syndrome (ARDS), and hypotension.

The late effects of TBI in bone marrow transplant recipients have been the focus of several reviews (18,22–27). Total body irradiation has been associated with the occurrence of cataracts, both restrictive and obstructive lung disease, as well as interstitial pneumonitis and leukoencephalopathy. Also, gonadal failure, short stature, and a multitude of endocrinopathies that include compensated and overt hypothyroidism and growth hormone deficiency may occur. TBI has been shown to produce primary gonadal failure in all patients who were postpubertal at the time of marrow transplantion. In one study, many of the children undergoing marrow transplant before puberty had irreversible gonadal damage. However, a small number of girls achieved menarche and some boys had normal (although delayed) gonadotrophin levels. Although growth retardation in these children is probably multifactorial, in etiology, total body irradiation may especially contribute to low growth hormone levels and epiphyseal injury.

We are now comparing the late effects of preparative regimens containing TBI with those containing no TBI in patients we have treated. While children receiving both cyclophosphamide and TBI have a blunted growth velocity and decreased final height, children receiving busulfan and cyclophosphamide demonstrate normal growth (88).

Busulfan

A bifunctional alkylating agent that is especially toxic to hematopoietic stem cells, busulfan induces fatal aplasia when given at high doses (over 15 mg/kg) (28,29). Pulmonary interstitial fibrosis, atypia of bronchiolar and alveolar epithelial cells, and hyperplasia of type II pneumatocytes may be seen after chronic administration of low doses of busulfan for treatment of chronic myelogenous leukemia (30,31). However, pulmonary fibrosis directly attributable to high-dose busulfan has not been verified in a study of over 100 patients given preparative therapy consisting of busulfan and cyclophosphamide before marrow transplant for treatment of acute nonlymphocytic leukemia. It is not known whether busulfan may contribute to the development of idiopathic interstitial pneumonitis (IP), which is a well-recognized complication related to marrow transplantation. The incidence of interstitial pneumonitis, however, is no higher in patients prepared with a busulfan containing regimen when compared to a regimen not containing busulfan. Indeed, 14 of 15 patients who developed interstitial pneumonitis after allogeneic bone marrow transplantation with use of a preparative regimen consisting of busulfan and cyclophosphamide also had evidence for disseminated viral infection, principally cytomegalovirus (CMV) or adenovirus (32).

At high doses, busulfan can cause hyperpigmentation of the skin, particularly in the intertiginous folds (33). On skin biopsy, there is an increased number of melanocytes and large mononuclear cells in the dermis. Furthermore, busulfan, like cyclophosphamide, causes destruction of spermatogonia and ovarian follicles with preservation of accessory gonadal cells (89). Hepatic abnormalities have also been reported with high-dose busulfan, including obliteration of the central vein lumen due to intimal fibrosis, centrilobular sinusoidal fibrosis with hepatocellular necrosis, and atrophy (34).

It has recently been suggested that patients with high serum levels of busulfan are significantly more likely to develop hepatic veno-occlusive disease (VOD).[90] However, the histopathological changes of sinusoidal scarring, hepatocellular damage, and centrilobular bile stasis that are consistent with high-dose busulfan are atypical features of veno-occlusive disease. These histopathological alterations associated with busulfan appear to be dose-dependent. Similar hepatic changes have been described after the administration of cytosine arabinoside and 6-thioguanine.

HEPATIC VENO-OCCLUSIVE DISEASE

Hepatic dysfunction after allogeneic bone marrow transplantation is common and may be due to many factors. Veno-occlusive disease, however, is a particular syndrome that is most commonly seen after marrow transplantation, although it may occur in patients receiving immunosuppressive agents in other clinical situations. Signs and symptoms of veno-occlusive disease appear within the first 21 days after bone marrow transplantation. The incidence of veno-occlusive disease may be as high as 22% with a mortality rate of 47%. At Johns Hopkins, hepatic veno-occlusive disease is the third leading cause of death in patients given allogeneic marrow transplants, and the second leading cause of death in patients given autologous marrow transplants (35). At the present time, there is no specific therapy for this complication. Supportive care usually consists of giving diuretic drugs and may include lactulose, heparinization, and protein restriction.

Veno-occlusive disease is characterized by hyperbilirubinemia with serum bilirubin above 2 mg/dl. There is ascites, weight gain (with weight increase of more than 5% above baseline), presence of a liver that is enlarged and tender to palpation, and refractoriness to platelet transfusions (35). Encephalopathy and azotemia are also common manifestations. A definite diagnosis can usually be made by clinical criteria alone. Because of the associated thrombocytopenia and impairment of coagulation, liver biopsies are routinely done. Histopathological examination of tissue obtained either from biopsy or at autopsy demonstrates concentric subintimal thickening and luminal narrowing of the terminal hepatic venules and small sublobular veins by either reticulin or collagen fibers (Figure 2). Atrophy of the perivenular hepatocytes, centrilobular necrosis, dilation of portal veins and sinusoids, and angiomatous dilation of portal venules and lymphatics have all been reported as being features of veno-occlusive disease (34,36,37). It is of interest that

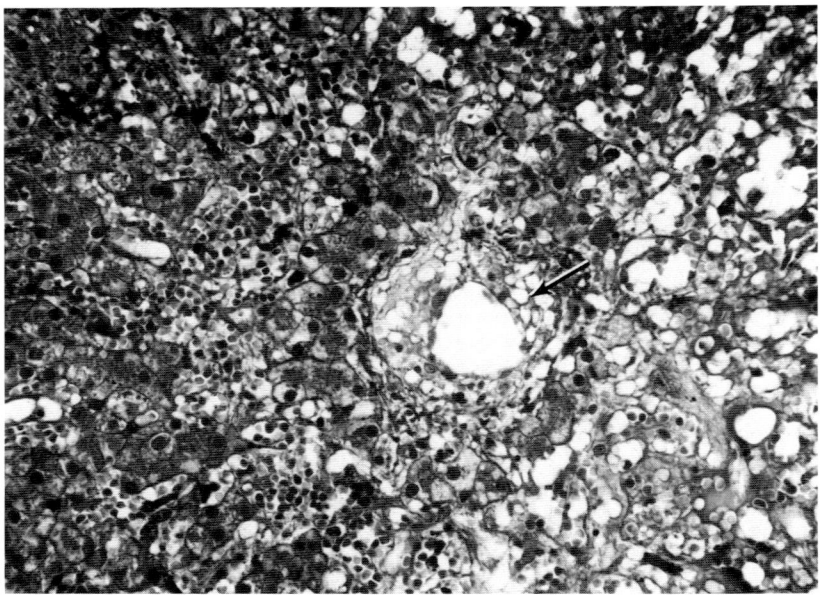

FIG. 2. Hepatic veno-occlusive disease. The terminal central veins have increased fibrosis with partial obliteration of the lumen (arrow). The surrounding centrilobular region shows hepatocellular necrosis and sinusoidal fibrosis. (Masson trichrome stain, ×250.)

studies have demonstrated that the intraluminal fibers are not fibrin or fibrinogen. This finding makes veno-occlusive disease an entity distinct from the Budd-Chiari syndrome, in which thrombus formation is the primary event. The histopathological changes noted in veno-occlusive disease are distinct from those of hepatic graft-vs.-host disease.

At least 2 factors contribute to the development of veno-occlusive disease. These are: (1) high-dose cytoreductive chemotherapy, and (2) a history of hepatitis preceding bone marrow transplantation. Veno-occlusive disease is relatively uncommon in patients undergoing marrow transplant for aplastic anemia or for genetic or immunodeficiency diseases. We were not able to show any differences in either the frequency or outcome of the disease to be associated with age. However, McDonald and colleagues (38) noted that patients under the age of 15 years had a decreased risk of veno-occlusive disease. Furthermore, patients with acute leukemia in first remission were found to be in a low risk category.

Chemoradiotherapy in the treatment of malignancy prior to bone marrow transplantation may be a significant contributing factor in the occurrence of veno-occlusive disease although such an association is not yet clearly defined. The centrilobular region appears to be the major site of injury in this disease. Perhaps the high concentrations of active cytotoxic metabolites in the pericentral zone of the liver lobules lead to hepatocyte damage and endothelial alterations. Active hepatitis may then further alter the metabolism and/or clearance of the antineoplastic agents and thus increase the risk of veno-occlusive disease.

OBLITERATIVE BRONCHIOLITIS

Interstitial pneumonitis is a well-recognized complication of bone marrow transplantation and is discussed in detail in chapter 22. Unlike interstitial pneumonitis, which generally occurs early, less than 100 days after bone marrow transplantation, obliterative bronchiolitis occurs late (39,40). Symptoms include progressive dyspnea, wheezing and cough. Chest x-rays may be completely normal or may demonstrate signs of hyperinflation, hyperlucencies consistent with bleb formation, interstitial pneumatosis, pneumothorax, or pneumomediastinum. Functional studies reveal a reduced expiratory flow rate, reduced vital capacity, and increased residual lung volume, findings which are all consistent with obstructive small airway disease. Unlike the chronic obstructive lung diseases, obliterative bronchiolitis is acute in onset and rapidly progressive.

Histopathological findings in this late-onset obstructive airway disease are best seen in the terminal bronchioles, where lymphocytic and mononuclear cell infiltrates and hyperplasia of bronchiolar smooth muscle may be noted. Transmural or focal necrosis of bronchioles and bronchi are present. The most

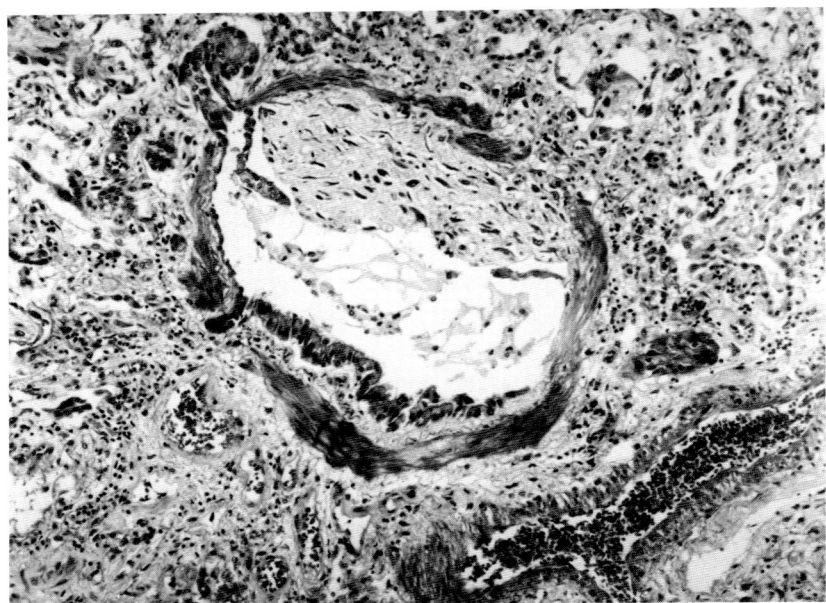

FIG. 3.   Obliterative bronchiolitis. The lumen of this small bronchiole is partially obliterated by submucosal granulation tissue and fibrosis. (Hematoxylin and eosin stain, ×110.)

striking feature is the intraluminal accumulation of inflammatory cells, fibroblasts and fibrin, which can completely occlude the bronchioles (Figure 3). Mucus plugging, together with atelectasis or emphysema of distal air spaces, may be present. Hyperplasia of bronchial mucus glands and destruction of alveoli, as seen in chronic bronchitis or emphysema, are absent in cases of obliterative bronchiolitis. Although focal interstitial inflammatory reactions may occur, the intensity and extent of these changes are minimal. In contrast, such lesions are extensive in interstitial pneumonitis.

Immunosuppression, alterations in immunoregulation, or both, may predispose patients to the development of obliterative bronchiolitis (41,42). Antecedent or coexistent chronic graft-vs.-host disease, a syndrome of immune dysregulation, is common in patients who develop obliterative bronchiolitis. Currently there is no specific therapy for this disorder. High-dose steroid therapy has been effective in reversing or stabilizing disease progression. The addition of bronchodilators or other immunosuppressive agents has been of little benefit.

INTERSTITIAL PNEUMONITIS

Interstitial pneumonitis (IP) occurs in approximately 40% of patients undergoing bone marrow transplantation and is fatal in about 60% of cases (32). The median time to onset of interstitial pneumonitis is 40 to 55 days post-marrow transplant, with the vast majority occurring between day 30 and day 100. Early-onset interstitial pneumonitis (at less than 100 days post-transplant) appears to differ in etiology and prognosis from late-onset type of the disease (cases appearing over 100 days following marrow transplant). Cases that appear in the first 4 weeks after bone marrow transplantation may represent acute alveolitis secondary to toxicity due to drugs and radiation (22,43,44). Interstitial pneumonitis occurring in the second 2 months, however, is usually caused by infection; cytomegalovirus (CMV) is the agent most often identified in these cases (45–49). Interstitial pneumonitis diagnosed after day 100 represents a minority of the cases (only 6%), but it is the second most common cause of death in patients surviving for more than 100 days after marrow transplant, being second only to leukemic relapse (32).

The etiologic agents responsible for interstitial pneumonitis include CMV, adenovirus, Herpes simplex virus, Varicella-zoster virus, *Pneumocystis carinii*, Mycoplasma, and Legionella. Yet, many cases of interstitial pneumonitis (at least 45%) are idiopathic in origin. The disease is characterized by diffuse bilateral interstitial infiltrates on chest x-ray. The disease may be rapidly progressive or it may follow an indolent course. The diagnosis is made by examination of lung tissue, obtained either by open lung biopsy, transbronchial biopsy or bronchial lavage (49–51). Tissue should be sent for culture (including bacterial, viral, mycobacterial, and fungal cultures), as well as for histopathologic examination.

Histologic examination typically reveals a mononuclear cell infiltrate in the interstitial space (Figure 4). Bacteria, fungi, and viral inclusions can usually be identified by special stains. Legionella, however, can often be identified by fluorescein-conjugated monoclonal antibodies. Diagnosis of the idiopathic type of interstitial pneumonitis is one of exclusion. This form of the disease may represent a delayed complication of chemoradiotherapy. The incidence of idiopathic interstitial pneumonitis is no different whether total body irradiation is given or not (51). Although interstitial pneumonitis occurs more frequently after allogeneic bone marrow transplantation, it has been noted to occur also after autologous and syngeneic marrow transplants.

GRAFT-VS.-HOST DISEASE

Graft-vs.-host disease (GVHD) continues to be a prominent cause of morbidity and mortality in human allogeneic bone marrow transplant recipients. Although patients and donors are matched for antigens of the major histocompatibility complex (MHC), it is thought that differences in minor histocompatibility antigens account for the disease (1,2,5,6). Clinically significant acute graft-vs.-host disease develops in 35 to 50% of patients receiving MHC-matched marrow within the first 100 days after marrow transplant. Of these patients, about 50% will die of GVH disease or from therapy-related

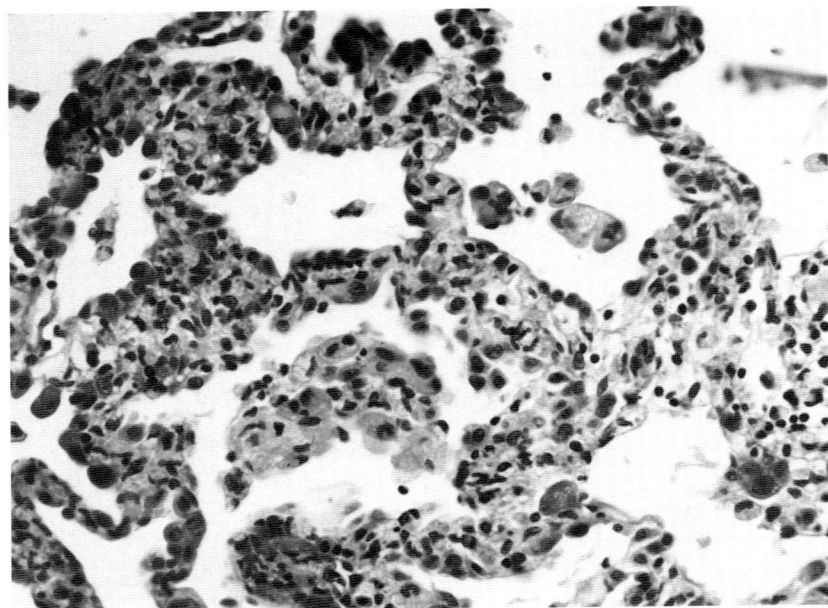

FIG. 4. Idiopathic interstitial pneumonitis. The alveolar septae are thickened with increased edema and fibrosis. There is hyperplasia of the type II alveolar cells and a variable amount of lymphocytic infiltration. (Hematoxylin and eosin stain, ×250.)

complications (52–55). Chronic graft-vs.-host disease, however, is characteristically a late complication. It develops 100 to 500 days after bone marrow transplantation. Chronic GVH disease affects about 45% of all long-term marrow transplant survivors (56–58).

Acute Graft-vs.-Host Disease

Acute graft-vs.-host disease is a complex clinical syndrome which is caused by an immunologic attack by donor T lymphocytes against host tissues. In addition, there are infectious complications due to the impaired immune response of the marrow transplant recipient. The principal target organs of acute GVH disease are the skin, liver, gastrointestinal tract, and lungs. Fever, rash, diarrhea, and dysfunction of the liver are the usual manifestations of the disease. Various systems for clinical and histopathological staging and grading of acute GVH disease have been devised (55).

Skin. On examination, cutaneous acute GVH disease may range from a mild maculopapular eruption to generalized erythroderma with formation of bullae and denudation of the epidermis. Differentiation of cutaneous acute graft-vs.-host disease from other processes, such as drug-induced eruptions and viral-associated exanthems, is often difficult by physical examination alone. Punch biopsy with excision of a piece of involved skin 4 mm in diameter will reveal focal vacuolar degeneration and perivenular lymphocytic infiltrates of the epidermal basal cell layer in mild acute GVH disease. In more advanced disease, dyskeratotic epidermal cells and a more extensive vacuolar degeneration may be noted (Figure 5). Severe cutaneous dermatopathologic changes characteristic of acute GVH disease include dermal-epidermal separation and frank loss of epidermal tissue (59,60).

Liver. Multiple factors may contribute to hepatic dysfunction in bone marrow transplant recipients. These contributing factors include drug-induced hepatic abnormalities, infections, parenteral hyperalimentation, and extrahepatic obstruction. As indicated earlier, hepatic veno-occlusive disease may cause mild elevations in hepatic transaminases (35). Differentiation between liver disease due to acute GVH disease and that due to other causes is often difficult on clinical grounds alone. Laboratory tests are not consistently diagnostic. Therefore, liver biopsy is especially helpful in the management of patients with hepatic disease associated with marrow transplant (34).

Histopathological changes of acute GVH disease include mild lymphocytic infiltration of the portal triads, with inflammation and necrosis of the small

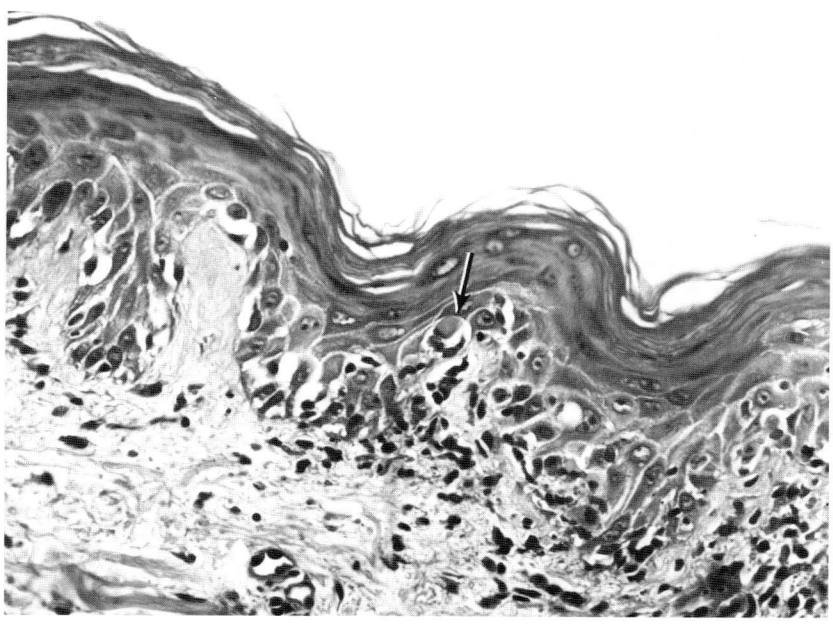

FIG. 5. Acute graft-vs.-host disease of the skin. The basal epithelium has a moderate infiltrate of lymphocytes with associated vacuolization of the basal cells and dyskeratotic cells (arrow). (Hematoxylin and eosin stain, ×250.)

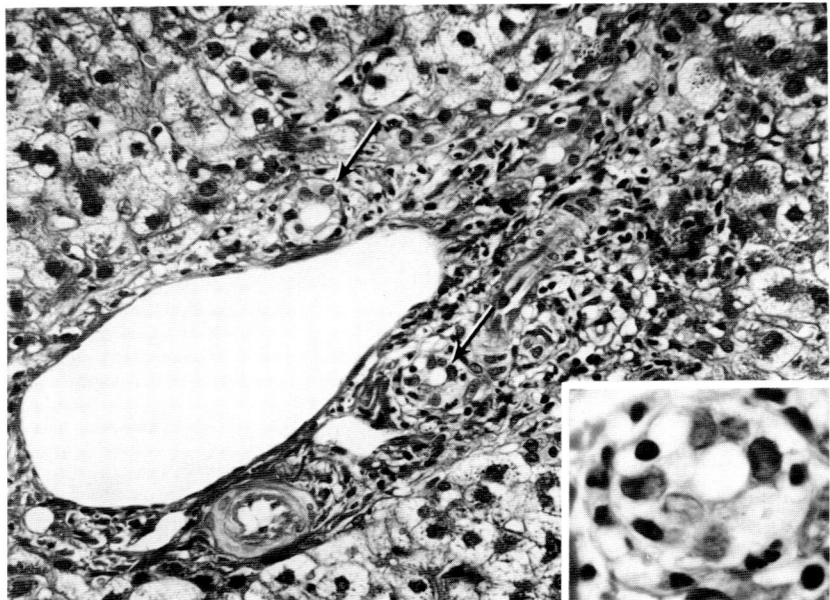

FIG. 6.   Acute graft-vs.-host disease of the liver. There is a moderate infiltrate of lymphocytes confined to the portal triads. Active GVH disease is indicated by the presence of lymphocytes within the bile duct basement membrane, associated with vacuolization and injury of the epithelium (arrows and inset). (Hematoxylin and eosin stain, ×250; inset, ×500.)

bile ducts (Figure 6). The injury is recognized by vacuolization, cellular debris and cytologic atypia of the duct epithelium. The epithelial changes remain long after other manifestations of GVH disease have resolved. Bile stasis and epithelial atypia alone, therefore, do not differentiate between active and residual GVH disease. The presence of lymphocytes within the duct basement membrane may be helpful in identifying active graft-vs.-host processes in the liver (61,62).

Gastrointestinal tract. Cramping abdominal pain and secretory diarrhea are the initial clinical manifestations of acute graft-vs.-host disease of the gastrointestinal tract. With progressive disease, there may be denudation of the mucosal layer, resulting in bloody diarrhea. Clinical staging of the gastrointestinal form of acute GVH disease is based on the volume of diarrhea. Diarrhea in these patients is certainly not diagnostic of GVH disease (63). The pre-BMT preparative therapy is a common cause of diarrhea occurring within the first 3 weeks after allogeneic bone marrow transplantation. Viral pathogens (such as enterovirus, adenovirus or rotavirus), bacterial pathogens (such as E. *coli,* Campylobacter, or *Clostridium difficile*) and protozoal organisms (such as *Giardia lamblia*) may also lead to enteritis in marrow transplant recipients (64).

The usefulness of radiographic studies (such as computed axial tomography and barium studies) to differentiate between acute GVH disease and infectious etiologies of diarrhea associated with marrow transplant is controversial (65). Examination of the gut following ingestion of barium may reveal a rapid transit time, a tubular appearance of the small and large intestine due to loss of mucosal folds, and "thumbprint" thickening of the bowel wall in patients with acute GVH disease. Pneumatosis cystoides intestinalis has also been observed (66). These findings are not specific for graft-vs.-host disease but may be useful adjuncts in following the response to therapy. Bowel biopsy is the most effective technique to establish the diagnosis of acute GVH disease in the gastrointestinal tract. Tissue samples may be obtained by small-bowel capsule biopsy, but rectal biopsy may provide similar information with a lower risk to the patient (67).

Signs of cutaneous GVH disease usually precede the onset of diarrhea by about one week. In the more severe cases, stool volume may approach 25 liters/day and consist of blood and sheets of sloughed mucosa. The gross appearance of the bowel depends on the severity and duration of graft-vs.-host disease. Sigmoidoscopy during the early stages of acute GVH disease may reveal little or no edema or inflammation, and only focal ulceration of the mucosa. Findings in more advanced forms of gastrointestinal acute GVH disease may include complete mucosal denudation, large ulcers, and edema and hemorrhage of the bowel wall.

Histopathological alterations are most striking in the terminal ileum, while the stomach tends to be only minimally affected. Histological studies of the small intestine and rectum demonstrate characteristic apoptotic crypt lesions. These lesions represent foci of necrosis and contain nuclear and cytoplasmic debris. Apoptotic lesions are most frequently found at the base of the crypts (Figure 7). Similar lesions in the gastrointestinal mucosa on occasion may be seen within the first 3 weeks after marrow transplantation. These lesions probably represent toxic effects of the cytoreductive regimens. Actually, these histopathological alterations have also been observed in the gastrointestinal mucosa of patients receiving intensive combination chemotherapy for induction of remission in acute leukemia. However, the finding of apoptotic lesions in gut biopsy specimens obtained after the first 14 to 21 days following marrow transplant is characteristic of acute graft-vs.-host disease.

Other histopathological findings that have been associated with acute GVH disease of the gastrointestinal tract include crypt abscesses, edema, variable numbers of lymphocytes and a marked decrease in the numbers of plasma cells in the lamina propria. Although the magnitude of crypt loss and the extent of mucosal denudation have been used to assess the severity of gastrointestinal GVH disease, it is important to realize that these changes are not specific for acute GVH disease.

The specific pathogenetic mechanisms of acute gastrointestinal GVH disease remain controversial and have been reviewed at length (68). Briefly, the

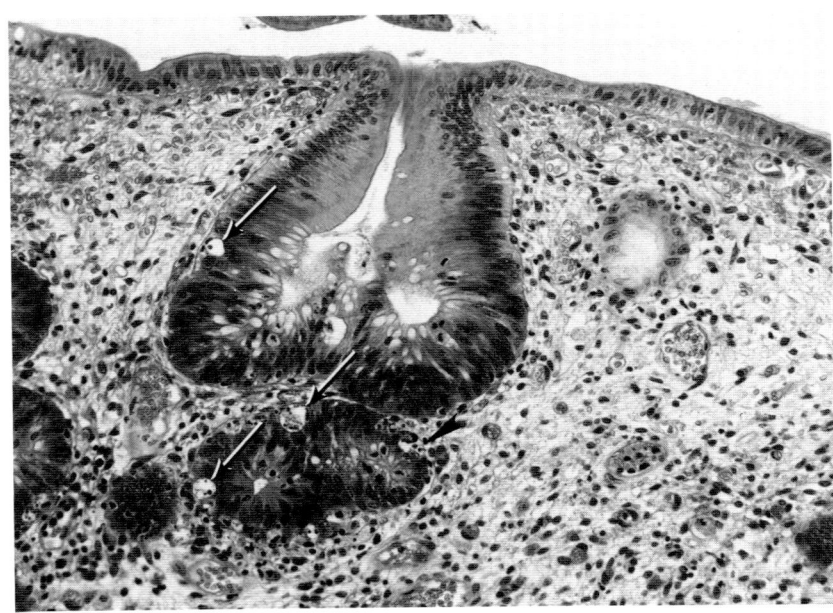

FIG. 7. Acute graft-vs.-host disease of the colon. The number of crypts is decreased. The lamina propria has numerous lymphocytes but few plasma cells. Multiple apoptotic lesions (arrows) are seen in the remaining crypts. (Hematoxylin and eosin stain, ×200.)

pathogenesis is based on 3 hypotheses: (1) the cytotoxic T lymphocytes in acute GVH disease interact directly with the intestinal epithelium (69); (2) the activity of these lymphocytes leads to the destruction of the leukocytes in the lamina propria with subsequent injury of the epithelium by infectious agents as an "innocent bystander" (70,71); and (3) acute graft-vs.-host disease leads to the depletion of plasma cells containing IgA and IgM (68). With a marked deficiency of intestinal immunity, the epithelium is then more vulnerable to injury by infectious agents. Intestinal microorganisms have long been recognized as a critical factor in the pathogenesis of intestinal GVH disease. Thus, experimental studies have shown that gnotobiotic rodents (that is animals raised in a controlled microbial environment) with the GVH reaction have minimal intestinal injury (172).

We believe that the mucosal sloughing results from both a deficiency of local intestinal immunity and the presence of epithelial injury associated with GVH disease. The apoptotic lesions are concentrated at the base of the crypts where most of the epithelial stem cells reside (68). As the surface epithelium is eliminated by intestinal microbes, crypt injury limits the regenerative capacity of the epithelium.

Jejunal and rectal biopsies are valuable in documenting acute GVH disease and may have additional value in prognosis. These biopsies reveal the presence or absence of apoptotic lesions that are characteristic of acute GVH disease. The biopsies also provide a means for evaluating residual intestinal immunity for detecting presence of intestinal infections, and assessing the regenerative capacity of the gut. For example, patients whose gut biopsies show the presence of increased mitotic figures, epithelial hyperplasia, and crypt distortion have significantly less diarrhea 3 weeks later (91).

Respiratory tract. Lymphocytic bronchitis is a pulmonary manifestation of acute GVH disease (72–75). The finding of cough and dyspnea that occurs 3 to 12 weeks after marrow transplant in patients previously diagnosed with graft-vs.-host disease are suggestive of pulmonary GVH disease. Although patients with lymphocytic bronchitis appear to have a higher incidence of interstitial pneumonitis, the two conditions are distinct and seem to have no cause-and-effect relationship. Lymphocytic bronchitis involves the larger bronchi, in contrast to obliterative bronchiolitis, which affects the terminal small airways. Lymphocytic infiltration of the mucosa, submucosa, and muscularis mucosa of proximal bronchi is observed (Figure 8).

Mucosal necrosis, loss of ciliated cells and a decrease in the number of goblet cells are all histopathological features of this disease. Because of the disruption in mucociliary clearance, it is not surprising that these patients are at high risk for symptomatic lower respiratory tract infections, such as bronchitis and bronchopneumonia. Animal models and clinical observations have

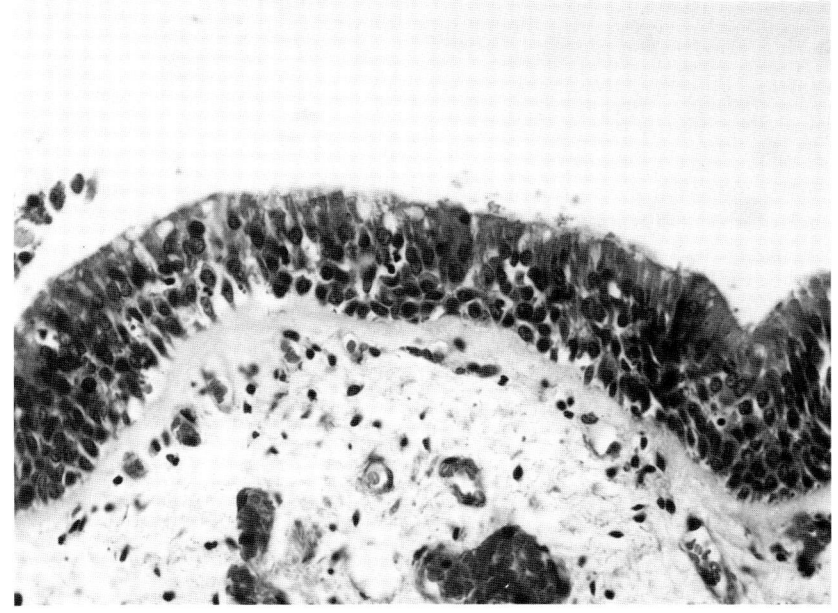

FIG. 8. Lymphocytic bronchitis in a bone marrow transplant patient with acute GVH disease. There is an infiltration of lymphocytes just beneath the basement membrane and within the mucosa. Many of the columnar cells have been injured. Elsewhere the mucosa has sloughed or has been replaced with squamous metaplasia. (Hematoxylin and eosin stain, ×250.)

recently shown that a similar pathologic process may take place in the proximal airways of patients with lung allografts which are being rejected after heart-lung transplantation (76,77).

Other organs. Ocular and oral lesions are most often associated with chronic graft-vs.-host disease, but may also be observed in patients with acute GVH reactions. For example, the "dry eye" syndrome, characteristically associated with chronic GVH disease, can also occur in acute GVH disease. In this setting, the dry eyes are most often secondary to stasis of flow of tears in the lacrimal glands (78,79), and may lead to corneal and conjunctival keratinization.

The oral mucosa is also commonly involved in acute GVH disease. Barrett and colleagues (80) describe 3 clinical patterns of oral acute GVH disease: (1) a fine papular exanthem, (2) a lichenoid or reticular eruption characterized by raised white striae, and (3) a desquamative process with exfoliation of whitish mucosal plaques.

Chronic Graft-vs.-Host Disease

Chronic GVH disease is a late complication of allogeneic bone marrow transplantation and typically occurs 3 to 6 months after transplantation. The incidence of chronic GVH disease appears to be in the range of 25 to 45% (56), with mortality as high as 80% when left untreated. Unlike acute graft-vs.-host disease, where there is an excess of cytotoxic donor-derived T lymphocytes, chronic GVH disease is immunologically characterized by an excess of nonspecific suppressor T cells (81). Clinically, chronic GVH disease is very similar to many connective tissue disorders. The organ systems primarily involved in chronic GVH disease are the integument, liver, gastrointestinal tract, and lungs (56). However, the eyes, oral mucosa, nasopharynx, and musculoskeletal system may also be affected. Moreover, there is a profound immunodeficiency associated with chronic graft-vs.-host disease. The impaired splenic function predisposes the patient to overwhelming sepsis by encapsulated microorganisms, such as *Streptococcus pneumoniae* and *Haemophilus influenzae*.

Skin. Cutaneous chronic GVH disease may present with poikiloderma, in which there is dermal atrophy that alternates with areas of telangiectasis and erythema, dermal sclerosis with contractures (similar to cutaneous scleroderma), and lichenoid papular lesions (especially on the palms and soles (82,83). The lichenoid phase of chronic graft-vs.-host disease usually precedes the sclerodermoid phase, although the phases may occur independently. End-stage cutaneous chronic GVH disease is characterized by progressive loss of skin elasticity, dermal atrophy, and fibrosis, hyperkeratosis, reticular hyperpigmentation, and limited joint mobility due to contractures. Periungual erythema, dystrophic nail changes, and persistent focal or generalized alopecia can occur.

The histopathological findings in lichenoid lesions of chronic GVH disease resemble those in idiopathic lichen planus (Figure 9A). There is hyperkeratosis, acanthosis, dyskeratosis, vacuolar alterations in the basal cell layer, and monocytic and lymphocytic infiltrates in the papillary dermis. The intensity of inflammation in lichenoid chronic GVH disease is less than that seen in idiopathic lichen planus. These lesions heal without dermal fibrosis or loss of elastic tissue.

In contrast, the sclerodermoid form of the disease is associated with sclerosis and thickening of the reticular dermis, loss of distinction between the papillary and reticular dermis, loss of rete pegs due to increased collagen deposition, and a mild perivascular lymphocytic infiltrate (Figure 9B). Characteristically, the sweat glands are infiltrated with lymphocytes, and melanophages may be seen in the subepidermal region. There is an increase in type III procollagen in the upper dermis, with a transition to type I procollagen in the later stages of disease (84). A similar process occurs in morphea but is limited to the lower reticular dermis and subcutis.

Liver. Liver involvement in chronic graft-vs.-host disease is associated with moderate elevations of alkaline phosphatase of the transaminases, and bili-

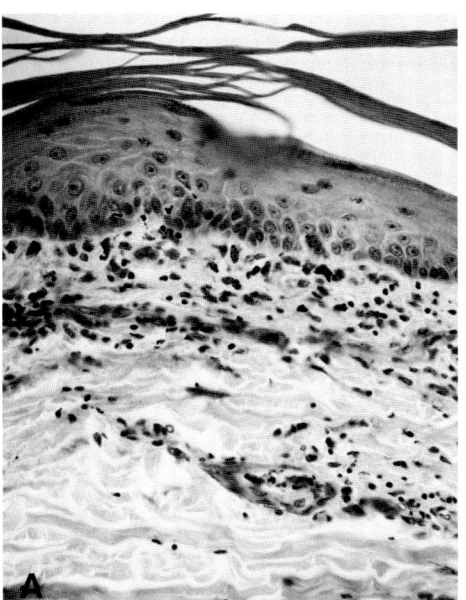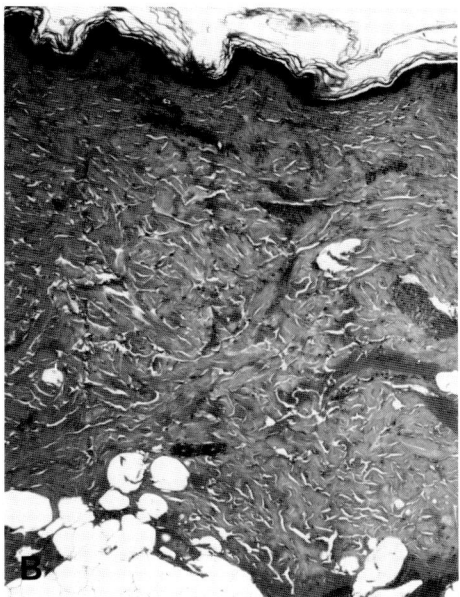

FIG. 9. Chronic cutaneous graft-vs.-host disease. A. Lichenoid form. In the early phase of chronic graft-vs.-host disease, the pattern resembles lichen planus with a bandlike infiltrate in the superficial dermis and variable acanthosis. In contrast to acute GVH disease (see Figure 5), there is little infiltration of the epidermis (hematoxylin and eosin stain, ×250). B. Sclerodermoid form. In the established phase, chronic graft-vs.-host disease resembles scleroderma with extension of the fibrosis into the subcutaneous fat, coarse fibrosis extending to the basal cell layer, and loss of the rete pegs and hair follicles. (Hematoxylin and eosin stain, ×50.)

rubin (56). The portal triads have a dense mixed infiltrate of lymphocytes and histocytes, and often there are also eosinophils and plasma cells. The infiltrate extends into the lobule with piecemeal necrosis. The bile ducts usually demonstrate lymphocyte-associated necrosis of the epithelium, and periportal bile stasis is prominent (Figure 10). There is increased portal fibrosis which can progress to micronodular cirrhosis. In long-standing cases, the triads have a decreased number or complete absence of ducts, leading to intrahepatic biliary atresia.

   Gastrointestinal tract. The gastrointestinal tract is involved less frequently and with less severity in chronic GVH disease than it is in acute GVH disease. Esophageal reflux, dysphagia, substernal pain, and impaired nutritional status may occur (85). Abnormal motility, mucosal desquamation, and web or stricture formation may be seen in the esophagus. Mucosal or submucosal fibrosis is most commonly observed in the esophagus but may occur anywhere along the upper gastrointestinal tract; it is rarely observed in the large intestine. Malabsorption may develop as a consequence of submucosal fibrosis and can cause steatorrhea and diarrhea. Lymphocytic infiltrates in the lamina propria may be seen anywhere along the gastrointestinal tract; shortening of villi and hyperplasia of crypts, however, may be especially evident in the small intestine (41,42).

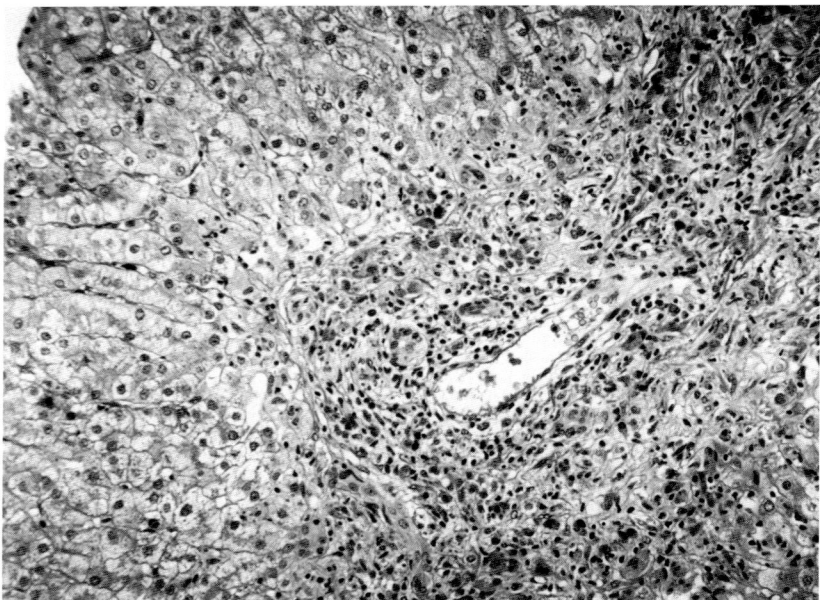

FIG. 10. Chronic hepatic graft-vs.-host disease. In contrast to acute GVH disease (Figure 6), the portal triad has a mixed cellular infiltrate which extends into the lobule. There is associated piecemeal necrosis of the hepatocytes and prominent bile duct injury. (Hematoxylin and eosin stain, ×250.)

Respiratory tract. Chronic sinopulmonary infections, cough, and broncho-spastic airway disease are observed in some patients with chronic graft-vs.-host disease. Histopathological findings are similar to those seen in acute GVH disease. Infiltration of submucosal glands with lymphocytes and plasma cells is common, but the bronchial and bronchiolar mucosa is spared. Obliterative bronchiolitis, which is associated with antecedent or concomitant chronic graft-vs.-host disease has been discussed.

Eyes. Photophobia, burning, and dry eyes are common symptoms in patients with extensive chronic GVH disease. Lymphocytic infiltration, fibrosis, and destruction of lacrimal glands result in decreased tear production, chemosis, and corneal scarring and ulceration. These pathological changes in the lacrimal apparatus resemble those seen in the sicca syndrome of Sjögren (78,79,86).

Mouth. Odynophagia (pain on swallowing) and xerostomia (dry mouth) are oral manifestations of chronic GVH disease. Decreased salivary pooling in the lower gingivolabial fold and dental caries occur with progressive disease. As in the skin, whitish plaques may appear on the buccal mucosa and can mimic oral lichen planus. Erythema, ulcerative lesions, and mucosal atrophy may develop. The histopathological features of these oral lesions are similar to those in lichenoid cutaneous chronic graft-vs.-host disease. Fibrosing sialadenitis, as seen in the Sjögren sicca syndrome, may be demonstrated by biopsy of a minor salivary gland (Figure 11) (56).

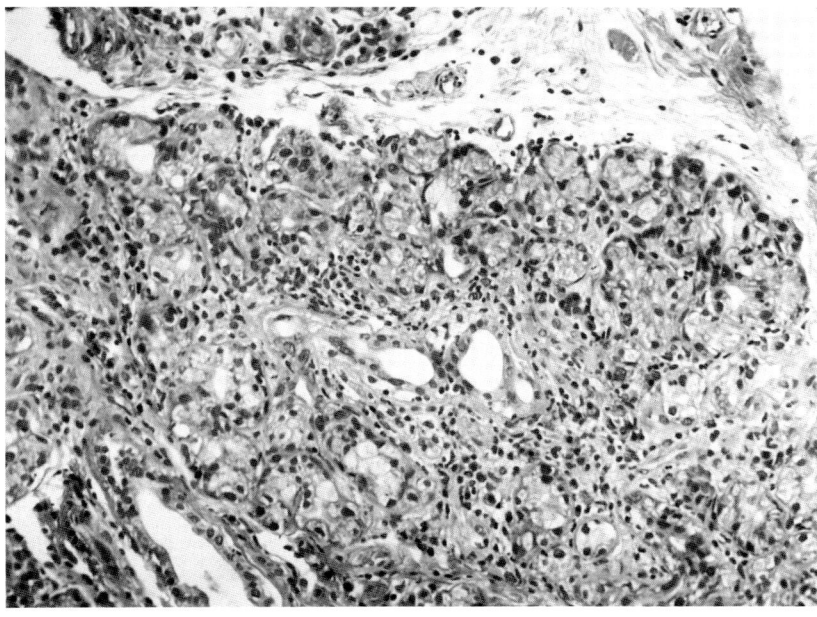

FIG. 11. Chronic graft-vs.-host disease in a minor salivary gland. There is extensive interstitial inflammation, injury of the ducts and loss of acini. (Hematoxylin and eosin stain, ×200.)

Other systems. Polyarthralgias and polyserositis with sterile effusions can occur in chronic graft-vs.-host disease. Myositis is a well-recognized feature of extensive disease. Mild involvement is manifested by interstitial perivascular inflammation and fibrosis, while severe cases demonstrate plasmacytic polymyositis with extensive myonecrosis (87). Eosinophilic fasciitis, leading to limitation in joint mobility and contractures, has been associated with chronic GVH disease. Eosinophilia, elevated immunoglobulins and the presence of auto-antibodies (including antinuclear antibody, antimitochrondrial antibody, and anti-erythrocyte antibody) are all features of chronic GVH disease (56).

SUMMARY AND CONCLUSIONS

Knowledge of the pathology associated with a particular complication provides useful clues as to its pathogenesis. The complications of allogeneic marrow transplantation are primarily the result of the high-dose chemoradiotherapy delivered prior to bone marrow transplantation, acute and chronic GVH disease, and infection. We have limited the discussion to the pathology of these complications and provide a brief description of the gross and microscopic morphology.

ACKNOWLEDGMENTS

The authors wish to thank Drs. Evan R. Farmer and George W. Santos for their helpful suggestions and constructive criticism of this manuscript. This work was supported in part by grant numbers PO1 CA15396, RO1 CA828701, and RO1 NS24097 from the National Institutes of Health, and by Institutional Research Grant number IN-11Y from the American Cancer Society.

REFERENCES

1. Santos GW. History of bone marrow transplantation. *Clin Haematol* 1983;12:3.
2. Santos GW. Bone marrow transplantation. In, Stollerman GH, (ed). *Advances in Internal Medicine.* Chicago, Year Book Publishers, 1979, p. 157.
3. Thomas ED. Bone marrow transplantation. In, Burchenal JH, Ochgen HR, (eds). *Achievements, Challenges and Prospects for the 1980s.* New York, Grune & Stratton, 1981; p. 625.
4. Mathe G. Bone marrow transplantation. In, Rappaport PT, Dausset J, (eds). *Human Transplantation.* New York, Grune & Stratton, 1968, p. 284.
5. Santos GW, Burke PJ, Sensenbrenner LL, Owens AH. Marrow transplantation and graft-vs.-host disease in acute monocytic leukemia. *Exp Hematol* 1969; 18:20.
6. Santos GW. The application of marrow grafts in human disease. Its problems and potential. In Hanna MG, (ed): *Contemporary Topics in Immunobiology.* New York, Plenum Publishers. 1972; p. 143.
7. Santos GW. Bone marrow transplantation in leukemia; current status. *Cancer* 1984;54:2732.
8. Santos GW, Sensenbrenner LL, Burke PJ, et al.: Allogeneic marrow grafts in men using cyclophosphamide. *Transplant Proceedings* 1974;6:345.

9. Storb R, Buckner CD, Dillingham LA, Thomas ED: Cyclophosphamide regimens in rhesus monkeys with and without marrow infusion. *Cancer Res* 1970;30:2195.

10. Santos GW, Sensenbrenner LL, Burke PJ, et al.: The use of cyclophosphamide for clinical marrow transplantation. *Transplant Proceedings* 1972;4:559.

11. Philips FS, Sternberg SS, Cronin AP, Vidal PM. Cyclophosphamide and urinary bladder toxicity. *Cancer Res* 1961;21:1577.

12. Link H, Neef V, Niethammer D, Wilms K. Prophylaxis of hemorrhagic cystitis due to cyclophosphamide-conditioning for bone marrow transplantation. *Blut* 1981;43:329.

13. Becher R, Kakati J, Sandberg AA: Mesna and bone marrow transplantation. *N Engl J Med* 1982;307:1152.

14. Ambinder RF, Burns W, Forman M, et al.: Hemorrhagic cystitis associated with adenovirus in bone marrow transplantation. *Arch Intern Med* 1986;146:1400.

15. Shields AF, Hackman RC, Fife KH, et al.: Adenovirus infections in patients undergoing bone marrow transplantation. *N Engl J Med* 1985;312:529.

16. Arthur RR, Keerti S, Baust SJ, et al.: Association of BK viruria with hemorrhagic cystitis in recipients of bone marrow transplants. *N Engl J Med* 1986;315:230.

17. DeFronzo RA, Braine H, Colvin OM, Davis PJ: Water intoxication in man after cyclophosphamide therapy. *Ann Intern Med* 1973;78:861.

18. Sanders JE, Buckner CD, Leonard JM, et al.: Late effects on gonadal function of cyclophosphamide, total body irradiation, and marrow transplantation. *Transplantation* 1983;36:252.

19. Kumar R, Biggart JD, McEvoy J, McGrown MG: Cyclophosphamide and reproductive function. *Lancet* 1972;1:1212.

20. Miller JJ, Williams GP, Leissring JC: Multiple late complications of therapy with cyclophosphamide, including ovarian destruction. *Am J Med* 1971;50:530.

21. Van Bekkum DW, de Vries MJ: *Radiation Chimeras.* London, Logos Press, 1967, pp. 1–277.

22. Khouri N, Saral R, Armstrong EM, et al.: Pulmonary interstitial changes following bone marrow transplantation. *Radiology* 1979;133:587.

23. Gross NJ: Pulmonary effects of radiation therapy. *Ann Intern Med* 1977;86:81.

24. Thompson CB, Sanders JE, Flournoy N, et al.: The risks of central nervous system relapse and leukoencephalopathy in patients receiving marrow transplants for acute leukemia. *Blood* 1986;67:195.

25. Sklar CA, Kim TH, Williamson TF, Ramsay NK; Ovarian function after successful bone marrow transplantation in post-menarcheal females. *Med Pediatr Oncol* 1983;11:361.

26. Richards GE, Wara WM, Grumbach MM, et al.: Delayed onset of hypopituitarism; sequelae of therapeutic irradiation of central nervous system, eye, and middle ear tumors. *J Pediatr* 1976;89:553.

27. Romshe CA, Zipf WB, Miser A, et al.: Evaluation of growth hormone release and human growth hormone treatment in children with cranial irradiation-associated short stature. *J Pediatr* 1984;104:177.

28. Tutschka PJ, Santos GW, Elfenbein GJ: Marrow transplantation in acute leukemia following busulfan and cyclophosphamide. *Blut* 1980;25:375.

29. Tutschka PJ, Elfenbein GJ, Sensenbrenner LL, et al.: Preparative regimens for marrow transplantation in acute leukemia and aplastic anemia; Baltimore experience. *Am J Pediatr Hematol Oncol* 1980;2:363.

30. Heard BE, Cooke RA: Busulfan lung thorax. *Thorax* 1968;23:187.

31. Ginsberg SJ, Comis RL: The pulmonary toxicity of antineoplastic agents. *Semin Oncol* 1982;9:34.

32. Wingard JR, Santos GW, Saral R: Late-onset interstitial pneumonia following allogeneic bone marrow transplantation. *Transplantation* 1985;39:21.

33. Hymes A, Simonton S, Farmer ER, et al.: Cutaneous busulfan effect in patients receiving bone marrow transplantation. *J Clin Pathol* 1985;12:125.

34. Beschorner WE, Pino J, Boitnott JK, et al.: Pathology of the liver with bone marrow transplantation; effects of busulfan, carmustine, acute graft-vs.-host disease and cytomegalovirus. *Am J Pathol* 1980;99:369.

35. Jones RJ, Lee KSK, Beschorner WE, et al.: Veno-occlusive disease of the liver following bone marrow transplantation. *Transplantation.* In press, 1987.

36. Shulman HM, McDonald GB, Matthews D, et al.: An analysis of hepatic veno-occlusive

disease and centrilobular hepatic degeneration following bone marrow transplantation. *Gastroenterology* 1980;179:1178.

37. McDonald GB, Sharma P, Matthews DE, et al.: Veno-occlusive disease of the liver after bone marrow transplantation; diagnosis, incidence and predisposing factors. *Hepatology* 1984;4:116.

38. McDonald GB, Sharma P, Matthews DE, et al.: The clinical course of 53 patients with veno-occlusive disease of the liver after marrow transplantation. *Transplantation* 1985; 36:603.

39. Krowka MJ, Rosenow EC III, Hoagland HC: Pulmonary complications of bone marrow transplantation. *Chest* 1985;87:237.

40. Johnson FL, Stokes DC, Ruggiero M, et al.: Chronic obstructive airways disease after bone marrow transplantation. *J Pediatr* 1984;105:370.

41. Ralph DD, Spingmeyer SC, Sullivan KM, et al.: Rapidly progressive airflow obstruction in marrow transplant recipients; possible association between obliterative bronchiolitis and chronic graft-vs.-host disease. *Am Rev Resp Dis* 1984;129:641.

42. Roca J, Granena A, Rodriquez-Roisim R, et al.: Fatal airway disease in an adult with chronic graft-vs.-host disease. *Thorax* 1982;37:77.

43. Bortin MM, Rimm AA: Interstitial pneumonitis; dose rate vs. total dose of irradiation. *Int J Radiat Biol* 1982;8:1815.

44. Kim TH, Rybka WB, Lebnert-Podgorsak EV, Freeman CR: Interstitial pneumonitis following total body irradiation for bone marrow transplantation using two different dose rates. *Int J Radiat Oncol Biol Phys* 1985;11:1285.

45. Elfenbein GJ, Saral R: Infectious disease during immune recovery after bone marrow transplantation. In, Allen JC (ed): *Infection and the Compromised Host.* Baltimore, Williams and Wilkens, 1981, p. 157.

46. Meyers JD, Flournoy N, Thomas ED: Nonbacterial pneumonia after allogeneic marrow transplantation; a review of 10 years' experience. *Rev Infect Disease* 1982;4:1119.

47. Meyers JD, Thomas ED: Infection complications in bone marrow transplantation. In, Rubin RH, Young LS (eds): *Clinical Approaches to Infection in the Compromised Host.* Plenum Publishers, New York, 1981, p. 507.

48. Singer C, Armstrong D, Rosen PP, et al.: Diffuse pulmonary infiltrates in immunosuppressed patients; prospective study of 80 cases. *Am J Med* 1979;66:110.

49. Armstrong D: Interstitial pneumonia in the immunosuppressed patient. *Transplant Proc* 1976;8:657.

50. Katzenstein AL, Askin FB: Surgical pathology of nonneoplastic lung disease. In, Bennington JL (ed): *Major Problems in Pathology Series* Vol 8. W. B. Saunders Company, Philadelphia, 1982.

51. Wingard JR, Mellits ED, Sostrin MB, et al.: Interstitial pneumonitis after allogeneic bone marrow transplantation; nine year experience at a single institution. *Blood.* Submitted for publication, 1987.

52. Bross DS, Tutschka PJ, Farmer ER, et al.: Predictive factors for acute GVHD in patients transplanted with HLA-identical bone marrow. *Blood* 1984;63:1265.

53. Santos GW, Tutschka PJ, Brookmeyer R, et al.: Cyclosporine plus methylprednisolone vs. cyclophosphamide plus methylprednisolone as prophylaxis for graft-vs.-host disease; a randomized double blind study in patients undergoing allogeneic marrow transplantation. *Clin Transplantation* 1987;1:21.

54. Storb R, Deeg HJ, Whitehead J, et al.: Methotrexate and cyclosporine compared with cyclosporine alone for prophylaxis of acute graft-vs.-host disease after marrow transplantation for leukemia. *N Engl J Med* 1986;314:729.

55. Storb R, Thomas ED: Graft-vs.-host disease in dog and man; the Seattle experience. *Immunol Rev* 1985;88:215.

56. Sullivan KM, Schulman HM, Storb R, et al.: Chronic graft-vs.-host disease in 52 patients; adverse natural cause and successful treatment with combination immunosuppression. *Blood* 1981;57:267.

57. Schulman HM, Sullivan KM, Weiden PL, et al.: Chronic graft-vs.-host syndrome in man; a long-term clinicopathologic study of 20 Seattle patients. *Am J Med* 1980;69:204.

58. Deeg HJ, et al.: Acute and chronic graft-vs.-host disease and treatment. *J Natl Cancer Inst* 1986;76:1325.

59. Sale GE, Lerner KG, Barker EA, et al.: The skin biopsy in the diagnosis of acute graft-vs.-host disease in man. *Am J Pathol* 1977;89:621.
60. Hymes SR, Farmer ER, Lewis PG, et al.: Cutaneous graft-vs.-host reaction; prognostic features seen by light microscopy. *J Am Acad Dermatol* 1985;12:30.
61. Lerner KG, Kao GF, Storb R, et al.: Histopathology of graft-vs.-host reaction (GVHR) in human recipients of marrow from HLA-matched sibling donor. *Transplant Proc* 1974; 6:367.
62. Slavin RE, Woodruff JM: The pathology of bone marrow transplantation. *Pathol Ann* 1974;9:291.
63. Sale GE, Schulman HM, McDonald GB, Thomas ED: Gastrointestinal graft-vs.-host disease in man; a clinicopathologic study of the rectal biopsy. *Ann J Surg Pathol* 1979;3:291.
64. McClelland DBL: Bacterial and viral infections of the gastrointestinal tract. In, Asquith P (ed): *Immunology of the Gastrointestinal Tract*, Churchill, Livingston, Edinburgh, Scotland, 1979, p. 214.
65. Fisk JD, Schulman HM, Greening RR, et al.: Radiographic features of human graft-vs.-host disease. *Radiology* 1981;138:371.
66. Yeager AM, Kanof ME, Kramer SS, et al.: Pneumotosis intestinalis in children after allogeneic bone marrow transplantation. *Pediatr Radiol* 1987;17:18.
67. Epstein RJ, McDonald GB, Sale GE, et al.: The diagnostic accuracy of the rectal biopsy in acute graft-vs.-host disease; a prospective study in 13 patients. *Gastroenterology* 1980;78:764.
68. Beschorner WE, Yardley JH, Tutschka P, Santos GW: Deficiency of intestinal immunity with graft-vs.-host disease in humans. *J Infect Dis* 1981;144:38.
69. Gallucci BB, Sale GE, McDonald GB, et al.: The fine structure of human rectal epithelium in acute graft-vs.-host disease. *Am J Surg Pathol* 1982;6:293.
70. Elson CO, O'Reilly RW, Rosenberg IH: Small intestinal injury in the graft-vs.-host reaction; an innocent-bystander phenomenon. *Gastroenterology* 1977;72:886.
71. Elkins WL, Guttmann RD: Pathogenesis of a local graft-vs.-host reaction; immunogenecity of circulating host leukocytes. *Science* 1968;159:1250.
72. Van Bekkum DW, Knaan S: Role of bacterial microflora in development of intestinal lesions from graft-vs.-host reaction. *J Natl Cancer Inst* 1977;58:787.
73. Beschorner WE, Saral R, Hutchins GM, et al.: Lymphocytic bronchitis associated with graft-vs.-host disease in recipients of bone marrow transplants. *N Engl J Med* 1978;299:1030.
74. Beschorner WE, Tutschka PJ, Santos GW: Sequential morphology of graft-vs.-host disease in the rat radiation chimera. *Clin Immunol Immunopathol* 1982;22:203.
75. Renkonen R, Hayry P: Bone marrow transplantation in the rat; quantitation of cellular infiltrates in parenchymal target organs in acute graft-vs.-host disease. *Scand J Immunol* 1986;23:351.
76. Yousem SA, Burke CM, Billingham ME: Pathologic pulmonary alterations in long-term heart-lung transplantation. *Hum Pathol* 1985;16:911.
77. Prop J, Tazelaar HD, Billingham ME: Rejection of combined heart-lung transplants in rats; function and pathology. *Am J Pathol* 1987;127:97.
78. Hirst LW, Jabs DA, Tutschka PJ, et al.: The eye in bone marrow transplantation. I. Clinical study. *Arch Ophthalmol* 1983;101:580.
79. Jabs DA, Hirst LW, Green WR, et al.: The eye in bone marrow transplantation. II. Histopathology. *Arch Ophthalmol* 1987;101:585.
80. Barrett AP, Bilous AM: Oral patterns of acute and chronic graft-vs.-host disease. *Arch Dermatol* 1984;120:1461.
81. Santos GW, Hess AD, and Vogelsang GB: Graft-vs.-host reaction and disease. *Immunol Rev* 1985;88:169.
82. Hood AF, Soter NA, Rappeport J, Gigli I: Graft-vs.-host reaction; cutaneous manifestations following bone marrow transplantation. *Arch Dermatol* 1977;113:1087.
83. Shulman HM, Sale GE, Lerner KG, et al.: Chronic cutaneous graft-vs.-host disease in man. *Am J Pathol* 1978;91:545.
84. Janin-Mercier A, Devergie A, Van Cauwenberge D, et al.: Immunohistologic and ultrastructural study of the sclerotic skin in chronic graft-vs.-host disease in man. *Am J Pathol* 1983;115:296.
85. McDonald GB, Sullivan KM, Schuffler MD, et al.: Esophageal abnormalities in chronic graft-vs.-host disease in humans. *Gastroenterology* 1981;80:914.

86. Moutsopoulos HM, Chused TM, Mann DL, et al.: Sjögren's syndrome (sicca syndrome); current issues. *Ann Intern Med* 1980;92:212.
87. Anderson BA, Young PV, Kean WF, et al.: Polymyositis in chronic graft-vs.-host disease; a case report. *Arch Neurol* 1982;39:188.
88. Wingard JR, Wagner JE Jr: Unpublished observations, 1987.
89. Wingard JR: Personal communication to the author, 1987.
90. Jones RJ, Grochow LB: Unpublished observations, 1987.
91. Beschorner WE: Unpublished observations, 1987.

Bone Marrow Transplantation in
Children, edited by F. Leonard Johnson
and Carl Pochedly. Raven Press, Ltd.,
New York © 1990.

Bone Marrow Transplantation for Correction of Primary Immunodeficiencies

Steven M.L. Neudorf, Gregory A. Yanik, and
Daniel W. Pietryga

*Children's Hospital Medical Center, College of Medicine, University of Cincinnati,
Cincinnati, Ohio 45229*

A. Severe combined immunodeficiency (SCID)
B. Wiskott–Aldrich syndrome
C. Chronic granulomatous disease
D. Kostmann's syndrome
E. Chediak–Higashi syndrome
F. Leukocyte adhesion deficiency
G. DiGeorge syndrome
Summary and conclusions

It has been over 20 years since the first case of successful bone marrow transplantation for the treatment of a child with congenital immunodeficiency was reported. Significant advances in the characterization of the various immune defects has led to the development of more effective marrow transplant protocols for severe congenital immunodeficiencies. There is improved understanding of the immune dysfunction and related hematologic abnormalities that occur in severe combined immunodeficiency, in Wiskott-Aldrich syndrome, and in other primary immunodeficiency diseases. This increased knowledge has influenced the design and selection of preparative regimens for bone marrow transplantation.

In this chapter, we will review approaches to use of marrow transplantation as well as the results of these studies in treating patients with primary immunodeficiencies. When possible, we will emphasize the results following use of mismatched marrow transplants.

SEVERE COMBINED IMMUNODEFICIENCY (SCID)

Severe combined immunodeficiency is a heterogeneous group of diseases characterized by severe dysfunction of both T lymphocytes and B lymphocytes. This results in a state of increased susceptibility to opportunistic infections and the occurrence of early death. There are several relatively well-defined etiologies for this syndrome. These include biochemical abnormalities, such as adenosine deaminase (ADA) deficiency and purine nucleoside deficiencies, as well as membrane abnormalities. However, in most cases, the specific etiology is not known.

Historically, use of marrow transplantation was restricted to patients who had an HLA-matched, MLC-identical sibling, in order to avoid the high incidence of severe, fatal graft-vs.-host disease which followed use of mismatched bone marrow (1). Methods were developed for depletion from the marrow of T lymphocytes which are responsible for causing graft-vs.-host disease. This technique has allowed the use of haplo-identical donors for patients with severe combined immunodeficiency. Although survival following use of mismatched marrow transplantation has improved, several problems associated with mismatched transplants remain. The most notable problems are a higher incidence of graft failure or graft rejection and delayed immunoreconstitution. These problems are best illustrated by comparing the results of using matched and mismatched donor marrow for treating patients with SCID.

A multinational European group reported a series of 41 patients with severe combined immunodeficiency who received a marrow transplant from a histocompatible, genotypically identical donor (2). These patients were not given pre-transplant cytoreductive conditioning, nor was T cell depletion of donor marrow performed. All 41 patients engrafted, and in the 28 patients who were evaluated for immunoreconstitution, all were noted to have developed T cell function. T cell reconstitution was defined as the presence of *in vitro* proliferation response to mitogens and a positive skin test in response to antigen. Reconstitution of both T and B lymphocyte function was achieved in 25 out of 28 cases (89.3%). Complete B cell reconstitution was defined as the presence of *in vivo* antibody response after immunization or infection. Three patients had reconstitution of T lymphocyte function; but only partial B lymphocyte reconstitution, which was defined as reduced or absent antibody response to a panel of antigens. Complete immunoreconstitution was achieved within 6 months post-transplant with the majority of cases having full immunoreconstitution within 2 to 4 months. Graft-vs.-host disease was infrequent, with an incidence of only 5.3% of grade II graft-vs.-host disease, and no cases of grade III or IV graft-vs.-host disease.

The actuarial survival rate in these patients was 68.1%, with a plateau in survival seen at 6 months post-transplant. Patients younger than 6 months of age had a better survival rate than older patients. The most frequent cause of death in all patients undergoing HLA-matched bone marrow transplant for severe combined immunodeficiency was infection. In many cases, the fatal infection was present prior to the transplant. This finding suggests that an earlier diagnosis of severe combined immunodeficiency, especially before the onset of severe infections, will improve the results of treatment with bone marrow transplantation. These findings also suggest that development of full immunoreconstitution does not require pre-transplant cytoreductive conditioning.

Neither the techniques used for marrow transplant in patients with a matched donor nor the favorable results can be extended to patients with SCID who lack an HLA identical marrow donor. Patients undergoing mismatched bone marrow transplantation require the use of T cell depletion of donor marrow. This marrow cell manipulation is needed in order to prevent severe or fatal graft-vs.-host disease which follows transplant of non-T cell depleted, mismatched marrow (1). Although T cell depletion of donor marrow has greatly reduced the incidence of graft-vs.-host disease, patients undergoing a mismatched marrow transplant have a higher incidence of graft failure or graft rejection.

The problem of increased graft failure and graft rejection was illustrated in a study by O'Reilly. This study reported the results of using mismatched T cell depleted bone marrow in 17 patients with severe combined immunodeficiency (3,4). All 17 patients were transplanted without preparative cytoreduction. Ten of these 17 patients showed sustained engraftment and immunoreconstitution, with no graft-vs.-host disease. Graft failure occurred in the remaining 7 patients, who were then retransplanted following use of cytoreductive preparative therapy. Five of these 7 patients who received a reinfusion of T cell depleted donor marrow were durably engrafted. It was noted that the patients who failed to engraft had high natural killer (NK) cell activity against K562 targets before marrow transplantation. On the other hand, those with sustained engraftment and immunoreconstitution had low natural killer activity. These observations, together with findings obtained using a murine model for mismatched marrow transplantation, suggest that NK cells may mediate bone marrow rejection (5,6,7). Residual T cell function in the recipient has also been implicated as a factor causing rejection of mismatched marrow (6).

In another study, bone marrow transplantation was used for treatment of 17 patients with various severe T cell dysfunctions (8) including 10 patients classified as having SCID with normal ADA activity (ADA+). All patients received haplo-identical, T cell depleted donor marrow without prior cytoreductive therapy. Seven out of 10 patients who had SCID and normal ADA activity had evidence of engraftment following a single transplant. In contrast to the frequency of graft failures in the previously noted series (3,4), NK activity was noted to be very low or absent in the 3 patients who failed to engraft. Two patients in this series who had normal natural killer activity engrafted. This finding suggested that preexisting normal NK activity did not correlate with failure to engraft.

In patients who engrafted, T cell reconstitution occurred between 100 and 215 days post-transplant. Delayed immunoreconstitution following use of mismatched donor marrow was also reported in the European survey (2). In that report, the mean time for return of T cell function was 6 months, whereas patients given matched donor marrow demonstrated immunoreconstitution within 2 to 4 months following transplant. Reconstitution of B cell function occurred between 6 and 18 months following transplant.

The etiology of delayed immunoreconstitution in patients undergoing mismatched bone marrow transplantation is not known, but there are several hypotheses that may help explain these observations. Although T cell depletion has reduced the incidence of clinically apparent graft-vs.-host disease, a subclinical form of graft-vs.-host disease may be present and may result in prolonged immunodeficiency (9). Another hypothesis is that HLA disparity between the patient and the donor marrow may result in suboptimal cell-cell interactions, which may led to delayed or incomplete immunoreconstitution. This hypothesis is based on findings derived from marrow transplant studies in mice in which lethal irradiation is required for the development of thymic antigen presenting cells (APC) of donor origin (10). It is proposed that disparity between the antigen presenting cells and the T cells may result in defective T cell dependent antigen responses (10).

Graft failure or graft rejection following use of mismatched bone marrow transplantation for severe combined immunodeficiency has an incidence of about 25% (2), and this incidence is probably higher in ADA-deficient patients. Out of 11 ADA-deficient patients transplanted without preparative therapy, 10 showed graft rejection (1,3,4,8,11,12). In contrast, 5 out of 6 ADA-deficient patients transplanted with prior cytoreductive conditioning showed marrow engraftment (12,13,14). The reason for the increased incidence of graft rejection in ADA-deficient patients is unclear (15). Perhaps transient engraftment may result in sufficient improvement in the biochemical abnormalities, and improvement in recipient immune function in patients with ADA deficiency, so as to allow rejection to occur.

The impact of pre-transplant conditioning on engraftment in patients with normal ADA activity is difficult to assess. This difficulty is due to the fact that a variety of conditioning regimens are used to treat patients with severe combined immunodeficiency, as well as the fact that the factors predicting rejection have not been clearly identified. In general, patients given pre-transplant cytoreductive preparative therapy had a higher rate of engraftment, but infectious complications secondary to neutropenia and mucositis were greater. The use of adjunctive immunosuppressive therapy may further facilitate engraftment, without necessarily increasing the severity of neutropenia or mucositis.

A series of 7 mismatched immunodeficient patients were conditioned with cyclophosphamide (given at 50 mg/kg/day for 4 days), antilymphocyte globulin, busulfan (given at 4 mg/kg/day for 4 days), and infusion of monoclonal anti-CD18. A group of historical control patients from the same institution were treated with the same regimen, but without the anti-CD18. Anti-CD18 has been shown to block the *in vitro* response of mixed lymphocyte culture; it also blocks T cell mediated cytotoxicity, natural killer function, antibody dependent T cell cytotoxicity, and antigen presentation (16,17). Seven patients who were given anti-CD18 engrafted. Five of these 7 survived; the other two died of infectious complications. In the control group, no evidence of engraftment was seen in 6 out of 7 patients. Although the number of patients reported is small, the results using anti-CD18 to facilitate hematopoietic engraftment and immunoreconstitution are encouraging. In addition to anti-CD18, we reported *in vitro* studies in which antithymocyte globulin (ATG) abrogated NK-mediated suppression of CFU-GM (18). It was proposed that ATG may be helpful in preventing graft rejection mediated by NK cells.

Further delineation of the causes of severe combined immunodeficiency should aid in predicting graft rejection. This improved knowledge has already led to the conclusion that preparative cytoreductive conditioning should be used in ADA-deficient patients who are given mismatched donor marrow because of the high incidence of graft rejection. Identification of the effector cells which cause rejection, and documenting their presence in patients with severe combined immunodeficiency, should also help predict rejection. In this regard, findings that support the role of NK cells in graft rejection are convincing, but they need to be confirmed by study of a larger series of patients.

In addition to facilitating engraftment, cytoreductive preparative therapy may also be indicated for treatment of certain complications of severe combined immunodeficiency. Preparative therapy has been effective in preventing the clinical manifestations of congenital graft-vs.-host disease in a neonate which was thought to have resulted from materno-fetal transfusions (11). Patients with significant autoimmune disease or lymphoproliferative disease should probably be given preparative therapy regardless of the nature of their underlying immunodeficiency.

However, there may be certain relative contraindications to the use of preparative therapy. Patients who have active infections at the time of transplant may be at higher risk for development of infectious or toxic complications due to therapy. Such patients may benefit from an initial bone marrow transplant performed without preparative therapy; this would be followed by a second transplant given in conjunction with preparative therapy if graft failure or graft rejection occurs. Similarly, in ADA-deficient patients who have active infections, temporary immunoreconstitution may be achieved by using partial exchange transfusions of red blood cells as a form of enzyme replacement therapy (19). This technique may allow the patient to sufficiently recover from the infections so that he or she may better tolerate the cytoreductive preparative regimen.

Another complication associated with use of mismatched marrow for transplant in patients with SCID is the development of lymphoproliferative malignancies. The majority of cases occur relatively soon after transplant (20,21,22). Many of the malignancies are B cell tumors, and a significant number of cases have evidence of the Epstein-Barr virus (EBV) genome present within the tumor. The pathogenesis of these tumors is poorly understood. Patients who were seropositive for EB virus and who received bone marrow from a seronegative donor have developed lymphoproliferative diseases (22), as did patients who were seronegative for EB virus and were given marrow from a seropositive donor (20). Thus, it is unclear whether the source of Epstein-Barr virus is from reactivation of latent virus or from acquisition of the virus from the marrow inoculum.

Most cases of lymphoproliferative malignancy occurred in patients who had rejected a transplant of mismatched marrow or had not reconstituted their immune function. However, 4 patients with lymphoproliferative disease associated with EB virus did have complete immunoreconstitution at the time when the lymphoproliferative disease was diagnosed (18). All 4 patients had normal NK activity and produced anti-EBV antibodies. Three of the 4 patients showed cytotoxic T lymphocyte activity against B cells infected by EB virus. One patient had a normal response to phytohemagglutinin and to alloantigens, while the remaining 3 had only suboptimal responses in these reactions. The survival rate is poor for patients who developed lymphoproliferative disease. However, recent studies suggest that treatment with alpha-interferon may be effective (23,24). It was also reported that prophylactic administration of acyclovir may reduce the incidence of post-marrow transplant lymphoproliferative disease (25,26). These preliminary findings support the presence of a viral etiology in many of these cases and offer new hope for prevention and treatment of lymphoproliferative malignancies.

WISKOTT–ALDRICH SYNDROME

The Wiskott–Aldrich syndrome is an X-linked disorder. The disease is characterized by eczema, thrombocytopenia, increased susceptibility to infection, and an increased incidence of lymphoreticular malignancies (27,28,29). The severity of the immune dysfunction in this syndrome is variable, and the immunodeficiency involves both humoral and cellular immunity (30). Bone marrow transplantation is a logical therapy for Wiskott-Aldrich syndrome since the clinical manifestations of the disease are due to abnormalities of function of lymphocytes, neutrophils, monocytes, and platelets. Replacement of the defective hematopoietic stem cell should, in theory, lead to both lymphoid reconstitution and hematopoietic engraftment, thereby correcting these underlying abnormalities.

Initial attempts in use of bone marrow transplantation for treatment of Wiskott–Aldrich syndrome resulted in only partial success (31,32,33). These early attempts in bone marrow transplantation apparently included adequate immunosuppression, but the preparative regimens were not sufficiently myeloablative to allow for the establishment of full engraftment. One patient (31) was initially prepared for transplantation by use of prednisone and procarbazine, but he failed to engraft. Cyclophosphamide alone was given prior to a second infusion of matched donor bone marrow. The patient became chimeric for peripheral blood T cells and, at the time of the published report, he had a mixed chimerism of the B cell population. However, his erythrocytes, neutrophils, monocytes, and platelets were all of recipient origin (32). Likewise, another patient (33) was prepared for transplant using only cyclophosphamide and showed improvement in platelet function; but there was no evidence of engraftment of other hematopoietic lineages.

HLA-matched bone marrow transplantation, resulting in full correction of thrombocytopenia and immunodeficiency, requires a more intensive myeloablative preparative regimen (34,35,36). In certain cases of severe combined immunodeficiency, severity of the immune dysfunction may minimize the possibility of rejection of donor marrow. However, experience with patients with Wiskott–Aldrich syndrome suggests the existence of an immune response adequate to prevent full engraftment. Whether this immune response is due to activity of intact NK cells in patients with Wiskott-Aldrich syndrome (37) is a matter of conjecture, in view of the conflicting data on the role of NK cells in graft rejection (5,6,7).

Correction of the immunologic and hematologic manifestations of Wiskott-Aldrich syndrome, following a bone marrow transplant using a more intensive preparative regimen, was first reported by Parkman (34). In this study, the first patient had only T cell engraftment following a preparative regimen consisting of cytosine arabinoside and cyclophosphamide. However, he had full reconstitution after a subsequent cytoreductive preparative regimen consisting of procarbazine, antithymocyte globulin, and total body irradiation (TBI). This same preparative regimen was used in a second patient, who showed prompt engraftment. Neither patient developed graft-vs.-host disease.

Concern for the potential toxicity of myeloablative doses of total body irradiation prompted others to design a preparative regimen using high-dose cyclophosphamide and moderate-dose busulfan alone (35). Three patients were treated with this regimen. They all showed prompt hematologic engraftment and rapid restoration of immunologic function. No treatment to prevent graft-vs.-host disease was given and only one patient developed mild graft-vs.-host disease. A slight variation of this regimen, utilizing busulfan at a dose of 3 mg/kg/day instead of 2 mg/kg/day, was used to successfully transplant 2 patients with Wiskott-Aldrich syndrome (36). In another study, a preparative regimen consisting of dimethylmyleran and cyclophosphamide was used for the transplantation of a patient with Wiskott-Aldrich syndrome (37). The patient engrafted and showed gradual correction of immune function. Methotrexate was used to prevent graft-vs.-host disease.

The use of HLA-mismatched donor marrow in treatment of patients with Wiskott–Aldrich syndrome has not been extensively examined. Prompt engraftment was obtained in a Wiskott-Aldrich patient who received T cell depleted mismatched donor marrow, following use of a preparative regimen consisting of busulfan and cyclophosphamide (38). Hong also used this regimen in a patient who was given donor marrow that was T cell depleted and mismatched at the HLA-B locus. The patient had evidence of initial engraftment, but he subsequently developed thrombocytopenia (39). This patient was given an additional infusion of non-T cell depleted bone marrow from the same donor without further myeloablative or immunosuppressive preparative therapy. Full hematologic engraftment was reestablished and only mild graft-vs.-host disease developed.

Other approaches leading to successful transplantation of mismatched donor marrow in patients with Wiskott-Aldrich syndrome have used more intensive myeloablative preparative regimens. Hong used a protocol consisting of cytosine arabinoside, cyclophosphamide, and total body irradiation in 2 patients who received T cell depleted, haplo-identical bone marrow from a parental donor (39). Both patients showed full hematopoietic engraftment and immunologic reconstitution. Graft-vs.-host disease developed in the patient who received no treatment for prevention of this complication, but graft-vs.-host disease did not develop in the second patient who was given cyclosporine A. Cytosine arabinoside, cyclophosphamide, and busulfan were used as the preparative regimen in a 1-year-old boy who was given mismatched donor marrow from his father. Full engraftment and normal immune function were promptly established and have persisted for the ensuing two years following the transplant. Gastrointestinal features of graft-vs.-host disease occurred, but the symptoms quickly resolved (40).

Fischer and colleagues (13) reported that *in vivo* administration of monoclonal anti-CD18 may facilitate engraftment following bone marrow transplantation. Anti-CD18 antibodies have been reported to block the mixed lymphocyte culture response, T cell mediated cytotoxicity, NK cell function, antibody dependent-T cell cytotoxicity, and antigen presentation (16,17). Three patients with Wiskott-Aldrich syndrome are included in their series of 7 patients who received busulfan, cyclophosphamide and antilymphocyte globulin as the preparative regimen prior to infusion of T cell depleted, mismatched bone marrow from a related donor. Murine anti-CD18 monoclonal antibody was infused for 2 days before and for 3 days following bone marrow infusion. Cyclosporine A was administered to prevent graft-vs.-host disease. All 3 patients had prompt engraftment.

Bone marrow transplantation has proved to be an effective treatment for both the hematologic and immune dysfunctions associated with Wiskott-Aldrich syndrome. The increased incidence of malignancy associated with this syndrome (41–44) may also be reduced following marrow transplant. Patients with Wiskott-Aldrich syndrome were reported to develop malignancies at a median age of about 6 years (44). A review of 15 patients who underwent bone marrow transplantation reported that 12 were alive at a median of 3.7 years post-transplant and at a median age of 5.3 years (44). None of these 12 patients developed malignancy, nor had malignancy contributed to the mortality of the three patients who died.

CHRONIC GRANULOMATOUS DISEASE

Chronic granulomatous disease (CGD) is characterized by recurrent suppurative infections. The infections most commonly involve the skin and reticuloendothelial system, but often the lungs, liver, and bones are affected. The severity of these infections often leads to death in early childhood, but occasionally a patient survives into adulthood. Whether this obvious clinical heterogeneity is due to the existence of variants of this disorder, or the prolonged survival is due to more aggressive management of these patients is unknown. It is unclear whether this disorder, which almost always affects young boys, is an X-linked disorder; an autosomal recessive variant may also exist (42). Common to all cases of chronic granulomatous disease is the inability of the patient's phagocytes to kill catalase-positive microorganisms. The nature of the primary metabolic defect is unclear. However, the defect is manifested by an absence of the postphagocytic respiratory burst of oxygen, lack of hexose monophosphate shunt activity, and failure of the phagocyte to produce hydrogen peroxide (45).

There is an intermediate defect in phagocyte function as measured by reduction of nitroblue tetrazolium (NBT) which is noted in the mothers and siblings of many affected males (45). Despite this fact, the potential improvement in cellular function which accompanies engraftment with HLA-matched bone marrow suggests that bone marrow transplantation is an appropriate form of treatment. However, there have been few reports of the use of bone marrow transplantation for treatment of chronic granulomatous disease aside from rare case studies. There has been no systematic study of preparative regimens designed to facilitate engraftment in these patients.

A 20-month-old boy who received conditioning with cyclophosphamide at a dose of 60 mg/kg/day for 4 days before transplant, was then given an infusion of histocompatible bone marrow from an unrelated donor (46). There was improvement in NBT reduction by his granulocytes and the patient had a decreased frequency of infections during the 3-year follow-up period, despite gradual development of mixed chimerism. In another study (47), busulfan (2 mg/kg/day for 4 days) and cyclophosphamide (50 mg/kg/day for 4 days) was used to prepare a 5-month-old boy for bone marrow transplantation. Histocompatible bone marrow from an unaffected brother was then given. Methotrexate was used to prevent GVHD. Although he showed good initial engraftment and the occurrence of normal neutrophil function, there was a gradual loss of the graft. Others used a more intensive preparative regimen consisting of procarbazine, total body irradiation, and antithymocyte serum, and obtained full hematologic reconstitution in a 15-year-old patient transplanted with HLA-matched donor marrow. Despite the use of prophylactic methotrexate, the patient developed severe graft-vs.-host disease and died 90 days after the transplant from sepsis (48).

KOSTMANN'S SYNDROME

Infantile genetic agranulocytosis (Kostmann's syndrome) is characterized by the presence of neutropenia associated with arrested myeloid maturation at the promyelocyte-myelocyte level (49). This results in severe pyogenic infections leading to early death.

Successful hematopoietic engraftment, and the establishment of normal neutrophil numbers and function, occurred in a patient given a transplant of HLA-matched donor marrow. This finding suggests that the etiology of Kostmann's syndrome is a defective hematopoietic stem cell, rather than an abnormal bone marrow microenvironment (50). In the case reported, procarbazine, antithymocyte serum and TBI were used to prepare the 20-month-old patient for bone marrow transplantation. Another patient was treated with a less intensive preparative regimen consisting of cyclophosphamide alone (51). Although there was initial engraftment, rejection occurred and there was return of agranulocytosis.

As in cases where bone marrow transplantation was used to correct other disorders of granulocyte function, use of an intensive preparative regimen consisting of chemotherapy and TBI is associated with successful engraftment (48,51). However, there is concern for the long-term sequelae of total body irradiation in young children, such as growth retardation, cataracts, and the possibility of malignant neoplasms. This concern for the delayed effects of the preparative regimen demands continued search for an efficient myeloablative therapy that entails less risk to the patient.

CHEDIAK–HIGASHI SYNDROME

Chediak–Higashi syndrome is an autosomal recessive disorder characterized by recurrent pyogenic infections and partial oculocutaneous albinism.

The leukocytes contain giant lysosomal inclusions, which are diagnostic of this disease (52). Phagocytes from patients with Chediak-Higashi syndrome have defective bactericidal activity, and they do not respond normally to chemotactic stimulants (53). In addition, patients often develop an accelerated phase of their disease. In this phase there is lymphohistiocytic proliferation, which results in lymphadenopathy, hepatosplenomegaly, pancytopenia, and peripheral neuropathy. Death is due to bleeding or infection.

Marrow transplant studies in mice showed that successful hematopoietic and immunologic reconstitution occur following transplant (54). A patient with Chediak–Higashi syndrome was transplanted in the accelerated phase of his disease (55). Conditioning with cyclophosphamide (50 mg/kg/day for 4 days) and TBI (700 cGy) resulted in full hematopoietic reconstitution, with loss of abnormal granules in the leukocytes and the return of NK cell activity. Also, a small series of patients with Chediak-Higashi syndrome were treated by transplantation of mismatched donor marrow following a conditioning regimen consisting of cyclophosphamide (50 mg/kg/day for 4 days) plus busulfan (4 mg/kg/day for 4 days) (56). Sustained engraftment did not occur. This finding suggested that patients with Chediak-Higashi syndrome have sufficient T cell function to enable them to reject mismatched bone marrow.

LEUKOCYTE ADHESION DEFICIENCY

In leukocyte adhesion deficiency (LAD) there is deficiency of a family of cell surface glycoproteins, consisting of a heterodimer in which the beta-subunit is common to all members. There are at least 3 different alpha-subunits, termed CD11a, CD11b and CD11c (57). All three subunits mediate adhesion of phagocytes or lymphocytes. Cell surface expression of alpha- and beta-subunits is deficient in leukocyte adhesion deficiency. The cell surface defect is believed to be the result of abnormalities in synthesis of the beta-subunit of the CD11 heterodimer (58). The CD11 deficiency results in defective cell-cell interactions which manifest an absence of chemotaxis and lack of adhesion by phagocytes. T lymphocytes from patients with leukocyte adhesion deficiency show impaired activity of cytotoxic T lymphocytes, and these cells respond poorly to suboptimal concentrations of mitogens.

Patients with leukocyte adhesion deficiency can be divided into 2 groups based on the level of expression of CD11 on the cell surface. Severely affected patients have less than 0.2% of normal expression of CD11. In its severe form, leukocyte adhesion deficiency becomes manifest in infancy with delayed umbilical cord separation, persistent leukocytosis (with leukocyte counts over 100,000/mm), (3) and impaired wound-healing. There are recurrent infections of the skin and respiratory tract resulting in death early in childhood. Moderately affected patients are less likely to develop severe life-threatening infections, presumably because of the greater cell surface expression of CD11. These less severely affected patients may survive into adulthood (57).

Bone marrow transplantation has been used for treatment of 6 patients with severe leukocyte adhesions deficiency (57,58). Three patients were given marrow from HLA identical donors and three patients had haplo-identical donors. All 6 patients engrafted following a conditioning regimen consisting of cyclophosphamide (50 mg/kg/day for 4 days) and busulfan (4 mg/kg/day for 4 days) or giving 800 cGy of total body irradiation. All 3 patients given HLA-matched donor marrow had improved function of phagocytes and lymphocytes. One patient is alive and well at least 6 years post-transplant. A second patient died at 7 months post-transplant due to chronic graft-vs.-host disease and a third patient died from an accident 15 months following marrow transplant.

Three mismatched patients also were given a conditioning regimen comprised of busulfan (4 mg/kg/day for 4 days) and cyclphosphamide (50 mg/kg/day for 4 days). The mismatched donor marrow was also treated for T cell depletion prior to infusion and cyclosporine A was given post-transplant. All 3 of these patients showed engraftment and achieved a stable mixed chimerism: there were more than 50% donor cells in 2 patients and 30% donor cells in the third patient (59). All three patients showed improvement in lymphocyte and neutrophil function. One patient developed grade II graft-vs.-host disease which responded to treatment with corticosteroids. All three patients were free of infections at from 19 months to 57 months following marrow transplantation.

The conditioning regimen consisting of cyclophosphamide and busulfan did not result in rejection in patients transplanted with mismatched donor marrow for treatment of leukocyte adhesion deficiency. This suggests that CD11 function may be involved in mediating graft rejection. Also, this concept is supported by the fact that anti-CD11 given *in vivo* may be useful in facilitating engraftment in other diseases (15).

DIGEORGE SYNDROME

The DiGeorge syndrome was first described in a patient who had hypo-parathyroidism associated with a deficiency in cellular immune function (60). Many variants of the syndrome have since been observed in which there are cardiovascular anomalies, a characteristic facies, and varying degrees of immunodeficiency. DiGeorge syndrome is caused by defective development of branchial pouches. The striking variability in clinical presentation of this syndrome is due to the degree of defective development in branchial pouches 1 through 6. Patients with total thymic aplasia will have absence of T cells and defective T cell dependent B cell function, which leads to an increased susceptibility to infection (61). In patients with an ectopic or hypoplastic thymus, spontaneous resolution of immunodeficiency may occur (62).

Only one case in which bone marrow transplantation was used to treat a patient with DiGeorge syndrome has been reported (63). The rationale for use of marrow transplant was to reconstitute the lymphoid system in a patient who had thymic aplasia. No preparative cytoreductive therapy was administered to this patient, who received an infusion of HLA-DR mismatched bone marrow from her brother. T cell engraftment and subsequent normal immune function were attained. There was no engraftment of other hematopoietic elements.

SUMMARY AND CONCLUSIONS

The techniques of bone marrow transplantation used for treating patients with severe combined immunodeficiency, Wiskott-Aldrich syndrome, and other primary immunodeficiencies, together with the results of these studies, are reviewed in this chapter.

Patients with severe combined immunodeficiency who received histocompatible donor marrow without preparative therapy showed immunoreconstitution within 2 to 4 months following marrow transplant. Patients with severe combined immunodeficiency who lack a histocompatible donor have successfully undergone bone marrow transplantation using T cell depleted donor marrow to prevent graft-vs.-host disease. In contrast to matched patients, the incidence of graft rejection and graft failure in patients with SCID who are given mismatched T cell depleted donor marrow is higher (approximately 25%). Factors predicting rejection include recipient natural killer (NK) cell activity and T cell activity as well as presence of adenosine deaminase (ADA) deficiency. In patients with such risk factors, the use of cytoreductive therapy may be indicated to facilitate engraftment.

Bone marrow transplantation has been used to treat patients with Wiskott-Aldrich syndrome, and has resulted in the correction of the thrombocytopenia and immunodeficiency associated with this disease. Bone marrow transplantation may also prevent the occurrence of lymphoreticular malignancies in patients with Wiskott-Aldrich syndrome. Graft rejection remains a problem of patients with Wiskott-Aldrich syndrome undergoing mismatched T cell depleted marrow transplant. However, preliminary results suggest that adjunct immunosuppressive therapy may be helpful in facilitating engraftment in such patients.

Bone marrow transplantation has been used to correct a variety of less severe immunodeficiencies including chronic granulomatous disease, Kostmann's neutropenia, and Chediak-Higashi syndrome. The indications for bone marrow transplantation for patients with these diseases need to be carefully determined since these patients, with supportive care alone, may survive into adulthood. The development of effective, less toxic preparative conditioning regimens may further encourage earlier use of marrow transplant in the treatment of patients with primary immunodeficiencies.

REFERENCES

1. Fischer A, Griscelli C, Friedrich W, et al.: Bone marrow transplantation for immunodeficiencies and osteopetrosis; European survey 1968–1985. *Lancet* 1986;2:1080–1084.
2. Kenny A, Hitzig W: Bone marrow transplantation for severe combined immunodeficiency disease. *Eur J Pediatr* 1979;131:155–177.
3. O'Reilly R, Brochstein J, Collins N, et al.: Evaluation of HLA-haplotype disparate parental marrow grafts depleted of T lymphocytes by differential agglutination with a soybean lectin and E-rosette depletion for the treatment of severe combined immunodeficiency. *Vox Sang* 1986;51 (Suppl 2):81–86.
4. O'Reilly R, Keever C, Kernan N, et al.: HLA nonidentical T cell depleted marrow transplants; a comparison of results in patients treated for leukemia and severe combined immunodeficiency disease. *Transplant Proc* 1987;19: (Suppl 7):55–60.
5. Murphy W, Kumar V, Bennett M: Rejection of bone marrow allografts by mice with severe combined immunodeficiency (SCID). *J Exp Med* 1987;165:1212–1217.
6. Murphy W, Kumar V, Bennett M: Acute rejection of murine bone marrow allografts by natural killer cells and T cells. *J Exp Med* 1987;166:1499–1509.
7. Warner J, Dennert G: Bone marrow graft rejection as a function of antibody-directed natural killer cells. *J Exp Med* 1985;161:563.
8. Buckley R, Schiff S, Sampson H, et al.: Development of immunity in human severe primary T cell deficiency following haploidentical bone marrow stem cell transplantation. *J Immunol* 1986;136:2398–2407.
9. Shearer G, Polisson R: Mutual recognition of parental and F_1 lymphocytes. *J Exp Med* 1980;151:20–31.
10. Longo D, Davis M: Early appearance of donor-type antigen presenting cell in the thymuses of 1200R radiation induced bone marrow chimeras correlates with self-recognition of donor I region gene products. *J Immunol* 1983;130:2525–2527.
11. Cowan M, Wara D, Weintraub P, et al.; Haplo-identical bone marrow transplantation for severe combined immunodeficiency disease using soybean agglutinin-negative, T-depleted marrow cells. *J Clin Immunol* 1985;5:370–376.
12. Friedrich W, Goldmann S, Ebell W, et al.: Severe combined immunodeficiency; treatment by bone marrow transplantation in 15 infants using HLA-haplo-identical donors. *Eur J Pediatr* 1985;144:125–130.
13. Morgan G, Linch D, Knott L, et al.: Successful haplo-identical mismatched bone marrow transplantation in severe combined immunodeficiency; T cell removal using CAMPATH-1 monoclonal antibody and E-rosetting. *Br J Hematol* 1986;62:421–430.
14. Blazar BR, Whitley CB, Desnick RJ, et al: Comparison of enzymatic activity with evidence of engraftment in patients with inborn errors of metabolism following allogeneic bone marrow transplantation. *March of Dimes Original Article Series* 1986;22:135–152.
15. Fischer A, Griscelli C, Blanche S, et al.: Prevention of graft failure by an anti-HLFA-1 monoclonal antibody in HLA-mismatched bone marrow transplantation. *Lancet* 1986;2:1058–1062.
16. Olive D, Charmot D, Dubreuil P, et al.: Human lymphocyte functional antigens. In, Feldmann M, (ed): *Human T Cell Clones; a New Approach to Immune Regulation*. Clifton, N.J., Humana Press, 1986, pp. 173–187.
17. Krensky AM, Robbins E, Springer TA, Burakoff SJ: LFA-1 and LFA-3 antigens are involved in CTL-target conjugation. *J Immunol* 1984;131:2180.
18. Neudorf S, Jones M: The effects of antithymocyte globulin (ATG) on natural killer (NK) cell activity. *Exp Hemat* 188;16:831–835.
19. Polmar S, Stern R, Schwartz A, et al.: Enzyme replacement therapy for adenosine deaminase deficiency and severe combined immunodeficiency. *N Engl J Med* 1976;295:1337–1343.
20. Shearer W, Ritz J, Finegold M, et al.: Epstein-Barr virus associated B cell lymphoproliferation of diverse clonal origins after bone marrow transplantation in a 12-year-old patient with severe combined immunodeficiency. *N Engl J Med* 1985;312:1151–1159.
21. Kapoor N, Jung L, Engelhard D, et al.: Lymphoma in a patient with severe combined immunodeficiency with adenosine deaminase deficiency, following unsustained engraftment of histoincompatible T cell depleted bone marrow. *J Pediatr* 1986;108:435–438.

22. Shapiro R, Pietryga D, Blazar B, et al.: B cell lymphoproliferative disorders following bone marrow transplantation. In, *Progress in Bone Marrow Transplantation*. Alan R. Liss, New York, 1987, pp. 647–657.
23. Shapiro R, Chauvenet A, McGuire W, et al.: Treatment of B cell lymphoproliferative disorders with interferon alpha and intravenous gamma globulin. *N Engl J Med* 1988;318:1334.
24. Shapiro R, Chauvenet A, Craft A, et al.: Successful alpha-interferon treatment of EBV-associated B cell lymphoproliferative disorders in immunodeficient patients. *Exp Hemat* 1988;16:Abstract #271.
25. Moen R, Horowitz S, Sondel P, et al.: Immunologic reconstitution after haplo-identical bone marrow transplantation for immune deficiency disorders; treatment of bone marrow cells with monoclonal antibody CT-2 and complement. *Blood* 1987;70:664–669.
26. Trigg M, Finlay J, Sondel P: Use of acyclovir in bone marrow transplant patients. *N Engl J Med* 1985;312:1708–1709.
27. Wiskott A: Familiarer, angeborener Morbus Werlhofii? *Monatsschr Kinderheitkd* 1937;68:212.
28. Aldrich RA, Steinberg AG, Campbell DC: Pedigree demonstrating a sex-linked recessive condition characterized by draining ears, eczematoid dermatitis, and bloody diarrhea. *Pediatrics* 1954;13:133.
29. Ammann AJ, Hong R: Disorders of the T cell system. In, Stiehm ER, Fulginiti VA, (eds): *Immunologic Disorders in Infants and Children*. Philadelphia, W.B. Saunders Company, 1980; p. 286.
30. Blaise RM, Strober W, Waldmann TA: Immunodeficiency in the Wiskott-Aldrich syndrome. In, Bergsma D, Good RA, Finstad J, Paul NW, (eds): *Immunodeficiency in Man and Animals*, vol 11. *Birth Defects Original Article Series*. New York, National Foundation, 1975, pp. 250–254.
31. Bach FH, Albertini RJ, Anderson JL, et al.: Bone marrow transplantation in a patient with the Wiskott-Aldrich syndrome. *Lancet* 1968;2:1364.
32. Neuwissen HJ, Bortin MM, Bach FH, et al.: Long-term survival after bone marrow transplantation; a 15-year follow-up report of a patient with Wiskott-Aldrich syndrome. *J Pediatr* 1984; 105:365.
33. August CS, Hathaway WE, Githens JH, et al.: Improved platelet function following bone marrow transplantation in an infant with the Wiskott-Aldrich syndrome. *J Pediatr* 1973;82:58.
34. Parkman R, Rappaport J, Geha R, Belli J, et al.: Complete correction of the Wiskott-Aldrich syndrome by allogeneic bone marrow transplantation. *N Engl J Med* 1978;298:921–927.
35. Kapoor N, Kirkpatrick D, Blaese RM, et al: Reconstitution of normal megakaryocytopoiesis and immunologic functions in Wiskott-Aldrich syndrome by marrow transplantation following myeloablation and immunosuppression with busulfan and cyclophosphamide. *Blood* 1981;57:692–696.
36. Goldsobel AB, Ehrlich RM, Mendoza GR, Stiehm ER: Bone marrow transplantation for Wiskott-Aldrich syndrome; report of 2 cases with use of 2-mercaptoethane sulfonate. *Transplantation* 1985;39:568–570.
37. Ochs HD, Lum LG, Johnson FL, et al.: Bone marrow transplantation in the Wiskott-Aldrich syndrome; complete hematological and immunological reconstitution. *Transplantation* 1982;34:284–287.
38. Kapoor N: Personal communication to the author, 1988.
39. Hong R: Personal communication to the author, 1988.
40. Trigg ME: Personal communication to the author, 1988.
41. Messina C, Kirkpatrick D, Fitzgerald PA, et al.: Natural killer cell function and interferon generation in patients with primary immunodeficiencies. *Clin Immunol Immunopathol* 1986;39:394–404.
42. tenBensel RW, Stadlan EM, Krivit W: The development of malignancy in the course of the Wiskott-Aldrich syndrome. *J Pediatr* 1966;68:761–767.
43. Cotelingam JD, Witebsky FG, Hsu SM, et al: Malignant lymphoma in patients with the Wiskott-Aldrich syndrome. *Cancer Invest* 1985;3:515–522.
44. Neudorf SML, Filipovich AH, Kersey JH: Immunoreconstitution by bone marrow transplantation decreases lymphoproliferative malignancies in Wiskott-Aldrich and severe combined immune deficiency syndrome. In, Purtilo DT, (ed): *Immune Deficiency and Cancer: Epstein-Barr Virus and Lymphoproliferative Malignancies*. Plenum Publishing, New York, 1984; pp. 471–480.

45. Johnston RB, Newman SL: Chronic granulomatous disease. In, *Pediat Clin N Am* 1977;24:365.
46. Westminster Hospitals Bone Marrow Transplant Team: Bone marrow transplant from an unrelated donor for chronic granulomatous disease. *Lancet* 1977;1:210–213.
47. Kamani N, August CS, Douglas Sd, et al.: Bone marrow transplantation in chronic granulomatous disease. *J Pediatr* 1984;105:42–46.
48. Rappaport J, Newburger PE, Goldblum RM, et al.: Allogeneic bone marrow transplantation for chronic granulomatous disease. *J Pediatr* 1982;101:952–955.
49. Nathan D, Oski F, (eds): *Hematology of Infancy and Childhood.* (3rd ed). W.B. Saunders Company, Philadelphia, 1987, p. 210.
50. Rappaport JM, Parkman R, Newburger PE, et al.: Correction of infantile agranulocytosis by allogeneic bone marrow transplantation. *Am J Med* 1980;68:605–609.
51. Pahwa RN, O'Reilly R, Broxmeyer HE: Partial correction of neutrophil deficiency in congenital neutropenia following bone marrow transplantation. *Exp Hematol* 1977;5(Suppl 2):45(Abstract).
52. Stiehm R, Fulginiti V, (eds): *Immunologic Disorders in Infants and Children.* W.B. Saunders, 1980, p. 361.
53. Clark RA, Kimball HR: Defective granulocyte chemotaxis in the Chediak-Higashi syndrome. *J Clin Invest* 1971;50:2645–2652.
54. Kazmierowski JA, Elin RJ, Reynolds HY: Chediak-Higashi syndrome; reversal of increased susceptibility to infection by bone marrow transplantation. *Blood* 1976;47:555–559.
55. Griscelli C, Virelizier JL: Bone marrow transplantation in a patient with Chediak-Higashi syndrome. In, Wedgewood RJ, Rosen FS, (eds): *Primary Immunodeficiency Diseases.* Alan R. Liss, New York, 1983, pp. 333–334.
56. Fischer A, Blanche S, Veber F, et al: Correction of immune disorders by HLA matched and mismatched bone marrow transplantation. In, Gale R, Champlin R, (eds): *Progress in Bone Marrow Transplantation.* UCLA Symposia on Molecular and Cellular Biology. New Series, Vol 53. Alan R. Liss, 1987, pp. 911–918.
57. Fischer A, Lisowska-Grosspiere B, Anderson C, Springer T: Leukocyte adhesion deficiency; molecular basis and functional consequences. *Immunodeficiency Rev* 1988;1:39–55.
58. Springer T, Thompson W, Miller L, et al.: Inherited deficiency of the Mac-1, LFA-1, p150,95 glycoprotein family and its molecular basis. *J Exp Med* 1984;160:1901–1918.
59. Fischer A, Trung PH, Descamps-Latscha B: Bone marrow transplantation for an inborn error of phagocytic cells associated with defective adherence, chemotaxis, and oxidative response during opsonised particle phagocytosis. *Lancet* 1983;1:473–479.
60. DiGeorge AM: Discussions on a new concept of the cellular base of immunology. *J Pediatr* 1965;67:907.
61. Conley ME, Beckwith JB, Mancer JFK, Tenckhoff L: The spectrum of DiGeorge syndrome. *J Pediatr* 1979;94:883–890.
62. Sieber OF, Durie BG, Hattler BG, et al.: Spontaneous evolution of immune competence in DiGeorge syndrome. *Pediatr Res* 1974;8:418.
63. Goldsobel AB, Haas A, Stiehm ER: Bone marrow transplantation in DiGeorge syndrome. *J Pediatr* 1987;111:40–44.

Bone Marrow Transplantation in Children, edited by F. Leonard Johnson and Carl Pochedly. Raven Press, Ltd., New York © 1990.

Use of Bone Marrow Transplantation in Bone Marrow Failure

Norma K. C. Ramsay

Pediatric Bone Marrow Transplantation Program, University of Minnesota Hospitals, and Department of Pediatrics, University of Minnesota Medical School, Minneapolis, Minnesota 55455

Introduction
A. Severe aplastic anemia
　　1. Etiology
　　2. Evaluation
B. Bone marrow transplantation for severe aplastic anemia
　　1. Early studies
　　2. Bone marrow transplantation in untranfused patients
C. Conditioning regimens
　　1. Preparation with cyclophosphamide alone
　　2. Preparation with cyclophosphamide and additional chemotherapy or immunosuppression
　　3. Preparation with cyclophosphamide and total body irradiation
　　4. Preparation with cyclophosphamide and total lymphoid irradiation
　　5. Preparation with cyclophosphamide and thoraco-abdominal irradiation
D. Graft-vs.-host disease
E. Syngeneic transplantation
F. Transplantation of patients with severe aplastic anemia who lack matched donors: use of mismatched donors
G. Late effects
H. Immunosuppression for treatment of patients with severe aplastic anemia
I. Bone marrow transplantation for treatment of other marrow failure states
　　1. Fanconi's anemia

INTRODUCTION

The effectiveness of bone marrow transplantation (BMT) for treatment of marrow failure states was first demonstrated for severe aplastic anemia (SAA) (1). Over the past decade improvements in preparative regimens, combined with transplantation early in the course of the disease, have increased survival rates substantially, such that bone marrow transplantation is currently the treatment of choice for children with severe aplastic anemia who have matched donors.

Because of the success of bone marrow transplantation for severe aplastic anemia, other conditions of marrow failure have been treated using this technique. Certain diseases such as severe neutropenia syndromes, platelet disorders, and thalassemia have recently been treated using marrow transplant.

This chapter will review the current status of marrow transplantation for treatment of severe aplastic anemia and other marrow failure states in children.

SEVERE APLASTIC ANEMIA

Severe aplastic anemia refers to a condition in which presence of pancytopenia is combined with bone marrow aplasia. The criteria for diagnosis of severe aplastic anemia as defined by the International Aplastic Anemia Study Group (IAASG) consists of at least two of the following peripheral blood findings: granulocyte count less than $500/mm^3$, platelets less than $20,000/mm^3$, anemia with total reticulocyte count less than $2000/mm^3$, combined with a bone marrow which has cellularity less than 25% or a marrow with less than 50% cellularity consisting of less than 30% hematopoietic cells (2). Although the exact incidence of severe aplastic anemia is not well documented, there are two recent population-based studies in the United States (3,4). Age-adjusted rates for incidence in males are 6.8 and 4.7 per million and incidence rates for females are 13.7 and 7.3 per million. These data are from studies done in South Carolina and Baltimore. A lower incidence (less than 3 per million per year) was recently reported from Israel and Europe (5).

Etiology

In children, most cases of severe aplastic anemia are acquired, although a constitutional form, Fanconi's anemia, often progresses to severe marrow aplasia (6). A number of etiologic agents have been associated with aplastic anemia including drugs, ionizing radiation, chemicals and infections (7–10). Certain drugs such as chloramphenicol produce a predictable dose-related myelosuppression which reverses upon withdrawal of the drug (7). Chloramphenicol may also be associated with an idiosyncratic reaction in which irreversible aplastic anemia occurs (10). Ionizing radiation produces myelosuppression and, if given in high enough doses, will result in permanent aplasia (8). Exposure to chemical agents such as benzene have also been reported to be associated with aplastic anemia (11). The infection most frequently followed by severe aplastic anemia is viral hepatitis (9). In spite of the many factors known to be associated with aplastic anemia, the majority of cases do not have a well-defined etiologic agent.

Regardless of the etiology, the pathophysiologic mechanisms responsible for aplasia may involve a defect in one or more areas of pluripotential cell maturation of differentiation, or may be a defect in the microenvironment. In addition, cellular or humoral regulating factors or cell-cell interaction may be involved in the development of severe aplastic anemia. Data supporting the different pathophysiologic mechanisms have been recently reviewed (12).

Evaluation

Children who present with decreased blood counts affecting two or more cell lineages should have a bone marrow aspiration and biopsy performed for assessment of cellularity. If a patient satisfies the criteria of the International Aplastic Anemia Study Group for diagnosis of severe aplastic anemia, HLA typing and mixed lymphocyte culture testing should be performed on all family members. If the patient has an HLA-matched donor, bone marrow transplantation should be performed immediately. However, family members should not be used as blood donors for patients prior to transplantation because of the risk of sensitization.

BONE MARROW TRANSPLANTATION FOR SEVERE APLASTIC ANEMIA

Early studies

Following successful bone marrow transplantation for treatment of severe combined immune deficiency in 1968 (13,14), severe aplastic anemia with marrow failure was a logical disease to be potentially cured by this technique. The first report of a successful bone marrow transplant in severe aplastic anemia was in 1972 (1). Since that time, marrow transplantation has become the preferred treatment for children and young adults with severe aplastic anemia who have matched donors.

Wide acceptance of this therapy, however, only followed reports from the International Aplastic Anemia Study Group (15). A multicenter prospective randomized study was performed in 110 newly diagnosed patients with severe aplastic anemia from 1974–1977. Patients with matched sibling donors underwent marrow transplant and were compared to severe aplastic anemia patients who did not have matched donors, who were randomized to receive supportive care and oral androgens, intramuscular androgens, or no androgens. The outcome for the patients on the nontransplant regimens was very poor. Only 30% of these patients were alive at one year, and more than 50% of the patients died of infection or hemorrhage within 6 months of diagnosis. Survival for the transplanted patients was significantly superior to that for nontransplant patients. This improvement in survival, as well as high mortality soon after diagnosis in the nontransplanted patients, argues for early transplantation for patients with severe aplastic anemia who have a matched donor (see Table 1).

Bone Marrow Transplantation in Untransfused Patients

The Seattle Transplant Team has published two reports of marrow transplant in untransfused patients (16,17). In the initial series of 30 patients reported in 1980, 25 patients were surviving 9 to 84 months after being transplanted using a conditioning regimen consisting of cyclophosphamide alone (16). This series has been expanded and a recent report (17) demonstrates the excellent long-term results in 50 untransfused patients undergoing bone marrow transplantation. Graft failure occurred in only 10% of the patients, and 42 of the 50 patients are surviving 1 to 12 years after transplantation with a median follow-up of 6.3 years. The actuarial 10-year probability of survival is 82%. This excellent long-term survival for untransfused patients should encourage the early transplantation of patients with severe aplastic anemia. For

TABLE 1. *Preparative regimens for bone marrow transplantation of transfused aplastic anemia patients*

Preparative regimen	N	% Survival	Rejection	Reference
CY Cyclophosphamide alone	60	43	21/60	25
CY + Buffy Coat Infusion	175		38/175	28
Patients with Sustained Engraftment	74			
Patients who Rejected Marrow	24			
CY + ATG and Procarbazine	40	64	4/40	37
CY + Cyclosporine	41	76	6/41	35
CY + Total Body Irradiation	46	62	1/46	40
CY + Total Lymphoid Irradiation	58	72	3/58	45
CY + Thoraco-abdominal Irradiation	40	85	1/40	46

the majority of aplastic anemia patients, however, this is not always practical and most patients have been transfused before marrow transplant.

CONDITIONING REGIMENS

The rate of long-term survival for patients transplanted for severe aplastic anemia in the 1970s was 40 to 45% in most series, and long-term survivors had successful reconstitution of hematopoiesis (18–22). In most early series, including that reported by the International Aplastic Anemia Study Group, patients were prepared by use of a standard immunosuppressive regimen consisting of cyclophosphamide 50 mg/kg/day for 4 days. Although this approach resulted in a number of long-term survivors, rejection of the marrow following transplant was a frequent occurrence, being as high as 30–60% in some series (18–22). This contrasts with the experience of patients undergoing marrow transplant for malignancies where graft failure rarely occurs. Although retransplantation was frequently attempted, the outcome was usually unfavorable because of the adverse effects of the prolonged period of pancytopenia. Likewise, long-term survival was poor for second transplants performed for treatment of a variety of diseases.[23] Second transplants were performed in 16 patients with severe aplastic anemia who rejected their grafts, with 40% of the patients becoming long-term survivors (24).

The adverse effect of marrow rejection on survival led to trials of several conditioning regimens. Each of these regimens was designed to decrease the rate of rejection and, therefore, to improve survival in patients with severe aplastic anemia undergoing marrow transplantation.

The new approaches to conditioning have involved either (1) increasing cell dose administered, or (2) increased immunosuppression by the use of radiation therapy, additional chemotherapy or immunosuppressive agents. The approach of increasing stem cell dose administered has been used by the Seattle group and is based on their analysis of factors associated with rejection (25). Other transplant investigators have used the approach of additional immunosuppression because the rejection rate in patients with malignancy undergoing bone marrow transplantation with matched donors has been extremely low.

Preparation with Cyclophosphamide Alone

The largest experience in using marrow transplant in severe aplastic anemia comes from the Seattle investigators. In their early series in the 1970s, approximately one-third of multiply-transfused patients conditioned for transplant with cyclophosphamide alone rejected their grafts (20). These patients had poorer survival than patients who had sustained engraftment following marrow transplant. An analysis of factors associated with graft rejection in these patients revealed two factors predictive of rejection, the unidirectional positive response with mixed lymphocyte culture and the marrow cell dose (26). The practice in Seattle has been to administer donor peripheral blood buffy coat cells in addition to the marrow. This is intended to overcome transfusion-induced sensitization and to decrease graft rejection. This practice was based on analysis of factors responsible for rejection as well as data obtained in their dog transplant model (27). With increasing numbers of cells transfused, the graft rejection rate decreased.

In a recent analysis of 175 patients with severe aplastic anemia, 5 factors predicted for graft rejection (28). These factors were: (1) previous blood transfusion, (2) a positive relative response in mixed leukocyte culture indicating sensitization of recipient against donor, (3) low number of marrow cells transplanted, (4) marrow grafts from male donors, and (5) lack of infusion of viable donor buffy coat cells in addition to marrow for transfused patients. Of the 175 patients, 7 died in the first two weeks; 130 patients had sustained engraftment of the first graft and 38 patients rejected their marrow grafts. The survival rate for the 130 patients with sustained engraftment was 74%, whereas only 24% of the patients survived who rejected their graft. Overall, 17% of the 168 patients died from complications associated with graft rejection, which was a decrease from earlier Seattle studies. The most recent update of these patients describes the changing impact of risk factors. The risk factors for rejection are now year of transplant, large number of platelet transfusions, positive relative response in mixed leukocyte culture, low marrow cell dose and omission of donor buffy coat cell infusion for transfused patients (29).

Even though sustained engraftment occurred in the majority of patients, a recent study demonstrated the persistence of host cells in certain patients when several techniques were used to evaluate patients post-transplant (30). Mixed hematologic chimerism was detected in 56 (58.3%) of 96 patients evaluated for chimerism. Only donor cells were present in 40 (41.7%) of the patients. Mixed chimerism was detected a median of 18 days post-transplant (range 14–68 days). Although the presence of mixed hematologic chimerism did not influence survival, it was predictive for graft rejection. Seventeen (30.4%) patients with mixed chimerism and 2 (5.0%) with complete chimerism rejected their grafts (p = .01). In addition, the incidence of grade II–IV acute graft-vs.-host disease (graft-vs.-host disease) was greater in the complete chimeras (57%) compared to the mixed chimeras (18%) (p = .03). The presence of mixed chimerism was independent of transfusion status prior to transplant and was also independent of the use of donor buffy coat infusions.

This large group of patients has also been evaluated for factors predictive of survival. In an analysis of 130 patients who had sustained engraftment, factors which were predictive of improved survival were laminar airflow isolation, absence of acute graft-vs.-host disease, younger patient age, and lack of refractoriness to random donor platelet transfusions (31).

Preparation with Cyclophosphamide and Additional Chemotherapy or Immunosuppression

Other groups have added immunosuppressive agents or chemotherapeutic agents to cyclophosphamide in the conditioning regimen to achieve reduced rejection rates. The group at Hammersmith Hospital in London has added cyclosporin to cyclophosphamide (32). In a series of 41 matched patients, 31 were alive from 3 to 38 months following transplant. Six of the 41 patients rejected their grafts, which is a rejection rate lower than their past experience, in which 6 out of 14 patients experienced graft rejection. Of interest is the fact that 4 patients experienced late graft failure at 6 to 9 months following transplant when the cyclosporine was withdrawn (33–35). The Boston group utilized a combination of antithymocyte globulin, procarbazine and cyclophosphamide in their conditioning regimen. This resulted in a decrease of the rejection rate to 10% in a series of 40 patients (36,37).

Preparation with Cyclophosphamide and Total Body Irradiation

The addition of radiation therapy to the preparative regimen was a logical step in that patients undergoing transplantation for malignancy rarely reject their graft. Initial studies at the University of California in Los Angeles (UCLA) used doses of total body irradiation (TBI) similar to that used for patients given marrow transplants for treatment of malignancies (38). Nine patients received 1000 cGy (rad) TBI combined with cyclophosphamide. Although graft rejection did not occur, the incidence of fatal interstitial pneumonitis was significant, such that overall survival was not improved when compared to preparation by use of cyclophosphamide alone. Therefore, the dose of total body irradiation subsequently was decreased to 300 cGy (39,40). Of 46 patients who were prepared for marrow transplant with 300 cGy TBI and cyclophosphamide, the 2-year actuarial survival was 62%. Rejection occurred in only one patient, indicating that his regimen could significantly overcome rejection in a transfused aplastic anemia patient. In this study the most important factor in predicting survival was age of the patient. The rate of 1-year survival for patients less than 25 years of age was 82% compared to a rate of 1-year survival of 31% for patients older than 25 years (p = .001). This difference in rate of survival was due in large part to the higher incidence of graft-vs.-host disease and interstitial pneumonitis in the older patients. The International Bone Marrow Transplant Registry also identified the use of total body irradiation to have an unfavorable influence on the risk of interstitial pneumonitis in SAA patients. Other unfavorable risk factors were age over 20 years, presence of moderate to severe acute graft-vs.-host disease and the use of methotrexate for graft-vs.-host disease prophylaxis as compared to cyclosporine (41).

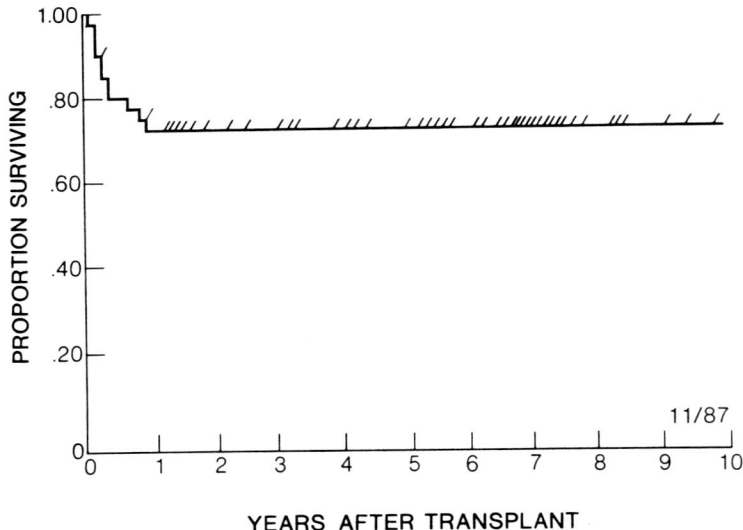

FIG. 1.   Survival of 64 multiply-transfused patients with severe aplastic anemia following preparation with 750 cGy total lymphoid irradiation and 200 mg/kg cyclophosphamide at the University of Minnesota.

Preparation with Cyclophosphamide and Total Lymphoid Irradiation

Although total body irradiation appears to overcome the problem of graft rejection, two centers have used more limited radiation for the same purpose. The University of Minnesota Transplant Team gave a combination of total lymphoid irradiation, giving a single dose of 750 cGy together with cyclophosphamide (200 mg/kg), in a series of children and adults (42,43). This preparative regimen was tried because studies in animals showed that total lymphoid irradiation could be successfully used to condition marrow transplant recipients (44). This regimen has resulted in a low rejection rate (3 out of 58) in a series of heavily transfused patients (45). As of November 1987, 45 of 64 patients are surviving with a median follow-up of 5.8 years and an actuarial survival of 72% (Figure 1).

Factors which predicted for survival in an earlier analysis of 40 patients with aplastic anemia were idiopathic etiology and younger donor age (43). In the expanded series of 58 patients with longer follow-up the factors which predicted for improved survival in multivariate analysis were: shorter interval from diagnosis to transplant and the absence of advanced graft-vs.-host disease (45). Unlike the UCLA series, patient age did not significantly influence survival. Of 30 patients under 18 years of age, 73% are surviving compared to 67% of 28 patients older than 18 years. Acute and chronic graft-vs.-host disease was significantly more common in adults than children.

Preparation with Cyclophosphamide and Thoraco-Abdominal Irradiation

A similar approach in the effort to decrease rejection, the use of single dose thoraco-abdominal irradiation (600 cGy) with lung shielding in combination with cyclophosphamide (150 mg/kg), has been used by Gluckman and colleagues at the Hopital St. Louis in Paris. The rejection rate was very low (1 out of 40) in a series of 40 patients and the survival was 85%, with a median follow-up of 18 months (46). The most commonly used conditioning regimens all have been effective in decreasing the rejection rate.

GRAFT-VS.-HOST DISEASE

Transplant related graft-vs.-host disease is the major problem in patients undergoing bone marrow transplantation for severe aplastic anemia now that graft rejection has been overcome. The survival rate of 130 patients transplanted in Seattle who achieved sustained engraftment correlated with the occurrence of graft-vs.-host disease. Thus, the survival rate of 86 patients with no graft-vs.-host disease or mild acute graft-vs.-host disease was greater than 80%, compared to a survival rate of only 40 to 50% in 44 patients who had grade II–IV acute graft-vs.-host disease (31). The incidence of graft-vs.-host disease was influenced by a number of factors. Patients housed in laminar airflow rooms had a lower incidence of grades II–IV graft-vs.-host disease compared to those patients treated in regular rooms. Certain conditioning regimens are associated with an increased risk of chronic graft-vs.-host disease. The use of viable donor buffy coat infusions in addition to marrow, as used by the Seattle group, has resulted in an increased incidence of chronic graft-vs.-host disease (47). The other factor associated with an increased risk of chronic graft-vs.-host disease was increased patient age at transplant. The dominant factor predicting for chronic graft-vs.-host disease, however, was the presence of acute graft-vs.-host disease. Likewise, the incidence of chronic graft-vs.-host disease increased with the grade of acute graft-vs.-host disease. The occurrence of chronic graft-vs.-host disease adversely affects not only quality of life but also long-term survival. Late deaths, more than 200 days following bone marrow transplant for severe aplastic anemia, are almost always associated with chronic graft-vs.-hose disease even though they are usually due to infectious complications. Control of graft-vs.-host disease will be necessary to improve the long-term survival in patients undergoing marrow transplant for aplastic anemia.

SYNGENEIC TRANSPLANTATION

Bone marrow transplantation using an identical twin donor (syngeneic marrow) offers the obvious advantage of lack of graft-vs.-host disease. If the cause of bone marrow failure is purely an absence or abnormality of stem cells, infusion of marrow from the normal donor without any immuno-suppression should restore hematopoiesis. In most cases, this occurs and engraftment follows an infusion of marrow cells from the identical twin with-out any prior immunosuppression. However, engraftment has failed to occur or has been only temporary in certain cases (48–50). This finding suggests either that factors in the microenvironment are important or that the original cause of the aplastic anemia persists.

In a review of syngeneic marrow transplantation for aplastic anemia, only 9 out of 21 patients had complete hematologic recovery following marrow infu-sion alone, while 12 patients failed to have sustained improvement in hematopoiesis following the infusion of bone marrow alone from their normal twin (48). When pre-transplant immunosuppression using cyclophosphamide (at a dose of 200 mg/kg) alone or combined with total body irradiation was subsequently used in 8 patients, all had complete recovery following rein-fusion of marrow from the same donor. Four patients had a second infusion of donor marrow without pre-transplant conditioning; one of these patients expe-rienced marrow recovery. Thus, sustained engraftment occurred following immunosuppression in this subset of patients. This finding suggests that immu-nologic or microenvironmental factors were overcome using pre-transplant immunosuppression. Based on the small numbers of reported cases, it is estimated that approximately half of the patients transplanted with syngeneic marrow alone will have hematologic recovery. The remainder of the patients should have a second transplant following immunosuppressive therapy; it is expected that the majority of these patients will have hematologic recovery.

TRANSPLANTATION OF PATIENTS WITH SEVERE APLASTIC ANEMIA WHO LACK MATCHED DONORS: USE OF MISMATCHED DONORS

Another approach to therapy of the two-thirds of patients who lack a matched sibling donor could be the use of histocompatible marrow from a nonrelated donor. Two patients with aplastic anemia have been successfully transplanted using marrow from volunteer donors unrelated to the recipient. The transplants were given following preparation with cyclophosphamide and cyclosporine and, in one case, additional antilymphocyte globulin and procar-bazine were used (51). Both patients engrafted and graft-vs.-host disease occurred in both patients.

Increased risks of graft-vs.-host disease will most likely be present when mismatched donors are used. A report comparing unrelated or mismatched family donors for patients with aplastic anemia and Fanconi's anemia demon-strated similar long-term results with 30% of patients surviving (52). How-ever, future improvements in areas of marrow transplantation such as preparative regimens and in control of graft-vs.-host disease should favorably affect the use of unrelated marrow donors.

LATE EFFECTS

Discussion of bone marrow transplantation in children, which includes the use of high-dose chemotherapy and in some cases radiation in the conditioning regimen, needs to address the potential late consequences of this therapy. It is encouraging that the rate of long-term survival for children with aplastic anemia treated with bone marrow transplantation is now greater than 70%, and there is an increasing population of long-term survivors. Medical centers performing bone marrow transplantation need to start now to evaluate prospectively the long-term effect of conditioning regimens.

Limited data are available for evaluating growth, endocrine function and thyroid function in long-term survivors of aplastic anemia treated with bone marrow transplantation. When cyclophosphamide alone was used in pre-transplant preparation, the majority of patients appear to be growing at a normal rate and most continue to grow along their pre-transplant height percentile curve (53). In a small number of children who received cyclophosphamide and 750 cGy single dose total lymphoid irradiation, growth also appears to be normal (54).

Thyroid dysfunction has been documented in a small series of patients conditioned with cyclophosphamide and single dose total lymphoid irradiation (55,56). Longer follow-up of these patients will be necessary to determine the incidence and impact of this transplant-related effect.

Evaluation of gonadal function will also be important, especially in young patients successfully transplanted for aplastic anemia. There is preliminary data on gonadal function available for both males and females. In males who received high-dose cyclophosphamide in their prepubertal years, spontaneous puberty occurred (53). Data in men receiving high-dose cyclophosphamide during or after puberty reveal a higher incidence of testicular dysfunction, compared to cases in which cyclophosphamide was given prior to the onset of puberty (57). Semen analysis has revealed variable degrees of spermatogenesis (53). In a small number of men who received cyclophosphamide and total lymphoid irradiation during adolescence, testosterone levels were normal; however, follicle stimulating hormone (FSH) and luteinizing hormone (LH) were transiently elevated in some of the males (58).

Females who were given only cyclophosphamide appear to have minimal ovarian dysfunction when treated as prepubertal females or adolescents. Also, pregnancy has been reported in females who are prolonged survivors after marrow transplantation for severe aplastic anemia using cyclophosphamide in the conditioning regimen (53). Ovarian function in 12 women treated postmenarche with cyclophosphamide and total lymphoid irradiation has resulted in elevated gonadotropins and either oligomenorrhea or amenorrhea in 11 out of the 12 patients (59).

Long-term follow-up will be necessary to evaluate more fully the adverse late effects of various preparative regimens used.

IMMUNOSUPPRESSION FOR TREATMENT OF PATIENTS WITH SEVERE APLASTIC ANEMIA

Although bone marrow transplantation is clearly the treatment of choice for patients with severe aplastic anemia who have matched donors, approximately two-thirds of patients do not have a matched sibling donor. The use of antilymphocyte serum, antilymphocyte globulin, or antithymocyte globulin has had some success. The use of antilymphocyte serum (ALS) was initiated by Mathe in 1979 (60) and has since been used by investigators in Europe and the United States. Early results of studies using antilymphocyte serum with therapy by Speck et al. (61,62), were very encouraging. Recently, a review of 72 patients treated with antilymphocyte serum by Speck and coworkers demonstrated a 65% survival rate (63). These patients remain on chronic low-dose androgen therapy and some of the patients have incomplete reconstitution of hematopoiesis. At 2 years, survival of the patients who were treated with antilymphocyte serum is significantly better than survival in a group of 28 patients with aplastic anemia who were transplanted. The transplanted patients had only a 46% survival rate. Although results of Speck et al., show an advantage for therapy with antilymphocyte serum, the transplant results of 46% are lower than those observed in most other recent transplant series.

The UCLA group has also compared use of bone marrow transplantation to antithymocyte globulin (ATG) therapy in a group of 57 patients under 25 years of age (64). In this study, the 2-year actuarial survival for the patients undergoing bone marrow transplant is 72%, as compared with 45% for those given ATG therapy. In the surviving patients, quality of life was better in the transplant patients who more commonly had a rapid return of peripheral blood counts to normal values.

A number of other centers have published nonrandomized studies using antilymphocyte globulin (ALG) or antithymocyte globulin for the treatment of aplastic anemia (65–68). In some of these studies infusion of haploidentical marrow (that is, marrow that is genetically only half identical), accompanied by steroids, androgens or both, have been combined with antilymphocyte globulin or antithymocyte globulin therapy. The survival rate varied from 30 to 60% in different series.

There have been two randomized studies performed which determine the relative effectiveness of giving immunosuppressive therapy with antilymphocyte globulin or antithymocyte globulin as compared to supportive care (69,70). In both studies survival was significantly better in those patients receiving antilymphocyte globulin or antithymocyte globulin as compared to those given only supportive care. In one study, 42 patients were randomized to receive antithymocyte globulin as compared to those given only supportive care. Eleven out of 21 patients had sustained improvement in hematopoiesis, none of 21 control patients who received supportive care alone showed sustained improvement in hematopoiesis (69). There was a trend for better survival for the patients who had a short duration of illness; however, the small numbers in this study limited statistical analysis of prognostic factors.

In a second multiinstitutional prospective study, newly diagnosed aplastic anemia patients were randomized to receive either standard therapy with androgens or antithoracic duct lymphocyte globulin (ATDLG), HLA-haploidentical marrow and androgens (70). At 2 years, life table analysis showed 76% of the patients who received ATDLG to be alive while only 31% of the concurrent control group were alive. In addition, greater improvement in hematologic factors occurred in the group treated with ATDLG, marrow infusion and androgens. Response to therapy was not predicted by any of the usual factors: age, sex, etiology of bone marrow failure, prior therapy, severity of pancytopenia, or duration of symptoms. As in all studies assessing therapy with antilymphocyte globulin or antithymocyte globulin, hematopoietic recovery was frequently incomplete. For these reasons long-term follow-up will be needed to determine the rate of long-term survival and quality of life.

The severity of the aplastic anemia was the major predictive factor in a series of 64 patients treated with antilymphocyte globulin (ALG Merieux) between 1980 and 1985. The actuarial survival at 6 years for all patients was 53%, but survival was 36% for patients with severe aplastic anemia compared to 79% for those with nonsevere aplastic anemia (71).

There have been no randomized studies comparing bone marrow transplant with therapy with ATG or ALG. Potential advantages exist for both approaches. Bone marrow transplantation is currently the therapy of choice in children with matched donors, where the risk for graft-vs.-host disease is low and the rate of prolonged survival is now greater than 70%. These survivors have complete hematopoietic recovery and rarely have recurrent aplasia, unlike patients, after therapy with ATG or ALG, who frequently have only partial hematopoietic recovery and more often have recurrence of aplasia.

Since immunosuppressive therapy using antithymocyte globulin or antilymphocyte globulin has been associated with hematopoietic recovery in aplastic anemia, it is logical that the immunosuppressive properties of corticosteroids may also be helpful. The effectiveness of high-dose methylprednisolone has been evaluated by Marmont and coworkers. Although some patients have responded to this drug, the results are not as promising as those seen after therapy with ATG or ALG (72,73).

The immunosuppressive agent, cyclosporine, evaluated in a small series of 12 patients with severe aplastic anemia, either alone or in combination with antilymphocyte serum produced disappointing results (74), although there are reports of responses in isolated cases (75). Currently, growth factors, such as GM-CSF, are being evaluated for the treatment of aplastic anemia (76).

BONE MARROW TRANSPLANTATION FOR TREATMENT OF OTHER MARROW FAILURE STATES

Fanconi's Anemia

Fanconi's anemia is a constitutional aplastic anemia in which patients have a variety of congenital malformations, characteristic chromosomal breaks, and slowly evolving bone marrow failure (77–80). Initially, patients with Fanconi's anemia have only mild aplasia, or involvement of one or two cell lines. Treatment with steroids, androgens, or both, results in improved peripheral blood counts for a variable period of time. Complications of androgen therapy may occur, the most serious being the development of malignant hepatic tumors which is associated with prolonged androgen therapy. Virtually all patients will eventually become unresponsive to androgen therapy and progress to severe aplastic anemia. An increased incidence of leukemia is also seen in patients with Fanconi's anemia.

Since bone marrow transplantation has been shown to be effective therapy for severe aplastic anemia of other etiologies, it was logical to treat patients with Fanconi's anemia with this technique. A number of centers have reported their experience (81–84).

Initially, conditioning regimens used to prepare these patients were similar to those used for other patients with severe aplastic anemia undergoing marrow transplantation. Patients with Fanconi's anemia experienced severe toxicity, due to the conditioning regimen, including skin sloughing, hemorrhagic cystitis, and severe mucositis. These abnormalities may be related to the underlying defect present in patients with Fanconi's anemia. It has been postulated that the abnormal findings may be related to a DNA repair defect (85,86). *In vitro* studies have demonstrated that cells from patients with Fanconi's anemia have increased sensitivity to alkylating agents such as cyclophosphamide, which is frequently used for pre-transplant conditioning. Gluckman proposed that the excessive toxicity experienced in patients with Fanconi's anemia undergoing bone marrow transplantation is because their cells are exquisitely sensitive to alkylating agents such as cyclophosphamide (87).

Gluckman devised a test to measure the *in vivo* radiosensitivity and rate of cell repair after skin contact radiotherapy in order to calculate the radiation dose which could be tolerated by patients with Fanconi's anemia (87). Of the 8 patients tested, one patient developed pigmentation and all patients had some desquamation. There was also a delayed skin response when compared to normal controls tested in the same manner. Based on these findings, a modified preparative regimen was used in 4 patients. The modified regimen consisted of 10% of the usual dose of cyclophosphamide (20 mg/kg total dose) and single dose of 400–500 cGy thoraco-abdominal radiation. All 4 patients engrafted and only one patient developed significant graft-vs.-host disease. Transplant complications were present, but they were not as severe as in patients with Fanconi's anemia transplanted following the standard doses of cyclophosphamide. An unusual complication was the presence of esophagitis in 3 out of 4 patients resulting in esophageal stenosis in 2 patients. All 4 patients were surviving longer than 2 months from transplant at the time of publication.

Deeg recently reported 8 Fanconi's anemia patients transplanted in Seattle (82). These patients experienced marked toxicity and only 4 of the 8 patients were long-term survivors. One of the patients who died after one year from transplant had received marrow from a donor who had chromosomal abnormalities similar to those seen in Fanconi's anemia. This emphasizes the need to test prospective donors for Fanconi's anemia with the mitomycin-C stress test, which may uncover patients with Fanconi's anemia that have not yet become manifest (88). Deeg also reviewed the published data on 12 patients with Fanconi's anemia reported from other centers. All patients had received large doses of cyclophosphamide in their preparative regimen, and 10 of the 12 patients experienced acute graft-vs.-host disease. This represents a high incidence of graft-vs.-host disease in this young group of patients who had a median age of only 10.5 years. Graft-vs.-host disease is usually less common in younger patients (89).

The optimal time for performing bone marrow transplantation in Fanconi's anemia is not clearly defined. Although androgens frequently cause temporary normalization of peripheral blood counts, severe complications to androgen therapy may occur. One of the most disturbing complications is the development of hepatic tumors, both benign and malignant. Marrow transplantation has been performed in at least two patients with known hepatic lesions. In both patients, the hepatic tumors resolved following successful transplantation (90). Now that an improved conditioning regimen is available for transplantation of patients with Fanconi's anemia, marrow transplantation should be performed earlier if a donor is available, before the onset of severe complications.

Thalassemia

Bone marrow transplantation has recently been explored as therapy for thalassemia major (91–92). The timing of marrow transplantation in the course of the disease is important. As in other diseases, long-term survival is better if patients are transplanted before developing complications of their disease and thus, are good-risk candidates for marrow transplant. However, the morbidity and mortality associated with marrow transplantation have to be considered when this procedure is performed in diseases such as thalassemia major where transfusion therapy will allow patients to survive for many years.

Reports from Seattle and Pesaro, Italy, describe the successful transplantation of patients with homozygous beta-thalassemia. The Italian investigators have had the largest experience to date. Lucarelli reported 30 patients (median age 3.5 years) with homozygous beta-thalassemia who have undergone allogeneic bone marrow transplantation. All patients were conditioned with busulphan and cyclophosphamide and received post-transplant immunosuppression with methotrexate or methotrexate and cyclophosphamide. Six patients received 16 mg/kg busulphan and 200 mg/kg cyclophosphamide. Three of these patients died of complications and three are surviving 2 years from the time of transplant. The 24 patients who were subsequently transplanted received a lower dose of busulphan (14 mg/kg) combined with 200 mg/kg cyclophosphamide as pre-transplant conditioning. Of the 24 patients, 23 are surviving; however, 4 patients have had return of thalassemia following failure of their graft. Marrow graft failure following busulphan and cyclophosphamide has also been reported in other diseases treated by bone marrow transplantation. In a recent report of a total of 70 patients transplanted, 80% are alive with functioning graft (93).

The early success of bone marrow transplantation for treatment of thalassemia in encouraging. The results suggest that marrow transplant is the treatment of choice for patients with homozygous beta-thalassemia.

Other Bone Marrow Failure States

Since improved survival has occurred following bone marrow transplantation of patients with severe aplastic anemia, this procedure has been tried in patients with other rare forms of bone marrow failure. In most of these rare diseases, either small numbers of patients or individual patients have been reported.

Paroxysmal nocturnal hemoglobinuria (PNH), which includes an acquired stem cell defect in some cases, results in bone marrow failure. Three patients with PNH accompanied by aplastic anemia had correction of their anemia following successful allogeneic marrow transplant. The conditioning regimen consisted of cyclophosphamide either alone or combined with procarbazine and antithymocyte globulin (94). A patient who received syngeneic bone marrow with no immunosuppression had persisting engraftment and a negative Ham's test at 3 years post-transplant. Ten years later, however, the patient's complement lysis sensitivity test was positive. But since no other genetic markers were available and the patient remains asymptomatic, one can only postulate that the reappearance of PNH cells signifies at least partial loss of the donor graft. Other cases of successful bone marrow transplantation in paroxysmal nocturnal hemoglobinuria have been reported (95–98).

Abnormalities of hemoglobin synthesis have also been corrected using bone marrow transplantation in sickle cell anemia. In the case of sickle cell anemia corrected by BMT, the primary reason for doing the transplant was the presence of acute nonlymphoid leukemia. However, the sickle cell disease that happened to be present also in this patient was corrected (98).

Selective deficiencies or abnormalities in specific cell lines have been corrected by bone marrow transplantation. An example of this is the correction of congenital hypoplastic anemia (Blackfan-Diamond syndrome), in which there is a deficiency of red cell precursors (99,100). Reports of two patients have occurred to date. Both patients had restoration of erythropoiesis and one patient was a long-term survivor. Correction of neutrophil deficiencies, such as infantile agranulocytosis (Kostmann's syndrome), have been reported (101).

A 4-year-old with Glanzmann's thrombasthenia was recently reported to have correction of his inherited platelet disorder following bone marrow transplantation (103). Of note is the fact that the first attempt at marrow transplantation, using cyclophosphamide (150 mg/kg total dose) and 600 cGy of thoraco-abdominal radiation for conditioning, resulted in rejection of the marrow graft. A sustained graft with correction of the platelet defect followed a successful second transplant.

SUMMARY

Bone marrow transplantation has emerged over the past decade as the treatment of choice for children with severe aplastic anemia who have a matched sibling donor. Rejection of the marrow occurred in early studies. The initial problem of rejection has been overcome with all of the commonly used conditioning regimens and over 70% of patients are long-term survivors. In order to improve the results further, the complications of graft-vs.-host disease and infections need to be addressed. For patients who do not have a matched sibling donor, immunosuppressive therapy with antithymocyte globulin or similar immunosuppressive agents currently offer improved survival compared to giving supportive care alone. The possibility exists of using less than fully matched donors for transplant more often in the future.

Application of the technique of bone marrow transplantation is now being applied to other bone marrow failure states and in thalassemia. Its use in these areas will increase in the future as the morbidity and mortality associated with the procedure declines. For long-term survivors, the late effects of the conditioning regimen need to be evaluated.

REFERENCES

1. Thomas ED, Buckner CD, Storb R, et al.: Aplastic anemia treated by marrow transplantation. *Lancet* 1972;1:284–289.

2. Camitta BM, Thomas ED, Nathan DG, et al.: Severe aplastic anemia: A prospective study of the effect of early marrow transplantation on acute mortality. *Blood* 1976;48:63–70.
3. Linet MS, McGaffrey LD, Morgan WF: Incidence of aplastic anemia in a three-county area of South Carolina. *Cancer Res* 1986; 46:426–429.
4. Szklo M, Sensenbrenner L, Markowitz J, et al.: Incidence of aplastic anemia in metropolitan Baltimore; a population-based study. *Blood* 1985; 66:115–119.
5. International agranulocytosis and aplastic anemia study: Incidence of aplastic anemia: the relevance of diagnostic criteria. *Blood* 1987; 70:1718–1721.
6. Alter BP, Potter NU, Li FP: Classification and etiology of aplastic anemias. *Clin Hæmat* 1978; 7(3):431–465.
7. Williams DM, Lynch RE, Cartwright GE: Drug induced aplastic anemia. *Semin Hematol* 1973; 10:195–223.
8. Kirshbaum JD, Matsuo T, Sato K, et al.: A study of aplastic anemia in an autopsy series with special reference to atomic bomb survivors in Hiroshima and Nagasaki. *Blood* 1971; 38:17–26.
9. Hagler L, Pastore RA, Bergin JJ: Aplastic anemia following viral hepatitis, report of two fatal cases and literature review. *Medicine* (Baltimore) 1975; 54:139–164.
10. Yunis AA: Chloramphenicol induced bone marrow suppression. *Semin Hematol* 1973; 10:225–234.
11. Huguley CM, Lea JW, Butts JA: Adverse hematologic reactions to drugs. *Progr Hematol* 1966; 5:105–136.
12. Rappeport JM, Nathan DG: Acquired aplastic anemia; pathophysiology and treatment. *Adv Intern Med* 1982; 547–590.
13. Gatti RA, Allen HD, Meuwissen JH, et al.: Immunological reconstitution of sex-linked lymphopenic immunological deficiency. *Lancet* 1968; 2:1366–1368.
14. Bach FH, Albertine RJ, Anderson JL, et al.: Bone marrow transplantation in a patient with Wiskott-Aldrich syndrome. *Lancet* 1968; 2:1364–1366.
15. Camitta BM, Thomas ED, Nathan DG, et al.: A prospective study of androgens and bone marrow transplantation for treatment of severe aplastic anemia. *Blood* 1979; 53:504–514.
16. Storb R, Thomas ED, Buckner CD, et al.: Marrow transplantation in 30 "untransfused" patients with severe aplastic anemia. *Ann Intern Med* 1980; 92:30–36.
17. Anasetti C, Doney KC, Storb R, et al.: Marrow transplantation for severe aplastic anemia: Long-term outcome in 50 "untransfused" patients. *Ann Intern Med* 1986; 104:461–466.
18. Advisory Committee of the Bone Marrow Transplant Registry: Bone marrow transplantation from histocompatible, allogeneic donors for aplastic anemia. A report from the ACS/NIH Bone Marrow Transplant Registry. *JAMA* 1979; 236:1131–1135.
19. Storb R, Thomas ED, Buckner CD, et al.: Allogeneic marrow grafting for treatment of aplastic anemia. *Blood* 1974; 43:157–180.
20. Storb R, Thomas ED, Weiden PL, et al.: Aplastic anemia treated by allogeneic bone marrow transplantation. A report of 49 new cases from Seattle. *Blood* 1976; 48:817–841.
21. UCLA Bone Marrow Transplant Team: Bone marrow transplantation in severe aplastic anemia. *Lancet* 1976; 2:921–923.
22. Kersey JH, Kim T, Levitt SH, et al.: Combined immunosuppression using cyclophosphamide plus total lymphoid irradiation in preparation for allogeneic marrow transplantation in humans. In: Thierfelder S (ed); *Immunobiology of Bone Marrow Transplantation*. New York, Springer-Verlag, 1980.
23. Wright SE, Thomas ED, Buckner CD, et al.: Experience with second marrow transplants. *Exp Hematol* 1976; 4:221–226.
24. Storb R, Weiden PL, Sullivan KM, et al.: Second marrow transplants in patients with aplastic anemia rejecting the first graft: Use of a conditioning regimen including cyclophosphamide and antithymocyte globulin. *Blood* 1987; 70:116–121.
25. Storb R, Doney KC, Thomas ED, et al.: Marrow transplantation with or without donor buffy coat cells for 65 transfused aplastic anemia patients. *Blood* 1982; 59:236–246.
26. Storb R, Prentice RL, Thomas ED: Marrow transplantation for treatment of aplastic anemia; an analysis of factors associated with graft rejection. *N Engl J Med* 1977; 296:61–66.
27. Deeg HJ, Storb R, Weiden PL: Abrogation of resistance to and enhancement of DLA-nonidentical unrelated marrow grafts in lethally irradiated dogs by thoracic duct lymphocytes. *Blood* 1979; 53:552–557.

28. Storb R, Prentice RL, Thomas ED, et al.: Factors associated with graft rejection after HLA-identical marrow transplantation for aplastic anemia. *Br J Haematol* 1983; 55:573–585.

29. Deeg HJ, Self S, Storb R, et al.: Decreased incidence of marrow graft rejection in patients with severe aplastic anemia: Changing impact of risk factors. *Blood* 1986; 68:1363–1368.

30. Hill RS, Petersen FB, Storb R, et al.: Mixed hematologic chimerism after allogeneic marrow transplantation for severe aplastic anemia is associated with a higher risk of graft rejection and a lessened incidence of acute graft-vs.-host disease. *Blood* 1986; 67:811–816.

31. Storb R, Prentice RL, Buckner CD, et al.: Graft-vs.-host disease and survival in patients with aplastic anemia treated by marrow grafts from HLA-identical siblings. *N Engl J Med* 1983; 308:302–307.

32. Hows J, Harris R, Palmer S, et al.: Immunosuppression with cyclosporin A in allogeneic bone marrow transplantation for severe aplastic anemia: Preliminary studies. *Br J Hæmatol* 1981; 48:227–236.

33. Hows JM, Palmer S, Gordon-Smith EC: Use of cyclosporin A in allogeneic bone marrow transplantation for severe aplastic anemia. *Transplantation* 1982; 33:382–386.

34. Hows J, Palmer S, Gordon-Smith EC: Cyclosporin and graft failure following bone marrow transplantation for severe aplastic anemia. *Br J Hæmatol* 1985; 60:611–617.

35. Gordon-Smith EC: Treatment of aplastic anemia. In: *Aplastic Anemia: Stem cell biology and advances in treatment.* pp. 335–341, Alan R. Liss, New York, 1984.

36. Parkman R, Rappeport J, Camitta B, et al.: Successful use of multiagent immunosuppression in the bone marrow transplantation of sensitized patients. *Blood* 1978; 52:1163–1169.

37. Ferrara J, Levey RH, Nathan DG, et al.: Efficacy of a cyclophosphamide-procarbazine-antithymocyte serum regimen for prevention of graft rejection following bone marrow transplantation for transfused patients with aplastic anemia. *Transplantation* 1985; 39:671–673.

38. UCLA Bone Marrow Transplantation Team for Aplastic Anemia: Conditioning with cyclophosphamide plus low-dose total body irradiation. In: Baum SJ, Ledney GD, eds; *Experimental Hematology Today,* pp. 185–191, Springer-Heidelberg, 1979.

39. Gale RP, Ho W, Feig S, et al.: Prevention of graft rejection following bone marrow transplantation. *Blood* 1981; 57:9–12.

40. Feig SA, Champlin R, Arenson E, et al.: Improved survival following bone marrow transplantation for aplastic anemia. *BR J Hæmatol* 1983; 54:509–517.

41. Weiner RS, Dicke KA: Risk factors for interstitial pneumonitis following allogeneic bone marrow transplantation for severe aplastic anemia: A preliminary report. *Transplantation Proc* 1987; 19:2639–2642.

42. Ramsay NKC, Kim T, Nesbit ME, et al.: Total lymphoid irradiation and cyclophosphamide as preparation for bone marrow transplantation in severe aplastic anemia. *Blood* 1980; 55:344–346.

43. Ramsay NKC, Kim TH, McGlave P, et al.: Total lymphoid irradiation and cyclophosphamide conditioning prior to bone marrow transplantation for patients with severe aplastic anemia. *Blood* 1983; 62:622–626.

44. Kersey JH, Kruger J, Song C, et al.: Prolonged bone marrow and skin allograft survival following pretransplant conditioning with cyclophosphamide and total lymphoid irradiation. *Transplantation* 1980; 29:388–391.

45. McGlave PB, Haake R, Miller W, et al.: Therapy of severe aplastic anemia in young adults and children with allogeneic bone marrow transplantation. *Blood* 1987; 1325–1330.

46. Gluckman E, Devergie A, Benbuman A, et al.: Bone marrow transplantation in severe aplastic anemia using cyclophosphamide and thoraco-abdominal radiation. In: *Aplastic anemia: Stem cell biology and advances in treatment.* Alan R. Liss, New York, 1984, pp. 325–333.

47. Storb R, Prentice RL, Sullivan KM, et al.: Predictive factors in chronic graft-vs.-host disease in patients with aplastic anemia treated by marrow transplantation from HLA-identical siblings. *Ann Intern Med* 1983; 98:461–466.

48. Champlin RE, Feig SA, Sparkles RS, et al.: Bone marrow transplantation for identical twins in the treatment of aplastic anemia: Implications for the pathogenesis of the disease. *BR J Hæmatol* 1984; 56:455–463.

49. Golembe BL, Ramsay NK, Krivit W, et al.: Rejection after bone marrow transplantation in aplastic anemia using an identical twin followed by permanent success using immunosuppression. *J Pediatr* 1979; 9:569–571.

50. Lu DP: Syngeneic bone marrow transplant for treatment of aplastic anemia: Report of a case and review of the literature. *Exp Hematol* 1981; 9:257–263.
51. Gordon-Smith EC, Fairhead SM, Shipping PM: Bone marrow transplantation for severe aplastic anemia using histocompatible unrelated volunteer donors. *Br Med J* 1982; 285:835–837.
52. Hows JM, Yin JL, Marsh J, et al.: Histocompatible unrelated volunteer donors compared with HLA nonidentical family donors in marrow transplantation for aplastic anemia and leukemia. *Blood* 1986; 68:1322–1328.
53. Sullivan KM, Deeg HJ, Sanders JE, et al.: Late complications after marrow transplantation. *Semin Hematol* 1984; 21:53–63.
54. Sklar CA, Ramsay NKC: Endocrine dysfunction after successful bone marrow transplantation. *Clin Oncol* 1985; 4:345–352.
55. Sklar CA, Kim TH, Ramsay NKC: Thyroid dysfunction among long-term survivors of bone marrow transplantation. *Am J Med* 1982; 73:688–694.
56. Shapiro RS, Robison LL, Kim TH, et al.: Thyroid dysfunction following bone marrow transplant: Long-term follow-up of 53 pediatric patients (Abstr). *J Cell Biochem* 1986; Suppl 10D:250.
57. Sanders JE, Buckner CD, Leonard JM, et al.: Late effects on gonadal function of cyclophosphamide, total body irradiation, and marrow transplantation. *Transplantation* 1983; 36:252–255.
58. Sklar CA, Kim TH, Ramsay NKC: Testicular function following bone marrow transplantation performed during or after puberty. *Cancer* 1984; 53:1498–1501.
59. Sklar CA, Kim TH, Williamson JF, et al.: Ovarian function after successful bone marrow transplantation in post-menarcheal females. *Med Pediatr Oncol* 1983; 11:361–364.
60. Mathe G, Amiel JL, Schwarzenberg L, et al.: Bone marrow graft in man after conditioning by antilymphocytic serum. *Br Med J* 1970; 2:131–136.
61. Speck B, Gluckman E, Haak HL, et al.: Treatment of aplastic anemia by antilymphocyte globulin with and without allogeneic bone marrow infusions. *Lancet* 1977; 2:1145–1148.
62. Speck B, Gratwohl A, Nissen C, et al.: Treatment of severe aplastic anemia with antilymphocyte globulin or bone marrow transplantation. *Br Med J* 1981; 282:860–863.
63. Speck B, Gratwohl A, Nissen C, et al.: Treatment of severe aplastic anemia. *Exp Hematol* 1986; 14:126–132.
64. Bayever E, Champlin R, Ho W, et al.: Comparison between bone marrow transplantation and antithymocyte globulin in treatment of young patients with severe aplastic anemia. *J Pediatr* 1984; 105:920–925.
65. Doney KC, Weiden PL, Buckner CP, et al.: Treatment of severe aplastic anemia using antithymocyte globulin with or without an infusion of HLA-haplo-identical marrow. *Exp Hematol* 1981; 9:829–834.
66. European Group of Bone Marrow Transplant (EGBMT): Results of immunosuppression of 170 cases of severe aplastic anemia. *Br J Hæmatol* 1982; 51:541–550.
67. Fairhead SM, Chipping PM, Gordon-Smith EC: Treatment of aplastic anemia with antilymphocyte globulin (ALG). *Br J Hæmatol* 1983; 55:7–16.
68. Miller WJ, Branda RF, Flynn PJ, et al.: Antithymocyte globulin treatment of severe aplastic anemia. *Br J Hæmatol* 1983; 55:17–25.
69. Champlin R, Ho W, Gale RP: Antilymphocyte globulin treatment in patients with aplastic anemia. *N Engl J Med* 1983; 308:113–118.
70. Camitta B, O'Reilly RJ, Sensenbrenner L, et al.: Antithoracic duct lymphocyte globulin therapy of severe aplastic anemia. *Blood* 1983; 62:883–888.
71. Marsh JCW, Hows JM, Bryett KA, et al.: Survival after antilymphocyte globulin therapy for aplastic anemia depends on disease severity. *Blood* 1987; 70:1046–1052.
72. Bacigalupo A, Giordano D, Van Lint MT, et al.: Bolus methylprednisolone in severe aplastic anemia. *N Engl J Med* 1979; 300:501–502.
73. Bacigalupo A, Podesta M, Van Lint MT, et al.: Severe aplastic anaemia: Correlation of *in vitro* tests with clinical response to immunosuppression in 20 patients. *Br J Hæaematol* 1981; 47:423–433.
74. Jacobs P, Wood L, Martell RW: Cyclosporin A in the treatment of severe aplastic anemia. *Br J Hæmatol* 1985; 61:267–272.

75. Bridges R, Pinea G, and Blahey W: Cyclosporin A for the treatment of aplastic anemia refractory to antithymocyte globulin. *Am J Hematol* 1987; 26:83–87.
76. Antin JH, Smith BR, Rosenthal DS, et al.: Phase I/II study of recombinant human granulocyte macrophage colony stimulating factor (GM-CSF) in bone marrow failure. *Blood* 1987; 70:129a.
77. Fanconi G: Familial constitutional panmyelocytopathy, Fanconi's anemia (FA). I. Clinical Aspects. *Semin Hematol* 1967; 4:233–240.
78. Schmid W: Familial constitutional panmyelocytopathy, Fanconi's anemia (FA). II. A discussion of the cytogenetic findings in Fanconi's anemia. *Semin Hematol* 1967; 4:241–249.
79. Swift MR, Hirschorn H: Fanconi's anemia inherited susceptibility to chromosome breakage in various tissues. *Ann Int Med* 1966; 65:496–503.
80. Barrett AJ, Brigden WD, Hobbs JR, et al.: Successful bone marrow transplant for Fanconi's anæmia. *Br Med J* 1977; 1:420–422.
81. Gluckman E, Devergie A, Schaison G, et al.: Bone marrow transplantation in Fanconi's anemia. *Br J Hæmatol* 1980; 45:557–564.
82. Deeg HJ, Storb R, Thomas ED, et al.: Fanconi's anemia treated by allogeneic marrow transplantation. *Blood* 1983; 61:954–959.
83. Bortin MM, Gale RP, Rimm AA for the Advisory Committee of the International Bone Marrow Transplant Registry: Allogeneic bone marrow transplantation for 144 patients with severe aplastic anemia. *JAMA* 1981; 245:1132–1139.
84. Sasaki MS: Is Fanconi's anæmia defective in a process essential to the repair of DNA-crosslinks? *Nature* 1975; 257:501–503.
85. Sasaki MS, Tonomura A: A high susceptibility of Fanconi's anemia to chromosome: Breakage by DNA cross-linking agents. *Cancer Res* 1973; 33:1829–1836.
86. Berger R, Bernheim A, Gluckman E, et al.: *In vitro* effect of cyclophosphamide metabolites on chromosomes of Fanconi's anæmia patients. *Br J Hæmatol* 1980; 45:565–568.
87. Gluckman E, Devergie A, Dutreix J: Radiosensitivity in Fanconi's anæmia: Application to the conditioning regimen for bone marrow transplantation. *Br J Hæmatol* 1983; 54:431–440.
88. Cervenka J, Arthur D, Yasis C: Mitomycin C test for diagnostic differentiation of idiopathic aplastic anemia and Fanconi's anemia. *Pediatrics* 1981; 67:119–135.
89. Ramsay NKC, Kersey JH, Robison LL, et al.: A randomized study for the prevention of acute graft-vs.-host disease. *N Engl J Med* 1982; 306:392–397.
90. Schmidt E, Deeg HJ, Storb R: Regression of androgen-related hepatic tumors in patients with Fanconi's anemia following marrow transplantation. *Transplantation* 1984; 37:452–455.
91. Lucarelli G, Polchi P, Galimberti M, et al.: Marrow transplantation for thalassemia following busulphan and cyclophosphamide. *Lancet* 1985; 1:1355–1357.
92. Thomas ED, Buckner CD, Sanders JE, et al.: Marrow transplantation for thalassemia. *Lancet* 1982; 2:227–229.
93. Lucarelli G, Galimberti M, Polchi P, et al.: Bone marrow transplantation in thalassemia after busulphan and cyclophosphamide: Report on 70 cases (abstr). *J Cell Biochem* 1986; Suppl 10D:216.
94. Szer J, Deeg HJ, Witherspoon RP, et al.: Long-term survival after marrow transplantation for paroxysmal nocturnal hemoglobinuria with aplastic anemia. *Ann Int Med* 1984; 101:193–195.
95. Hows JM, Palmer S, Gordon-Smith EC: Use of cyclosporin A in allogeneic bone marrow transplantation for severe aplastic anemia. *Transplantation* 1982; 33:382–386.
96. Gluckman E, Devergie A, Dutreix A: Bone marrow grafting in aplastic anemia after conditioning with cyclophosphamide and total body irradiation with lung shielding. In: Thierfelder S, Rodt H, Kolb HJ (eds); *Immunobiology of Bone Marrow Transplantation*, Berlin, Springer-Verlag, 339–347, 1980.
97. Hershko C, Gale RP, Ho WG, et al.: Cure of aplastic anemia in paroxysmal nocturnal hemoglobinuria by marrow infusion from identical twin; failure of peripheral-leukocyte transfusion to correct marrow aplasia. *Lancet* 1979; 1:945–947.
98. Johnson FL, Look AT, Gockerman J, et al.: Bone marrow transplantation in a patient with sickle cell anemia. *N Engl J Med* 1984; 31:780–783.
99. Iriondo A, Garijo J, Baro J, et al.: Complete recovery of hemopoiesis following bone marrow transplant in a patient with unresponsive congenital hypoplastic anemia (Blackfan-Diamond syndrome). *Blood* 1984; 64:348–351.

100. August CS, King E, Githens JH, et al.: Establishment of erythropoiesis following bone marrow transplantation in a patient with congenital hypoplastic anemia (Blackfan-Diamond syndrome). *Blood* 1976; 48:491–498.
101. Rappaport JM, Parkman R, Newburger P, et al.: Correction of infantile agranulocytosis (Kostmann's syndrome) by allogeneic bone marrow transplantation. *Am J Med* 1980; 68:605–609.
102. Bellucci S, Divergie A, Gluckman E, et al.: Complete correction of Glanzmann's thrombasthenia by allogeneic bone marrow transplantation. *Br J Hæmatol* 1985; 59:635–641.

Bone Marrow Transplantation in
Children, edited by F. Leonard Johnson
and Carl Pochedly. Raven Press, Ltd.,
New York © 1990.

Use of Bone Marrow Transplantation in the Leukemias

Howard J. Weinstein

Department of Pediatrics, Harvard Medical School, Pediatric Bone Marrow Transplant Unit, The Children's Hospital and the Dana-Farber Cancer Institute, Boston, Massachusetts 02115

Introduction
A. Principles of bone marrow transplantation for leukemia
B. Acute lymphoblastic leukemia
  1. Allogeneic transplants
  2. Autotransplants
C. Acute nonlymphoblastic leukemia
  1. Chemotherapy vs. bone marrow transplantation in first remission
  2. Autotransplants
D. Chronic myeloid leukemia (Ph[1] chromosome positive and juvenile types)
E. Myelodysplastic syndromes
F. T cell depletion and bone marrow transplantation
G. Alternative donors
Summary

INTRODUCTION

Bone marrow transplantation (BMT) has played an increasingly important role in the treatment of various hematologic malignancies (1–3). Children who are likely to benefit from marrow transplantation include those with: (1) acute lymphoblastic leukemia (ALL) in second or subsequent remission, (2) acute nonlymphoid leukemia (ANLL) in first or subsequent remission or in early relapse, (3) Philadelphia (Ph[1]) chromosome positive chronic myeloid leukemia (CML) in chronic phase, (4) juvenile chronic myeloid leukemia, and

(5) myelodysplastic (preleukemic) syndromes. Overall survival following bone marrow transplantation is adversely affected by the presence of leukemic relapse, graft-vs.-host disease (GVHD), and interstitial pneumonitis. Among factors that influence the incidence of leukemic relapse are the type of leukemia, remission status, the preparative regimen used, and length of the initial remission. Acute and chronic graft-vs.-host disease increases in frequency and severity with advancing age of the patient.

Approximately one-third of children who might benefit from bone marrow transplantation have histocompatible donors. Autologous transplants and transplants from a partial HLA-matched family member or from an unrelated donor have been performed for children who did not have fully matched donors. Current results and applications of bone marrow transplantation for leukemia in children are summarized in this chapter.

PRINCIPLES OF BONE MARROW TRANSPLANTATION FOR LEUKEMIA

A general strategy used in attempting curative treatment of leukemia is to increase the doses of active cytotoxic agents to the limit of normal tissue tolerance. In many instances this limit of toxicity is manifested by suppression of the hematopoietic system. The use of marrow grafting in patients with leukemia allows for the administration of doses of drugs or radiation that are lethal to the host hematopoietic system. The obliterated hematopoietic system is then restored by infusion of HLA-identical bone marrow from a normal donor. In addition to the enhanced antileukemic efficacy of the ultraintense chemoradiotherapy regimen used in preparation for the grafting, there is the possibility of a graft-vs.-leukemia effect from the transplanted immunocompetent cells. Support for the existence of an antileukemic effect of allogeneic marrow comes from studies in identical twins and studies in patients with moderate or severe graft-vs.-host disease. The relapse rate in genetically identical twins who receive transplants from their twin for treatment of acute myeloid leukemia in first remission is 3 times greater than that in recipients of grafts from HLA identical donors (4). The risk of leukemic relapse is lower in patients who develop moderate or severe graft-vs.-host disease (5).

In leukemic disorders, preparation of the recipient must involve not only immunosuppression but also therapy designed to eradicate the leukemia. Early studies in dogs showed that 950 cGy of total body irradiation (TBI) was sufficiently immunosuppressive to permit successful grafting of allogeneic marrow with production of complete chimeras (6). Dogs prepared with cyclophosphamide were mixed chimeras, that is, both donor and host cells were present (7). Preparation for bone marrow transplant with cyclophosphamide or irradiation alone for grafting patients with refractory leukemia resulted in early recurrence of leukemia (8–10); in one study, there was lack of complete engraftment after cyclophosphamide (9). The combination of cyclophosphamide and total body irradiation has been extensively studied by the Seattle group and was associated with successful engraftment (in 99%), and fewer relapses of leukemia compared to either agent used alone (1).

The Johns Hopkins transplant team has shown that preparation with cyclophosphamide and busulfan (Bu-Cy) results in high-level chimerism. Furthermore, the results of treatment of patients with acute myeloid leukemia, using preparation with Bu-Cy, are comparable to the Seattle data (11).

The administration of total body irradiation varies significantly between transplant centers. Total radiation doses range from 750 to 1400 cGy. Many centers give fractionated total body irradiation (giving 4 to 8 fractions over 2 to 4 days) at lower dose rates. Fractionation of radiation appears to reduce toxicity to normal tissues but does not reduce the antileukemic effect (12).

A few transplant groups have added other drugs to cyclophosphamide and total body irradiation in an attempt to reduce the rate of leukemic relapse. In several of these early studies toxicity outweighed any potential therapeutic advantage (13). Recent trials employing VP-16 (Etoposide) and total body irradiation (14), or high-dose cytosine arabinoside (ara-C) and total body irradiation (15) have proved to be sufficiently immunosuppressive to ensure engraftment, and preliminary results suggest that they are highly effective preparative regimens for acute lymphoblastic leukemia.

ACUTE LYMPHOBLASTIC LEUKEMIA

Allogeneic Transplants

The early candidates for bone marrow transplantation were patients with advanced leukemia which was resistant to therapy, patients who had failed conventional and experimental chemotherapy. Transplantation resulted in long-term survival in 10 to 20% of patients (1). The major cause of treatment failure was relapse, which occurred in more than 60% of patients but infection early in the course of bone marrow transplantation, graft-vs.-host disease, and interstitial pneumonia also accounted for a significant number of deaths. These results, however, were superior to those of existing alternative therapies.

Since some patients with end-stage acute lymphoblastic leukemia (ALL) could be cured by bone marrow transplantation, it seemed logical to attempt transplantation earlier in the course of the disease, but at a time when the prognosis was known to be poor. Therefore, bone marrow transplantation was undertaken during second or subsequent remission, and the results were compared to those of concurrent patients with acute lymphoblastic leukemia who were transplanted in relapse. Results from an early Seattle study showed a survival rate of 27% for the patients transplanted in remission, compared to a rate of 15% for patients transplanted in relapse (16).

In 1976, another study by Johnson and colleagues compared the use of combination chemotherapy with use of bone marrow transplantation in treatment of ALL. This study was done in children with acute lymphoblastic leukemia who had had a bone marrow relapse while receiving maintenance chemotherapy, but were in a second or subsequent remission (17). Patients were given a marrow transplant if a matched sibling donor was available. After a minimum follow-up of 3 years, 8 out of 24 transplant recipients compared to none of 21 patients treated with chemotherapy were leukemia-free survivors (18). However, these two groups of patients were not entirely comparable with regard to possible risk factors. The chemotherapy group was unfavorably biased since it contained both patients who had high-risk features at diagnosis and shorter initial durations of remission compared to the group treated by transplant. The marrow transplant recipients who continue to survive all had initial durations of continuous complete remission of more than 20 months and 4 had continuous complete remission of over 3 years. In this study, leukemic relapse was the most frequent cause of failure after either chemotherapy or marrow transplantation.

The University of Minnesota transplant group conducted a similar study. They showed that the transplanted patients also had a significantly increased chance of leukemia-free survival compared to a conventionally treated group of patients (19). In the Minnesota study, significant risk factors for predicting relapse after bone marrow transplantation included an initial leukocyte count of over 50,000/mm^3 and presence of extramedullary leukemia. The authors of the Seattle and Minnesota bone marrow transplantation studies agreed in their conclusions. They concluded that marrow transplantation offered the best chance of long-term remission and cure after a patient with acute lymphoblastic leukemia had a relapse in the bone marrow while still receiving chemotherapy. In these 2 studies the patients were treated between 1976 and 1980.

However, not all studies suggest that bone marrow transplantation is more effective than chemotherapy for children with acute lymphoblastic leukemia in second marrow remission. Chessels recently reported a study comparing bone marrow transplantation with chemotherapy in 53 children in a single center with ALL whose first complete remission ended in bone marrow relapse (20). Five out of 13 patients (39%) who had HLA-compatible donors and who were eligible for bone marrow transplantation survive, compared with 16 out of 40 (40%) who received further chemotherapy. There is no statistically significant difference in survival rate between the groups. The lengths of first and second remissions in both groups were similar.

A literature review, including data from the International Bone Marrow Transplant Registry, also shows that outcome after treatment with either bone marrow transplantation or chemotherapy is correlated with risk factors present at diagnosis and with length of the first remission (21). Bone marrow transplantation seemed superior only in patients who relapsed within 18 months of first remission.

Since 1980, newer multidrug chemotherapy regimens have been used in treating children with refractory acute lymphoblastic leukemia. Results from one of these studies showed that for patients whose initial remission was less than 18 months the 2-year probability of maintaining remission was less than 10%. But for patients whose initial remission lasted more than 18 months, the probability of achieving a 2-year remission was 55%. (22). Controlled trials are needed to compare the results of chemotherapy with marrow transplantation in patients who are stratified for various prognostic variables. Such trials are needed to clarify the relative efficacy of chemotherapy and bone marrow transplantation in children with acute lymphoblastic leukemia in second remission (Table 1).

The major obstacle to success in marrow grafting for treatment of acute lymphoblastic leukemia in second or subsequent remission is relapse, which occurs in 30 to 50% of patients. (23,24). Therefore, recent therapeutic efforts have focused on improving the antileukemic efficacy of the pre-transplant chemoradiotherapy regimen. Hyperfractionated total body irradiation followed by cyclophosphamide used at the Memorial Sloan-Kettering Cancer Center (25), and high-dose cytosine arabinoside (15) combined with fractionated total body irradiation as used in Cleveland, appear to have resulted in an improvement in leukemia-free survival for children with acute lymphoblastic leukemia transplanted in second remission. It remains to be seen if these results will be confirmed by studies carried out by other groups.

Children in several other subsets of acute lymphoblastic leukemia might benefit from bone marrow transplantation. Boys with acute lymphoblastic leukemia who develop an isolated testicular relapse while on chemotherapy have a very poor rate of long-term survival after treatment with additional chemotherapy and testicular irradiation (26). The majority of such patients experience marrow relapse within 1 year of testicular relapse, and eventually die from their disease. Bone marrow transplantation should be considered for these patients, but there is insufficient data to indicate whether this approach would be beneficial.

Children with acute lymphoblastic leukemia in first bone marrow remission

TABLE 1. *Comparison of results of chemotherapy and bone marrow transplantation in children with acute lymphoblastic leukemia**

Disease status	Chemotherapy (survival rate)	Bone marrow transplantation (survival rate)
Second remission		
Total group	10–30%	30–60%
If first remission lasted		
less than 18 months	0–10%	20%
more than 18 months	10–55%	30–60%

*Approximate range of leukemia-free survival determined from literature review

who experience an isolated CNS relapse usually cannot be successfully treated. Re-treatment with intensive systemic chemotherapy and another course of CNS irradiation results in only a 30% likelihood of long-term leukemia-free survival (27). The most frequent site of subsequent relapse after an aggressive re-treatment approach is in the bone marrow. Results from a study of acute lymphoblastic leukemia carried out by the Children's Cancer Study Group suggest that children who had inadequate primary CNS prophylaxis, such as intrathecal methotrexate alone, may have a somewhat better prognosis than those children whose initial CNS prophylaxis included cranial irradiation (28).

Some groups have recommended use of bone marrow transplantation for patients who have had an isolated CNS relapse. In several transplant studies, however, the presence of extramedullary leukemia prior to bone marrow transplantation was associated with a high risk of relapse (19,29). Many of these patients had combined CNS and bone marrow relapse before transplant, and therefore are not totally comparable. Since the risk of CNS relapse following transplant is highest in patients with prior CNS leukemia, the Seattle group has recommended giving intrathecal chemotherapy after marrow transplant (30). Giving intrathecal methotrexate following bone marrow transplantation may reduce the incidence of CNS relapse, but it has occasionally been associated with severe leukoencephalopathy. At present, there is insufficient data to decide whether bone marrow transplantation or intensive chemotherapy together with repeat irradiation of the CNS is better for the child with acute lymphoblastic leukemia who has an isolated CNS relapse.

Bone marrow transplantation is usually not recommended for children with acute lymphoblastic leukemia in first remission because with current chemotherapy regimens more than 70% of these patients are expected to remain in long-term continuous remission. (31). Even children with high-risk acute lymphoblastic leukemia have at least a 50% chance of cure with chemotherapy.

Several prognostic factors predict a very poor outcome for children with acute lymphoblastic leukemia. (32). These include the B cell type of ALL, the presence of the Ph^1 chromosome or other chromosomal translocations, such as t (4,11), and age less than 12 months at the time of diagnosis. Bone marrow transplantation has been recommended by some investigators for treatment of these very high-risk patients. There is little published data with respect to the post-transplant survival rate for this group of patients. However, the European experience regarding transplantation in patients with the B cell type of acute lymphoblastic leukemia in first remission is promising (33).

The survival rate of patients who relapse after bone marrow transplantation is extremely low. However, some patients with acute lymphoblastic leukemia who relapsed after transplantation have been successfully reinduced into complete remission using a chemotherapy regimen consisting of vincristine, prednisone, L-asparaginase, and daunorubicin. (34). The median length of survival was 4 months, with a range from 3 to 22 months. Interestingly, there was a positive correlation between the disease-free interval from bone marrow transplantation to relapse and the overall duration of survival following relapse.

Autotransplants

Autologous transplants have been performed in children with acute lymphoblastic leukemia who did not have HLA-matched donors (35). Various techniques have been developed to purge or remove contaminating leukemic cells present in the patient's marrow harvested during remission. Most of these approaches to purging the marrow include the *in vitro* use of monoclonal antibodies or drugs. Monoclonal antibodies can be used: (1) with rabbit complement to lyse leukemic cells, (2) as conjugates of antibody and a toxin, such as antibody-ricin conjugates, and (3) use of antibodies with magnetic beads (immunophysical separation). Pharmacologic approaches using *ex vivo* treatment of the bone marrow with the cyclophosphamide derivatives, 4-hydroperoxycyclophosphamide (4-HC) or ASTA-Z, have also been studied.

Autotransplants using monoclonal antibodies have been carried out at the Dana-Farber Cancer Institute and The Children's Hospital Medical Center in Boston (36). Patients with acute lymphoblastic leukemia were eligible if their leukemic cells expressed CALLA (common ALL antigen), if they were in second or third remission, and did not have HLA-identical donors. The following protocol was used. Remission marrow was harvested and treated with two anti-CALLA (J5 and J2) monoclonal antibodies and complement, then the marrow was cryopreserved. Following marrow harvest, patients were given pre-transplant conditioning with VM-26 (teniposide), cyclophosphamide, cytosine arabinoside and total body irradiation. At first, TBI was given as 850 cGy in a single fraction, but now we use a dose of 1400 cGy given as fractionated total body irradiation. A total of 30 children were transplanted between 1980 and 1986. The probability of leukemia-free survival at 5 years after transplant is 27%. Twelve patients relapsed between 2 months and 14 months after transplantation, and 9 patients have died of infection or bleeding following transplant. As noted with some trials comparing chemotherapy and allogeneic bone marrow transplantation for relapsed acute lymphoblastic leukemia, the duration of initial remission strongly influences the post-transplant outcome. Children who had initial bone marrow remissions of less than 24 months duration had significantly shorter leukemia-free survival following transplant.

The University of Minnesota bone marrow transplant team has also been studying use of autologous marrow transplants in children with CALLA positive acute lymphoblastic leukemia in second or subsequent remission (37). In their technique, harvested bone marrow is treated with three monoclonal antibodies (BA-1, BA-2 and BA-3), and complement. Preparation of patients for bone marrow transplantation included use of cyclophosphamide and a dose of 1320 cGy of fractionated total body irradiation, or high-dose cytosine arabinoside and a single dose of 850 cGy of total body irradiation. The outcome was similar for the patients prepared with the two regimens, with leukemia-free survivals of 22% to 30%. The majority of treatment failures were due to leukemic relapse.

The autotransplant results using *ex vivo* treatment (purging) of marrow with 4-HC in patients with acute lymphoblastic leukemia also show a very high relapse rate (38). Since allogeneic bone marrow transplantation performed in second or subsequent remission of acute lymphoblastic leukemia is associated with a high risk of leukemic relapse, the high relapse rates after autotransplants are not surprising. It is impossible to tell if relapse results from residual leukemia in the patient or from presence of occult leukemia in the infused autologous marrow. Therefore, it is difficult to determine whether *ex vivo* marrow purging methods with either monoclonal antibodies or pharmacologic agents are useful in these transplants.

ACUTE NONLYMPHOBLASTIC LEUKEMIA

Bone marrow transplantation in the treatment of acute nonlymphoid leukemia (ANLL), like that for acute lymphoblastic leukemia, was initially reserved for patients with relapsed or refractory disease. Most patients were treated with preparatory regimens including high-dose cyclophosphamide (120 to 200 mg/kg) and a dose of 800–1000 cGy of total body irradiation. As in acute lymphoblastic leukemia, approximately 10% of patients given allogeneic transplants for treatment of refractory ANLL achieved long-term survival, that is, more than 10 years of leukemia-free survival (1). These results were superior to those of patients given alternative therapies. More intensive chemotherapy regimens combined with total body irradiation were associated with increased toxicity, but there was no improvement in overall survival (13).

Chemotherapy vs. Bone Marrow Transplantation in First Remission

In the mid-1970s, bone marrow transplantation was first applied to patients with acute myeloid leukemia in first remission (39). The use of bone marrow transplantation in pediatrics was mainly limited to patients older than 2 years of age who had HLA-identical donors. Approximately 70 to 80% of children with ANLL achieve complete remission with chemotherapy regimens employing cytosine arabinoside and an anthracycline, with or without the addition of 6-thioguanine (32). From this pool of patients approximately one-third are likely to have an HLA compatible donor and be eligible for bone marrow transplantation. Most studies of bone marrow transplantation for children with acute nonlymphoblastic leukemia grafted in first remission show actuar-

TABLE 2. *Comparison of results of chemotherapy and bone marrow transplantation in children with acute nonlymphoid leukemia**

Disease status	Chemotherapy (survival rate)	Transplantation (survival rate)
First remission	30–50%	50–65%
Second remission	less than 10%	20–45%
Early relapse	—	30–40%
Relapse	—	10–20%

*Approximate range of leukemia-free survival determined from literature review

ial relapse rates ranging from 15 to 25%, and actuarial leukemia-free survival rates ranging from 50 to 65% (Table 2) (11,25,40–42). Mortality is primarily due to graft-vs.-host disease and interstitial pneumonitis.

At nearly the same time that bone marrow transplantation was applied to patients with ANLL in first remission, several clinical studies using novel chemotherapeutic protocols were begun (43–45). Prior to these trials, the median duration of remission of children with ANLL had been 8 to 12 months (46). Less than 20% of patients remained in complete remission for 5 years or more. These new protocols employed early intensification or consolidation chemotherapy. The median duration of remission was extended to 18 to 24 months, with 5 year actuarial leukemia-free survival rates of 40 to 50% (43–45).

Data from these uncontrolled trials of bone marrow transplantation and chemotherapy show a decreased risk of recurrent leukemia following transplantation, but there was a less significant survival advantage in the transplanted patients. It is difficult to compare the results of chemotherapy with those of marrow transplant because of the numerous variables that influence outcome. For example, early bone marrow transplant trials did not include children younger than 2 years of age. Also, in these trials the interval between achieving remission and performing bone marrow transplantation varied between 1 and 9 months, and therefore some individuals who relapsed within the first several months may have been excluded from transplant studies. There has been only one large prospective controlled pediatric trial designed to compare the efficacy of chemotherapy and bone marrow transplantation in first remission of ANLL. The results of this trial, carried out by the Children's Cancer Study Group, show that marrow transplantation has a statistically significant better disease-free survival rate (49% vs. 36%) than chemotherapy.

Bone marrow transplantation should be seriously considered as first-line therapy for children with ANLL in first remission and an HLA-identical donor. Another strategy is to treat with chemotherapy and to withhold transplantation for children who relapse following an initial complete remission. The overall results with chemotherapy followed by transplantation in second remission or early relapse should be comparable to transplantation in first remission. Another alternative might be to reserve transplantation for those patients likely to have an inferior outcome with use of chemotherapy.

Unfortunately there are few clinical or laboratory parameters that indicate those children who are at significant risk of leukemic relapse following chemotherapy. The presence of the M4 and M5 FAB cytologic subtypes of acute leukemia have been shown to be adverse prognostic factors in several chemotherapy trials (43,44). Interestingly, several transplant studies have also reported similar prognostic significance for the M4 and M5 subtypes of acute nonlymphoid leukemia (41,42). It may be that factors which predict a poor outcome with use of one treatment modality have similar prognostic value for assessing an alternative therapy. Further studies will be required to confirm this hypothesis.

There is little doubt about the superiority of bone marrow transplantation compared to chemotherapy for the treatment of a patient with acute nonlymphoid leukemia who has suffered a relapse. Second remissions that are maintained with chemotherapy usually last only from several weeks to a few months (46). This contrasts with the 20 to 45% leukemia-free survival rates observed in patients who are transplanted in second remission (1,41).

A matter of controversy is the timing of bone marrow transplantation for the patient with ANLL who has had a relapse. Should one attempt to induce a second remission prior to transplant or should one proceed directly to bone marrow transplantation? There are few reports that address this issue. Retrospective analysis of data from the Seattle transplant experience indicate similar outcomes for patients who are transplanted either in second remission or in early relapse (47). The poorest outcome was observed in patients who failed to enter a second remission after induction chemotherapy and then had a transplant.

Autotransplants

Several centers have tried the use of autologous bone marrow transplantation in patients with ANLL (48). In contrast to the use of autotransplantation for acute lymphoblastic leukemia, most immunologic approaches for purging marrow have been limited by cross-reactivity of most anti-ANLL monoclonal antibodies with normal hematopoietic progenitors and precursors. However, several autotransplant protocols for treatment of ANLL utilizing anti-ANLL monoclonal antibodies and complement are currently being tried. As an alternative approach, pharmacologic purging of leukemic cells from remission marrow has been attempted. Preliminary results of an autotransplant study using 4-hydroperoxycyclophosphamide (4-HC) to treat marrow that was harvested from children and adults with acute nonlymphoid leukemia in second or third remission have been encouraging (49). The actuarial relapse rate was

46% and the actuarial survival rate at 2 years was 43%. As in autologous bone marrow transplantation for acute lymphoblastic leukemia, the clinical efficacy of *ex vivo* purging of remission marrow remains undetermined.

Other centers are evaluating use of purged and nonpurged autologous bone marrow for autologous transplantation of patients with acute nonlymphoid leukemia in first complete remission (48). Bone marrow is harvested and cryopreserved early in the first remission usually after several months of consolidation chemotherapy. Then the patient receives supralethal preparatory therapy and reinfusion of autologous marrow. This precedure may be viewed as another course of intensive consolidation therapy. There is no data to support the proposal that freezing and thawing of the marrow may be lethal to residual leukemic cells. Results are too preliminary for a fair critique of this treatment method.

CHRONIC MYELOID LEUKEMIA (PH[1] CHROMOSOME POSITIVE AND JUVENILE TYPES)

Chronic myeloid leukemia (CML) in children can be separated into the Ph[1] chromosome positive and the juvenile types. The biology and natural history of Ph[1] chromosome positive CML in children is virtually indistinguishable from the disease in an adult. The median survival of children with chronic myeloid leukemia is 3 to 4 years. The disease is usually fatal when conventional treatment is used (50).

Juvenile chronic myeloid leukemia has its peak incidence in the first 2 years of life. It is initially characterized by splenomegaly, rash, lymphadenopathy, a moderately elevated leukocyte count (with presence of immature granulocytic precursors and monocytosis), thrombocytopenia, anemia, and an increased level of fetal hemoglobin (51). Approximately one-third of patients progress to a blast phase, whereas the others succumb to infection or hemorrhage. The median survival is approximately 1 year and there is no curative chemotherapy.

It is unclear if juvenile chronic myeloid leukemia is a disease originating in a multipotent or pluripotent stem cell. Nevertheless, therapy designed for ANLL usually fails to induce complete remissions of the blood and bone marrow. Chemotherapy is considered to be only palliative for both the Ph[1] chromosomal positive and the juvenile types of chronic myeloid leukemia.

Several transplant centers have now evaluated use of bone marrow transplantation for patients with Ph[1] chromosome positive chronic myeloid leukemia (52–54). Patients transplanted in an accelerated phase or in blast crisis have fared poorly. Only 15 to 20% of this group have survived free of disease for more than 5 years. For patients transplanted in the chronic phase, actuarial survival rates range from 55 to 70%. The best results have been achieved in young patients transplanted early in the chronic phase (before 1 year), or in recipients of syngeneic grafts. For patients who enter blast crisis, but then enter a second chronic phase, transplantation offers a surprisingly good out-come, with a survival rate of approximately 50% (52). It appears that the presence or absence of a spleen prior to transplant for treatment of Ph^1 chromosome positive chronic myeloid leukemia does not significantly affect post-transplant survival.

The success of bone marrow transplantation in Ph^1 chromosome positive chronic myeloid leukemia led investigators to transplant children with juve-nile chronic myeloid leukemia. There have been too few patients transplanted to give actuarial survival figures, but it appears that juvenile chronic myeloid leukemia responds favorably to high dose chemoradiotherapy followed by infusion of allogeneic marrow (55).

MYELODYSPLASTIC SYNDROMES

The myelodysplastic or preleukemia syndromes are rare in childhood. Most children with these bone marrow stem cell disorders either die of complica-tions related to thrombocytopenia or leukopenia, or develop acute myeloid leukemia (56). Monosomy 7 is the most common chromosomal change associ-ated with the myelodysplastic syndromes in children (57). Complete remission following chemotherapy is rare. In those cases where initial remission was achieved, the response was short-lived.

Bone marrow transplantation has recently been used in children and young adults with preleukemia after conditioning with cyclophosphamide and total body irradiation (58). In combined experience with both children and adults in Seattle overall survival was approximately 60%. Eight children with myelodysplastic syndromes have undergone transplants at the Children's Hos-pital Medical Center in Boston (58a). Preparation before transplant included cyclophosphamide and total body irradiation, with or without cytosine ara-binoside. Four out of 8 children survive in remission, including 1 child who had a preleukemic syndrome induced by alkylating agents. Based upon these results, use of bone marrow transplantation should be considered early in the course of preleukemia for a child who has an HLA-identical sibling.

T CELL DEPLETION AND BONE MARROW TRANSPLANTATION

Moderate or severe graft-vs.-host disease (grades 2 to 4) occurs in approxi-mately 40% of young recipients of HLA-identical grafts and in 75% of recipi-ents of HLA-mismatched transplants (59). Graft-vs.-host disease is an impor-tant determinant of survival after bone marrow transplantation. Attempts to prevent graft-vs.-host disease with methotrexate, corticosteroids, antithymo-cyte globulin, and cyclosporine have been only partially successful.

Studies in animals established that graft-vs.-host disease is initiated by thymus-derived lymphocytes, and that depletion of T cells *in vitro* and *in vivo* can modify or prevent graft-vs.-host disease and graft rejection in animals given transplants from donors that are mismatched for major and minor HLA antigens (60). Several methods have been developed to remove T cells from donor marrow. T cells have been removed by use of monoclonal anti-T antibodies and complement; T cells may also be removed by linking anti-T antibodies to immunotoxins such as ricin, or by physical techniques, such as use of lectins and E-rosette formation with sheep erythrocytes.

There is mounting evidence that T cell depletion of marrow prevents or markedly reduces the incidence and severity of graft-vs.-host disease in humans (61–64). However, the incidence of graft rejection in HLA-identical grafts increases from an expected incidence of 1% to approximately 10% after T cell depletion of donor marrow. The pathogenesis of graft rejection is not known, but it may be in part due to residual cytotoxic T cells of the host (recipient) (65). There is some evidence to suggest that increasing host immunosuppression (i.e., by use of higher doses of total body irradiation) reduces the risk of graft rejection (62). Recent observations also indicate that the likelihood of leukemic relapse is higher in recipients of T cell depleted grafts (66). Thus, although T cell depletion reduces the severity of graft-vs.-host disease, it has not been associated with an increase in survival because of the greater risk of graft rejection and leukemic relapse.

Similar protocols employing T cell depletion of the donor marrow have been used in transplanting HLA-mismatched marrow. Results of these trials have been poor because of the occurrence of an even higher rate of graft rejection, the rejection rate being from 30 to 50% (62,67).

ALTERNATIVE DONORS

Several centers have performed transplants using matched or partially matched unrelated donors when HLA-identical family members were unavailable (68,69). The process of identifying a well-matched unrelated donor is costly and time-consuming. Graft rejection and severe graft-vs.-host disease have also limited the success of these transplants. Bone marrow transplantation from mismatched family donors (with mismatch of more than one HLA antigen) or from unrelated matched donors should be considered as highly investigational therapy for patients with leukemia.

SUMMARY

Bone marrow transplantation from an HLA-identical sibling is useful in children with acute lymphoblastic leukemia who are in a second or subsequent remission. The results of both chemotherapy and bone marrow transplantation for children with acute lymphoblastic leukemia in second remission are highly dependent on the length of the initial remission. The data suggest an advantage for bone marrow transplantation in children whose initial remissions are less than 18 months. Recurrent leukemia remains a major problem for these patients.

The timing of marrow transplantation in children with acute nonlymphoid leukemia remains controversial. The likelihood of leukemic relapse is substantially reduced by bone marrow transplantation in children with acute nonlymphoid leukemia in first remission, but there is a less significant improvement in overall survival because of transplant-related complications. Allogeneic bone marrow transplantation is recommended therapy for children with acute nonlymphoid leukemia in second remission.

Chemotherapy has only a palliative role in children with Ph^1 chromosome positive chronic myeloid leukemia, juvenile CML, and in preleukemia or myelodysplastic syndromes. Bone marrow transplantation is useful in these diseases and should be attempted early in their course.

Further progress in bone marrow transplantation will depend upon the development of more effective antileukemic conditioning regimens and an improved understanding of the pathophysiology of graft-vs.-host disease, the graft-vs.-leukemia reaction, and graft rejection.

REFERENCES

1. Thomas ED: Marrow transplantation for malignant disease (Karnofsky Memorial Lecture). *J Clin Oncol* 1983; 1:517–531.
2. Champlin R, Gale RP: Bone marrow transplantation for acute leukemia: Recent advances and comparison with alternative therapies. *Seminars in Hematology* 1987; 24, 1:55–67.
3. O'Reilly R: Allogeneic bone marrow transplantation. Current status and future directions. *Blood* 1983; 62, 5:941–964.
4. Gale RP, Champlin RE: How does bone marrow transplantation cure leukemia? *Lancet* 1984; 2, 28–30.
5. Weiden PL, Sullivan KM, Flournoy N, et al.: Antileukemic effect of chronic graft-vs.-host disease: Contribution of improved survival after allogeneic marrow transplantation. *N Engl J Med* 1981: 304:1529–1532.
6. Storb R, Thomas ED: Bone marrow transplantation in randomly bred animal species and in man. *Proceedings of the Sixth Leucocyte Culture Conference*. Edited by MR Schwarz. New York, Academic Press, 1972, 805–840.
7. Storb R, Epstein RB, Rudolph RH, et al.: Allogeneic canine bone marrow transplantation following cyclophosphamide. *Transplantation* 1969; 7:378–386.
8. Thomas ED, Storb R, Clift RA, et al.: Bone marrow transplantation (first of two parts). *N Engl J Med* 175; 292:832–843.
9. Graw RG, Yankee RA, Rogentine GN, et al.: Bone marrow transplantation from HLA-matched donors to patients with acute leukemia: Toxicity and antileukemic effects. *Transplantation* 1972;14:79–90.
10. Santos GW, Sensenbrenner LL, Burke PJ, et al.: Marrow transplantation in man following cyclophosphamide. *Transplant Proc* 1971; 3:400–404.
11. Santos GW, Tutschka PJ, Brookmeyer R, et al.: Marrow transplantation for acute non-lymphocytic leukemia after treatment with busulfan and cyclophosphamide. *N Engl J Med* 1983; 309:1347–1353.

12. Peters LJ, Withers R, Cundiff JH, et al.: Radiobiologic considerations in the use of total body irradiation for bone marrow transplantation. *Radiology* 1979; 131:243.
13. UCLA Bone Marrow Transplantation Group. Bone marrow transplantation with intensive combination chemotherapy/radiation therapy (SCARI) in acute leukemia. *Annals of Int Med* 1977; 86:155–161.
14. Blume K, Forman S. O'Donnell et al.: Total body irradiation and high-dose etoposide: A new preparatory regimen for bone marrow transplantation in patients with advanced hematologic malignancies. *Blood* 1987; 69:1015.
15. Coccia P, Strandjord S, Warkentin P et al.: High-dose cytosine arabinoside and fractionated total body irradiation: An improved preparative regimen for bone marrow transplantation of children with acute lymphoblastic leukemia in remission. *Blood* 1988; 71, 888–893.
16. Thomas ED, Sanders JE, Flournoy N, et al.: Marrow transplantation for patients with acute lymphoblastic leukemia: A long-term follow-up. *Blood* 1983; 62:1139–1141.
17. Johnson FL, Thomas ED, Clark BS, et al.: A comparison of marrow transplantation with chemotherapy for children with acute lymphoblastic leukemia in second or subsequent remission, *N Engl J Med* 1981; 305:846–851.
18. Johnson FL, Thomas ED: Treatment of relapsed acute lymphoblastic leukemia in childhood. *N Engl J Med* 1984; 310:263–264.
19. Woods WG, Nesbit ME, Ramsay NKC, et al.: Intensive therapy followed by bone marrow transplantation for patients with acute lymphocytic leukemia in second or subsequent remission. Determination of prognostic factors. *Blood* 1983; 61:1182–1189.
20. Chessels JM, Leiper AD, Plowman PN, et al.: Bone marrow transplantation has a limited role in prolonging second marrow remission in childhood lymphoblastic leukemia. *Lancet* 1986; 1239–1241.
21. Butturini A, Bortin MM, Rivera GK, et al.: Which treatment for childhood acute lymphoblastic leukemia in second remission? *Lancet* 1987; 429–432.
22. Rivera GK, Buchanan G, Boyett JM, et al.: Intensive retreatment of childhood acute lymphoblastic leukemia in first bone marrow relapse. *N Engl J Med* 1986; 315:273–278.
23. Sanders JE, Flournoy N, Thomas ED, et al.: Marrow transplantation experience in children with acute lymphoblastic leukemia: An analysis of factors associated with survival, relapse and graft-vs.-host disease. *Med Ped Onc* 1985; 13:165–172.
24. Barrett AJ, Joshi R, Kendra JR, et al.: Prediction and prevention of relapse of acute lymphoblastic leukemia after bone marrow transplantation. *Brit J Hæm* 1986; 64:179–186.
25. Brochstein J, Kernan N, Groshen S et al.: Allogeneic bone marrow transplantation after hyperfractionated total body irradiation and cyclophosphamide in children with acute leukemia. *N Engl J Med* 1987; 317, 1618.
26. Bowman WP, Aur RJA, Hustu HO, et al.: Isolated testicular relapse in acute lymphocytic leukemia of childhood. Categories and influence in survival. *J Clin Oncol* 1984; 2:924–929.
27. Kun LE, Camitta BM, Mulhern RH, et al.: Treatment of meningeal relapse in childhood acute lymphoblastic leukemia. Results of craniospinal irradiation. *J Clin Oncol* 1984; 2:359–364.
28. Nesbit ME, D'Angio GJ, Sather HN, et al.: Effect of isolated central nervous system leukemia on bone marrow remission and survival in childhood acute lymphoblastic leukemia. *Lancet* 1981; 1386–1391.
29. Spruce WE, Forman SJ, Krance RA, et al.: Outcome of bone marrow transplantation in patients with extramedullary involvement of acute leukemia. *Blut* 1983; 48:75–79.
30. Thompson CB, Sanders JE, Flournoy N, et al.: The risks of central nervous system relapse and leukoencephalopathy in patients receiving marrow transplants for acute leukemia. *Blood* 1986; 67:195–199.
31. Clavell LA, Gelber RD, Cohen HJ, et al.: Four-agent induction and intensive asparaginase therapy for treatment of childhood acute lymphoblastic leukemia. *N Engl J Med* 1986; 315:657–662.
32. Chessels JM: Acute leukemia in children. *Clinics in Hæmatology* 1986; 15:727–753.
33. Zwann FE, Hermans J: Factors associated with relapse following allogeneic bone marrow transplantation for acute leukemia in remission. In: Hagenbeck A, Lowenberg B, eds. *Minimal residual disease in acute leukemia.* Martinus Nijhoff Publishers; 1984, 293–310.
34. Barrett AJ, Joshi R, Tew C: How should acute lymphoblastic leukemia relapsing after bone marrow transplantation be treated? *Lancet* 1985; 1188–1190.

35. Dicke KA, Spitzer G: Clinical studies of autografting in acute lymphocytic leukemia. *Clinics in Hæmatology* 1986; 15:85–103.
36. Niemeyer C, Donahue K, Ritz J, et al.: Antibody purged autologous bone marrow transplantation for relapsed non-T cell acute lymphoblastic leukemia (ALL) in childhood. *Blood* 1986; 68:291a (abstract #1039).
37. Ramsay N, LeBien T, Nesbit M, et al.: Autologous bone marrow transplantation for patients with acute lymphoblastic leukemia in second or subsequent remission: Results of bone marrow treated with monoclonal antibodies BA-1, BA-2 and BA-3 plus complement. *Blood* 1985; 66:508–513.
38. Kaizer H, Stuart RK, Brookmeyer R, et al.: Autologous bone marrow transplantation in acute leukemia: A phase II study of *in vitro* treatment with 4-hydroperoxycyclophosphamide to purge tumor cells. *Blood* 1985; 65:1504–1510.
39. Thomas ED, Buckner CD, Clift RA, et al.: Marrow transplantation for acute nonlymphoblastic leukemia in first remission. *N Engl J Med* 1979; 301:597–599.
40. Sanders JE, Thomas ED, Buckner CD, et al.: Marrow transplantation for children in first remission of acute nonlymphocytic leukemia. An update. *Blood* 1985; 66:460–462.
41. Zwaan FE, Hermans J, Barrett AJ, et al.: Bone marrow transplantation for acute non-lymphoblastic leukemia: A survey of the European Group for bone marrow transplantation (E.G.B.M.T.). *Brit J Hæmat* 1984; 56:645–653.
42. Bostrom B, Brunning RD, McGlave P, et al.: Bone marrow transplantation for acute nonlymphocytic leukemia in first remission. Analysis of prognostic factors. *Blood* 1985; 65:1191–1196.
43. Weinstein HJ, Mayer RJ, Rosenthal DS, et al.: Chemotherapy for acute myelogenous leukemia in children and adults: VAPA update. *Blood* 1983; 62:315–319.
44. Grier HE, Gelber RD, Camitta BM et al.: Prognostic factors in childhood acute myelogenous leukemia. *J Clin Oncol* 1987; 5:1026–1032.
45. Creutzig U, Ritter J, Riehm H, et al.: Improved results in childhood acute myelogenous leukemia. A report of the German Cooperative Study AML-BFM-78. *Blood* 1985; 65:298–304.
45a. Nesbit M, Buckley J, Lampkin B et al.: Comparison of allogeneic bone marrow transplantation (BMT) with maintenance chemotherapy in previously untreated childhood acute nonlymphocytic leukemia (ANLL). *Proc Amer Soc Clin Oncol,* 1987; 6, 163 (abst. 640).
46. Lampkin BC, Woods W, Strauss R et al.: Current status of the biology and treatment of acute nonlymphocytic leukemia in children (Report from The Children's Cancer Study Group). *Blood* 1983; 61,215–228.
47. Applebaum FR, Clift RA, Badner CD et al.: Allogeneic marrow transplantation for acute nonlymphoblastic leukemia after first relapse. *Blood* 1983; 61, 949–953.
48. Linch DC, Burnett AK: Clinical studies of ABMT in Acute Myeloid Leukemia. *Clinics in Hæmatology* 1986; 15, 167–186.
49. Yeager AM, Kaiser H, Santos G et al.: Autologous bone marrow transplantation in patients with acute nonlymphocytic leuekmia, using *ex vivo* marrow treated with 4-hydroperoxycyclophosphamide. *N Engl J Med* 1986; 315, 141–147.
50. Castro-Malaspina H, Schaison G, Briere J et al.: Philadelphia Chromosome-Positive Chronic Myelocytic Leukemia in Children (Survival and Prognostic Factors). *Cancer* 1983; 52, 721–727.
51. Castro-Malaspina H, Schaison G, Passe S et al.: Subacute and Chronic Myelomonocytic Leukemia in Children (Juvenile CML). *Cancer* 1984; 54, 675–686.
52. Thomas ED, Clift RA, Fefer A et al.: Marrow transplantation for the treatment of chronic myelogenous leukemia. *Annals of Int Med* 1986; 104, 155–163.
53. Speck B, Bortin MM, Champlin R et al.: Allogeneic bone marrow transplantation for chronic myelogenous leukemia. *Lancet* 1984; 1, 665–668.
54. Goldman JM, Apperley JF, Jones L et al.: Bone marrow transplantation for patients with chronic myeloid leukemia. *N Engl J Med* 1986; 314:202–207.
55. Sanders J, Buckner D, Thomas E, et al.: Allogeneic marrow transplantation for children with juvenile chronic myelogenous leukemia. *Blood* 1988; 71; 1144–1146.
56. Blank J, Lange B: Preleukemia in children. *J Ped* 1981; 98, 565–568.
57. Nowell P, Wilmoth D, Lange B: Cytogenetics of childhood preleukemia. *Cancer Genetics and Cytogenetics* 1983, 261–266.

58. Applebaum FR, Storb R, Ramberg RE et al.: Treatment of preleukemic syndromes with marrow transplantation. *Blood* 1987; 69, 92–96.

58a. Guinan E, Tarbell N, Tantravahi R, et al.: Bone marrow transplantation for children with myelodysplastic syndromes. *Blood* 1989; 73, 619–622.

59. Gale RP: Graft-vs.-host disease. *Immunologic Reviews* 1985; 87, 1–22.

60. Cobbold S, Martin G, Waldmann H: Monoclonal antibodies for the prevention of graft-vs.-host disease and marrow graft rejection. Transplantation 1986; 42, 239–247.

61. Kersey JH, LeBien T, Vallera D et al.: Allogeneic and autologous marrow transplantation: *ex vivo* purging with monoclonal antibody or immunotoxins to remove leukemic cells or to prevent graft-vs.-host disease. In: Hagenbeek A, Lowenberg B, eds. *Minimal residual disease in acute leukemia.* Boston: Martinus Nijhoff Publishers 1986; 275–281.

62. O'Reilly RJ, Kernan N, Collins N et al.: Abrogation of both acute and chronic GVHD following transplant of lectin-agglutinated, E-rosette depleted (SBA-E) marrow for leukemia. (Abstract) *Blood* 1986;68 (suppl 1):291a.

63. Smith BR, Burakoff SJ, Weinstein H et al.: Differential outcome of histocompatible vs. histoincompatible Leu-1 depleted bone marrow transplants (Abstract). *Blood* 1986; 68 (suppl 1):292a.

64. Prentice HG, Blacklock HA, Janossy G, et al.: Depletion of T lymphocytes in donor marrow prevents significant graft-vs.-host disease in matched allogeneic leukemic marrow transplant recipients. *Lancet* 1984; 1:472–476.

65. Butturini A, Seeger R, Gale RP: Recipient immune-competent T lymphocytes can survive intensive conditioning for bone marrow transplantation. *Blood* 1986; 68, 954–956.

66. Goldman J, Gale R, Horowitz M, et al.: Bone marrow transplantation for chronic myelogenous leukemia in chronic phase (increased risk for relapse associated with T-cell depletion). *Annals of Int Med* 1988; 108:806–814.

67. Bozdech MJ, Sondel PM, Trigg ME et al.: Transplantation of HLA-haploidentical T-cell depleted marrow for leukemia: addition of cytosine arabinoside to the pretransplant conditioning prevents rejection. *Exp Hematol.* 1985, 13:1201–1210.

68. Gingrich R, Howe C, Goekin N et al.: Successful bone marrow transplantation with partially matched unrelated donors. *Transplantation Proceedings.* 1985; 17, 450–452.

69. Hows JM, Yin JL, Marsh et al.: Histocompatible unrelated volunteer donors compared with HLA nonidentical family donors in marrow transplantation for aplastic anemia and leukemia. *Blood* 1986;68:1322–1328.

Bone Marrow Transplantation in Children, edited by F. Leonard Johnson and Carl Pochedly. Raven Press, Ltd., New York © 1990.

Bone Marrow Transplantation for Treatment of Solid Tumors

Thomas E. Williams and Shahrokh Safarimaryaki

Division of Hematology/Oncology, The University of Texas Health Science Center at San Antonio, San Antonio, Texas 78284

Introduction
A. Neuroblastoma
B. Rhabdomyosarcoma and other soft tissue sarcomas
C. Ewing's sarcoma
D. Lymphomas
    1. Hodgkin's disease
    2. Burkitt's lymphoma
    3. Non-Burkitt's, non-Hodgkin's lymphomas
E. Other tumors
    1. Brain tumors
    2. Wilms' tumor
    3. Osteosarcoma
    4. Germ cell tumors
    5. Retinoblastoma
    6. Peripheral neuroepithelioma
    7. Histiocytic tumors
Summary

INTRODUCTION

Dose-response relationships between radiotherapy and between numerous chemotherapeutic modalities and most solid tumors in childhood are often linear across a wide dose range. However, myelotoxicity is frequently dose-limiting, making bone marrow reconstitution a rational procedure for allowing the larger doses of chemotherapy and radiotherapy to be given. Two facts limit the application of bone marrow reconstitution: (1) metastasis to the bone marrow is a common early complication of many childhood solid tumors and (2) only an estimated one-fourth to one-third of patients have a suitable sibling bone marrow donor.

Autologous reinfusion of marrow would be preferable to allogeneic bone marrow transplantation if the reinfused marrow could be made free of malignant cells. Consequently, numerous investigators have developed novel methods of purging the marrow of tumor cells. In this situation, allogeneic transplants of bone marrow appear to be less desirable because graft rejection and graft-vs.-host disease are possible complications.

Bone marrow reconstitution is primarily the technique that allows an extension of the range of dosages of radiotherapy and chemotherapy. Thus, it follows that the entire treatment program is no better than the regimen of high dose chemotherapy and radiotherapy chosen (30). Therefore, if the dose-limiting toxicity of a useful drug in the therapy of a particular tumor is not myelosuppressive, it could not ordinarily be escalated beyond its already established maximally tolerated dose. Consequently, the technique of high-dose chemoradiotherapy and autologous marrow rescue is best applied to those tumors in which effective antitumor drugs include one or more agents which have myelosuppression as the only, or at least the primary, dose-limiting toxicity.

Experience in marrow transplanted in childhood solid tumors is limited and numerous questions remain which lend themselves well to prospective studies of high-dose chemotherapy and radiotherapy regimens, bone marrow purging, and graft-vs.-tumor effect (1).

NEUROBLASTOMA

Neuroblastoma is the most frequently encountered nonhematologic childhood malignancy outside the central nervous system. Unfortunately, little progress has been made in its therapy over the past 30 years. At best only 20% of patients survive following current treatment methods. The tumor usually presents in an advanced stage, frequently with bone marrow metastases. The tumor's heterogeneity is shown by the fact that it usually responds initially to radiotherapy, to alkylating agents, vinca alkaloids, anthracyclines, podophyllotoxins, and antimetabolites. However, neuroblastomas usually recur in the primary site, or in distant sites, despite the use of many rigorous treatment methods aimed at preventing relapse. Consequently, the tumor has been the childhood malignancy most often treated with high-dose chemoradiotherapy and bone marrow rescue. As in treatment of most other childhood solid tumors, more experience has been accumulated with autologous marrow reinfusion than with allogeneic transplantation. A number of clinical studies using autologous reconstitution for treatment of neuroblastomas are noted in Table 1.

TABLE 1. *Treatment of neuroblastoma using autologous (nonpurged) bone marrow rescue*

Extent of disease pre massive therapy	Number of patients	Type of massive therapy	Responses	Duration of response	References
Clinical Remission	12	L-PAM	7 PR	3 CCR 18–35+ months	2
Stages III & IV	13	L-PAM ±CTX		7 CCR 1–37+ months	3
Refractory	10	L-PAM	5 CR 2 PR	0 CCR median response of 6 months	4,63,64
Advanced PR (7)	7	L-PAM	NR among PR patients	0 CCR	5
CR (8)	15	L-PAM		8 CCR	57
Relapse (3)	5	L-PAM/TBI	1 CR 1 PR	3 CCR 5+–12 months	8
Stages III & IV (marrow negative)	19	L-PAM/VM26/ DOXO/ TBI/L-XRT		11 CCR 6–22+ months, 2 NR, 5 ED	9,10
Stage IV	4	VCR/DTIC/CTX/ ± DOXO/± ARA-C	1 CR 2 PR	1 CCR 4 months	20

CR   = complete response
PR   = partial response
NR   = no response
ED   = early death due to therapy related toxicity
CCR   = continuous complete remission
L-PAM = phenylalanine mustard

CTX   = cyclophosphamide
VM26   = teniposide
DOXO   = doxorubicin (Adriamycin)
ARA-C   = cytosine arabinoside
DTIC   = diaminotriimidazole carboximide
TBI   = total body irradiation
L-XRT   = localized radiotherapy

McElwain was among the first to study the use of high-dose melphalan and autologous bone marrow rescue in neuroblastoma. Melphalan appeared particularly promising in this setting because it is short-acting and has few nonhematologic toxicities. In these initial studies (2), 12 children were given melphalan in a single dose of 140 mg/m^2 followed by infusion of nonpurged, noncryopreserved bone marrow. Seven had evidence of tumor regression, and 3 were long-term survivors of more than 18 months. Subsequently, investigators in the Netherlands tried high-dose melphalan (with or without cyclophosphamide priming) at a dose of 140 to 180 mg/m^2. They noted that 7 of 13 patients with stage III and IV disease were alive with no evidence of disease at 1, 3, 5, 6, 10, 24, and 37 months respectively, after receiving high-dose melphalan (3). Using somewhat higher doses of melphalan, 10 children in Cleveland (4,63,64) and 7 in Houston (5) were rescued with nonpurged marrow but none became long-term survivors.

All of McElwain's patients were in their initial clinical remission at the time that high-dose melphalan and autologous rescue were given. Thus, it is possible that their tumor burden was less than in the patients treated in Cleveland and Houston, who showed less favorable results. This possibility appeared to be confirmed by French workers (57,67) who noted no long-term survivors among 7 patients treated while in partial remission (PR), but 5 among 8 patients treated while in complete remission (CR) were long-term survivors.

Following the observations of D'Angio and Evans (7), low-dose total body irradiation (TBI) was included as a useful "fourth drug" along wih cyclophosphamide, vincristine, and DTIC for treatment of metastatic neuroblastoma. Also, using techniques largely derived from earlier leukemia protocols, other investigators have combined TBI and melphalan with bone marrow reconstitution. Graham-Pole presented initial results in 3 patients who were treated while in relapse using melphalan, TBI and autologous bone marrow (8). One complete remission and one partial remission, each lasting 12 months before recurrence of the disease, were noted. One of two patients treated in second remission remained in remission more than 5 months.

Other investigators have chosen to combine other chemotherapeutic agents with either high-dose melphalan, or with high-dose melphalan and TBI followed by autologous marrow rescue (61,68). August combined VM-26 (teniposide) and doxorubicin (adriamycin) with high-dose melphalan, fractionated TBI, together with local irradiation to involved bones and to tumors greater than 5.0 cm in greatest diameter, in treatment of 4 children with advanced neuroblastoma (9). Two remain in complete clinical remission 35+ and 22+ months later. The others died early of fungal pneumonia. Later, these same investigators reported that 10 children with stage III and IV neuroblastomas were treated with VM-26, adriamycin, high-dose melphalan, TBI, and autologous bone marrow. In 4 other children, adriamycin alone was withheld, and in one additional child VM-26 alone was not given. Nine of the 15 patients achieved a complete remission, but 4 relapsed 6 to 9 months after being given chemoradiotherapy and autologous bone marrow. Two did not respond and three died in the first months of fungal infections and cardiorespiratory problems of uncertain etiology (10). Ekert in Australia treated 4 patients with vincristine, DTIC, and cyclophosphamide. One patient received adriamycin as well, while one received adriamycin and cytosine arabinoside. All received nonpurged autologous marrow. One complete remission and 2 partial remissions were observed, but the longest patient survived only 4 months (20).

More recently, investigators have turned to purging autologous bone marrow of tumor cells (Table 2). Purging has taken several forms. Murine monoclonal antibodies when absorbed by anti-mouse immunoglobulin-coated magnetic beads (immunomagnetic purging) have been shown to be useful in removing tumor cells from the bone marrow (11,12). Another method is chemical purging, such as with Asta-Z (13), a derivative of cyclophosphamide, or with the combination of 6-hydroxy-dopamine and ascorbic acid (14). Other promising purging methods include differential agglutination with lectin (15) and dye-mediated photolysis (16).

Fourteen patients with stage III and IV neuroblastomas with various degrees of tumor burden were treated with a program of 5-day continuous infusion vincristine, high-dose melphalan, fractionated TBI, and purged or nonpurged autologous marrow reconstitution. Eight patients were evaluable with a mean observation time since bone marrow reinfusion of 5 months (13,66,67). Six patients were transplanted in relapse; 3 responded to therapy and in 2 no further progression was observed. Four were treated while their disease was stable and only 1 has progressed. Of 4 transplanted in complete remission only 1 has relapsed. It was not possible for these authors to evaluate the effect of marrow purging in general or in any of the three methods they used; however, they favored use of immunomagnetic purging.

The marrows of 11 stage IV neuroblastoma patients were purged with Asta-Z and reinfused following high-dose chemotherapy with BCNU, VM-26 (teniposide), and melphalan. As in a previous study by the same authors, there was no measurable response to high-dose chemotherapy in patients reconstituted in partial remission. However, 8 out of 9 patients who were in complete remission remained without evidence of neuroblastoma for periods ranging from 2+ to 11+ months at the time of their report (6). These investigators also treated 10 patients with high-dose busulfan and cyclophosphamide. Six received Asta-Z-purged autologous marrow and 4 were not purged. None were treated while in complete remission. Tumor regression was observed in 8; all but one eventually died with persistent neuroblastoma. Nonetheless, this well-tolerated regimen appears promising enough to be tried in patients with less residual tumor. The median duration of neutropenia and thrombocytopenia following this double alkylating agent approach did not differ among patients given purged or nonpurged bone marrow (17).

Helson used 6-hydroxy-dopamine and ascorbic acid to purge the marrows of 17 children that he treated with high-dose melphalan and dianhydrogalac-

TABLE 2. *Treatment of neuroblastoma using autologous (purged) bone marrow reconstitution*

Extent of disease pre massive therapy	Number of patients	Type of massive therapy	Response	Duration of response	References
Stage III & IV 6-relapse 4-CR 4-SD	14	L-PAM/VCR/fx-TBI (IM beads/ASTA-Z) 60H dopamine)	3 OR 5 SD 3 PD	9 CCR median observation of 5 months	13,66,71
Stage IV 9-CR	11	L-PAM/BCNU/VM26 (ASTA-Z)		8 CCR 2+–11+ months	6
Stage IV	6	BU/CY (ASTA-Z)	1 CR 3 PR 2 PD	0 CCR	17
Stage III & IV 11 in relapse 6 in remission	17	L-PAM/±TBI/ dianhydrogalactitol (6 OH dopamine & ascorbic acid)		9 CCR median FU of 12 months	18
Stage III & IV	4	L-PAM/VM26/ DOXO/CP/ TBI (IM beads)		2 CCR	19

CR = complete response
PR = partial response
OR = objective response
SD = stable disease
PD = progressive disease
CCR = continuous complete remission
IM = immunomagnetic beads
OH = hydroxy

L-PAM = phenylalanine mustard
CP   = cisplatin
CY   = cyclophosphamide
VCR   = vincristine
VM26 = teniposide
BU   = busulfan
BCNU = bis-chloro-nitrosourea

titol, with or without TBI. Eleven were treated in relapse and 6 were treated in remission. Survivors (median follow-up of 12 months) included 5 among those treated while in relapse and 4 of the 6 who were in remission (18).

Moss treated 13 stage III and IV patients with teniposide (VM-26), adriamycin, melphalan, and cisplatin (VAMP) with fractionated TBI followed by autologous bone marrow rescue. Four were purged by an 8-monoclonal antibody immunomagnetic bead technique. Eight did not receive immunomagnetically purged marrow. Six patients had survived 14 to 48 months at the time of their report. All were given VAMP/TBI and autologous bone marrow rescue after initial chemotherapy but before recurrence of their disease (19).

Fewer patients have been treated with allogeneic transplantation following intensive chemotherapy or both chemotherapy and radiotherapy for advanced neuroblastoma (Table 3). While the possibility of infusion of malignant cells is practically nil, that advantage relative to autologous reinfusion is balanced by the morbidity associated with graft-vs.-host disease. A theoretical advantage may accrue to the recipient of allogeneic marrow, namely the graft-vs.-tumor effect. In August's series two patients received teniposide, adriamycin, high-dose melphalan and fractionated TBI (MAT-TBI) followed by allogeneic bone marrow transplantation. Both are long-term survivors at 36+ and 54+ months. Notable is the patient with the longest survival. This 3-year-old girl presented with stage II neuroblastoma which initially responded completely to treatment with local radiotherapy, cyclophosphamide, DTIC, vincristine, teniposide, adriamycin, and cisplatin. However, she relapsed with metastases in the skull, left femur and lymph nodes. She received MAT-TBI followed by a bone marrow transplant from her 7-year-old brother. Mild chronic graft-vs.-host disease attended her continuous complete remission (9).

In another study, 2 out of 9 patients given VAMP-TBI and allogeneic bone marrow transplants were survivors of more than 14 months (19). The authors attributed these inferior results, when compared to their experience with VAMP-TBI and autologous marrow, to be due to methotrexate (given to prevent GVH disease) and graft-vs.-host disease. For that reason, they do not recommend use of VAMP-TBI together with allogeneic bone marrow transplantation. Graham-Pole reported that none of the 3 patients given high-dose melphalan and TBI followed by reconstitution with allogeneic marrow were long-term survivors (8).

These experiences with intensive chemotherapy and radiotherapy given in association with bone marrow transplantation have shown that it is possible to cure some patients with neuroblastoma even when the patient has relapsed following initial surgery and chemotherapy. Collectively, these results appear to some authors to be better than those following current conventional therapy (19). Nonetheless, numerous questions remain. It is hoped that these questions will be answered at least in part by larger randomized clinical trials: What is the best intensive therapy? (59) What is the role of marrow purging? Is reconstitution with purged autologous marrow better than allogeneic trans-

TABLE 3. *Treatment of neuroblastomas with allogeneic bone marrow transplantation*

Extent of disease pre massive therapy	Number of patients	Type of massive therapy	Response	Duration of response	References
Stage IV	4	L-PAM/VM26/ DOXO/ TBI/L-XRT	2 CR 2 ED	2 CCR 36+ & 54+ months	9
Stage III & IV	9	L-PAM/VM26/ DOXO/ CP/TBI		2 CCR 14+ months	19
Relapse	3	L-PAM/TBI	2 CR	0 CCR	8

CR = complete response
ED = early death
CCR = continuous complete remission
L-PAM = phenylalanine mustard
VM26 = teniposide

DOXO = doxurubicin (Adriamycin)
CP = cisplatin
TBI = total body irradiation
L-XRT = localized radiotherapy

plantation? What is the best time for doing the procedure? These questions will not be resolved in a static environment as progress in the initial therapy of neuroblastoma is expected to improve as well.

RHABDOMYOSARCOMA AND OTHER SOFT TISSUE SARCOMAS

Sporadic reports of the use of bone marrow transplantation in rhabdomyosarcoma and in other soft tissue sarcomas have appeared (Table 4) (4,17,20–22). The results at the National Cancer Institute are presented in chapter 7 by Miser. Four patients with stages III and IV rhabdomyosarcoma were given high-dose cyclophosphamide, DTIC, adriamycin, and nonpurged autologous marrow. Two patients achieved a complete remission lasting 3+ and 6+ months at the time of the report. Two patients achieved a partial remission, one lasting 14 months (20). Another patient with advanced rhabdomyosarcoma was treated with busulfan, cyclophosphamide and autologous nonpurged marrow. Although a complete remission was observed, the patient died of hepatic veno-occlusive disease and systemic fungal infection (17).

Herzig (4) and Phillips (21) have each reported the results of using high-dose BCNU and nonpurged autologous marrow in the treatment of 4 patients with advanced soft tissue sarcomas. In each instance, 3 responses were observed. Miser was able to induce a complete remission in 14 out of 17 patients using vincristine, adriamycin, cyclophosphamide and local irradiation. These patients were then given these 3 drugs and TBI along with autologous bone marrow reinfusion. Eleven were in continuous complete remission at the time of the report (22).

EWING'S SARCOMA

Although it is an uncommon tumor in children, there has been sufficient experience with Ewing's sarcoma so that now it can be expected that about 50% of patients will respond to treatment with surgery together with chemotherapy, radiotherapy, or both, for localized lesions. Progress, however, has been slow for patients who present with metastatic tumors or who have tumors that recur locally within the first year. Fortunately, bone marrow involvement is found in only one-third of such patients, thereby making them excellent candidates for high-dose chemotherapy with autologous bone marrow rescue. The initial reports and those that followed document that the response to high doses of single drugs or treatment with multiple agents, based primarily on alkylating agents, is 50% or more (23) (Table 5).

Among 42 patients from 7 reports (3–5,23,51,58,63–65,72) who were treated with melphalan as a single agent, approximately half had complete responses. Recently, Miser treated 10 patients with stage III and 12 with stage IV disease with a combination of vincristine, adriamycin, cyclophosphamide

TABLE 4. *Treatment of rhabdomyosarcomas and other soft tissue sarcomas with bone marrow transplantation*

Extent of disease pre massive therapy	Number of patients	Type of massive therapy	Response	Duration of response	References
Stage III & IV	4	CY/DTIC/DOXO	2 CR 2 PR	2 CCR 3+, 6+ months	20
Advanced Alveolar	1	BU/CY	1 CR	1 CCR 1.5 months	17
Soft Tissue Sarcomas	8	BCNU	6 PR		4,21
All Stages 14-CR	14	VCR/DOXO/CY/TBI		11 CCR	22

CR = complete response
PR = partial response
CCR = continuous complete remission
CY = cyclophosphamide
DTIC = diaminotriimidazole carboxamide

DOXO = doxorubicin (Adriamycin)
BU   = busulfan
BCNU = bis-chloro-nitrosourea
TBI = total body irradiation
VCR = vincristine

TABLE 5. *Treatment of Ewing's sarcoma with bone marrow transplantation*

Extent of disease pre massive therapy	Number of patients	Type of massive therapy	Response	Duration of response	References
All Stages	42	L-PAM	10 CR 13 PR 19 ND	9 CCR 2+−30+ months	3,4,5,23,51,58,63,64,65,72
Stages III & IV 22-CR	22	VCR/DOXO/CY/TBI		14 CCR 8 for 12+ months	53

CR = complete response
PR = partial response
ND = not designated
CCR = continuous complete remission
CY = cyclophosphamide

DOXO = doxorubicin (Adriamycin)
TBI = total body irradiation
VCR = vincrisinte
L-PAM = phenylalanine mustard

and local radiation during the initial 15 weeks of therapy. Twenty-two achieved a complete remission and were then treated with an intensification program consisting of TBI, vincristine, adriamycin, cyclophosphamide and unpurged autologous bone marrow rescue. At the time of the report, 14 patients were surviving disease-free, 8 for over 12 months (53). An update on this study is given in Chapter 7.

LYMPHOMAS

Hodgkin's disease and non-Hodgkin's lymphomas in children are a diverse group of tumors with variable prognosis. High-dose chemotherapy or chemotherapy combined with radiotherapy followed by allogeneic or autologous bone marrow rescue has been used in a limited number of children and its efficacy remains largely unknown. The experience in adults, however, is more extensive (32). While the prognosis of Hodgkin's disease in children and in adults is similar for like stage and histologic type, there are significant differences between adults and children with non-Hodgkin's lymphomas. Therefore, while experience with high-dose chemotherapy or chemoradiotherapy and bone marrow transplantation among adults with Hodgkin's disease might be extended to children, the results in non-Hodgkin's lymphomas may not be applicable.

Hodgkin's Disease

Experience with use of allogeneic bone marrow transplantation in Hodgkin's disease in children is limited. Among 3 patients from St. Louis and Cleveland ranging in age from 19 to 25 years, the combination of high-dose cyclophosphamide, fractionated total body irradiation (fx TBI) and allogeneic reconstitution achieved a complete remission in all. However, one patient died of acute graft-vs.-host disease. The others are surviving more than 17 months following transplantation (24). Also, there were no children among 8 patients with advanced recurrent disease reported by the Seattle group. Their patients received high-dose cyclophosphamide and TBI prior to allogeneic bone marrow transplantation. Two remained in continuous complete remission in excess of 38 months, while 4 died of complications of the procedure and 2 died following relapse. (25).

The experience with autologous bone marrow rescue following high-dose chemotherapy or chemoradiotherapy is more extensive, however (Table 6). The preparative regimens are varied. Use of a single drug as chemotherapy has been advocated by some (26,27). Among 15 patients treated with high-dose melphalan and autologous bone marrow rescue, 4 are surviving after 9+ to 61+ months. Multiple-drug chemotherapy together with TBI had been given prior to autologous bone marrow rescue to 6 patients (28,29), and two patients

TABLE 6. Treatment of Hodgkin's disease using autologous bone marrow rescue

Extent of disease pre massive therapy	Number of patients	Type of massive therapy	Response	Duration of response	Reference
Stages II, III, IV MOPP and/or ABVD resistant	15	L-PAM	4 CR 8 PR 2 NR	4 CCR 9+–61+ months	26,27
All Stages 3-PR	6	ARA-C CY/TBI CCNU/CY/VCR/ DOXO/Carolysin/ TBI VP16/CY/TBI	2 CR 2 PR 2 NR	2 CCR 7+–25+ months	28,29
All Stages MOPP and/or ABVD resistant	9	CY/VP16	5 CR 1 PR 1 NR 2 NE	4 CCR 1+–8+ months	26,33
All Stages MOPP and/or ABVD resistant	30	BCNU/ CY/ VP16	15 CR 10 PR 5 NR	11 CCR 1+–44+ months	35
All Stages MOPP and/or ABVD resistant	5	TACC	2 CR 1 NR 2 NE	2 CCR 66+ months	38
All Stages MOPP and/or ABVD resistant	10	BACT	9 CR 1 NE	4 CCR 18+–43+ months	29,40

CR = complete response
PR = partial response
NR = no response
NE = not evaluable
CCR = continuous complete remission
DOXO = doxorubicin (Adriamycin)
BCNU = bis-chloro-nitrosourea

CY = cyclophosphamide
L-PAM = phenylalanine mustard
ARA-C = cytosine arabinoside
CCNU = cis-chloro-nitrosourea
VCR = vincristine
VP16 = etoposide
TACC = thioguannine, cytosine arabinoside, CCNU, cyclophosphamide

TBI = total body irradiation
BACT = BCNU, cytosine arabinoside, cyclophosphamide, thioguanine

were surviving 232+ and 754+ days. The largest experience has been among MOPP-resistant and/or ABVD-resistant patients who received 2-, 3-, 4- or 5-drug regimens before autologous bone marrow reinfusion (26,27,28,29–33,35,38,40). Overall, about 35% achieved a durable remission.

Consequently, many questions remain unanswered about the role of high-dose chemotherapy or giving both chemotherapy and radiotherapy followed by bone marrow reconstitution in the treatment of Hodgkin's disease in general, and in the treatment of Hodgkin's disease in children in particular. These questions include: Is autologous rescue better than allogeneic bone marrow transplantation? What is the role of TBI? What is the optimal regimen of chemotherapy? Only controlled randomized clinical trials will answer these questions.

Burkitt's Lymphoma

Both allogeneic marrow transplantation and autologous reconstitution have been used in the therapy of poor prognosis Burkitt's lymphoma following various preparative regimens.

In one study 5 patients were treated. Three were in remission at the time of allogeneic bone marrow transplantation following a preparative regimen consisting of the combination of BCNU, cytosine arabinoside, cyclophosphamide and TBI consisting of a dose of 750 cGy delivered in one day. All engrafted. Those transplanted in remission continued in remission from 18+ to 73+ months at the time of the report (34). Two patients transplanted while in relapse died of graft-vs.-host disease, and interstitial pneumonia and with bone marrow and CNS relapse respectively. Phillips treated three patients with high-dose cyclophosphamide and fractionated TBI (1200 cGy given as 200 cGy twice a day for 3 days) followed by allogeneic bone marrow transplantation. Two are alive in remission 17+ and 21+ months respectively. The other patient died of acute graft-vs.-host disease but without evidence of tumor (35).

Appelbaum was the first to report successful application of autologous marrow rescue following multiple-drug chemotherapy with the BACT regimen (BCNU, cytosine arabinoside, cyclophosphamide, and 6-thioguanine) for treatment of Burkitt's lymphoma in children and young adults. Among 8 patients treated in this manner, 5 responded and three achieved durable remissions lasting from 9+ to 29+ months. These patients may be cured, because no relapses have occurred among the responders 2 months after BACT therapy (36).

A total of 51 Burkitt's lymphoma patients were treated with the BACT regimen (43 patients) or the BEAM regimen (BCNU, etoposide, cytosine arabinoside, and melphalan) (8 patients). This was followed by nonpurged (39 patients) and immunologically purged (12 patients) autologous bone marrow rescue. Fifty-two percent were long-term survivors. But prolonged survival was observed only among those patients treated while in initial complete remission (CR) or following successful reinduction of remission with salvage chemotherapy. While the response rate to BACT or BEAM for patients with measurable disease was impressive (70%), the durations of remissions were short (median 100 days). In a later study, 12 patients were treated with BACT and nonpurged autologous marrow. Among 10 who had been followed for more than 3 months, four were in durable remissions of more than 3 months including 2 who were not treated while in complete remission (37). Hartmann and his coworkers used the BACT regimen and autologous bone marrow infusion to treat 10 patients. Four attained a durable remission lasting more than 2 years (38).

Baumgartner treated 5 patients with abdominal presentation with vincristine, adriamycin, high-dose cyclophosphamide, and TBI (600 cGy in one day) followed by autologous nonpurged marrow. Four were in complete remission and one in a partial remission. Four are alive without disease 5+ to 35+ months later. However, 3 of these patients have continued to receive chemotherapy after autologous bone marrow reconstitution (39). Others have reported results of therapy of Burkitt's lymphoma with either fractionated or single-dose TBI and high-dose cyclophosphamide (CY/TBI) and autologous marrow rescue (40,41). Among 11 patients treated with CY/TBI, 5 have achieved durable unmaintained remissions lasting over 20 months at the times of their reports.

Non-Burkitt's, Non-Hodgkin's Lymphomas

In this category of non-Hodgkin's lymphomas are included lymphoblastic (primarily T cell) and nonlymphoblastic histologic types. The experience is limited both in the allogeneic and autologous marrow reconstitution settings in children.

Four children with T cell lymphoblastic lymphomas (three in remission and one in relapse) were given BCNU, cyclophosphamide, cytosine arabinoside and total body irradiation followed by allogeneic bone marrow transplantation (34). Two achieved durable remissions of 29+ and 49+ months. Death in the others was due to sepsis and relapse. When 7 children and young adults were given high-dose cyclophosphamide, fractionated TBI and allogeneic bone marrow transplantation, only one achieved a durable remission. The others died of acute graft-vs.-host disease, interstitial pneumonia and progressive disease (35). CY/TBI and allogeneic marrow transplantation was also used to treat 3 children with chemotherapy-resistant lymphoblastic lymphoma. None achieved a durable remission. All 3 died of either acute graft-vs.-host disease or progressive tumor (42).

As with other lymphoma types, the experience with autologous marrow reconstitution is more extensive in children. Chemotherapy has been given either with or without TBI.

High-dose cyclophosphamide and TBI have been given to 9 children from two series (31,41). Five achieved a durable remission. Vincristine, adria-mycin, cyclophosphamide and TBI were given with autologous bone marrow rescue to 5 children and one was a long-term survivor (24). Following Appel-baum's lead, 3 series comprising the experience with 26 children have re-ported the results of using the non-TBI containing BACT regimen (43,44,73). Nineteen achieved a complete remission, and 7 of these remained disease-free at the time of the reports. Lastly, 3 children received vincristine, cytosine arabinoside, adriamycin, and methotrexate (given both systemically and in-trathecally) followed by autologous marrow rescue. All achieved a complete remission, but only one was a long-term survivor (45).

OTHER TUMORS

A group of children with other miscellaneous tumor types have been treated primarily with autologous, nonpurged, marrow rescue following prepa-ration with various combinations of chemotherapy with or without radiother-apy. The numbers treated are too small to draw any definite conclusions about the efficacy of these methods. Nonetheless, some promising results noted below suggest the value of continuing to study the use of this method of therapy for these tumors.

Brain Tumors

Wolff (46,48) gave both high-dose etoposide and high-dose BCNU with autologous marrow rescue to patients of ages 8 to 68 years with recurrent or progressive glioblastoma multiforme and anaplastic astrocytoma. Among those treated with etoposide, one-half had responses lasting 4 to 8 months. Twelve out of 27 who were given BCNU responded, one in excess of 84 months. Nine patients, ranging in age from 20 to 64 years, were treated with high-dose BCNU and autologous bone marrow rescue immediately following primary surgery and initial radiotherapy, with or without chemotherapy but before tumor progression. At the time of their report (47), 3 patients were alive without progression at 27+, 48+, and 70+ months after autologous marrow infusion. These observations were subsequently confirmed by these authors. They noted that survival did not substantially differ from that follow-ing conventional therapy, but they added that severe encephalopathy and diffuse pulmonary infiltrates with hypoxemia were formidable late sequelae (48).

High-dose aziridinylbenzoquinone (AZQ) was given to 4 children with re-fractory CNS tumors followed by cryopreserved autologous bone marrow rescue. Two, one each with grade II astrocytoma and pineal teratoma, re-sponded for 6+ and 4+ months respectively. Two patients, both with brain stem gliomas, did not respond (49).

Wilms' Tumor

Among 6 patients with progressive Wilms' tumor, all responded to high-dose melphalan alone and two are long-term survivors (50). Another child with metastatic Wilms' tumor was reported to have achieved a complete remission lasting 180 days (51).

Osteosarcoma

The Lyon (France) group have given either high-dose melphalan or high-dose busulfan to 3 patients with osteosarcoma, but the overall response rate was less than 50% and no complete responses were observed (37). Miser reported that 12 out of 24 relapsed osteosarcoma patients given a high-dose, 7-drug regimen over a 21-day period followed by autologous bone marrow reconstitution were long-term survivors of more than 2 years (52).

Germ Cell Tumors

Only a small number of children with advanced malignant germ cell tumors have received high-dose chemotherapy and autologous bone marrow rescue. However, a few examples may be illustrative. French workers have reported that a 4-year-old child with a pretreated and localized yolk sac tumor of the retroperitoneum was given high doses of melphalan and etoposide prior to autologous bone marrow rescue. The patient achieved a complete remission with normal serum alpha-fetoprotein determinations lasting one month (74). Baumgartner treated 3 children with advanced metastatic yolk sac tumors. One was in complete remission, one in partial remission, and one had progressive disease prior to treatment with vincristine, adriamycin, high-dose cyclophosphamide, and TBI. The patient in partial remission achieved a complete response, while the patient with progressive disease achieved a partial remission. However, only the patient treated in complete remission became a long-term survivor (39).

Retinoblastoma

Two patients with stage IV retinoblastoma were given a combination of vincristine, cyclophosphamide, DTIC, and adriamycin followed by cryopreserved autologous bone marrow rescue. A complete remission was observed in both but lasted only 5 months in one (45).

Peripheral Neuroepithelioma

This primitive neural tumor arises outside the central nervous system. It usually occurs in the chest wall and histologically resembles several small round-cell tumors, such as Ewing's sarcoma and neuroblastoma. It may be distinguished from these tumors, however, by characteristic cytogenetic, biochemical, and oncogenic markers. A total of 17 children and young adults were treated with vincristine, adriamycin, and cyclophosphamide and 16 achieved a complete remission (53). Eight of these then received TBI followed by vincristine, adriamycin, and high-dose cyclophosphamide with autologous bone marrow rescue. Five are long-term survivors.

Histiocytic Tumors

High-dose cyclophosphamide and TBI were given to a preadolescent child with progressive and chemotherapy-resistant histiocytosis-X. Thereafter, he received an allogeneic bone marrow transplant from his HLA/MLC compatible sister. At the time of the report, the child was alive without disease 2½ years later (54).

A patient with familial erythrophagocytic lymphohistiocytosis was prepared for allogeneic bone marrow transplantation with high-dose etoposide, cytosine arabinoside, busulfan, and cyclophosphamide. He achieved a complete remission lasting more than one year at the time of the report (75).

A 9-year-old girl with recurrent malignant histiocytosis in remission was prepared for allogeneic bone marrow transplantation with high-dose etoposide, cyclophosphamide and TBI. The patient had remained in remission more than 4 years at the time of the report (76).

SUMMARY

Bone marrow transplantation of malignant childhood solid tumors, both allogeneic and autologous, is a technique which takes advantage of the observation that tumors unresponsive to standard dosing of chemotherapy will respond to higher doses, doses which could not otherwise be given in the absence of marrow rescue. However, when this technique is applied to children with advanced tumor burdens, responses are usually short-lived and transplant associated mortality and morbidity is high. Preliminary information suggests however that when this technique is applied earlier in the course of the child's disease and at a time of less tumor burden, durable tumor control is often observed. It is expected that further studies will seek to develop cytoreductive regimens of greater efficacy than those currently in use and that more children will be offered the technique at an earlier time before tumor progression. Last, improvements in supportive care of these transplant recipients should lower transplant associated complications and make the method more acceptable.

REFERENCES

1. Stinner G, Souverein M, Dettmer R: Graft-vs.-tumor. Model for autologous bone marrow transplantation in murine tumor systems. In, McVie JG, Dalesio O, Smith IE, (eds): *Autologous Bone Marrow Transplantation in Murine Systems.* New York, Raven Press, 1984.
2. Pritchard J, McElwain TJ, Graham-Pole J: Treatment of advanced neuroblastoma with supralethal chemotherapy, radiation, and allogeneic or autologous marrow reconstitution. *Br J Cancer* 1982;45:86–94.
3. Alvegerd T: Data presented at the EORTC Workshop on Autologous Bone Marrow Transplantation in Solid Tumors, Amsterdam, 1983.
4. Herzig RA, Phillips RL, Lazarus HM, et al.: Extensive chemotherapy and autologous BMT for the treatment of refractory malignancies. In, Dicke K, Spitzer G, Zander A, Gorin N, (eds): *Autologous Bone Marrow Transplantation.* Proceedings of the First International Symposium. The University of Texas M.D. Anderson Hospital and Tumor Institute at Houston, 1985, pp. 197–202.
5. Culbert S, Cangir A, Jaffe N, et al.: Therapeutic potential of high-dose phenylalanine mustard in pediatric solid tumors. *Proc Am Soc Clin Oncol* 1981;22:400.
6. Hartman O, Kalifa C, Beaujean F, et al.: Treatment of advanced neuroblastoma with two consecutive high-dose chemotherapy and autologous bone marrow transplants. In, Evans A (ed): *Advances in Neuroblastoma Research.* New York, Alan R. Liss, Inc. 1985: pp. 565–568.
7. D'Angio GJ, Evans AE: Experience with cyclic low-dose total body irradiation for metastatic neuroblastoma. *Proc Am Soc Clin Oncol* 1982;23:52.
8. Graham-Pole J: Autologous bone marrow transplantation for patients with neuroblastoma. In, Dicke KA, Spitzer G, Zander AR, Gorin NC, (eds): *Autologous Bone Marrow Transplantation.* Proceedings of the First International Symposium. The University of Texas M.D. Anderson Hospital and Tumor Institute at Houston, 1985, pp. 173–176.
9. August C, Serota F, Koch P, et al.: Treatment of advanced neuroblastoma with supralethal chemotherapy, radiation, and allogeneic or autologous bone marrow reconstitution., *J Clin Oncol* 1984;2:609–616.
10. August CS, Elkins WL, Burkey E, et al.: Treatment of advanced metastatic neuroblastoma with supralethal chemotherapy, total body irradiation and reconstitution with autologous bone marrow. In, Dicke KA, Spitzer G, Zander AR, Gorin NC, (eds): *Autologous Bone Marrow Transplantation.* Proceedings of the First International Symposium. The University of Texas M.D. Anderson Hospital and Tumor Institute at Houston, 1985, pp. 167–171.
11. Treleaven JG, Gibson FM, Ugustad J, et al.: Removal of neuroblastoma cells from bone marrow with monoclonal antibodies conjugated to magnetic microspheres. *Lancet* 1984;11:70.
12. Reynolds CP, Seeger RC, Vo DD, et al.: Model system for remaining neuroblastoma cells from bone marrow monoclonal antibodies and immunobeads. *Cancer Res* 1986;46(11):5882–5886.
13. Philip T, Biron P, Philip I, et al.: Autologous bone marrow transplantation for very bad prognosis neuroblastoma. In, Evans A (ed): *Advances in Neuroblastoma Research,* New York, Alan R. Liss, Inc., 1985; pp. 569–586.
14. Helson L, Clarkson B, Langleben A, et al.: Purging neuroblastoma cells from bone marrow. XIVth Meeting of The International Society of Pediatric Oncology. September 21–25, 1982.
15. Reisni Y, Gan J: Differential binding of soybean agglutinin to human neuroblastoma cell lines; potential application to autologous bone marrow transplantation. *Cancer Res* 1985;45:4025–4031.
16. Sieber F, Rao S, Rowley SD, Sieber-Blum M: Dye-mediated photolysis of human neuroblastoma cells; implications for autologous bone marrow transplantation. *Blood* 1986;68(1):32–36.
17. Hartman O, Benhamon E, Beaujean F, et al.: High-dose busulfan and cyclophosphamide with autologous bone marrow transplantation support in advanced malignancies in children; a phase II study. *J Clin Oncol* 1;4(12):1804–1810.
18. Helson L, Guloti S, O'Reilly R, et al.: Autologous bone marrow transplantation in neuroblastoma. Presented at the Third Conference on Advances in Neuroblastoma Research, Children's Hospital of Philadelphia, 1984.
19. Moss TJ, Fonkalsrud EW, Feig ST, et al.: Delayed surgery and bone marrow transplantation for widespread neuroblastoma. *Ann Surg* 1987;206(4):514–520.

20. Ekert H, Ellis WM, Waters KD, Tauro KP: Autologous bone marrow rescue in the treatment of advanced tumors of childhood. *Cancer* 1982;49:(3):603–609.
21. Phillips GL, Fay JW, Herzig GP, et al.: Intensive 1, 3-bis (2-chloroethyl)-1-nitrosourea (BCNU), NSC number 4366650 and cryopreserved autologous marrow transplantation for refractory cancer; a phase I–II study. *Cancer* 1983;52:1792–1802.
22. Miser J: High-dose therapy and autologous bone marrow transplantation in pediatric solid tumors. In, deBernard B (ed): *Novel Therapeutic Approaches in Pediatric Oncology.* Boston, Martinus Nijhoff. In press, 1988.
23. Cornbleet M, Corringham R, Prentice H, Bolsen E, McElwain TJ: Treatment of Ewing's sarcoma with high-dose melphalan and autologous bone marrow transplantation. *Cancer Treat Rep* 1981;63:241–244.
24. Phillips GL, Herzig RH, Lazarus HM, et al.: High-dose chemotherapy, fractionated total body irradiation and allogeneic marrow transplantation for malignant lymphoma. *J Clin Oncol* 1986;4(4):480–488.
25. Appelbaum FR, Sullivan KM, Thomas ED, et al.: Allogeneic marrow transplantation in the treatment of MOPP-resistant Hodgkin's disease. *J Clin Oncol* 1985;3(11):1490–1494.
26. Ascensao JL, Ahmed T, Arlin ZA: Autologous and allogeneic bone marrow transplantation. *NY State J Med* 1986;86:178–183.
27. Russell JA, Berry J, Blahey WB, et al.: Bone marrow transplantation for Hodgkin's disease. *J Clin Oncol* 1986;4(4):610–611.
28. Armitage JO, Gingrich RD, Klarsen LW, et al.: Trial of high-dose cytarabine, cyclophosphamide, total body irradiation and autologous bone marrow transplantation for refractory lymphoma. *Cancer Treat Rep* 1986;70(7):871–875.
29. Philip T, Dumont J, Teillet F, et al.: High-dose chemotherapy and autologous bone marrow transplantation in refractory Hodgkin's disease. *Br J Cancer* 1986;53:737–742.
30. Verdonck LF, Dekker AW, Vendrick PJ, et al.: Intensive cytoreductive therapy followed by autologous bone marrow transplantation for patients with hematologic malignancies or solid tumors. *Cancer* 1987;60:289–295.
31. Verdonck LF, Dekker AW, von Kampen MK, et al.: Intensive cytotoxic therapy followed by autologous bone marrow transplantation for non-Hodgkin's lymphoma of high-grade malignancy. *Blood* 1985;65(4):984–989.
32. Jagannath S, Dicke KA, Armitage JO, et al.: High-dose cyclophosphamide, carmustine, and etoposide and autologous bone marrow transplantation for relapsed Hodgkin's disease. *Ann Int Med* 1986;104:163–168.
33. Takvorin T, Canellos GP, Ritz J, et al.: Prolonged disease-free survival after autologous bone marrow transplantation in patients with non-Hodgkin's lymphoma with poor prognosis. *N Engl J Med* 1987;316:1499–1505.
34. O'Leary M, Ramsay NKC, Nesbit ME, et al.: Bone marrow transplantation for non-Hodgkin's lymphoma in children and young adults. *Am J Med* 1983;74(3):497–501.
35. Phillips GL, Herzig RH, Lazarus HM, et al.: High-dose chemotherapy, fractionated total body irradiation, and autologous marrow transplantation for malignant lymphoma. *J Clin Oncol* 1986;4(4):480–488.
36. Appelbaum FR, Deisseroth AB, Graw RG, et al.: Prolonged complete remission following high-dose chemotherapy of Burkitt's lymphoma in relapse. *Cancer* 1978;41:1059–1063.
37. Philip T, Biron B, Philip I, et al.: Aggressive chemotherapy and autologous bone marrow transplantation in nonleukemic lymphomas and solid tumors. In, McVie JG, Dalesio O, Smith IE, (eds): *Autologous Bone Marrow Transplantation and Solid Tumors.* New York, Raven Press, 1984; pp. 137–144.
38. Dumont J, Teillet F: Autologous bone marrow transplantation in Hodgkin's disease. *Blood Transfus Immunohematol* 1985;28(5):531–538.
39. Baumgartner C, Bleher EA, Brun de Re G, et al.: Autologous bone marrow transplantation in the treatment of children and adolescents with advanced malignant tumors. *Med Pediatr Oncol* 1984;12:104–111.
40. Phillips GL, Herzig RH, Lazarus HM, et al.: Treatment of resistant malignant lymphoma with cyclophosphamide, total body irradiation, and transplantation of cryopreserved autologous marrow. *N Engl J Med* 1984;310(24):1557–1561.
41. Braine HG, Santos GW, Kaiser H, et al.: Treatment of poor prognosis non-Hodgkin's

lymphoma using cyclophosphamide and total body irradiation regimens with autologous bone marrow rescue. *Bone Marrow Transplantation* 1987;2:7–14.

42. Mascret B, Maraninchi D, Gastaut JA, et al.: Treatment of malignant lymphoma with high dose of chemo- or chemoradiotherapy and bone marrow transplantation. *Eur J Cancer* 1986;22(4):461–471.

43. Philip T, Biron P, Maraninchi D, et al.: Massive chemotherapy with autologous bone marrow transplantation in 50 cases of non-Hodgkin's lymphoma with poor prognosis. In, Dicke KA, Spitzer, G, Zander AR, Gorin NC, (eds): *Autologous Bone Marrow Transplantation*, Proceedings of the First International Symposium. The University of Texas M.D. Anderson Hospital and Tumor Institute at Houston, 1985, pp. 89–107.

44. Hartman O, Pein F, Beaujean F, et al.: High-dose polychemotherapy with autologous bone marrow transplantation in children with relapsed non-Hodgkin's lymphoma. *J Clin Oncol* 1984;2:979–985.

45. Ekert H, Ellis WM, Water KD, Tauro GP: Autologous bone marrow rescue in the treatment of advanced tumors of childhood. *Cancer* 1982;49:603–609.

46. Wolff SN, Phillips GL, Fay JW, et al.: High-dose chemotherapy with autologous bone marrow transplantation for primary tumors of the central nervous system; phase II and III studies of the Southeastern Cancer Study Group. In, Dicke, KA, Spitzer G, Zander AR, Gorin NC, (eds): *Autologous Bone Marrow Transplantation*. Proceedings of the First International Symposium. The University of Texas M.D. Anderson Hospital and Tumor Institute at Houston, 1985; pp. 255–259.

47. Phillips GL, Wolff SN, Fay JW, et al.: Intensive 1,3-bis (2'-chlorethyl)-1-nitrosurea (BCNU) monochemotherapy and autologous marrow transplantation for malignant glioma. *J Clin Oncol* 1986;4(5):639–645.

48. Wolff SN, Phillips GL, Herzig GP: High-dose carmustine with autologous bone marrow transplantation for the adjuvant treatment of high-grade gliomas of the central nervous system. *Cancer Treat Rep* 1987;71:183–187.

49. Abrams RA, Casper J, Kine L, et al.: High-dose aziridinylbenzoquinone for preliminary analysis in ABMT. In, Dicke, KA, Spitzer G, Zander AR, Gorin NC, (eds): *Autologous Bone Marrow Transplantation*. Proceedings of the First International Symposium. The University of Texas M.D. Anderson Hospital and Tumor Institute at Houston, 1985; pp. 227–230.

50. Barrett, 1985, (personal communication) quoted by Pinkerton R, Philip T, Bouffet E, Lashford L, Kemshead J: Autologous bone marrow transplantation in pediatric solid tumors. *Clinics in Hematology* 1986;15(1):187–203.

51. Slav I, Urban CH, Kaulfersch W, Teubi I: Die Anwendung der Autologen Knochenmarkstransplantation A(KMT) Bei Pädiatrischen Malignen Erkrankungen-Ergebnisse und Schlussfolgerungen. *Wien Klin Wochenschr* 1987;99(3):74–79.

52. Miser J: High-dose therapy and autologous bone marrow transplantation in pediatric solid tumors. In, de Bernardi B, (ed): *Novel Therapeutic Approaches in Pediatric Oncology*. Boston, Martinus Nijhoff, 1987. In press.

53. Miser JS, Kinsella TJ, Triche TT, et al.: Treatment of peripheral neuroepithelioma in children and young adults. *J Clin Oncol* 1987;5(11):1752–1755.

54. Ringden O, Ahhstrom L, Lonnqvist B, et al.: Allogeneic bone marrow transplantation in a patient with chemotherapy-resistant progressive histiocytosis-X. *N Engl J Med* 1987;312:(12):735–737.

55. August CS, Serota FT, Koch PA, et al.: Bone marrow transplantation for relapsed stage IV neuroblastoma. *Proceed. Am. Assoc. Cancer Research* 23; 122, 1982.

56. August C, Elkin W, Evans A, et al.: Metastatic neuroblastoma managed by supralethal therapy and bone marrow reconstitution. Results of a four institution Children's Cancer Study Group pilot study. Presented at the Third Conference on Advances in Neuroblastoma Research, May 1984.

57. Hartman O, Kalifa C, Benhamon E, et al.: Treatment of advanced neuroblastoma with high-dose melphalan and autologous bone marrow transplantation. *Cancer Chem and Pharm* 1986;16:165–169.

58. Wist E: The Norwegian Radium Hospital, Oslo, 1983: Data presented at the EORTC workshop: Autologous Bone Marrow Transplantation in Solid Tumors. Amsterdam.

59. Franzone P, Corvo R, Dine G, et al.: Treatment of neuroblastoma: Role of total body irradiation. *Radiol. Med.* (Torino) 1986;72(12):959–962.
60. Dini G, Garaventa A, Lanino E, et al.: Total body irradiation, continuous infusion vincristine, and high-dose melphalan followed by autologous bone marrow transplantation in the treatment of neuroblastoma. *Pediatr. Med. Chir.* 1987;9(1):1–7.
61. Gee AP, Graham-Pole J, Elfenbein G, et al.: Disseminated (Stage D) neuroblastoma: Engraftment and toxicity following autologous or allogeneic bone marrow transplantation. Proceed. Am. Assoc. Cancer Research 1986;27:202.
62. Tranconi L, Riccardi R, Montemaygi, P, et al.: Treatment of neuroblastoma with 131 I-metadiodobenzyl-guanidine. *Med. Pediatr. Oncol.* 1987;15(4):220–223.
63. Graham-Pole J, Lazarus HM, Herzig RH, et al.: High-dose melphalan therapy for the treatment of children with refractory neuroblastoma and Ewing's sarcoma. *Am J. Pediatr. Hematol. Oncol.* 1984;6:17–26.
64. Lazarus HM, Herzig RH, Graham-Pole J, et al.: Intensive melphalan chemotherapy and cyropreserved autologous bone marrow transplantation for the treatment of refractory cancer. *J. Clin. Oncol.* 1983;1:359–367.
65. Alvegard TA, Berg ND, Willen H: Pulmonary bone marrow embolisation after unfiltered autologous bone marrow transplantation. *Acta. Pathol. Microbiol. Immunol. Scand.* (A) 1984;92:81–82.
66. Philip T, Bernard JL, Zucker JM, et al.: High-dose chemoradiotherapy with bone marrow transplantation as consolidation treatment in neuroblastoma: an unselected group of stage IV patients over one year of age. *J. Clin. Oncol.* 1987;5(2):266–271.
67. de Kraker J, Hartman O, Voute PA, et al.: The effect of high-dose melphalan with autologous bone marrow transplantation in neuroblastoma patients with advanced disease. In, Raybaud C, Clement R, Lebreuil G, and Bernard JL, (eds): *Pediatric Oncology.* International Congress Series 570, Excerpta Medica, Amsterdam, 1982, pp. 165–170.
68. Hartman O, Zucker JM, Pinkerton R, et al.: Metastatic neuroblastoma in children older than one year old at diagnosis. Treatment with intensive chemoradiotherapy and autologous bone marrow transplant. *Revue Française de Transfusion et Immunohematologie* 1985; 28(5):539–546.
69. Frappaz D, Philip T, Philip I, et al.: Chimiothérapie massive et autogreffe de moelle purgee dans les neuroblastomes graves. *Pediatrie* 1985; 40(7):539–551.
70. Treuner J, Klingebiel T, Bruchelt G, et al.: Treatment of neuroblastoma with metaiodo-benzylguanidine: results and side effects. *Med. Ped. Oncol.* 1987;15(4):199–202.
71. Philip T, Bernard JL, Zucker JM, et al.: Purged autologous bone marrow transplantation in 25 cases of very poor prognosis neuroblastoma. *Lancet* 1985;1(8425):576–577.
72. Kingston JE, McElwain TJ, Malpas JS: Childhood rhabdomyosarcoma: experience of the children' solid tumor group. *Brit J. Cancer* 1983;48: 195–207.
73. Appelbaum FR, Herzig GP, Ziegler JL, et al.: Successful engraftment of cryopreserved autologous bone marrow in patients with malignant lymphoma. *Blood* 1978;52(1):85–95.
74. Biron P, Philip T, Maraninchi D, et al.: Massive chemotherapy and autologous bone marrow transplantation in progressive disease of nonseminomatous testicular cancer. A Phase II study of 15 patients. In Dicke K, Spitzer G, Zander A, Gorin N, (eds): *Autologous Bone Marrow Transplantation.* Proceeding of the First International Symposium. The University of Texas, M.D. Anderson Hospital and Tumor Institute at Houston, 1985, pp. 203–210.
75. Fischer A, Cerf-Bensussan N, Blanche S, Le Deist F, Bremard-Oury C, Levenger G, Schaison G, Durandy A, Griscelli C: Allogeneic bone marrow transplantation for erythro-phagocytic lymphohistiocytosis. *J Pediatr* 1986;108(2):267–270.
76. Vowels MR, Lam-Po-Tang R, Mameghan H, Heller E, Ford D, Ziegler J, O'Gorman, Hughes D: Bone marrow transplantation for malignant histiocytosis in childhood. *Cancer* 1985;56:2786–2788.

Bone Marrow Transplantation in Children, edited by F. Leonard Johnson and Carl Pochedly. Raven Press, Ltd., New York © 1990.

Bone Marrow Transplantation for Genetic Diseases

Kenneth I. Weinberg and Robertson Parkman

Division of Research Immunology/Bone Marrow Transplantation, Children's Hospital of Los Angeles, and Department of Pediatrics, University of Southern California School of Medicine, Los Angeles, California.

Introduction
A. Classification of genetic diseases
B. Class 1 diseases
C. Class 2 diseases
    1. Myeloid restricted defects
    2. Monocyte restricted defects
    3. Erythroid restricted defects
    4. Megakaryocyte restricted defects
    5. Multilineage defects
D. Class 4 diseases
E. Class 5 diseases
F. Class 6 diseases
G. The future

INTRODUCTION

Histocompatible bone marrow transplantation (BMT) has been an effective therapy for pediatric patients with hematologic, immunologic and oncologic disorders for more than 15 years. However, bone marrow transplantation was first used to successfully treat nonimmunologic genetic disorders less than 10

Preparation of this chapter was supported in part by United States Public Health Services Grant CA-35972, National Cancer Institute, Bethesda, MD.

years ago when patients with the Wiskott-Aldrich syndrome were first completely corrected (1–3). Since 1977 more than 15 genetic diseases have been corrected or stabilized by allogeneic bone marrow transplantation (Table 1). The purpose of this chapter is to review the present status of bone marrow transplantation in the treatment of genetic diseases.

Normal bone marrow contains both hematopoietic and lymphoid stem cells which differentiate into peripheral lymphoid and hematopoietic elements (Figure 1). Although a totipotential stem cell exists in early fetal life, its existence in postnatal life is still debated. Therefore, bone marrow transplantation functionally consists of the transplantation of two separate stem cell pools. The lack of interchange between the lymphoid and hematopoietic stem cell pools has clinical significance since engraftment of both lymphoid and hematopoietic stem cells is necessary to assure complete donor lymphoid and hematopoietic engraftment. Most genetic diseases are characterized by the presence of defective stem cells, rather than by the absence of stem cells, as in patients with aplastic anemia. Thus, pre-transplant preparative regimens for correction of genetic diseases must ablate the patient's abnormal lymphoid and hematopoietic stem cells.

At present no single agent can eradicate both stem cell populations; therefore, a combination of agents must be used to ensure the complete eradication of the patient's stem cells. If the patient's (or recipient's) lymphoid stem cells survive, they will ultimately cause the immunological rejection of the donor bone marrow graft. Cyclophosphamide or antithymocyte serum (or antithym-

TABLE 1. *Genetic diseases for which bone marrow transplantation has been attempted to provide correction or stabilization*

Disease	References
Severe combined immune deficiency	2
Wiskott-Aldrich syndrome	7, 11, 12
Granulocytic actin deficiency	17
Infantile agranulocytosis	24
Osteopetrosis	26, 27
Chronic granulomatous disease	20, 21
Thalassemia	28, 29, 30
Hurler's disease	39, 40
Hunter's disease	
gpL-115 deficiency	
Gaucher's disease	38
Sanfilippo B disease	42
Sickle cell disease	31
Metachromatic leukodystrophy	49
Adrenoleukodystrophy	50
Lesch-Nyhan syndrome	45
Maroteaux-Lamy syndrome	43

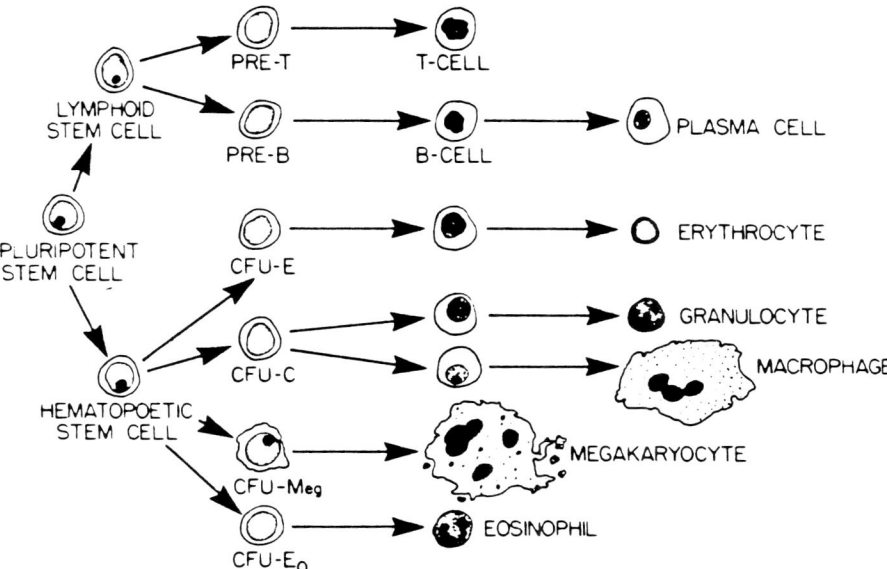

FIG. 1. Diagram of normal bone marrow differentiation: stages in maturation of lymphoid and hematopoietic cells.

ocyte globulin) are used as immunosuppressive agents. Inadequate eradication of the hematopoietic stem cells in recipients of bone marrow transplants will result in regrowth of those cells even if the recipient's lymphoid stem cells are ablated. Total body irradiation (TBI) or busulfan and its analogues can eradicate hematopoietic stem cells (4,5). Other chemotherapeutic drugs like cyclophosphamide and cytosine arabinoside are ineffective in ablating hematopoietic stem cells in bone marrow recipients (6,7).

CLASSIFICATION OF GENETIC DISEASES

Evaluation of the role of bone marrow transplantation in the treatment of genetic diseases is aided by using a simple classification. Genetic diseases classified as *restricted* are those in which the expression of the genetic defect is restricted to the lymphoid or hematopoietic system; diseases classified as *generalized* are those in which the defect is found in multiple tissues. The restricted diseases can be further divided into those in which the expression of the genetic defect is limited to lymphoid cells, to hematopoietic cells, or is found in both lymphoid and hematopoietic cells (Table 2).

TABLE 2. *Classification of genetic diseases*

Clinical Parameters	Class 1	Class 2	Class 3	Class 4	Class 5	Class 6
Expression of genetic defect	Restricted to lymphoid and hematopoietic cells	Restricted to hematopoietic cells	Restricted to lymphoid cells	Generalized; clinical symptomatology restricted to lympho-hematopoietic cells	Generalized; clinical symptomatology generalized with CNS involvement	Bone marrow leukocyte cells do not contain normal gene product
Treatment	Correctable by BMT	Correctable by BMT	Correctable by BMT	Correctable by BMT	May be correctable by BMT	Not correctable by BMT
Disease included	Wiskott-Aldrich syndrome Chediak-Higashi syndrome	Thalassemia Actin deficiency Chronic granulocyte disease Infantile agranulocytosis Sickle cell disease Osteopetrosis	Severe combined immune deficiency gpL-115 deficiency Agammaglobulinemia	Gaucher's disease Adenosine deaminase deficiency Nucleotide phosphorylase deficiency	Adrenoleukodystrophy Metachromatic leukodystrophy Krabbe's Disease	Cystic fibrosis Hemophila Phenylketonuria

Class 1 diseases are those in which the expression of the disease is found in both lymphoid-derived and hematopoietic-derived cells, but not in nonlymphoid and nonhematopoietic cells. Class 1 diseases include the Wiskott-Aldrich syndrome and the Chediak-Higashi syndrome. Class 2 diseases are those in which the clinical expression of the genetic abnormality is restricted to hematopoietic-derived cells. This class includes abnormalities of hemoglobin synthesis (such as thalassemia, sickle cell disease, and other hemoglobinopathies), abnormalities of granulocyte function (such as chronic granulomatous disease, actin deficiency, etc.), and abnormalities of monocyte function (as in osteopetrosis). Class 3 diseases are those which are restricted to the lymphoid stem cells and include combined immune deficiency, gpL-115 deficiency, and other immune deficiency diseases such as X-linked agammaglobulinemia. The treatment of Class 3 diseases by bone marrow transplantation will not be discussed in this chapter since it is discussed elsewhere (see Chapter 7 on immunodeficiency syndromes).

All Class 1, Class 2 and Class 3 diseases are potentially correctable by bone marrow transplantation. Such correction will occur if the abnormal hematopoietic stem cells, lymphoid stem cells, or both, are eradicated by the pretransplant preparation and if successful donor lymphoid and hematopoietic stem cell engraftment is achieved.

Class 4 diseases are generalized diseases. The genetic defect is found in multiple tissues, but the clinical manifestations are restricted to lymphoid or hematopoietic cells or are present in both. Nonneuronotropic Gaucher's disease is an example of a generalized defect in which the clinical symptomatology is primarily in hematopoietic cells. Most Class 5 diseases are characterized by absent or defective enzymes. In Class 5 diseases, the generalized defect is manifested in non-lymphoid and hematopoietic cells, including the central nervous system. In some of these diseases, previous clinical research has demonstrated that passively administered enzyme can ameliorate the symptoms. Bone marrow transplantation has a potential role in the treatment of both Class 4 and Class 5 diseases, either by replacing the affected hematopoietic derived cells or by providing a continuing source of normal enzyme.

Class 6 diseases are generalized diseases which are probably not treatable by transplantation. Bone marrow transplantation is not a therapeutic possibility because either (1) the bone marrow-derived cells do not contain the missing gene product or (2) circulating enzyme is not able to gain access to the site of the enzyme deficiency. The ability of circulating normal enzyme to gain access to the site of disease is of particular importance in efforts to correct central nervous system storage diseases by use of bone marrow transplantation.

CLASS 1 DISEASES

Wiskott-Aldrich syndrome is the prototype of Class 1 diseases in which the primary genetic abnormality is expressed in both lymphoid and hematopoietic cells. For a long time, a unitarian hypothesis to explain the multifaceted nature of the Wiskott-Aldrich syndrome did not exist (8,9). The constellation of widespread abnormalities including immunodeficiency, eczema, and thrombocytopenia with platelets of decreased size and function frustrated attempts to define a primary defect. Recent evidence, however, indicates that there is a primary defect in glycoprotein structure in both T lymphocytes and platelets (3,10). Abnormalities of a T lymphocyte glycoprotein (gpL-115) and platelet glycoproteins GP Ia-Ib have been found and explain the observed clinical abnormalities.

Wiskott-Aldrich syndrome was one of the first diseases whose correction was attempted by histocompatible bone marrow transplantation (11,12). Early attempts were only partially successful since sustained donor hematopoietic engraftment was not achieved, and therefore, the platelet abnormalities were not corrected. However, sustained donor lymphoid engraftment was achieved with improvement of the immunological components of the syndrome.

The first complete correction of the Wiskott-Aldrich syndrome by allogeneic bone marrow transplantation was achieved in 1977 following two transplants (7). A 4-year-old boy was prepared for his first transplant with cyclophosphamide for immunosuppression and cytosine arabinoside to destroy hematopoietic stem cells. A temporary donor T lymphocyte graft was achieved; however, no evidence of engraftment of donor hematopoietic cells was noted (Table 3). When donor T lymphocyte engraftment was no longer detectable, the patient was re-transplanted. He was prepared with rabbit antihuman thymocyte serum (ATS) and procarbazine as immunosuppressive agents and total body irradiation (TBI) to destroy the hematopoietic stem cells. Utilizing the same female donor, complete engraftment by donor hematopoietic and lymphoid cells was achieved with correction of all of the patient's clinical and laboratory abnormalities. Additional patients were successfully transplanted after preparation with regimens that included both antithymocyte serum and total body irradiation.

Because of the potential side effects associated with the use of total body irradiation, investigators explored the use of busulfan as an alternative antihematopoietic stem cell agent based upon canine and rodent animal studies (5,13). The use of busulfan as an antihematopoietic stem cell agent and cyclophosphamide with or without antithymocyte serum for immunosuppression has proved to be an effective preparatory regimen which regularly produces lymphoid and hematopoietic engraftment. The main difference observed between the use of total body irradiation and the use of busulfan is that with the dose of busulfan originally used, 2 mg/kg/day for 4 days, complete hematopoietic ablation was not achieved in 10 to 20% of cases. In these cases there was recovery of the patient's own abnormal hematopoietic cells (14). Increase in the busulfan dose to 3.0 to 3.5 mg/kg/day for 4 days resulted in consistent hematopoietic engraftment, even though this busulfan dose is lower than that used as preparation for patients with bone marrow transplantation in acute myeloid leukemia (15).

TABLE 3. *Summary of markers for the transplantation of a patient with Wiskott-Aldrich syndrome*

Clinical parameters	Pre-transplant	Post-transplant 1	Post-transplant 2
Preparation	—	Ara-C Cyclophosphamide	Antithymocyte serum Procarbazine TBI
ABO blood type	O	O	A
Bone marrow karyotype	XY	XY	XX
Platelet count	20–50,000/mm^3	20–50,000/mm^3	>200,000/mm^3
PHA stimulated lymphocyte karyotype	XY	XX→XY	XX
Isohemagglutinin titer			
Anti-A	1:4	1:64→1:2	0
Anti-B	1:2	1:32→1:2	1:8

Patient was a male who was blood group O, and donor was a female who was blood group A.

Ara-C = cytosine arabinoside TBI = total body irradiation

CLASS 2 DISEASES

Bone marrow transplantation can successfully correct a wide variety of primary hematopoietic stem cell defects. Genetic diseases can be restricted to single lineage (myeloid, monocyte, erythroid or megakaryocytic) or can affect all cell lines.

Myeloid restricted defects

The first hematopoietic restricted genetic diseases to be corrected by bone marrow transplantation were the myeloid-restricted type. Both defects of differentiation (as in infantile agranulocytosis) as well as intrinsic functional defects (such as actin deficiency and chronic granulomatous disease) have been corrected. Patients with abnormal granulocytic actin have dysfunctional granulocytes that predispose them to overwhelming bacterial sepsis (16). Affected patients have been successfully engrafted with normal donor granulocytes following a preparative regimen including antithymocyte serum and procarbazine as immunosuppressive agents and use of total body irradiation to eliminate the abnormal hematopoietic stem cells (17). The preparative regimen for the initial transplant of one patient achieved inadequate hematopoietic ablation and resulted in no donor hematopoietic stem cell engraftment. Re-transplantation of the patient with use of the same immunosuppressive drugs, and total body irradiation to destroy the hematopoietic stem cells, resulted in complete engraftment with donor hematopoietic and lymphoid stem cells. Successful granulocyte engraftment was demonstrated by normal skin Rebuck windows and normal *in vitro* granulocyte function studies, including phagocytosis and killing.

In chronic granulomatous disease, phagocytic cells (neutrophils, eosinophils, and macrophage/monocytes) have defects in oxidative metabolism which can be detected *in vitro* by their inability to reduce nitroblue tetrazolium (NBT) dye (18,19). Initial attempts to correct chronic granulomatous disease by allogeneic bone marrow transplantation failed due to the lack of sustained hematopoietic engraftment (20). A 15-year-old boy, however, was successfully transplanted following preparation with antithymocyte serum, procarbazine, and TBI (21). He was successfully engrafted with donor hematopoietic cells. Engraftment was demonstrated both by a change in the karyotype of his spontaneously dividing bone marrow cells and by normalization of the capacity of his circulating granulocytes and monocytes to reduce NBT. However, the patient died 6 months following transplant of progressive interstitial pneumonitis, which was a complication of chronic graft-vs.-host disease. Chronic graft-vs.-host disease is the primary limitation to increased use of allogeneic bone marrow transplantation for treatment of genetic diseases (22).

Besides intrinsic defects of granulocyte function, defects in granulocyte differentiation also exist. Patients can be completely lacking in circulating granulocytes due to a block in myeloid differentiation at the metamyelocyte stage, as in cases of infantile agranulocytosis (23). The precise defect cannot be defined; however, normal CFU-C growth by the marrow of affected patients is observed. Following the eradication of the abnormal recipient hematopoietic stem cells with total body irradiation and immunosuppression with antithymocyte serum and procarbazine, patients have had the establishment of normal numbers of circulating granulocytes of donor origin (24). Patients have been followed for up to 7 years after transplantation and have shown sustained production of normal donor granulocytes.

Monocyte restricted defects

Osteopetrosis is due to defective osteoclast activity resulting in the lack of reabsorption of ossified cartilage. The persistence of ossified cartilage results in brittle, nonlamellar long bones with a reduced marrow cavity and secondary extramedullary hematopoiesis (25). Patients with osteopetrosis have been completely engrafted following the ablation of their lymphoid and hematopoietic stem cells (24,27). Development of normal osteoclastic activity was detected by an increase in urinary calcium excretion secondary to osseous remodeling and increased marrow hematopoiesis. The presence of normal osteoclast activity following bone marrow transplantation shows (1) that osteoclasts are hematopoietic-derived cells and (2) that the normal half-life of osteoclasts is 4 months. Children with osteopetrosis should be transplanted immediately if a histocompatible donor exists, to correct the disease before irreversible neurological damage (such as blindness and deafness) occurs.

Erythroid restricted defects

Genetic defects of erythroid cells can be divided into two principal categories: (1) defects in the regulation of hemoglobin synthesis (as in thalassemia) and (2) defects in the primary structure of hemoglobin (as in sickle cell disease and other hemoglobinopathies). β-thalassemia, the most common defect of the regulation of hemoglobin synthesis, was the first erythroid restricted disease to be successfully treated by bone marrow transplantation (28). Following preparation with antithymocyte serum and dimethyl-myleran, an analogue of busulfan, sustained engraftment of donor hematopoietic stem cells was achieved which resulted in the establishment of normal erythropoiesis.

Bone marrow transplantation of the first patient with thalassemia was done in Seattle. Thereafter, most of the bone marrow transplants for thalassemia were done in Italy where thalassemia has its greatest incidence. Initial transplant attempts frequently resulted in regrowth of the patient's own abnormal hematopoietic cells or death of the patient (29). Some deaths were due to cardiac failure, possibly due to the combined effects of excessive cardiac iron accumulation (hemosiderosis) and irradiation. Because the patients had been given many transfusions before transplantation, there was an increased incidence of immunological rejections. Recent results with younger patients (6 months to 10 years of age) have led to improved clinical results with a 73% actuarial survival rate (30). The improved clinical results are based on fewer deaths due to toxicity and a decreased incidence of immunologic rejections, both of these factors being related to the decreased number of transfusions given to these patients.

If the incidence of graft-vs.-host disease, particularly chronic graft-vs.-host disease, could be reduced, the early use of bone marrow transplantation as therapy for β-thalassemia would have greater application. Children as young as 2 months of age with primary hematopoietic defects have been successfully transplanted, suggesting that patients with genetic defects could be transplanted before any significant clinical symptomatology occurred. Also the incidence of chronic graft-vs.-host disease is less in younger patients (22).

So far no patients have been transplanted primarily for treatment of a hemoglobinopathy. However, a patient with acute myeloid leukemia, who also had sickle cell disease, was successfully transplanted from a histocompatible sibling who had sickle cell trait (31). The favorable result confirms that bone marrow transplantation has a potential therapeutic role for selected patients with sickle cell disease if their severe symptoms do not respond to standard therapy.

In addition to genetic defects in hemoglobin synthesis or hemoglobin structure, patients with primary defects in red cell differentiation have been treated with bone marrow transplantation. Patients with pure red cell aplasia, who had normal production of leukocytes and platelets, have been successfully transplanted. Their abnormal hematopoietic stem cells were ablated with total body irradiation or busulfan, and cyclophosphamide, antithymocyte serum, or both, were used for immunosuppression (32). The patients, like the hypertransfused patients with thalassemia, are probably best transplanted before they develop clinical symptoms due to their iron overload and before they become sensitized to the non-HLA antigens of their donors.

Patients with hemolytic anemia due to enzyme deficiencies (such as G-6-PD deficiency) are also potentially correctable if the risk/benefit ratio is appropriate. Successful treatments would protect them from the long-term sequellae of increased hemoglobin degradation, such as hemosiderosis, bone marrow hypertrophy, and cholelithiasis.

Megakaryocyte restricted defects

As yet no patients with defects restricted to megakaryocytic function or megakaryocytic differentiation have been treated with bone marrow transplantation. However, the experience with use of marrow transplantation for both intrinsic defects and differentiation defects of erythroid and myeloid cells clearly indicate that such defects (such as amegakaryocytosis or Bernard-Soulier syndrome) would be correctable if adequate preparation were used. At present it is not clear whether secondary defects of platelet function due to autoantibody production (as in idiopathic thrombocytopenic purpura) are correctable by bone marrow transplantation.

Multilineage defects

Bone marrow transplantation was established early to be an effective form of therapy for patients with severe aplastic anemia, in which the total phagocytic cells are less than $500/mm^3$, corrected reticulocyte count is less than 1%, and platelet count is less than $20,000/mm^3$. However, the use of marrow transplantation for treatment of congenital aplastic anemia, as in Fanconi's anemia, was less certain. Since these diseases are usually slowly progressive, the patients had received many transfusions before being transplanted, which increased the probability of immune rejection. The finding that certain preparative regimens, such as multiagent immunosuppression, use of low-dose total body irradiation, or the use of donor buffy coat transfusion, permitted the successful engraftment of sensitized patients has increased the use of bone marrow transplantation for Fanconi's anemia (33–35). An unexpected problem, however, was the increased sensitivity of patients to the toxicity of the preparatory drugs (36,37). The increased fragility of the chromosomes of patients with Fanconi's anemia is well known. The agents used in the preparatory regimen (cyclophosphamide, total body irradiation and busulfan) all have the capacity to produce chromosome damage, and some patients died from toxicity of the preparatory regimen. At present the magnitude of the toxicity associated with the standard preparatory regimens is not clear. Many centers use reduced doses of total body irradiation, cyclophosphamide, and busulfan in the preparation of these patients.

CLASS 4 DISEASES

Class 4 diseases are characterized by generalized enzymatic deficiencies in which the manifestations of disease are restricted to lymphoid and hematopoietic cells. Diseases in this class are Gaucher's disease (which is due to a functional deficiency of the enzyme beta-glucocerebrosidase), adenosine deaminase (ADA) deficiency and nucleotide phosphorylase (NP) deficiency (in which affected patients have impaired T lymphocyte function). The symptoms of Gaucher's disease are caused by the accumulation of glucocerebroside in phagocytic cells, including monocytes, bone marrow macrophages, Kupffer cells, etc. Thus, it was proposed that the elimination of the abnormal hematopoietic cells and their replacement with normal hematopoietic cells containing normal beta-glucocerebrosidase might diminish the patient's symptoms.

The first patient with Gaucher's disease successfully transplanted was an 8-year-old boy with type 3 subacute neuronopathic Gaucher's disease who was prepared with antithymocyte serum, procarbazine, and busulfan (38). Three months following transplantation, all of the patient's peripheral blood elements were of donor origin as demonstrated by karyotypic analysis and enzyme levels. However, a bone marrow biopsy at that time showed no improvement, with the continued presence of lipid-laden macrophages. Repeated marrow aspirates revealed no improvement in hematopoietic function until 6 months following transplantation when the bone marrow examination revealed 50% normal hematopoietic cells and 50% Gaucher's cells. The continued presence of Gaucher's cells in the patient's bone marrow for 6 months indicates that the turnover of bone marrow derived mononuclear cells varies from tissue to tissue. Whereas all circulating mononuclear cells are of donor origin by one month following transplantation and Kupffer cells are of donor origin by two months, the turnover of bone marrow macrophages is much slower, with a half-life of at least 6 months. Therefore, the minimum time in which bone marrow hematopoietic function can be expected to improve following transplantation of patients with Gaucher's disease is much longer than the length of time expected for improvement of primary hematopoietic defects, like hemoglobinopathies, thalassemia, aplastic anemia, and acute myeloid leukemia.

Of particular importance in the treatment of both Class 4 and Class 5 diseases is whether bone marrow-derived cells are a normal component of the central nervous system, in particular whether microglial cells are of bone marrow origin. If microglial cells are of hematopoietic origin, then abnormal microglial cells might be expected to be replaced by normal microglial cells following their normal cellular turnover. At present the degree of improvement that may be expected in patients with neuronotropic Gaucher's disease is unclear.

CLASS 5 DISEASES

Class 5 diseases represent the area of greatest clinical interest in bone marrow transplantation for genetic diseases at present. Class 5 diseases are diseases characterized by a generalized enzymatic deficiency in which there is accumulation of abnormal products in non-lympho-hematopoietic cells or in which abnormalities are found in non-lympho-hematopoietic cells. The greatest clinical experience in the use of bone marrow transplantation to correct generalized enzymatic deficiencies is in the treatment of patients with Hurler's syndrome. Patients with this disease lack the enzyme iduronidase, which degrades dextran sulfate and heparan sulfate (39,40).

Most of the patient's symptoms are due to the extra-central nervous system collection of abnormal products which causes hepatosplenomegaly and corneal clouding. As the disease progresses, the patients also develop mental retardation due to central nervous system mucopolysaccharide accumulation. Clinical research has established that exogenous administration of enzyme causes a temporary increase in urinary excretion of mucopolysaccharide (41). The Westminster Group has pioneered the use of bone marrow transplantation in patients with Hurler's syndrome following preparation with busulfan and cyclophosphamide. Engraftment of donor bone marrow cells with normalization of circulating leukocyte enzyme levels has been followed by clinical improvement of noncentral nervous system symptoms, including hepatosplenomegaly and corneal clouding. The primary question, however, is whether there is stabilization or improvement of the patient's central nervous system function and level of intelligence. At this time, documentation of the patient's long-term intellectual and neurological function following transplantation is not available. The question of whether engraftment of normal bone marrow permits stabilization of central nervous system function is crucial in deciding if bone marrow transplantation should be used for the treatment of genetic diseases.

There are two mechanisms by which bone marrow transplantation may be able to improve the central nervous system function of patients with Class 5 diseases. First, the circulating enzyme released by peripheral blood leukocytes may enter the central nervous system. Second, microglial cells, a normal component of the central nervous system, may be of hematopoietic origin. If microglial cells were of hematopoietic origin, the abnormal microglial cells would be replaced by normal microglial cells of donor origin containing normal enzyme. The enzyme released by the *in situ* microglial cells could then gain access to the intraneural accumulations.

In addition to Hurler's syndrome, Hunter's syndrome, Sanfilippo B disease, and Maroteaux-Lamy syndrome have been treated with bone marrow transplantation, with the establishment of normal peripheral blood leukocyte enzyme levels (42,43). In all cases the effects of bone marrow transplantation on central nervous system function awaits long-term follow-up.

Patients with Lesch-Nyhan syndrome are deficient in the enzyme hypoxanthine guanine-phosphoribosyl transferase (HGPRT) (44). Heterozygotes or patients with partial defects who have greater than 1.5% of normal enzyme activity are protected from the self-mutilation that characterizes patients with the full-blown syndrome; such patients still have the athetoid movements and increased uric acid levels that characterize the full Lesch-Nyhan syndrome. Following bone marrow transplantation, approximately 8 to 10% of the cellular mass of the body is of donor origin. Therefore, if a homozygous normal donor is used, the maximum amount of normal enzyme that could be expected would be 8 to 10% of the normal total body enzyme level, assuming that the enzyme is found equally in all cells. If symptoms are observed when enzyme levels in heterozygotes or partial defects are 30 to 40% of normal, then bone marrow transplantation is unlikely to make a significant clinical impact on the disease. However, if low levels of enzyme (less than 10% of normal) produce clinical stabilization, then bone marrow transplantation may be expected to be beneficial.

Because presence of low levels of normal enzyme relieves the self-mutilating behavior of HGPRT-deficient patients, a patient with Lesch-Nyhan syndrome was transplanted following preparation with cyclophosphamide, antithymocyte serum, and busulfan. Following transplantation there was normalization of his peripheral leukocyte enzyme levels but with no improvement in his self-mutilating behavior. This suggested either that circulating HGPRT does not enter the central nervous system to normalize brain metabolism or that undetectable anatomic damage occurred prior to the transplant (45). The transplantation of younger patients may be necessary before a firm statement can be made about the potential role of bone marrow transplantation in the treatment of Lesch-Nyhan syndrome.

If young patients with Lesch-Nyhan syndrome have their symptoms stabilized or improved by transplantation of allogeneic bone marrow, it raises the possibility that the transplantation of autologous bone marrow following insertion of the cloned DNA for the missing enzyme may be therapeutic. The gene for human HGPRT has been cloned and has been inserted into murine hematopoietic stem cells (46).

If allogeneic bone marrow transplantation is successful, it is possible that autologous bone marrow transplantation of patients without histocompatible donors could be undertaken. After the patient's bone marrow has been removed, the normal HGPRT gene wold then be transfected with high efficiency viral vectors into the patient's hematopoietic stem cells. Following the vector insertion of the HGPRT gene, the bone marrow would be cryopreserved. Following preparation with busulfan to eliminate the abnormal hematopoietic stem cells, the treated autologous bone marrow together with the inserted HGPRT gene would be transplanted. If the introduced gene results in normal amounts of enzyme production, the establishment of hematopoiesis derived from transfected hematopoietic stem cells would permit production of circulating enzyme levels similar to those achieved with allogeneic bone marrow transplantation. Patients with Lesch-Nyhan syndrome and adenosine deaminase deficiency are the most likely candidates for the first clinical use of autologous bone marrow transplantation using transfected cloned genes.

Another group of Class 5 diseases that may be treated by bone marrow transplantation are the central nervous system storage diseases in which the symptoms are limited primarily to the central nervous system. Metachromatic leukodystrophy and adrenoleukodystrophy are two such diseases. Animal studies with the twitcher mouse, a model for Krabbe's disease, a central nervous system storage disease, have demonstrated that circulating enzyme degrades intraneural accumulations of abnormal products, but only after a significant lag period (47,48). Two months following transplantation of abnormal twitcher nerves into histocompatible littermates, there was still absence of intraneural enzyme and no reduction in abnormal metachromatic material. However, 6 months following transplantation, normal intraneural enzyme levels were detected, and the amount of metachromatic material was diminished. These animal experiments suggest that circulating enzyme can only slowly gain access to intraneural sites; thus, improvement of central nervous system storage diseases may only slowly occur following bone marrow transplantation.

Metachromatic leukodystrophy is characterized by demyelination and the accumulation of galactosyl-sulfatide in central nervous system white matter and peripheral nerves. A patient with metachromatic leukodystrophy was successfully engrafted with histocompatible bone marrow after preparation with cyclophosphamide and total body irradiation (49). Besides evidence of peripheral engraftment, as shown by karyotypic analysis and normalization of enzyme levels, lymphocytes of donor origin were detected in the cerebrospinal fluid of the recipient. Longitudinal evaluation of the patient's development showed that the patient's clinical condition stabilized in about 4 to 6 months following transplantation. Since that time, the patient has developed and maintained a IQ of 70. The engraftment of normal bone marrow permitted stabilization of the patient's central nervous system function although no relative improvement of his neurological or neuromuscular function occurred. Thus, the presence of normal enzyme cannot reverse preexisting neurological damage. The results observed in the patient with metachromatic leukodystrophy are consistent with the findings in the twitcher mouse. They show that a lag period of 4 to 6 months exists between the establishment of normal circulating enzyme levels and the degradation of intraneural accumulations of abnormal metachromatic material.

Patients with adrenoleukodystrophy have elevated plasma long-chain fatty acids and white matter demyelination, but the exact nature of the primary defect is unknown. Transplantation of a patient with adrenoleukodystrophy was followed by normalization of the long-chain (C26) fatty acids levels. This showed that the engrafted lymphohematopoietic cells were able to normalize the patient's peripheral long-chain fatty acid metabolism (50). However, the patient died 140 days following transplantation, a time at which the initial stabilization of the patient's intellectual and neuromuscular function might have been expected. Thus, the role of bone marrow transplantation in the treatment of adrenoleukodystrophy is unclear.

The transplantation of patients with genetic diseases that involve neurological and intellectual function is both medically and ethically complex. At present it is not clear whether bone marrow transplantation can stabilize or improve the patient's central nervous system function. However, it is possible to stabilize or improve many of the patient's noncentral nervous system symptoms. Long-term neurological and intellectual evaluation of the patients already transplanted will be necessary before the potential role of bone marrow transplantation in treatment of Class 5 diseases can be clearly defined.

CLASS 6 DISEASES

Class 6 diseases are a heterogenous group, all of which cannot be corrected or stabilized by bone marrow transplantation. Diseases in which the abnormal or missing gene product is not contained in bone marrow-derived cells (such as cystic fibrosis, hemophilia, etc.) are not correctable by bone marrow transplantation. It is possible that some central nervous system diseases will not be correctable, even if normal peripheral leukocyte enzyme levels are achieved and substrate levels are normalized, because inadequate amounts of enzyme will reach the intraneural accumulations.

THE FUTURE

Ultimately, histocompatible bone marrow transplantation may only be an intermediate step in the primary correction of genetic diseases. If histocompatible bone marrow transplantation is successful in curing or stabilizing genetic diseases due to enzyme deficiencies, it indicates that producing normal enzyme levels in only a minority of the body's cells (approximately 10%) is adequate to cure the patient. However, histocompatible bone marrow can be applied to only the 25 to 35% of patients who have a donor. Therefore, ultimately the use of allogeneic bone marrow transplantation may be replaced by autologous bone marrow transplantation, following the insertion of the appropriate gene for the missing enzyme or gene product. If normal genes can be inserted into the patient's own hematopoietic stem cells with the production of normal gene products, then all patients could be potentially cured. Recent evidence in transgenic mice, however, has suggested that the transcription or translation of the transfected genes may be suppressed by *cis*-acting regulatory genes (51,52). Thus, more information about the control of inserted genes will be necessary before autologous transplantation with inserted genes will have clinical use.

It may be possible that certain CNS storage diseases will not be treatable by allogeneic or autologous bone marrow transplantation since the circulating enzyme will not be able to gain adequate entry to the CNS. In the future, it may be possible to construct vectors with specificity for cells other than the hematopoietic stem cells. If it were possible to target the appropriate gene by coupling it to a vector with specificity for a specific cell type (such as oligodendrocytes, hepatocytes, etc.), it might be possible to cure some genetic diseases by the intravenous infusion of vector linked genes targeted for a specific organ. Thus, bone marrow transplantation, whether allogeneic or autologous, may only be a single step in our attempts to cure rather than to treat patients with genetic diseases.

REFERENCES

1. Thomas ED, Storb R, Clift RA, et al.: Bone marrow transplantation. *N Engl J Med* 1975;49:511–533.
2. Parkman R: The present status of bone marrow transplantation in pediatrics. In, Moss A, (Ed.): *Pediatric Update* Elseveier Science Publishing New York, 1986. pp. 73–92.
3. Parkman R: Genetic Disorders. In, Blume KG and Petz LD (Eds.): *Clinical Bone Marrow Transplantation*, Churchill Livingstone Publishers, New York, 1983. pp. 241–270.
4. Storb R, Weiden PL, Graham TC, et al.: Hematopoietic grafts between DLA-identical canine littermates following dimethyl myleran: evidence for resistance to grafts not associated with DLA and abrogated by antithymocyte serum. *Transplantation* 1977;24:349–357.
5. Tutschka PJ, Santos FW: Bone marrow transplantation in the busulfan treated rat. III. Relationship between myelosuppression and immunosuppression for conditioning bone marrow recipients. *Transplantation* 1977;24:52–62.
6. Botnick LE, Hannon EC, Hellman S: Limited proliferation of stem cells surviving alkylating agents. *Nature* 1976;262:68–70.
7. Parkman R, Rappeport J, Geha R: Complete correction of the Wiskott-Aldrich syndrome by allogeneic bone marrow transplantation. *N Engl J Med* 1978;298:921–927.
8. Aldrich RA, Steinberg AG, Campbell DC: Pedigree demonstrating a sex-linked recessive condition characterized by draining ears, eczematoid dermatitis and bloody diarrhea. *Pediatrics* 1954;13:133–138.

9. Wiskott A: Familiarer, angeborener Morbus Werlhofii. *Monatsschr Kinderheilkd* 1937;68:212–216.
10. Remold-O'Donnell E, Kenney DM, Parkman R, et al.: Characterization of a human lymphocyte surface sialoglycoprotein that is defective in Wiskott-Aldrich syndrome. *J Exp Med* 1984;159:1705–1723.
11. August CS, Hathaway WE, Githens JH, et al.: Improved platelet function following bone marrow transplantation in an infant with the Wiskott-Aldrich syndrome. *J Pediatr* 1973;82:58–64.
12. Bach FH, Albertini RJ, Anderson JL, et al.: Bone marrow transplantation in a patient with the Wiskott-Aldrich syndrome. *Lancet* 1968;ii:1364–1366.
13. Boggs DR, Boggs SS: The effect of graded single doses of busulfan on murine erythropoiesis. *Proc Soc Exp biol Med* 1980;163:181.
14. Parkman R, Rappeport JM, Hellman S, et al.: Busulfan and total body irradiation as antihematopoietic stem cell agents in the preparation of patients with congenital bone marrow disorders for allogeneic bone marrow trnasplantation. *Blood* 1984;64:852–857.
15. Santos GW, Tutschka PJ, Brookmeyer R, et al.: Marrow transplantation for acute non-lymphoblastic leukemia after treatment with busulfan and cyclophosphamide. *N Engl J Med* 1983;309:1347–1353.
16. Boxer LA, Hedley-Whyte ET, Stossel TP: Neutrophil actin dysfunction and abnormal neutrophil behavior. *N Engl J Med* 1974;291:1093–1099.
17. Camitta BM, Quesenberry PJ, Parkman R, et al.: Bone marrow transplantation for an infant with neutrophil dysfunction. *Exp Hematol* 1977;5:109–116.
18. Newberger PF, Kruskall MS, Rappeport JM, et al.: Chronic granulomatous disease: Expression of the metabolic defect by *in vitro* culture of bone marrow progenitors. *J Clin Invest* 1980;66:599–602.
19. Zakhireh B, Root RK: Development of oxidase activity by human bone marrow granulocytes. *Blood* 1979;54:429–439.
20. The Westminster Hospitals Bone Marrow Transplant Team: Bone marrow transplantation from an unrelated donor for chronic granulomatous disease. *Lancet* 1977;i:210–212.
21. Rappeport JM, Newberger PE, Goldblum RM: Allogeneic bone marrow transplantation for chronic granulomatous disease. *J Pediatr* 1984;101:952–955.
22. Sullivan KM, Parkman R: The pathophysiology and treatment of graft-vs.-host disease. *Clin Haematol* 1983;12:775–789.
23. Amato D, Freedman MH, Saunders EF: Granulopoiesis in severe congenital neutropenia. *Blood* 1976;47:531–538.
24. Rappeport JM, Parkman R, Newberger P, et al.: Correction of infantile agranulocytosis (Kostmann's syndrome) by allogeneic bone marrow transplantation. *Am J Med* 1980;68:605–609.
25. Dent CE, Smellie JM, Watson L. Studies in osteopetrosis. *Arch Dis Child* 1965;40:7–15.
26. Coccia PF, Krivit W, Cervenka J, et al.: Successful bone marrow transplantation for infantile malignant osteopetrosis. *N Engl J Med* 1980;302:701–708.
27. Sorell M, Kapoor N, Kirkpatrick D, et al.: Marrow transplantation for juvenile osteopetrosis. *Am J Med* 1981;70:1280–1287.
28. Thomas ED, Buckner CD, Sanders JE, et al.: Marrow transplantation for thalassemia. *Lancet* 1982;ii:227–229.
29. Lucarelli G, Polchi P, Izzi T, et al.: Allogeneic marrow transplantation for thalassemia. *Exp Hematol* 1984;12:676–681.
30. Lucarelli G, Galimberti M, Delfini C, et al.: Marrow transplantation for thalassemia following busulfan and cyclophosphamide. *Lancet* 1985;i:1355–1357.
31. Johnson FL, Look AT, Gockerman J, et al.: Bone marrow transplantation in a patient with sickle cell anemia. *N Engl J Med* 1984;311:780–783.
32. Iriondo A, Garijo J, Baro J, et al.: Complete recovery of hematopoiesis following bone marrow transplantation in a patient with unresponsive congenital hypoplastic anemia (Blackfan-Diamond syndrome). *Blood* 1984;64:348–351.
33. Parkman R, Rappeport J, Camitta B, et al.: Successful use of multiagent immunosuppression for bone marrow transplantation of sensitized patients. *Blood* 1978;52:1163–1169.
34. Storb R, Doney KC, Thomas ED, et al.: Marrow transplantation with or without donor buffy coat cells from 65 transfused aplastic anemia patients. *Blood* 1982;59:236–246.

35. UCLA Bone Marrow Transplant Team. Prevention of graft rejection following bone marrow transplantation. *Blood* 1981;57:9–12.
36. Barrett AJ, Brigden WD, Hobbs JR, et al.: Successful bone marrow transplant for Fanconi's anæmia. *Br Med J* 1977;i:420–422.
37. Storb R, Thomas ED, Weiden PL, et al.: Allogeneic bone marrow grafting for treatment of aplastic anemia: A follow-up on 49 new cases from Seattle. *Blood* 1976;48:817–841.
38. Rappeport JM, Ginns EI: Bone marrow transplantation in severe Gaucher's disease. *N Engl J Med* 1984;311:880–888.
39. Hobbs JR, Barrett AJ, Chambers D, et al.: Reversal of clinical features of Hurler's disease and biochemical improvement after treatment by bone marrow transplantation. *Lancet* 1981;ii:709–712.
40. Hobbs JR, Hugh-Jones K, James DCO, et al.: Bone marrow transplantation has corrected the systemic disease of 3 patients with Hurler's mucopolysaccharidosis. *Exp Hematol* 1982;10(Suppl.10):48–49.
41. Dean MF, Muir H, Benson PF, et al.: Increased breakdown of glycosaminoglycans and appearance of corrective enzyme after skin transplant in Hunter syndrome. *Nature* 1975;257:609–611.
42. Hugh-Jones K, Kendra J, James DCO, et al.: Treatment of Sanfilippo B disease (MPS 111B) by bone marrow transplant. *Exp Hematol* 1982;10(Suppl.10):50–51.
43. Krivit W, Pierpont ME, Ayaz K, et al.: Bone marrow transplantation in the Maroteaux-Lamy syndrome (mucopolysaccharidosis Type VI). *N Engl J Med* 1984;311:1606–1611.
44. Kelley WN: Hypoxanthine-guanine phosphoribosyl transferase deficiency in the Lesch-Nyhan syndrome and gout. *Fed Proc* 1968;27:1047.
45. Nyhan WL, Parkman R, Page T: Bone marrow transplantation in Lesch-Nyhan disease. *Proc. 5th Symposium on Murine and Pyrimadine Metabolism in Man.* July 28–Aug 1, 1985, San Diego. Plenum Pres, NY. In press.
46. Miller AD, Eckner RJ, Jolly DJ: Expression of a retrovirus encoding human HPRT in mice. *Science* 1984;225:630–632.
47. Caravilli B, Jacobs JM: Peripheral nerve grafts in hereditary leukodystrophic mutant mice (twitcher). *Nature* 1981;290:56–58.
48. Scaravilli F, Suzuki K: Enzyme replacement in grafted nerve of twitcher mouse. *Nature* 1983;305:713–715.
49. Bayever E, Phillippart M, Nuwer M, et al.: Bone marrow transplantation for metachromatic leucodystrophy. *Lancet* 1985;i:471–473.
50. Moser HW, Tutschka PJ, Brown FR, et al.: Bone marrow transplant in adrenoleuko-dystrophy. *Neurology* (Cleveland) 1983;34:1410–1417.
51. Stout TJ, Chen HY, Brennand J, et al.: Expression of human HPRT in the central nervous system of transgenic mice. *Nature* 1985;317:250–252.
52. Swanson LW, Simmons DM, Arriza J, et al.: Novel developmental specificity in the nervous system of transgenic animals expressing growth hormone fusion genes. *Nature* 1985;317:363–365.

Bone Marrow Transplantation in Children, edited by F. Leonard Johnson and Carl Pochedly. Raven Press, Ltd., New York © 1990.

Lysosomal Storage Diseases Treated by Bone Marrow Transplantation: Review of 21 Patients*

William Krivit, Chester B. Whitley, Pi-Nian Chang, Elsa Shapiro, Kumar G. Belani, Dale Snover, C. Gail Summers, and Bruce Blazar

University of Minnesota Medical School, Minneapolis, Minnesota 55455

A. Rationale
    1. Cross-correction *in vitro*
    2. Derivation of new reticuloendothelial system by bone marrow transplant in humans
    3. Origin of brain microglial cell
    4. Animal experiments
B. Clinical results: HLA-identical nonreactive MLC sibling donors
    1. Leukodystrophy (3 types)
    2. Mucopolysaccharidosis (MPS) I (Hurler syndrome)
    3. Hunter syndrome (MPS II)
    4. Sanfilippo syndrome (MPS III)
    5. MPS VI
C. Clinical results: nonsibling donors
D. Bone marrow transplant procedures
    1. prevention of graft-vs.-host disease

Supported by Grants from NCI (CA-21737) Children's Cancer Research Fund, Minnesota Medical Foundation, Graduate School, Preston Arnold Research Fund, Viking Children's Fund, Eagles KROC, Minneapolis, Minnesota

These clinical studies were carried out by the University of Minnesota Pediatric Bone Marrow Transplant Team which included J.H. Kersey, Norma K.C. Ramsay, L.A. Lockman, S. Smith, J. Bass, M.Y. Tsai, and R. Brunning. These people represent the Departments of Pediatrics, Laboratory Medicine and Pathology, Neurology, Ophthalmology, Otolaryngology, Anesthesia and the Institute of Human Genetics, University of Minnesota Variety Club Children's Hospital.

*This report was written in January 1988 and accepted with revisions in May 1988. The total number of patients with lysosomal storage diseases treated with bone marrow transplantation at the University of Minnesota is now 33 as of September 1, 1989.

E.   Discussion
Summary

Twenty-one children, representing a spectrum of lethal lysosomal storage diseases, have been treated by bone marrow transplantation at the University of Minnesota in a pilot study. This is a review of the experience to date.

This chapter will provide the rationale for use of bone marrow transplantation in lysosomal storage diseases. This will include review of *in vitro* tissue co-culture changes and the results of animal experiments in which bone marrow transplantation was used to replace deficient lysosomal enzymes. The pre-transplant preparative regimen and the regimen given to prevent graft-vs.-host disease will be described. Measurement of intellectual capacity as well as other clinical observations in our patients treated with bone marrow transplantation will be compared to those of untreated children. Studies planned for the future will be outlined.

RATIONALE

Cross-Correction In Vitro (Figure 1).

The seminal observations by Neufeld and colleagues are the cornerstone for the concept of using enzyme replacement in treating children with these diseases (1). They demonstrated that *in vitro* cross-correction of fibroblast tissue

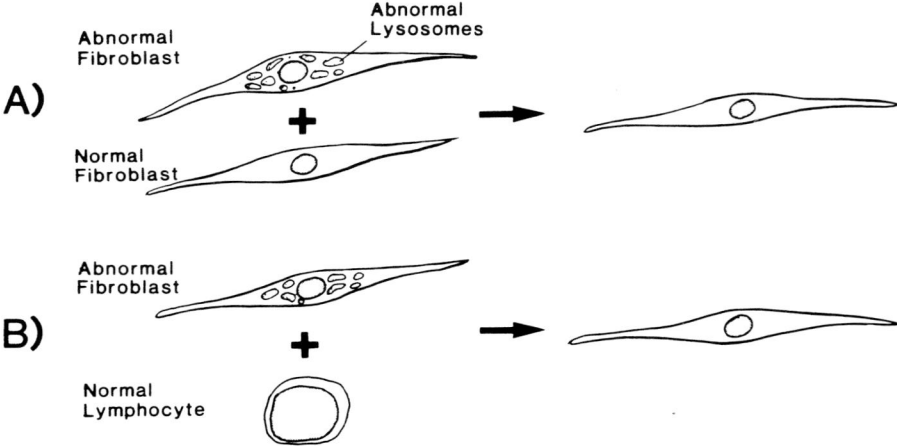

FIG. 1. Diagram indicating that both normal fibroblasts (A) and normal lymphocytes (B) cross-correct the metabolic defect in enzyme deficient cells (in patients with Hurler syndrome, Hunter syndrome, or metachromatic leukodystrophy).

cultures has produced reduction of abnormal substrate and repletion of enzymes. Correction of Hurler fibroblasts after co-culture with either normal fibroblasts or by Hunter fibroblasts has been reported. Subsequently, *in vitro* cross-correction has been noted using the same systems with tissue from patients with metachromatic leukodystrophy (2,3). Sandhoff and others have noted that cross-correction can be accomplished even though there may be only a minimal amount of enzyme in the culture (4). The *in vitro* cross-correction studies are not restricted to fibroblasts; normal lymphocytes have been shown to be capable of similar enzyme transfer *in vitro* and can correct the metabolic abnormality (5,6). Of special interest is the observation that enzyme deficient glial cells also exhibit metabolic correction when co-cultured with normal cells (7,8).

Derivation of New Reticuloendothelial System by Bone Marrow Transplantation in Humans (Figure 2).

The macrophage system of the liver (Kupffer cell), lung, peritoneal and lymphoid system, as well as osteoclasts of bone marrow and Langerhans cells of skin, have all been proved to be derived from bone marrow derived monocyte system. These cellular components of the donor reticuloendothelial system (RES) become that of the engrafted recipient system following bone marrow transplantation. These experiments designed to identify origin of cell types have relied upon differences between sex chromosomes from donor to recipients and the resultant karyotype changes following marrow transplant.

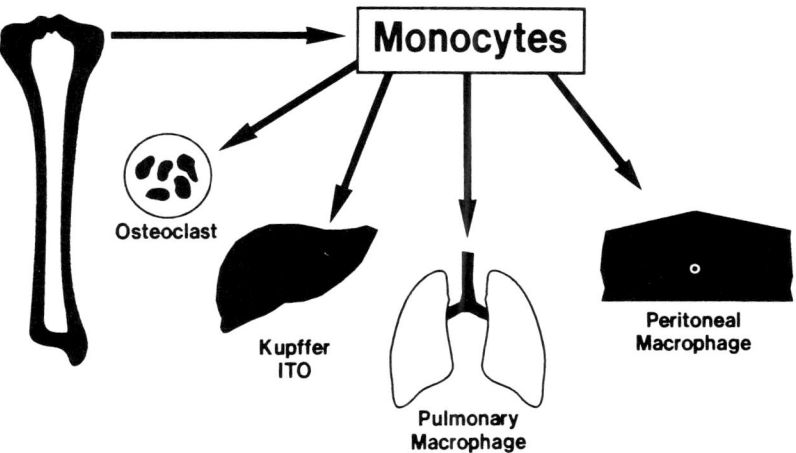

FIG. 2. Diagram showing that monocytes derived from donor bone marrow repopulate the reticuloendothelial system of recipient.

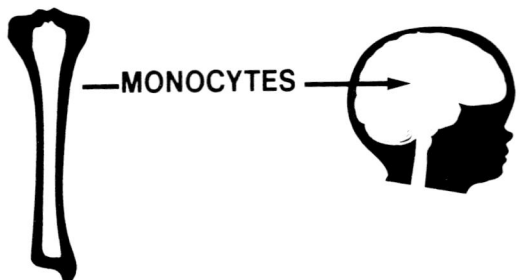

FIG. 3. Schema indicating that monocytes derived from donor bone marrow might potentially repopulate the microglial cells of the recipient's brain.

Origin of Brain Microglial Cell (Figure 3).

The brain microglial cell appears to originate from the circulating monocyte (9–13). Experiments to identify the cell of origin used donor monocyte cells labeled with tritium which were injected into experimental animals which had sustained brain inflammation and trauma. The cellular infiltrate of the recipient then becomes labeled with donor monocytes. A recent study has shown that "perivascular microglial cells" are bone marrow derived (14). This study showed that "perivascular microglial cells" have cell membrane features of marrow derivation. But additional proof is needed, such as by showing conversion of sex chromosomal karyotype similar to other documented RES changes following marrow transplant. The macrophage cell in globoid cell leukodystrophy in the brain has been shown to be of bone marrow origin (15,16). Whether or not there is a normal marrow population within the brain has been debated (17–19; 59–61).

Animal Experiments (Table 1).

The most conclusive animal studies to date have been done by Shull et al. (20), in dogs with mucopolysaccharidosis type I-H, as defined by morphologic, enzymologic, and biochemical methods. Conversion to normal morphology in blood vessels (pericytes), neurons and glial cells has occurred subsequent to engraftment by bone marrow transplantation. Repletion of the deficient enzyme, α-L-iduronidase, and reductions of accumulated substrate of glycosaminoglycan are clearly noted in these studies in dogs.

Taylor studied animals deficient in enzyme fucosidase (21,22). In the untreated animal, progressive accumulation of substrate (oligosaccharides) occurs in the CNS as well as in the viscera. The clinical spectrum in these animals includes severe deterioration of CNS function. After bone marrow transplantation, the fucosidase enzyme activity in the cerebrum, cerebellum, midbrain and peripheral nerve is significantly increased. The enzyme activity was found in the central nervous system in amounts comparable to that in the

TABLE 1. *Animal model trials of bone marrow transplantation: experiences with lysosomal storage disorders*

Year	Reference	Disease defect	Animal model	Comments subsequent to BMT
1987	20	MPS I-H α-L-iduronidase	Platt hounds	1. Brain morphology in BMT revealed disappearance of abnormal vesicle, Zebra bodies and neuronal degeneration. 2. Enzyme noted in brain. 3. Biochemical changes noted in brain.
1986	21,22	Fucosidosis α-L fucosidase	English springer spaniels	1. Enzyme noted in CNS tissue. 2. Accumulated oligosaccharides in brain decreased post-BMT. 3. Absence of neurological deterioration.
1984 1986	26	arylsulfatase B MPS VI	Siamese cats	1. In addition to resolution of corneal clouding and facial dysmorphia, there was evidence of clinical improvement of CNS symptoms. 2. Sensitivity of enzyme system to detect an increase in brain not commented upon in specific areas of brain.
1984 1987	23	Globoid cell leukodystrophy galactosyl ceramidase	Twitcher mouse	1. Increased survival was noted to be associated with delay in onset of CNS symptoms. 2. Psychosine levels in brain were less in BMT animals compared to littermates. 3. Peripheral nerve demyelination repaired. 4. Globoid cells in brain identified as bone marrow derived macrophage.
1983	24	Niemann-Pick disease	Spin mice	1. BMT not started until after 5 weeks of age. Demise of animals usually occurred at 10 weeks. Highly unlikely to have expected CNS changes since damage had already been done. 2. Clearing of substrate in liver and spleen was quite complete.
1987	27	MPS VII β-glucuronidase mice Mucopolysaccharidosis	Gusa mice	1. Enzyme activity at end of experiment in brain was 6% (this level is different from and greater than nontreated littermates).
1976	25	Mannosidosis (α-L mannosidosis)	Freemartin Angus calves	1. Decrease in both visceral and *CNS* substrate accumulated by biochemical measurement. 2. Chimera: chimeric female lymphocytes were present. 3. Animal sacrificed early in life. 4. Detailed clinical results and precise comparison to controls not given.

liver. One dog that had bone marrow transplantation at 8 months of age, before clinical signs were evident, showed only mild abnormalities 14 months later. This was at a time well past the usual time of onset of serious neurological disease. Two other dogs who were treated by bone marrow transplantation before 5 months of age are now normal without signs and symptoms of neurological disease 2 years later.

In both of these experimental studies, in dogs with either MPS I or fucosidosis, the long-term clinical outcome needs to be elucidated. Repletion of enzyme activity and disappearance of toxic metabolites appear to predict greater longevity, as well as improved quality of the outcome, if the bone marrow transplant is done very early in the animal's life span.

Yeager, in his studies of bone marrow transplantation in the twitcher mouse, succinctly provides evidence for the presence in the brain of galactocerebrosidase, and a concomitant decrease in the accumulated toxic metabolite psychosine (23). Despite these salutary changes, the animals treated by bone marrow transplantation did not gain weight differently from controls. However, the onset of CNS symptoms in those treated by bone marrow transplant occurred at a later time than in the untreated animals. Thus: "Gait, foraging and grooming behavior were qualitatively less impaired in twitcher mice which did develop the characteristic hindlimb paralysis observed in untreated animals." "The subnormal but stable motor conduction velocities in transplanted animals were sufficient to allow neuromuscular transmission and prevent paralysis." Yeager showed that the timing of marrow transplantation is critical in the mouse model. He noted marked differences in results clinically and biochemically when bone marrow transplantation is done at day 7 or 14 or at 30 days. The earlier in life the marrow transplant is done, the greater the neurologic improvement.

Bone marrow transplantation was successful in treatment of visceral accumulation of sphingomyelin mice with Niemann-Pick disease (24). The animals were transplanted at 4 to 5 weeks of age, by which time the CNS disease must be assumed to have already been firmly established. The animals died by 8 to 10 weeks of age. Obviously, once neurons are destroyed by nuclear disorganization, fibrosis or damage to cytoplasm with dysmetabolism, no recovery is possible. Repair of neurons and return to normal function will require exposure to normal enzyme and hematopoietic cells. Timing of enzyme entrance and presence in brain cells must occur before irreparable harm is done and must be present for many months before final conclusions can be made as to the beneficial effects of the enzyme and the hematopoietic cells.

The observation by Jolly and colleagues on a single animal are often quoted to support the concept that bone marrow transplantation in mannosidosis cannot affect the CNS (25). However, Jolly did note a substantial decrease in substrate that accumulated in the brain. Lymphocytes, monocytes and bone marrow derived cells had to be those of the enzyme deficient animal. Jolly sacrificed animals early in life, at 1 year of age, while a full life span of many years might be anticipated. Whether or not the relatively small number of normal lymphocyte (monocyte and macrophages) would have eventually made a more significant impact upon function and appearance is not known because of the limited follow-up period. This experimental animal model needs to be more fully explored.

Clinical improvement is locomotion and gait following bone marrow transplant was seen in cats with arysulfatase B deficiency (26). This clinical improvement may be due to improved joint mobility since no arysulfatase B was found in the brain 12 months post-marrow transplant. Lack of sensitivity of enzyme detection may have precluded observations of only a slight increase. Also, later observations of the cat after more years of enzyme presence may allow for detection of greater changes.

Treatment of glucuronidase deficiency with bone marrow transplantation is revealing in this discussion even though in this model there is no CNS pathology with excessive substrate (27). There was an increase of glucuronidase into the CNS. The CNS enzyme level was greater at the end of study and was above littermate levels. In catalase studies (28), brain contamination by peripheral blood from transplanted marrow citations confounded the issue of whether enzyme entered the CNS.

CLINICAL RESULTS: HLA-IDENTICAL NONREACTIVE MLC SIBLING DONORS

Leukodystrophy (3 types) (Table 2)

We have transplanted 6 patients from within the broad diagnostic category of leukodystrophy. Two had metachromatic leukodystrophy, three had Krabbe disease, and one child had Niemann-Pick disease type A. The patient with metachromatic leukodystrophy is now 10 years of age and is 5 years post-bone marrow transplant. Her clinical course since the transplant has allowed development and growth consistent with her age. The intellectual growth and development is improving. This is not what would have been predicted by the history of her sister (Figure 4). The affected sibling had the usual inexorable course of the disease. As the disease progressed, she had to be fed by gastrostomy at 5 years of age, she became decerebrate at 6 years, she became comatose and then finally died at 7½ years of age. The enzymatic activity of the leukocytes in both siblings were the same, being 8 nmoles/mg protein/hr in leukocytes of arylsulfatase A. Early signs of disease in both were identical and were present in both at 2½ years of age.

Following transplant in the second child, the enzymatic activity of leukocyte arylsulfatase A has been normal for the past 5 years. Our patient's clinical course has been one of continued school activity. Neurologic effect, as as-

TABLE 2. *Clinical trials of histocompatible bone marrow transplantation for leukodystrophy storage diseases at the University of Minnesota*

Patient number	BMT date	Diagnosis	GVH disease	Age at time of BMT studies	Latest engraftment status*	Clinical status
217	8/1/84	Metachromatic Leukodystrophy	None	4 years	1,2,3	Alive and well with neurologic signs and symptoms
400	8/1/86	Krabbe disease	None	6 months	1,2,3	Died at 3 years of age
758	7/1/87	Krabbe disease	None	8 weeks	1,2,3	Significantly delayed; Graft lost at 2 years
794	10/15/87	Niemann-Pick disease Type A	Acute & chronic Grade III	8 months	1,2,3,4	Severely impaired

*Criteria for engraftment:
1. Restriction Fragment Length Polymorphism (RFLP) (100% donor cells by RFLP in peripheral blood and marrow) (Blood 66:1436–1444, 1985)
2. Donor Enzyme Activity
3. Red Cell Phenotype
4. Karyotype conversion of donor
Note: In addition to the above, we have had engraftment in a 13 year old with juvenile globoid cell leukodystrophy and in a 16 year old with juvenile metachromatic leukodystrophy in 1989.

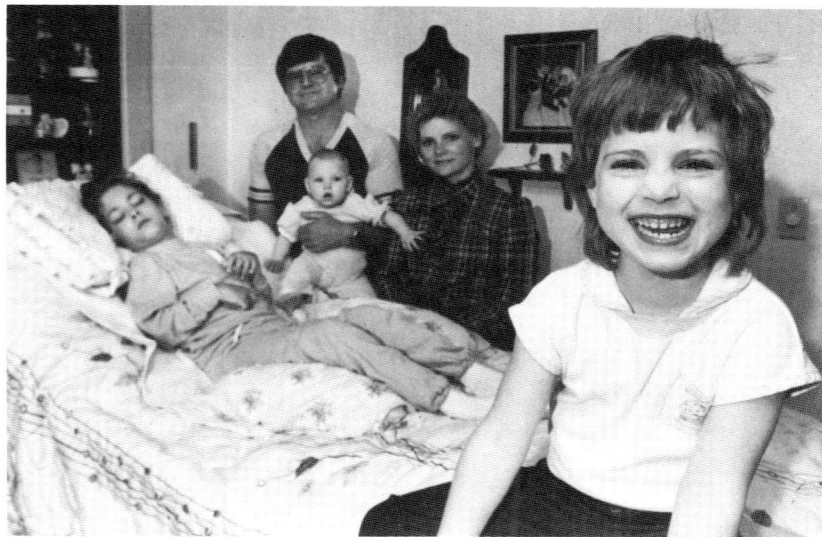

FIG. 4. Family of a patient with metachromatic leukodystrophy. The propositus who received bone marrow transplantation is on the right. The sister who is lying in bed, died 1½ years later. The infant is the normal bone marrow donor.

assessed by brain stem auditory response, has shown no deterioration over a 5 year period. Psychometric measurements have been totally consistent with continued normal life activity (Figure 5) (29–31). The radiologic evidence of demyelination, cerebral atrophy and ventricular dilatation that is seen in metachromatic leukodystrophy has not occurred. Indeed, the areas of demyelination noted earlier have diminished markedly (Figure 6). The myelin basic protein, total protein and sulfatide levels of the spinal fluid have remained normal. The motor nerve conduction has become stabilized at 20 meters/sec in upper extremities and continues to show decreases in lower extremities (17–19 m/dec). Ophthalmologic examination continues to show a fine horizontal nystagmus which increases with monocular occlusion and diminishes with left head turn and chin elevation. Vision remains stable at 20/30–40, and no corneal clouding or strabismus has developed. The mild perifoveal greyness is unchanged and no optic atrophy is detected on clinical examination 5 years following marrow transplantation. However, patterned visual evoked potentials show increasingly prolonged latencies.

The clinical heterogeneity of metachromatic leukodystrophy from family to family is well known (32). However, among siblings in the same family with the same levels of enzyme activity, the disease course may be different (33). This concordancy is a matter of concern in all families. In one unusual report, affected siblings' clinical courses were different from each other (34). One

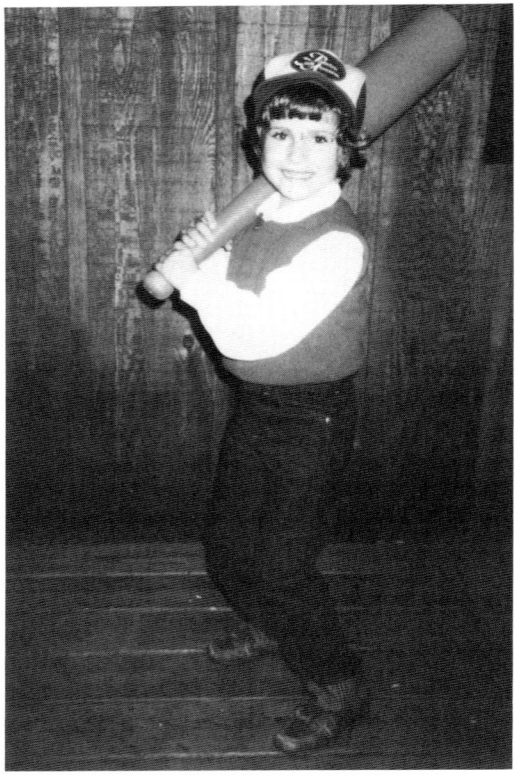

FIG. 5. Our patient with metachromatic leukodystrophy who is now 10 years old and 5 years post-bone marrow transplant. She is attending regular school.

explanation of this disparity in the same family might be related to the fact that the turnover of sulfatide in fibroblast culture was higher than in the least affected sibling, perhaps indicating inherent differences in arylsulfatase A enzyme activity.

Clearly, future cases of metachromatic leukodystrophy who are treated with bone marrow transplantation should have fibroblast culture studies prior to transplant.

In two other families with metachromatic leukodystrophy, observations following bone marrow transplant have indicated marked differences in the clinical course from that of untreated siblings (35,36,55). In our patient, as well as in the other reported families, the radiologic and neurophysiologic measurements revealed much more nervous system damage than had been suspected from the clinical examination. Earlier treatment, beginning long before any signs or symptoms are present, is needed. By comparison to animal experiments, when severe neuronal damage is already present, one can expect only minimal correction or stabilization of neurologic function as a result of normalization of enzymatic activity after bone marrow transplantation.

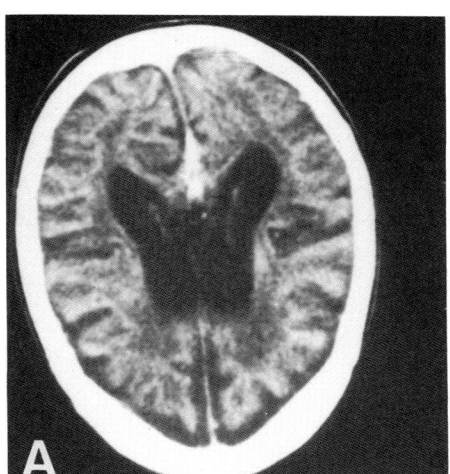
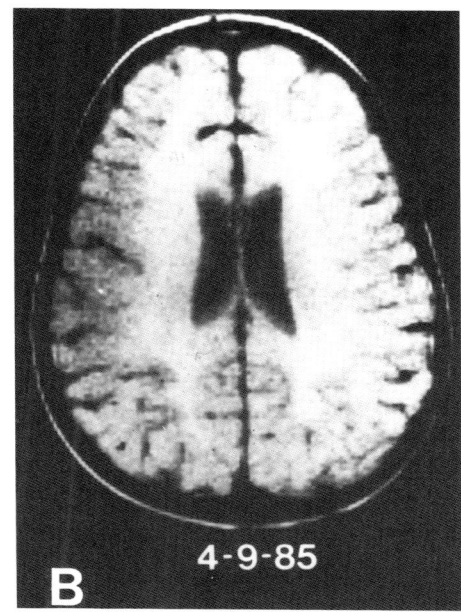

FIG. 6. Cranial CT scan. Differences between two sisters with metachromatic leukodystrophy. In **A**, the untreated sister (7 years of age) has severe ventricular dilatation and atrophy. In **B**, the propositus (5 years of age) who was bone marrow transplanted has only slight degree of dilatation and atrophy. Further radiologic studies by MRI at 7 years of age show amelioration of disease process. (Ref. 31)

In both of our patients with infantile Krabbe disease full engraftment of bone marrow produced the anticipated normalization of leukocyte enzymatic activity, the enzyme being galactocerebrosidase. This normal leukocyte galactocerebrosidase level had been present for 2 years in one patient and for 1½ years in the second. In the second patient, the cerebrospinal fluid protein was 284 mg% before bone marrow transplantation, 194 mg% 1 month post-transplant, and 119 mg% at 4 months post-transplant. The myelin basic protein remained normal. The motor nerve conduction velocity improved (from 19 meters/sec to 28 meters/sec). Developmental milestones have been markedly delayed in this latter patient. However, the severity of the course appears to be different from that of an older sibling, who had been similarly affected with Krabbe disease. Opisthotonos had not developed and the infantile responsiveness was improving. This patient had received a T cell depleted marrow 2 years ago. The loss of graft was documented by enzyme level returning to pre-transplant level and by loss of donor cells as measured by RFLP data in July 1989.

The first patient with Krabbe disease had an episode of severe cerebral hypoxia related to an attack of encephalitis due to Epstein-Barr virus infection which occurred during the transplant process. The EB virus etiology was confirmed by viral serology and culture. The effects of cerebral hypoxia were demonstrated radiologically as severe cerebral atrophy. This infant continues to be severely impaired. A sudden onset of respiratory illness caused demise in August 1989. Examination of brain by biochemical and morphological methods will be reported at a later date. The cerebrospinal fluid protein remained elevated but the myelin basic protein was normal.

Our patient with Niemann-Pick disease quickly engrafted and had severe acute and chronic graft-vs.-host disease which abated. Engraftment has been present with normal enzymatic activity and RFLP data for the past 22 months. Although the cerebrospinal fluid levels of protein and basic myelin protein have not changed, there has been no clinical improvement. The neurological status has not improved beyond that noted at end of transplant and no gains in development have been present. Patient has to be fed by gastrostomy tube.

Mucopolysaccharidosis (MPS) I (Hurler Syndrome) (Table 3)

Many aspects of central nervous system function have been continuously monitored on a serial basis on all of our patients. This has included careful repeated psychometric tests and developmental assessments, CT scan and MRI (37).

We have monitored Type I-H patients' intelligence in a serial manner, utilizing individually administered Stanford-Binet and Minnesota Child Inventory Developmental and the Bailey Scale of Infant Development. In our three oldest patients with mucopolysaccharidosis type I-H, continued gains and skills in intellectual development have been observed. These gains include improvement in language, comprehension and verbal capability. Attendance at school in appropriate classes and review by teacher indicates improvement each year following the bone marrow transplant. Our observations give credence to the results of the longer observations reported by Hugh-Jones (38). Gains in intellectual capacity with each passing year noted by these observers can be confirmed by our observations. Some amelioration of the typical facial characteristics of Hurler syndrome is apparent (Figure 7).

Enzymatic activity: All patients who are permanently engrafted retain leucocyte α-L-iduronidase activity at levels appropriate to those that would be present in the donor.

Bone marrow changes: The typical accumulations of glycosaminoglycan shown as metachromatic inclusions in mucopolysaccharidosis has been noted in all our patients. These are readily seen in bone marrow specimens obtained both from bone marrow aspiration and from trephine biopsy. By day 28 post-transplant, these accumulations of glycosaminoglycan are markedly diminished in all who have had bone marrow engraftment. By day 100, and thereafter, there is absence of metachromatic inclusions. This has been observed in

TABLE 3. *Clinical trial of histocompatible bone marrow transplantation for mucopolysaccharidosis storage diseases at the University of Minnesota*

Patient number	BMT date	Diagnosis (syndrome)	GVH disease	Age at BMT	Latest engraftment status*	Clinical status
217	4/21/82	Maroteaux-Lamy	None	12.9	2,3	Alive
330	9/16/83	Hurler	None	2.1	1,2,3	Alive
453	1/18/85	Hurler	Grade I	2.8	1,2,3,4	Alive
463	2/18/85	Hurler	Grade I	3.1	1,2,3,4	Alive
503	8/12/85	Sanfilippo (A)	Graft IV (chronic)	5.8	1,2,3	Alive
618	8/15/86	Hurler	None	1.0	Nonengrafted	Deceased 2/22/87
628	9/15/86	Hurler	None	1.7	Engraftment declining	Alive
659	11/13/86	Sanfilippo (B)	Grade I	1.9	1,2,3,4	Alive
677	12/18/86	Hurler	Grade II	1.3	Engrafted	Deceased 12/4/87
699	2/11/87	Hurler	Grade II (chronic)	1.1	1,2,3	Alive
729	3/1/87	Hurler	Grade I	1	Varying level of engraftment	Alive
759	6/11/87	Hunter	Grade II (chronic)	4	1,2,3	Alive
819	11/10/87	Hurler	None	0.8	1,2,3,4	Alive
926	7/8/88	Hurler				
950	8/24/88	Sanfilippo (A)				
977	10/14/88	Hurler				
1130	8/2/89	Maroteaux-Lamy				

*Criteria for engraftment: see Table 2.

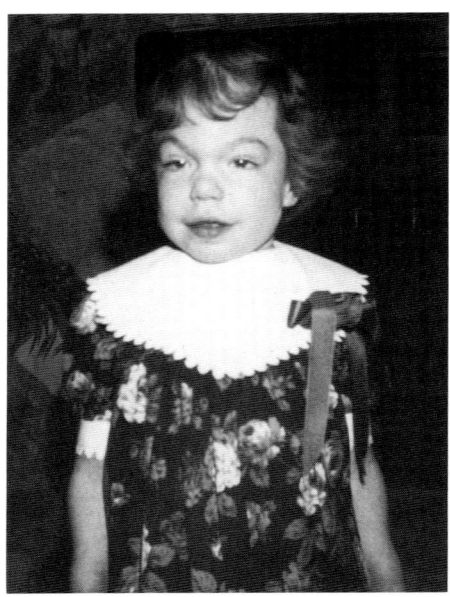

FIG. 7.   Picture of one of our two oldest patients with Hurler syndrome at 2½ years post-bone marrow transplant. She is now 4 years post transplant and 7 years of age.

all of our patients. However, if engraftment is lost, the inclusions reaccumulate in the bone marrow. The evidence from this study indicates that bone marrow histopathology is concordant with other markers of engraftment in mucopolysaccharidosis.

Liver biopsy: Biopsies of liver have been done before the transplant, at 30 days post-transplant, at 100 days and at longer intervals post-transplant in our patients. During full engraftment, enzyme activity is in the range of 10 to 15% of normal. Glycosaminoglycan activity, as observed by histochemical and ultrastructural techniques in hepatocytes as well as Kupffer cells, is also diminished and the liver cells show clearing of lysosomal abnormalities (Figure 8). Levels of hepatic glycosaminoglycan quantitated by biochemical methods show return to normal (37).

The CSF glycosaminoglycan levels have fallen to normal levels or have remained at pre-transplant levels. Total protein of the cerebrospinal fluid has not changed (39,40).

In all patients, the urinary glycosaminoglycan levels have fallen to almost normal after a period of several months.

Growth pattern: The growth rate of children has been consistent. One of our longest engrafted patients (UPN453), who is now 5 years 8 months of age, has a weight of 42 pounds (25th percentile) and a height of 41 inches (10th percentile). Even though the original gibbus deformity has persisted, growth of the vertebral column above and below the deformity has significantly reduced apparent clinical kyphosis.

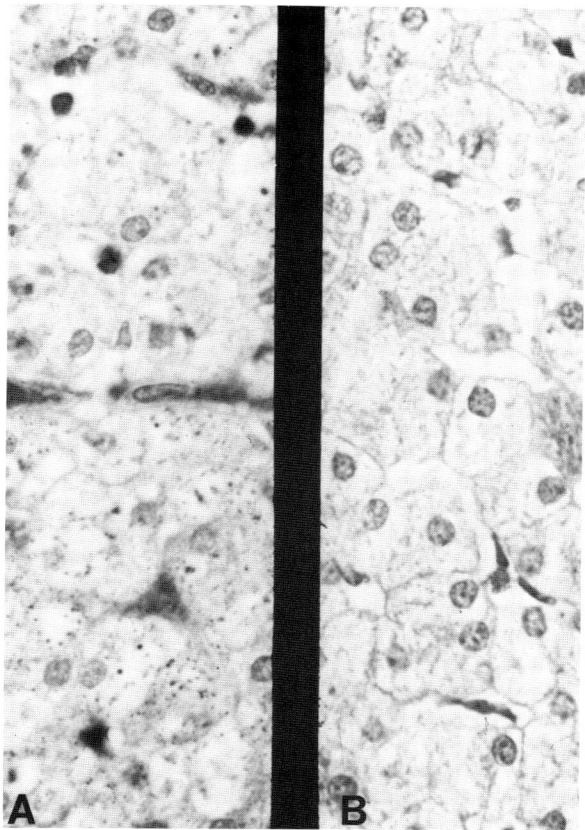

FIG. 8. Histochemical study of liver biopsy before (A) and after (B) bone marrow transplantation. Clearing of accumulated intracellular and intercellular substrate in both Kupffer cells and hepatocytes is noted.

Ophthalmic studies: A rapid decrease in the lysosomal inclusions in the adjacent conjunctiva follows engraftment. Three patients have shown a significant decrease in corneal clouding and improved media clarity. No change in the corneal clouding was detected prior to one year following bone marrow transplantation, and in one patient, significant improvement in corneal clouding did not occur until 2½ years after marrow transplant.

At the young ages of these patients, funduscopic evidence of retinal pigmentary degeneration is minimal or absent prior to marrow transplantation. Progressive retinal changes following marrow transplantation have not been detected with ophthalmoscopy. Electroretinography (ERG) recorded under photopic and scotopic conditions before marrow transplantation showed evidence of early retinal degeneration (delayed implicit times, decreased amplitudes). In some patients, the ERG changes have stabilized or improved over several months following marrow transplantation (41). The earliest improvement in the ERG is a decrease in the implicit time, followed by an improvement in amplitude.

This finding is to be compared to previous reports in which no improvement occurred in patients who received amniotic membrane implants (42).

Special attention has been made in assessing the need for monitoring for sleep apnea. Immediately after receiving preparative regimen containing busulfan in one patient and busulfan and cyclophosphamide in another patient, sleep apnea disappeared (43).

Two patients with Hurler syndrome (mucopolysaccharidosis type I) have died. The first patient had a cerebral hypoxic event 4 weeks after marrow transplant. The other patient had lost initial engrafted marrow and was successfully engrafted a second time. A sudden episode of overwhelming pneumonia was cause of death at 6 weeks post-transplant. Medial hyperplasia of coronary arteries as in advanced cases of mucopolysaccharidosis type I was quite apparent.

Hunter Syndrome (MPS II)

We have transplanted one patient with Hunter syndrome. The psychometric development was carefully monitored and has shown no loss of mental capabilities. Other neurophysiologic measurements show no evidence of deterioration at the present time. Similarly, spinal fluid protein levels remain as before.

Sanfilippo Syndrome (MPS III)

Our first patient with Sanfilippo syndrome (MPS III) (type A) is now 4 years postengraftment. He has had acute and chronic graft-vs.-host disease and is still on medication for treatment of chronic graft-vs.-host disease. He has recently entered a special school. One major difficulty was his hyperactivity and inattentiveness. The slow intellectual development may be secondary, in part, to his chronic graft-vs.-host disease, although moderate developmental delay was present before transplantation. His mental function is subjectively considered by the family to be better than other older patients with Sanfilippo syndrome. Measurements of his cognitive function have recently been shown to be at values present before the bone marrow transplant.

The second patient with Sanfilippo syndrome (type B) continues to show no loss of intellectual ability. His electroretinogram remains stable 2½ years following bone marrow transplantation. These two patients corroborate the clinical impression noted by Hugh-Jones in the twins with mucopolysaccharidosis type III A treated by bone marrow transplantation. In these latter two instances, the results of intelligence testing remains the same as before transplantation. The children are attending special schools (44,56).

MPS VI

Our initial patient with mucopolysaccharidosis type VI, now 7 years post-marrow transplant, has recently graduated from high school as valedictorian. She still has normal leukocyte enzyme levels and is on no medication. MPS VI is different in that the central nervous system is not usually involved. Our patient at the time of transplant was in severe congestive heart failure, and she had such a severe sleep apnea (with episodes of 30 to 40 seconds) that her life expectancy was considered limited to a few months. Other mucopolysaccharidosis type VI patients with similar apnea have had tracheotomy, as in our patient, but without relief of congestive heart failure and other symptoms. Indeed, our experience with sleep apnea would indicate tracheotomy to be contraindicated (43). The cardiopulmonary status of our patient is now markedly improved (46,57). Other MPS VI patients have progressed in later teen years so that shunt procedures have been required for hydrocephalus.

CLINICAL RESULTS: NONSIBLING DONORS (Table 4)

Early in our bone marrow transplant program, we treated a patient with Wolman disease using the mother (who was a haplo-identical match) as donor. This patient never engrafted and died 6 weeks after the transplant. Similarly, a patient with Gaucher disease (nonneuronopathic type) with hepatosplenomegaly was transplanted from the father. He died within several weeks following the transplant.

In two patients with Hurler syndrome, haplo-identical transplants were attempted. In one, grandfather's marrow was used and, in the other a nonrelated HLA, nonidentical MLC slightly reactive donor was used. T cell depletion was employed in all these 4 patients. Autoengraftment occurred in the latter two patients and neither have shown any improvement in hepatosplenomegaly or in the signs and symptoms of the disease process.

These and other similar autografted patients demonstrate that preparative regimen and graft-vs.-host prophylaxis per se are not responsible for salutory effects noted postengraftment.

BONE MARROW TRANSPLANT PROCEDURES

In the HLA-identical, MLC nonreactive sibling donor matches, we have continuing engraftment at the present time in 15 out of 17 patients. If 100% of cells were of donor origin at 100 days post-transplant, none have lost engraftment. We were able to detect changes very early in transplant indicative of engraftment by all techniques of measurement: by restriction fragment length polymorphisms, enzyme assays, red cell antigens, HLA type, and chromosomal analysis.

Busulfan and cyclophosphamide have remained the primary preparative

TABLE 4. Clinical trials of nonsibling marrow transplants

Patient number	Donor	Transplant date	Regimens for preparation and GVH disease prophylaxis	Primary diagnosis	MLC reactivity D→TR: R→D	Clinical status
375	Mother	9/10/84	Cyt + TBI TuT Ricin T cell depleted	Wolman disease	20:10	Nonengrafted: died
497	Father	12/1/84	Cyt + TBI ATB, Pred, MTX, T cell depleted	Gaucher disease	0:8	Nonengrafted: died
641	Grandfather	10/1/86	Cyt + TBI Pred, ATG, MTX, T cell depleted	Hurler (MPS type I) syndrome	0:8	Nonengrafted: autologous recovery
793	Nonrelated Red Cross Donor	11/1/87	BU + Cyt CS + MP T cell depleted	Hurler (MPS type I) syndrome	9:0	Nonengrafted: autologous recovery

CY = cyclophosphamide
TBI = total body irradiation
BU = busulfan
CS = cyclosporine A
MP = methylprednisolone
MTX = methotrexate
ATG = antithymocyte globulin
Note: In addition to above we have transplanted 3 additional patients with unrelated matched donors (1104,1101,1125) and 3 additional patients with related matched donors other than histocompatible sibling (1040,1052,1089).

regimen throughout this pilot study in all HLA identical, MLC nonreactive, sibling donor transplants.

The dosage of busulfan of 20 mg/kg is given orally in four daily dosage during a 4 day period (on days -12 to -9). We originally began with a total dosage of 8 to 12 mg/kg of busulfan and we have gradually increased the dosage with no apparent evidence of toxicity. The cyclophosphamide dose has remained the same, at a total dosage of 240 mg/kg given intravenously in a one hour infusion for 4 days (on days -6 to -3).

The dose of donor bone marrow cells has remained at 5.0×10^8 nucleated cells/kg of recipient body weight. We have utilized higher doses of bone marrow cells when these are readily available. The marrow is infused over a one hour period on day 0. In the HLA identical, MLC nonreactive series we have not had an ABO incompatibility between donor and recipient.

Prevention of Graft-vs.-Host Disease

Measures used to prevent graft-vs.-host disease have been of two types. The first 11 patients received Minnesota anti-graft-vs.-host prevention (methotrexate, anti-thymocyte globulin, and steroids). The last 6 patients have received cyclosporine A (CSA) and methylprednisolone (MP). The graft-vs.-host disease has been relatively nonsevere (Table 5).

Of those who have lost their original engraftment, 3 have been retransplanted. All three received cyclophosphamide and total body irradiation (TBI), at a dose of 750 cGy as the preparative regimen and to prevent graft-vs.-host disease, the first had Minnesota prophylaxis and the other two had cyclosporine and methylprednisolone prophylaxis. The first patient has remained engrafted for 3 years. The second died as a result of acute respiratory disease syndrome on day 30 post-marrow transplant but full engraftment was noted prior to the sudden demise. The third is now engrafted 10 months after transplant.

Busulfan and cyclophosphamide have been used instead of TBI and cyclophosphamide as preparation for all our sibling matched transplants. The rationale was that TBI potentially could have a deleterious effect on continu-

TABLE 5. *Graft-vs.-host disease in BMT for lysosomal storage diseases using HLA-identical histocompatible MLC nonreactive sibling donors*

Acute GVH disease grade	Number
0	8
I	4
II	3
III–IV	2

ing brain development. Also, the pulmonary toxicity of busulfan was considered to be less when compared to TBI. Busulfan, however, appears to be metabolized at a different rate in infants and children from that in adults (58). Busulfan in larger dosages could cause an increasing toxicity to lungs. There have been reports of toxicity to the CNS, in the form of seizures, with increasing dosages of busulfan.

The possibility of using a different preparative regimen in initial therapy must be carefully considered. Total lymphoid irradiation conceivably could cause growth retardation in patients who are already destined to be stunted because of their primary disease.

Use of total body irradiation still might be considered despite reservations noted above. TBI may also be given in split dosages and then may have less tissue toxicity than if it were given as a single dose. For instance, cataracts are present in 80% of patients when single dose TBI is used as compared to an incidence of only 18% when split dosages of irradiation are used (47).

Our experience in use of busulfan and cyclophosphamide as the preparative regimen has been reported (48,49). Our present plan is to increase busulfan to 24 mg/kg. We will review our data concerning the "rest period" between busulfan and cyclophosphamide and between cyclophosphamide and marrow infusion. We will use cyclosporine A and methylprednisolone as prophylaxis for graft-vs.-host disease, but we will retain the option to compare this with the Minnesota method of graft-vs.-host disease prevention. Careful and frequent monitoring of cyclosporine levels will be required to maintain levels at an effective range, especially in infants.

DISCUSSION

The fact that the natural course of the several lysosomal storage diseases includes severe morbidity and certain death is well known. The unabated neurological regression leads to inability to walk, swallow or speak. The intelligence or development of these infants and children leads inexorably to severe and incapacitating regression of mentation. Death from infection, aspiration and hypoxia in these conditions is certain. Throughout their short life span, these children and infants are considered chronically ill. They require much-needed medical and surgical support. On the other hand, we must analyze and compare the problems and burdens of conventional care of these patients to the cost effectiveness of bone marrow transplantation.

The morbidity of bone marrow transplantation procedures in our patients needs to be noted. The 13 days used to myeloablate and immunosuppress patients are associated with nausea and vomiting. Temporary total marrow asplasia occurs. Return of marrow function (defined as having a peripheral leucocyte count above $1000/m^3$ for 3 consecutive days) occurs on the average by day 20. Acute and chronic graft-vs.-host disease are the main reasons for severe morbidity.

Clinical improvement caused by bone marrow transplantation has been noted by disappearance of severe sleep apnea within days of beginning treatment. After engraftment is achieved at day 28, there is a very gradual decrease of hepatosplenomegaly, and biochemical and morphologic abnormalities decrease considerably. In 887 of our HLA identical, MLC histocompatible sibling matches, engraftment has so far been permanent. Loss of engraftment had occurred in 3 patients. Two patients had been retransplanted and engraftment has continued following the second transplant.

The cognitive changes and neurological improvement are more apparent at one year post-transplant. Cellular changes in liver and bone marrow due to enzyme activity during this period of time indicate penetration of tissue and improved physiologic function.

Patients who have had bone marrow engraftment have done better according to all aspects of clinical scrutiny when compared to those who are untreated. This clinical improvement has been specifically measured in cases where previous siblings have had the same disease. In these cases, the positive improvement in the marrow transplanted children is quite obvious (Table 6).

In many patients who have been treated, considerable damage had already occurred in multiple organs prior to transplant. Patients treated earliest do better than those treated later. However, the inability to replace damaged neurons, and to repair "scars" or tissue disorganization, is an obvious limitation. In future patients, the transplant needs to be given earlier.

Many consider that the "blood-brain barrier" will prevent the entrance of appropriate enzyme into the brain (54). However, the data provided to date in the experimental animal studies clearly indicate the contrary. There is ample evidence in these latter studies of sufficient enzyme in the brain to provide normal function and morphology and prevention of neurologic disease. The entry into the brain post bone marrow transplantation need not be across the blood-brain barrier. The monocytes derived from the new marrow following transplantation do enter the brain through the capillary wall by diapedesis. Moreover, now that there are methods of controlling monocyte proliferation by use of recombinant hematopoietic growth factors, we can test in experimental animals whether or not we can enhance monocyte entrance into brain. This could be of major importance in improving the outcome of bone marrow transplant in treatment of patients with lysosomal storage diseases.

There are opportunities to borrow useful information from prior experience in other clinical studies. It is important to characterize different phases of a clinical study and to view bone marrow transplantation in the evolving progression.

In a phase I study of a procedure, the toxic or other adverse effects of the procedure are quantitatively measured and the relative degree of safety is determined. According to this definition, a phase I study was accomplished by early reports of bone marrow transplantation in lysosomal storage diseases as well as from reference to the longer history of marrow transplantation for treatment of hematopoietic diseases. The associated morbidity and mortality were carefully documented in each report.

TABLE 6. *Bone marrow transplant results improvement and/or prevention of deterioration in course of disease as compared to siblings with same disease not treated by bone marrow transplantation.*

Disease process	Hospital	BMT sibling	Untreated sibling
Metachromatic Leukodystrophy Case 1 (Patient number 217)	University of Minnesota	BMT 4 yrs. alive and attending school 8 yrs; ataxic tremulous	Same symptoms as at 4 yrs. Decerebrate 6 yrs; Coma 7 yrs; Died 8 yrs
Case 2 (Personal Communication)	Johns Hopkins	BMT 4 yrs; alive but retarded 10 yrs	Same signs and symptoms, but progressive to death at 14 yrs
Case 3 (References 35,36)	UCLA	BMT 2 yrs; alive but moderately retarded 7 yrs	Same signs and symptoms in 2 previous sibs, both died at 3 years
MPS III Twins (Reference 44)	Westminster	BMT 8 yrs; alive but retarded	Same signs and symptoms in 2 previous siblings, both died at 3 years of age
Krabbe (Patient number 758)	University of Minnesota	Alive at 9 months of age; Nerve conduction improved	Sibling was decorticate at same age, died at 12 months

A phase II study is the next step in which new treatments are compared to an existing procedure, or the procedure is used for specific diagnostic categories not previously treated. A phase II study is done to determine if responsiveness can occur. A phase II study does not analyze total effectiveness of care. A phase II study has now been done in the case of bone marrow transplantation for treatment of lysosomal storage diseases. We do know there are longterm remissions from the expected progressive course of the disease. Positive improvements have been obtained in patients so far studied.

A phase III study is aimed at defining the better methods of obtaining improved clinical result. The comparisons to be made include changes noted above in methods of preparation for transplant, prevention of graft-vs-host disease and infection. A wider use of unrelated matched donors has become feasible within the past two years because of the establishment of bone marrow donor registries. In future, the use of hematopoietic growth factors might add another dimension to improvement in engraftment as well as more rapid and extensive entrance of enzyme through monocyte proliferation.

SUMMARY

Enzyme repletion can now be accomplished by bone marrow transplantation. The new enzyme provided by bone marrow transplantation is maintained in the recipient at the level found in a normal donor and will last for a lifetime. The new enzyme is qualitatively normal and is replenished in the recipient at the same rate as in a normal donor. The new enzyme is present equally in neutrophils, lymphocytes, platelets and monocytes. The new enzyme by transport through wandering monocytes can enter into liver, lung, lymph nodes, tonsils, pulmonary, peritoneal and brain (microglial) reticuloendothelial system. The new set of reticuloendothelial cells then can provide clearance of previously accumulated substrate and prevent further deleterious damage.

Enzyme repletion as noted above has been accomplished in several mucopolysaccharidosis disease entities. Patients with Hurlers (I-H), Sanfilippo (A and B III), Hunters (II), and Maroteaux-Lamy have been engrafted permanently. Patients with sphingolipidosis also have had enzyme repletion provided by bone marrow transplantation. Cases of Gaucher's disease, both nonneuropathic and neuropathic, Krabbe disease, Niemann-Pick Disease A and adrenoleukodystrophy and metachromatic leukodystrophy have also been permanently engrafted.

The clinical resultant in each patient, of necessity, will vary because of previous accumulation of substrate and accompanying preexisting organ damage. But, in each case in which engraftment is permanently present with enzyme repletion, there has been marked improvement. Further, mental retardation has been prevented and in some instances average intelligence has been obtained. Since enzyme repletion has been present for 7 years in the patient with the longest engraftment, the full effect cannot be assessed.

The visceral (cardiac, lung, liver, spleen, and tonsil) component by enzyme repletion has reversed the pathophysiologic effects which had in the past caused death of these individuals. Death had occurred previously in such patients as mucopolysaccharidosis Hurler type I-H by 4–10 years of age. With remission of the disease process by enzyme repletion, the life span of such engrafted individuals should be extended manyfold.

Growth impairment resulting in dwarf status had been the typical fate of patients. Physical disfigurement, for which the term gargoyle was used for the description of this disease, has been a striking feature. Subsequent to enzyme repletion by bone marrow transplantation, growth and loss of severity of abnormal facies can now be expected.

Mortality and morbidity of bone marrow transplantation procedure depend upon advances being made in developing science of preparative regimens and prevention of graft-vs.-host disease.

Graft-vs.-host disease, acute and chronic failure of the graft, infection, and central nervous system crises are problems which need to be overcome. In the very near future, one can anticipate further decreases in morbidity and mortality. The use of unrelated donors from the National Bone Marrow Registry has been increasing rapidly in the past two years. This source of donors will increase the opportunities for bone marrow transplantation since only a third of the patients have either a sibling HLA genotypically identical or a matched related donor other than sibling. The experience in use of the unrelated donors for lysosomal storage disease has already proven of great interest (62). The use of unrelated matched donors for lysosomal storage diseases is based upon the success noted in treatment of leukemia and other malignancies (63–65).

A new epoch has arrived relative to lysosomal storage defects. There are numerous other diseases for which bone marrow transplantation is feasible. *In utero* transplantation in animals is now being successfully done. Transgenic accomplishments are also successfully achieved. Truly, we have entered a new and exciting era of therapeutic endeavors for these otherwise sad, unfortunate, and heretofore untreatable patients.

REFERENCES

1. Neufeld EF: Replacement of genotype specific proteins in mucopolysaccharidosis enzyme therapy in genetic disease. In, Desnick RJ, Bernlohr RW, Krivit W (eds): *Birth Defects March of Dimes Original Series* Vol. IX, No. 2. New York, Alan R. Liss, 1973, pp. 27–30.
2. Kihara H, Porter MT, Fluharty AL: Enzyme replacement in cultured fibroblasts from metachromatic leukodystrophy. (Ibid), pp. 19–26.
3. Weismann VN, Rosi EE, Hirschowitz NN: Treatment of metachromatic leukodystrophy fibroblasts by enzyme replacement. *N Engl J Med* 1971;204:672–673.
4. Conzelmann E, Sandhoff K: Partial enzyme deficiencies; residual activities and the development of neurological disorders. *Dev Neurosci* 1983/1984;6:58–71.

5. Olsen I, Muir H, Smith R, et al.: Direct enzyme transfer from lymphocytes is specific. *Nature* 1983;306:75–77.

6. Abraham D, Muir H, Olsen I, Winchester B. Direct enzyme transfer from lymphocytes corrects a lysosomal storage. *Biochem Biophys Res Comm* 1985;129:415–417.

7. Brooks SE, Adachi M, Hoffman LM, et al.: Enzymatic biochemical and morphological correction of Tay-Sachs disease glial cells *in vitro*. In, Calahan W, Lowden JL (eds): *Lysosomes and Lysosomal Storage Diseases*. New York, Raven Press, 1981, pp. 195–203.

8. Gruber HE, Koienker R, Lichtman A, et al.: Glial cells metabolically cooperate: Potential requirements for gene replacement therapy. *Proc Natl Acad Sci USA* 1985;82:6662–6666.

9. Konigsmark BW, Sidman RL. Origin of brain macrophages in the mouse. *J Neuropathol Exp Neurol* 1983;22:643–648.

10. Kosunen TV, Wahsman BH, Samuelsson IK: Radioautograph study of cellular mechanisms in delayed hypersensitivity. *J Neuropathol Exp Neurol* 1963;22:367–374.

11. Hoogerbrugge PM, Suzuki K, et al.: Donor derived cells in the central nervous system of twitcher mice after bone marrow transplantation, *Science* 1988, 239: 1035–1039.

12. Oehmichen M: Mononuclear phagocytes in the central nervous system. New York: Springer-Verlag, 1978.

13. Oehmichen M: Are resting and/or reactive microglia macrophages? *Immunobiology* 1982;161:246–254.

14. Hickey NF, Kimura H: Perivascular Microglial Cells of the CNS Are Bone Marrow Derived and Present Antigen *In Vivo*. *Science* 1988;239:290–292.

15. Kobayashi S, Katayama M, Bourque E, et al.: The twitcher mouse: Positive immuno-histochemical staining of globoid cells with monoclonal antibody against Mac-1-antigen. *Develop Brain Res* 1985;20:49–54.

16. Ting JPY, Nixon DF, Weiner LP, Frelinger JA: Brain Ia Antigen Have a Bone Marrow Origin. *Immunogenetics* 1983;17:295–301.

17. Bartlett PF: Pluripotential hemopoietic stem cells in adult mouse brain. *Proc Natl Acad Sci USA* 1982;79:2722.

18. Hoogerbrugge PM, Wagemaker G, Van Bekkum DW: Failure to demonstrate pluripotential hemopoietic stem cells in mouse brain. *Proc Natl Acad Sci* 1985;82:4268.

19. Choi BH: Hematogenous cells in the central nervous system of developing human embryos and fetuses. *J Compar Neurol* 1981;196:683–694.

20. Shull RM, Hastings, NE, Selcer RR, *et al:* Bone marrow transplantation in canine mucopolysaccharidosis I: Effects within the central nervous system. *J Clin Invest* 1987;79:435–443.

21. Taylor RM, Stewart GJ, Farrow BRH: Enzyme replacement in nervous tissue after alloge-neic bone marrow transplantation for fucosidosis in dogs. *Lancet* 1986;2:722.

22. Taylor RM, Farrow BRH, Stewart GJ: Correction of enzyme deficiency by allogeneic bone marrow transplantation following total lymphoid irradiation in dogs with lysosomal storage disease (Fucosidosis). *Transpl Proc XVIII* 1986;2:326–329.

23. Yeager AM, Ichioka T, Toyoshima Y, et al.: The twitcher mouse; a model of a human sphingolipidosis (Krabbe disease) in murine globoid cell leukodystrophy. In, Baum SJ, Santos GW, Takaku (eds): Recent Advances and Future Directions in Bone Marrow Transplantation. *Experimental Hematology Today*. New York, Springer-Verlag, 1987, pp. 36–44.

24. Sakiyama T, Tsuda M, Jok K, et al.: Bone marrow transplantation for Niemann-Pick mice. *Biochem Biophys Res Commun* 1983;113:605–610.

25. Jolly RD, Thompson KG, Murphy CE, et al.: Enzyme replacement therapy; an experiment of nature in a chimeric mannosidosis calf. *Pediatr Res* 1976;224:10219.

26. Wenger DA, Gasper PW, Thrall MA: Feline arylsulfatase B deficiency (mucopolysac-charidosis VI); correction by bone marrow transplantation. *Am J Hum Genet* 1984;36(Suppl 1):80S.

27. Hoogerbrugge PM, Poorthius BJHM, Wagemaker G, Van Bekkum DW: Bone marrow correction of lysosomal enzyme deficiency in various organs of β-glucuronidase deficient mice by allogeneic bone marrow transplantation. *Transplantation* 1987;43(5):609–614.

28. Tuchman M, Blazar BR, Krivit W: Brain catalase activity following syngeneic bone marrow transplantation in acatalasemic mice. March of Dimes Birth Defects Original Article Series, Vol. 22, No. 1. In, Krivit W, Paul NW (eds): *Bone Marrow Transplantation for Treatment of Lysosomal Storage Diseases*. Alan R. Liss, Inc., New York, 1986, pp. 165–176.

29. Krivit W, Lipton ME, Lockman LA, et al.: Prevention of deterioration in metachromatic leukodystrophy by bone marrow transplantation. *Amer J Med Sci* 1987; pp. 80–85.
30. Lipton M, Lockman LA, Ramsay NKC, et al.: Bone marrow transplantation in metachromatic leukodystrophy. March of Dimes Original Birth Defects Series, Vol. 22, No. 1. In, Krivit W, Paul NW (eds): *Bone Marrow Transplantation for Treatment of Lysosomal Storage Diseases.* New York, Alan R. Liss, 1986, pp. 57–69.
31. Krivit W, Whitley CB, Lund G, et al.: Improvement of clinical expression of central nervous system manifestations in lysosomal storage diseases treated by bone marrow transplantation. Experimental Hematology. In, Baum SJ, Santos GW, Takaku F (eds): *Recent Advances and Future Directions in Bone Marrow Transplantation.* New York, Springer-Verlag, 1987, pp. 189–194.
32. Kihara H: Genetic heterogeneity in metachromatic leukodystrophy. *Am J Hum Genet* 1982;34:171–181.
33. MacFaul R, Cavanaugh N, Lake BD, et al.: Metachromatic leukodystrophy: review of 38 cases. *Arch Dis Child* 1982;57:168–175.
34. Clarke JTR, Skomorowski MA, and Chang PL: Marked clinical difference between two sibs affected with juvenile metachromatic leukodystrophy. *Am J of Med Genet* 1986;33:10–13.
35. Bayever E, Ladisch S, Phillipart M, et al.: Bone marrow transplantation for metachromatic leukodystrophy. *Lancet* 1985;1:471–473.
36. Ladisch S, Bayever E, Phillippart M, Feig S: Biochemical findings after bone marrow transplantation for metachromatic leukodystrophy. In, Krivit W (ed): Birth Defects: March of Dimes: Original Article Series. New York, Alan R. Liss, 1986;22:7–24.
37. Whitley CB, Ramsay NKC, Kersey JH, Krivit W: Bone marrow transplantation for Hurler syndrome; assessment of metabolic correction. March of Dimes Original Birth Defects Series, Vol. 22, No. 1. In, Krivit W, Paul NW (eds): *Bone Marrow Transplantation for Treatment of Lysosomal Storage Diseases.* New York, Alan R. Liss, Inc., 1986, pp. 57–69.
38. Hugh-Jones K: Psychomotor development of children with mucopolysaccharidosis I-H following bone marrow transplantation. In, Krivit W (ed): Birth Defects: Original Article Series, New York, Alan R. Liss, 1986;22:25–29.
39. Whitley CB, Ramsay NKC, Kersey JH, Krivit W: Progressive elevation of CSF glycosaminoglycan in neuropathic mucopolysaccharidosis and normal levels after bone marrow transplantation. *Am J Hum Genet* 1986;38:A87.
40. Whitley CB, Lockman LA, Lipton ME, et al.: A blood brain gateway; access to the central nervous system after bone marrow transplantation for lysosomal storage disease. *Clin Res* 1986;34:964A.
41. Summers CG, Purple LR, Krivit W, et al.: Ocular changes in the mucopolysaccaridoses after bone marrow transplantation: a preliminary report. *Ophthalmology,* 1989;96:977–985.
42. Caruso RC, Kaiser-Kupfer MI, Meunzer J, et al.: Electroretinographic findings in the mucopolysaccharidoses. *Ophthalmology* 1986;93:1612–1616.
43. Malone BM, Whitley CB, Duvall AJ, et al.: Resolution of sleep apnea in Hurler disease after bone marrow transplantation. *J Pediatr Otolaryngol* 1988;15:23–31.
44. Hugh-Jones K, Kendra J, James DCO, Hobbs JR: Treatment of Sanfilippo disease (MPS IIIA) by bone marrow transplantation. *Exper Hematol* 1983;19(10):50–51.
45. Krivit W, Pierpont ME, Ayaz T, et al.: Bone marrow transplantation in the Maroteaux-Lamy syndrome (mucopolysaccharidosis Type VI); biochemical and clinical status 24 months after transplantation. *N Eng J Med* 1983;311:1606–1611.
46. McGovern MM, Ludman MD, Short MP, et al.: Bone marrow transplantation in Maroteaux-Lamy syndrome (MPS type 6); status 40 months after marrow transplant. In, *Bone Marrow Transplantation for Treatment of Lysosomal Storage Diseases.* Birth Defects: Original Article Series, Vol. 22, No. 1, New York, Alan R. Liss, 1986; pp. 41–53.
47. Deeg JH, Storb R, Thomas ED, et al.: Cataracts after total body irradiation and bone marrow transplantation; a sparing effect of dose fractionation. *Int J Radiat Oncol Biol Phy* 1984;10:957–964.
48. Blazar BR, Ramsay NKC, Kersey JH, et al.: Pretransplant conditioning with busulfan (myleran) and cyclophosphamide for nonmalignant diseases; failure of complete engraftment following histocompatible allogeneic bone marrow transplantation. *Transplantation* 1985;39:597–603.
49. Blazar BR, Whitley CB, Desnick RJ, et al.: Correlation of enzymatic analysis with evidence

of engraftment in patients with congenital enzymatic deficiency disorders receiving allogeneic marrow transplantation. In, Krivit W, Paul J, (eds): March of Dimes Original Birth Defects Series, Vol. 22, No. 1. New York, Alan R. Liss, 1986.

50. Krivit W: Introduction and conclusions on ethics, cost and future of bone marrow transplantation for lysosomal storage diseases. In, Krivit W, Paul J (eds): March of Dimes Original Birth Defects Series, Vol 23, No. 1, 1986, pp. 1–6, and pp. 189–194.

51. Krivit W: Inborn errors of metabolism treated by bone marrow transplantation. In, Hollaender A, Lashen A, Rogers P (eds): *Basic Biology of New Developments in Biotechnology.* New York, Plenum Publishing Corp., 1986, pp. 63–76.

52. Krivit W, Whitley CB: Bone marrow transplantation for genetic diseases. *N Engl J Med* 1986;316:1085–1087.

53. Hobbs JR, Hugh-Jones K, Chambers JD, et al.: Lysosomal enzyme replacement therapy by displacement bone marrow transplantation with immunoprophylaxis. *Adv Clin Enzymol* 1986;3:184–201.

54. Desnick RJ, et al.: In, Kabach MM, Shapiro S, (eds): *Bone Marrow Transplantation in Genetic Diseases; A Status Report.* 92nd Ross Conference on Pediatric Research, Frontiers in Genetic Medicine, June 1–4, 1986. 1987, pp. 71–97.

55. Yeager AM: Personal communication to the author, 1988.

56. Hugh-Jones K: Personal communication to the author, 1988.

57. Desnick RJ: Personal communication to the author, 1988.

58. Blazar BR, Krivit, W, Grachow LB: Personal communication to the author, 1988 (submitted to *Blood*).

59. Unger E, Krivit W, Sung JH, et al.: Determination by Y chromosome in-situ hybrization of origin of donor derived microglia cells in the central nervous system of humans after bone marrow transplantation. 1989 (submitted to *Science*).

60. Hoogerbrugge PM, Suzuki K, Poorthuis BJHM, et al.: Donor derived cells in the central nervous system of twitcher mice after bone marrow transplantation. *Science* 1988;239:1035–1039.

61. Perry VH, Gordon S: Macrophages and microglia in the nervous system. *Trends in Neuroscience* 1988;11:273–277.

62. Krivit W, et al.: A summary of 75 patients with lysosomal storage diseases treated by bone marrow transplantation in the United States in eighteen institutions. In Press: Hobbs J: Transaction of the COGENT International Meeting, Westminster Medical School, July 29–30, 1989.

63. Beatty PG, Clift RA, Mickelson EM, et al.: Marrow transplantation from related donors other than HLA-identical siblings. *N Engl J Med* 313(13):765–771.

64. Anasetti C, Amos D, Beatty PG, et al: Effect of HLA compatability on engraftment of bone marrow transplants in patients with leukemia or lymphoma. *N Engl J Med* 320(4):197–204.

Bone Marrow Transplantation in Children, edited by F. Leonard Johnson and Carl Pochedly. Raven Press, Ltd., New York © 1990.

Autologous Bone Marrow Transplantation for the Treatment of Sarcomas

James S. Miser

Division of Pediatric Hematology/Oncology, Mayo Clinic, Department of Pediatrics, Mayo Medical School, Rochester, Minnesota 55905

Introduction
A. Autologous bone marrow transplantation for recurrent disease
B. Autologous bone marrow transplantation as end intensification therapy
Summary

INTRODUCTION

The use of autologous bone marrow transplantation has allowed the development of high-dose chemotherapeutic regimens and regimens using total body irradiation with chemotherapy. These regimens would otherwise result in prolonged or permanent bone marrow hypoplasia if administered without reconstitution with cryopreserved autologous bone marrow. Dose response curves have not been established for chemotherapeutic agents in the treatment of sarcomas. However, it has recently been observed that the complete remission rate for advanced small cell sarcomas of children and young adults can be improved from 50 to 70%, using conventional doses and schedules, to a remission rate of over 90% using a dose intensity that is 50 to 100% higher. These observations support the concept of a dose response curve for chemotherapy of these high-risk and metastatic sarcomas (1).

The majority of small cell sarcomas have been shown to be responsive to both radiotherapy and chemotherapy. This conclusion is based on the lack of local recurrence for most small cell sarcomas at the primary site when radiation therapy at conventional fractionation has been used in combination with chemotherapy, but without surgical excision of the tumor (2,3). Also, recurrent small cell sarcomas respond favorably to radiation therapy alone given for local control of the tumor. Based on this clinical experience, the use of total body irradiation, delivered in a single fraction or in a limited number of fractions, appears to be an additional systemic therapy to be used to treat micrometastases.

AUTOLOGOUS BONE MARROW TRANSPLANTATION FOR RECURRENT DISEASE

The use of autologous bone marrow transplantation as a means to allow the administration of high-dose chemotherapy or total body irradiation has increased in the past 5 years. Its use in the treatment of patients with sarcomas has been primarily restricted to patients who have suffered a relapse or are refractory to conventional therapy (4–13). The important information that has been derived from this approach is that (1) intensive therapy can be delivered without excessive toxicity and (2) this therapy can result in significant regression of measurable tumor (4–13). Unfortunately, virtually all of the responses in patients with overt recurrence of malignant disease have been transient (6–13). Nevertheless, the failure of this approach in permanently controlling gross recurrent tumors does not lessen importance of the observation that giving total body irradiation and high-dose chemotherapy have significant activity against various malignant tumors.

Limited studies in recurrent rhabdomyosarcomas have been undertaken. Use of the combination of high-dose busulphan and cyclophosphamide in one patient with recurrent rhabdomyosarcoma showed a complete remission of the tumor (8). Similarly, Eckert used high-dose cyclophosphamide, DTIC (Decarbazine) and Doxorubicin (adriamycin) for patients with advanced rhabdomyosarcoma and achieved complete remissions in 2 out of the 4 patients (10). In another study using high-dose BCNU, 3 out of 4 patients showed favorable responses (11).

The responsiveness of recurrent Ewing's sarcoma to high-dose chemotherapy has also been explored with use of high doses of melphalan (6,7,12,13). A number of investigators have observed excellent initial responses to this agent, but the responses have been brief. However, the important conclusion is that melphalan administered at high doses is active in the treatment of Ewing's sarcoma (6,7,12,13).

AUTOLOGOUS BONE MARROW TRANSPLANTATION AS END INTENSIFICATION THERAPY

The effectiveness of total body irradiation in preventing the occurrence of metastases has been suggested by 2 different clinical observations. First, Jenkin observed that a single dose of 300 cGy of total body irradiation when combined with chemotherapy resulted in long-term remissions in a small number of patients who had metastases (14). Second, the first Intergroup Ewing's Sarcoma Study showed the effectiveness of pulmonary irradiation in preventing subsequent pulmonary metastases (3). Use of a regimen including hemibody irradiation in patients with recurrent Ewing's sarcoma also showed that this tumor is responsive to total body irradiation (15). In another study, however, hemibody irradiation delivered as a systemic adjuvant therapy showed no lasting benefit (16).

Based on these observations in patients with recurrent tumors, others evaluated total body irradiation as systemic adjuvant therapy of Ewing's sarcoma. The initial approach used a low dose fractionated schedule of 300 cGy per week for 5 weeks in patients with high-risk Ewing's sarcomas, that is, patients with central axis primaries or those with metastases (17). The radiation was delivered without autologous bone marrow reinfusion to patients who received a standard chemotherapy regimen (consisting of vincristine, dactinomycin, adriamycin, cyclophosphamide, and DTIC) together with irradiation therapy to the primary site. The long-term disease-free survival of these patients is now 25% at 7 to 10 years following their initial diagnosis.

Based on the results of *in vitro* radiation, survival and repair studies of tumor cell lines established from patients with recurrent Ewing's sarcoma, a high-dose radiation regimen was subsequently developed (1,18). It was believed that these cell lines represent a "resistant" subpopulation of Ewing's sarcoma cells that persist as subclinical disease in patients treated initially with both radiation and chemotherapy. The *in vitro* radiation survival curve for these Ewing's cells showed a large shoulder, implying that these cells have a significant capacity to repair sublethal radiation damage when exposed to a single dose of less than 400 cGy (18). Furthermore, experiments on plateau phase cells showed no repair of potentially lethal damage after exposure to 450 cGy of irradiation (18). As a result of these *in vitro* studies, a high-dose schedule consisting of two 400 cGy fractions separated by 24 hours and delivered at 10 to 15 cGy per minute was evaluated as a systemic adjuvant in patients who had achieved complete remission (1). Radiation survival curves of normal bone marrow cells exposed to the two 400 cGy fractions suggested that prolonged myelosuppression would occur if autologous bone marrow reconstitution is not provided. Thus, previously extracted, unpurged, cryopreserved bone marrow was reinfused into these patients after the total body irradiation was delivered (18).

Pilot studies in patients in relapse showed that high-dose chemotherapy and total body irradiation could induce only short-lived responses in patients with overt, grossly measurable tumors. As a result, this protocol was designed to be delivered only to patients who by clinical examination were in complete remission or who had at most only microscopic residual disease (1).

Although the outcome for many children and adolescents with sarcomas has significantly improved over the past 15 years, a large proportion of patients still have a poor long-term outcome (2,19–26). Patients with stage III rhabdomyosarcoma, who have large tumors of the retroperitoneum, chest wall, perineum, or extremities, have a significantly lower rate of disease-free survival than (1) those with stage I or II rhabdomyosarcomas, or (2) those with stage III tumors at selected sites of the head or in the paratesticular region (2,19–21). Similarly, Ewing's sarcoma is associated with a poorer prognosis when it arises in a central axis site or is associated with a large soft tissue mass (22,23,25,26). Furthermore, patients who have sarcomas with metastases at the time of diagnosis have had a very low rate of disease-free survival, especially when the metastases involve the bone or bone marrow (2,21,24).

With the improvements in chemotherapy and local radiation therapy, the rate of complete remission for this group of patients has improved; however, the relapse rate has remained high. Thus, the results are poor when standard therapy consisting of chemotherapy and local irradiation is used. Because of these poor results, a group of newly diagnosed patients with high-risk sarcomas, who had a projected overall rate of prolonged disease-free survival of less than 25% when treated with standard therapy, was used to evaluate the effectiveness of adjuvant total body irradiation (27). These patients had either (1) stage III rhabdomyosarcomas of the perineum, retroperitoneum extremity or trunk; (2) stage IV rhabdomyosarcomas at any site; (3) a Ewing's sarcoma of the central axis (humerus, femur, chest wall or pelvis); or (4) a Ewing's sarcoma at any site with presence of metastases. Subsequent review of the histopathology of these sarcomas suggested that diagnostic variants of rhabdomyosarcoma and Ewing's sarcoma existed, which included primitive sarcomas of bone and soft tissue (28) and primitive tumors with evidence of neural differentiation of both bone and soft tissue (29). These other soft tissue tumors were staged as rhabdomyosarcomas and the other bone tumors were staged as Ewing's sarcomas. Use of this experimental approach was justified because of the high risk of relapse of these patients when treated with standard therapy alone, and because treatment failure in this group of high-risk patients is usually in the form of systemic metastases.

Ninety-four patients who had high risk sarcomas or primitive neural tumors were treated according to two chemotherapy induction programs from 1981 to 1986 (27). Of these patients, 80 achieved a complete remission and were eligible for treatment with autologous bone marrow transplantation. Twelve patients did not undergo the procedure: 6 of these refused further therapy, 4 relapsed just prior to the procedure, and 2 had major toxicity that precluded further chemotherapy or radiotherapy. The remaining 68 patients underwent autologous bone marrow transplantation as a form of consolidation. All of these 68 patients were in clinical complete remission as determined by computerized tomography, chest radiograph, bone scan, and physical examination. Thirty patients had Ewing's sarcoma, 18 had rhabdomyosarcoma, 10 had primitive sarcomas, and 10 had primitive neural tumor (9 being identified as peripheral neuroepithelioma and 1 as neuroblastoma). Thirty-five of the pa-

TABLE 1. *Treatment schema for autologous bone marrow transplantation**

Day	Treatment
1	TBI
2	TBI
3	VCR, Adria, Cyclo
4	Adria, Cyclo
5	Rest
6	Bone Marrow Infusion

*See text.
TBI   = total body irradiation
VCR   = vincristine
Adria   = adriamycin
Cyclo = cyclophosphamide

tients had metastases at diagnosis: 15 of these had involvement of the bone marrow and only 4 patients had solitary metastases (2 in bone and 2 in lung).

The consolidation therapy schedule is outlined in Table 1. The two daily doses of total body irradiation (given at 400 cGy/day) were followed by two days of chemotherapy consisting of vincristine (2.0 mg/m^2 given on day 3, maximum total dose 2.0 mg), adriamycin (35 mg/m^2/day given on days 3 and 4), and cyclophosphamide (1200 mg/m^2/day given on days 3 and 4). The autologous bone marrow was reinfused on day 6, two days following completion of chemotherapy.

At 30 months following the autologous bone marrow transplantation in these patients, the overall survival rate was 51%, the rate of disease-free survival was 41%, and adverse events (relapse or death) occurred in 65% of cases (Figure 1). Furthermore, the pattern of relapse was not different from that seen in patients treated in a conventional fashion without autologous reconstitution. This observation suggested that the main cause of relapse was not reinfusion of tumor cells, but rather, failure to eradicate the micrometastases with the preparative regimen.

The most important factor influencing the overall outcome of this therapy was the extent of disease at diagnosis (Figure 2). The rate of adverse event-free survival of those patients who had no metastases at diagnosis was 50% at 30 months, compared to a rate of event-free survival of only 20% for those who had metastases at the time of diagnosis. This difference in event-free survival rates was independent of histologic type of the tumor. The significantly worse outcome for patients who had metastases at the time of diagnosis suggests that, even when clinical complete remission is achieved, complete remission, as defined by the presently available imaging studies, is in fact a very crude estimate of the amount of residual disease. Furthermore, the results of this study suggest that the patient who has metastases at the time of diagnosis probably has a larger and more resistant tumor cell burden when

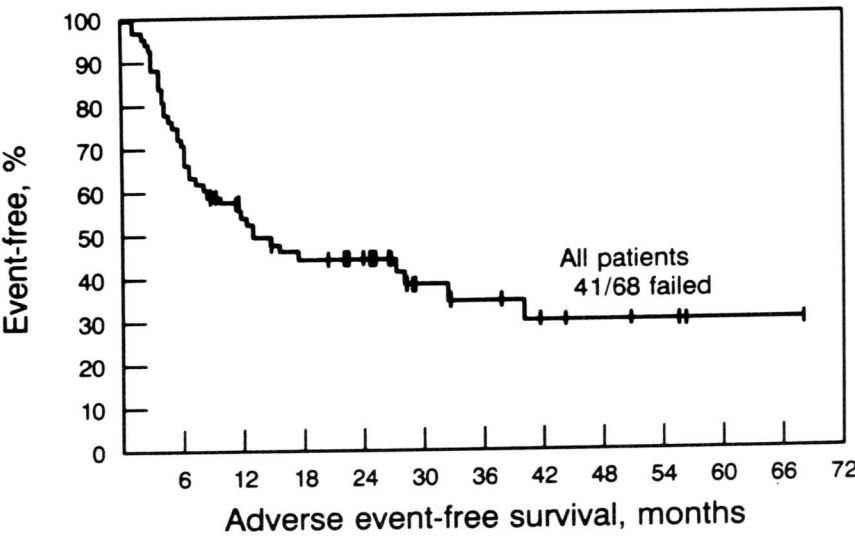

FIG. 1. The adverse event-free survival of all 68 patients.

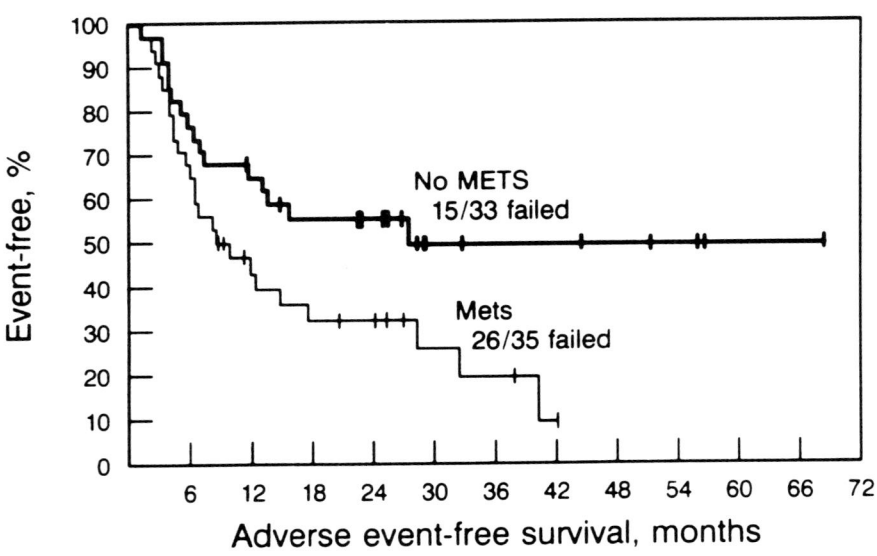

FIG. 2. A comparison of the rate of adverse event-free survival of 35 patients who had metastases at the time of diagnosis to that of 33 patients who had no metastases at diagnosis.

"clinical complete remission" is achieved than a patient who did not have metastases at diagnosis. Moreover, the results of this study suggest that the therapeutic strategies used in regimens that include autologous bone marrow transplantation should be different for patients with metastases at diagnosis compared to those who have no evidence of metastases at diagnosis.

This program of therapy was originally designed for the treatment of patients with Ewing's sarcoma and was based on *in vitro* and *in vivo* experience with this tumor. Thus, it was of interest to compare the outcome of therapy for patients with Ewing's sarcoma with the outcome of patients with other diagnoses treated according to this program (Figure 3). The adverse event-free survival rate for the patients with Ewing's sarcoma was approximately 50% at 30 months. This was compared to a rate of adverse event-free survival of only 25% for all other histologic categories, including rhabdomyosarcoma, primitive sarcoma, and primitive neural tumors. However, when corrected for extent of disease, the only trend was that in favor of the Ewing's group. This program of therapy was employed in 10 additional patients with Ewing's sarcoma, resulting in an actuarial 2-year relapse-free survival rate of 85% (30). This result compared favorably to previous experience in which melphalan was used in 10 patients as an end intensification therapy where the rate of 2-year relapse-free survival was only 20%.

The combined experience in treatment of these 40 patients using this regimen suggests that (1) total body irradiation may play an important role in the

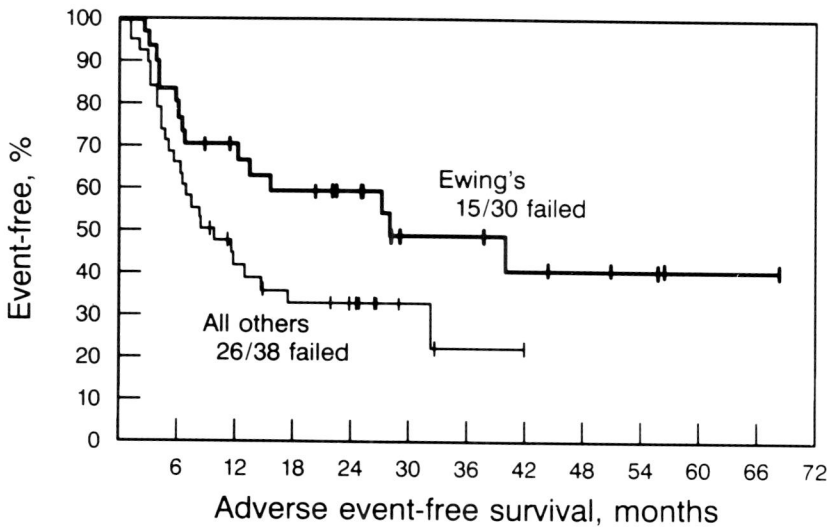

FIG. 3. A comparison of the rate of adverse event-free survival of 30 patients with Ewing's sarcoma compared to that of 38 patients who had other histologic diagnoses.

treatment of high-risk Ewing's sarcoma and (2) further clinical trials evaluating this modality are warranted. The role of total body irradiation in treatment of patients with other types of tumors is less well established. However, the results following use of this therapy in patients who have metastases in the bone marrow compare favorably to the results of the Intergroup Rhabdomyosarcoma Study (21).

Reduction of tumor bulk by surgery is included as a part of several programs of therapy, being carried out before the patient is given intensive anticancer therapy and autologous bone marrow transplantation. When surgery is required to achieve complete remission, however, it is likely that the complete remission thus achieved is different from that achieved with chemotherapy and radiation. Furthermore, incomplete response to the chemotherapy, radiation, or to the combination of the two, indicates that the tumor will be relatively resistant to subsequent total body irradiation. This resistance to TBI may be due either to an intrinsic tumor cell resistance or to a higher tumor cell burden with quantitative resistance to therapy. The 5 patients who required "debulking" surgery in order to eradicate tumor that had been incompletely responsive to chemotherapy, did poorly (Figure 4). The experience with these 5 patients at least raises the question as to whether surgical debulking before intensive therapy is an effective strategy, especially if the residual tumor is relatively resistant to intensive combined therapy with irradiation and chemotherapy.

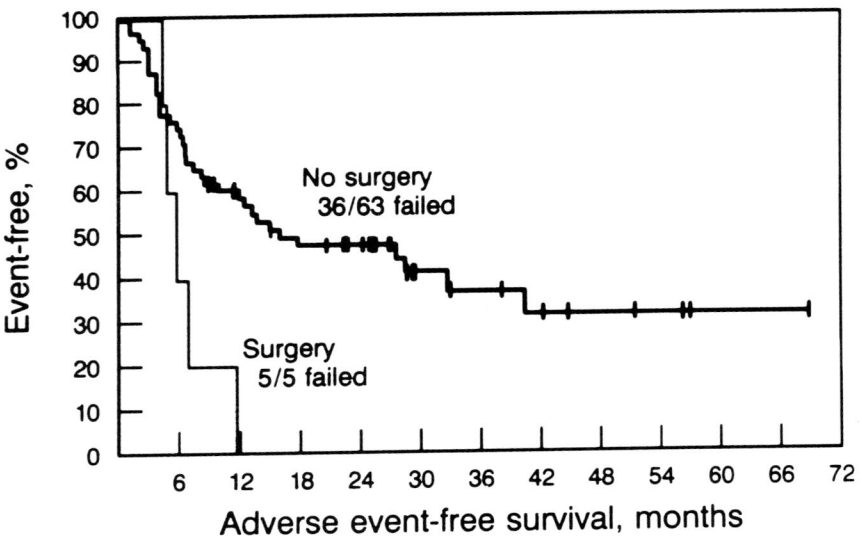

FIG. 4. A comparison of the rate of adverse event-free survival of 5 patients who required surgery with or without intraoperative irradiation to achieve complete remission to that of the 63 patients who achieved complete remission following use of chemotherapy and irradiation alone.

The majority of patients treated with an intensive therapy program followed by autologous bone marrow transplantation, even those who are in their first remission, can still be expected to relapse. Thus, it is clear that more effective induction and consolidation therapies need to be developed. It is likely that intensive therapies used in conjunction with autologous bone marrow transplantation will need to be variable depending on both the histologic diagnosis of the tumor and the extent of tumor growth and presence of metastases.

Also, with the marked improvements in supportive care and the advances in the technology of marrow transplantation, the major limitation in applying autologous bone marrow transplantation in treatment of high-risk sarcomas is the availability of effective regimens to eradicate the residual tumor. Further development of effective consolidation regimens and their evaluation in subsequent randomized studies will be required, however, before the use of intensive therapy and autologous bone marrow transplantation in first or second remission can be generally advocated in the treatment of sarcomas.

SUMMARY

Although small cell sarcomas are both chemosensitive and radioresponsive, patients with extensive local or systemic disease continue to have a high rate of recurrence. The use of high-dose chemotherapy following relapse has demonstrated that these recurrent tumors are responsive to high-dose therapy. Based on this experience, as well as on *in vitro* and *in vivo* studies of total body irradiation, use of intensive therapy with total body irradiation combined with autologous marrow transplantation, was evaluated in first remission in an attempt to prevent relapse. The outcome of this approach was related to the extent of disease at diagnosis, the histologic diagnosis and the initial responsiveness to induction therapy. New regimens evaluated in randomized trials will be required before the use of intensive therapy can be generally advocated for the treatment of sarcomas.

REFERENCES

1. Miser JS, Steis RG, Longo DL, et al.: Treatment of newly diagnosed high risk sarcomas and primitive neuroectodermal tumors (PNET) in children and young adults. *Proc Am Soc Clin Oncol* 1985;4:240(C-935).
2. Maurer HM: The Intergroup Rhabdomyosarcoma Study. *Cancer Bull* 1982;34:108–110.
3. Nesbit ME, Perez CA, Tefft M, et al.: Multimodal therapy for the management of primary nonmetastatic Ewing's sarcoma of bone; an intergroup study. *Natl Cancer Inst Monogr* 1981;56:255–262.
4. Philip T, Armitage JO, Spitzer G, et al.: High-dose therapy and autologous bone marrow transplantation after failure of conventional chemotherapy in adults with intermediate-grade or high-grade non-Hodgkin's lymphoma. *N Engl J Med* 1987;316:1493–1498.
5. Seeger R, Lenarsky C, Moss T, et al.: Bone marrow transplantation of poor prognosis neuroblastoma. *Proc Am Soc Clin Oncol* 1987;6:221.
6. Graham-Pole J, Lazarus HM, Herzig RM, et al.: High-dose melphalan therapy for the

treatment of children with refractory neuroblastoma and Ewing's sarcoma. *Am J Pediatr Hematol Oncol* 1984;6:17–26.

7. Cornbleet MA, Corringham RET, Prentice HG, et al.: Treatment of Ewing's sarcoma with high-dose melphalan and autologous bone marrow transplantation. *Cancer Treat Rep* 1981; 65;241–244.

8. Hartman O, Benhamon E, Beaujean F, et al.: High-dose busulphan and cyclophosphamide with autologous bone marrow transplantation support in advanced malignancies in children. A phase II study. *J Clin Oncol* 1986;4:1804–1820.

9. Kingston JE, McElwain TJ, Malpas JS: Childhood rhabdomyosarcoma; experience of the Children's Solid Tumor Group. *Br J Cancer* 1983;48:195–207.

10. Ekert H, Ellis WM, Waters KD, et al.: Autologous bone marrow rescue in the treatment of advanced tumors of childhood. *Cancer* 1982;49:603–609.

11. Phillips GL, Fay JW, Herzig GP, et al.: Intensive 1,3 bis (2-chloroethyl)-nitrosourea (BCNU), NSC#4366650, and cryopreserved autologous bone marrow transplantation for refractory cancer. A phase I–II study. *Cancer* 1983;52:1792–1802.

12. Herzig RA, Phillips RL, Lazarus HM, et al.: Extensive chemotherapy and autologous bone marrow transplantation for the treatment of refractory malignancies. In Dicke KA, Spitzer G, Zander AR, et al., (eds): *Autologous Bone Marrow Transplantation*. Proceedings of the First International Symposium. The University of Texas M.D. Anderson Hospital and Tumor Institute, Houston, 1985, pp. 197–202.

13. Lazarus HM, Herzig RH, Graham-Pole J, et al.: Intensive melphalan chemotherapy and cryopreserved autologous bone marrow transplantation for the treatment of refractory cancer. *J Clin Oncol* 1983;1:359–362.

14. Jenkin RDT, Rider WD, Sonley MJ: Ewing's sarcoma; adjuvant total body irradiation, cyclophosphamide and vincristine. *Int J Radiat Oncol Biol Phys* 1976;1:407–413.

15. Evans RG, Burgert EO, Gilchrist GS, et al.: Sequential half-body irradiation and combination chemotherapy as salvage treatment for failed Ewing's sarcoma. A pilot study. *Int J Radiat Oncol Biol Phys* 1984;10:2363–2368.

16. Berry MP, Jenkin RDT, Harwood AR, et al.: Ewing's sarcoma; a trial of adjuvant chemotherapy and sequential half-body irradiation. *Int J Radiat Oncol Biol Phys* 1976;1:407–413.

17. Kinsella TJ, Glaubiger D, Deisseroth A, et al.: Intensive combined modality therapy including low-dose TBI in high-risk Ewing's sarcoma patients. *Int J Radiat Oncol Biol Phys* 1983;9:1955–1960.

18. Kinsella TJ, Mitchell JB, McPerson S, et al.: *In vitro* radiation studies on Ewing's sarcoma cell lines and human bone marrow; application to the clinical use of total body irradiation (TBI). *Int J Radiat Oncol Biol Phys* 1984;10:1005–1011.

19. Ransom JL, Pratt CB, Hustu HO, et al.: Retroperitoneal rhabdomyosarcoma in children. *Cancer* 1980;45:845–850.

20. Raney RB, Regab AH, Ruymann FB, et al.: Soft tissue sarcoma of the trunk in childhood. *Cancer* 1982;49:2612–2616.

21. Ruymann FB, Newton WA, Ragab AH, et al.: Bone marrow metastases at diagnosis in children and adolescents with rhabdomyosarcoma; a report from the Intergroup Rhabdomyosarcoma Study. *Cancer* 1984;53:368–373.

22. Gehan EA, Nesbit ME, Burgert EO, et al.: Prognostic factors in children with Ewing's sarcoma. *Natl Cancer Inst Monogr* 1981;56:273–278.

23. Glaubiger DL, Makuch R, Schwarz J, et al.: Determination of prognostic factors and their influence on therapeutic results in patients with Ewing's sarcoma. *Cancer* 1980;45:2213–2219.

24. Vietti TJ, Gehan EA, Nesbit ME, et al.: Multimodal therapy in metastatic Ewing's sarcoma; an intergroup study. *Natl Cancer Inst Monogr* 1981;56:279–284.

25. Mendenhall CM, Marcus RB, Enneking WF, et al.: The prognostic significance of soft tissue extension in Ewing's sarcoma. *Cancer* 1985;51:913–917.

26. Göbel U, Jurgens H, Etspuler M, et al.: Prognostic significance of tumor volume in localized Ewing's sarcoma of bone in children and adolescents. *J Cancer Res (Clin Oncol)* 1987;113:187–191.

27. Miser JS, Kinsella TJ, Triche TJ, et al.: Autologous bone marrow transplantation in first remission; consolidation therapy of high-risk sarcomas in children and young adults. (Submitted for publication, 1988.)

28. Tsokos M, Miser JS, Horowitz M, et al.: Primitive sarcoma of bone; a group of tumors resembling Ewing's sarcoma by light microscopy but with distinctive ultrastructural features. *Lab Invest* 1988;58:96A(570).
29. Miser JS, Kinsella TJ, Triche TJ, et al.: Treatment of peripheral neuroepithelioma in children and young adults. *J Clin Oncol* 1987;5:1752–1758.
30. Marcus RB, Graham-Pole JR, Springfield DS, et al.: High-risk Ewing's sarcoma; end intensification using bone marrow transplantation. *Int J Radiat Oncol Biol Phys* 1987;13S:181 (Abstra #176).

Bone Marrow Transplantation in
Children, edited by F. Leonard Johnson
and Carl Pochedly. Raven Press, Ltd.,
New York © 1990.

Pediatric Bone Marrow Transplantation Utilizing Unrelated Donors*

*James T. Casper, **Nancy Bunin, *Robert Truitt, *Bruce Camitta, and *Robert Ash

*Medical College of Wisconsin and Midwest Children's Cancer Center, Children's Hospital of Wisconsin, Milwaukee, Wisconsin 53201, and **Children's Hospital of Philadelphia and School of Medicine, University of Pennsylvania, Philadelphia, Pennsylvania

Introduction
A. Donor selection
B. Indications
C. Supportive measures
D. Conditioning regimen
E. Graft-vs.-host disease
F. Immune reconstitution
G. Current survival
Summary

INTRODUCTION

Bone marrow transplantation is now considered the treatment of choice for selected patients suffering from a number of diseases including severe aplastic anemia, immune deficiency disorders, and the leukemias (1–3). Lack of matched donors however is a limiting factor in further application of marrow transplantation in these disorders. Most patients will have only a 30 to 40% chance of having an HLA-compatible sibling to serve as a donor for marrow transplantation (4). However, transplants performed using related donors

*Preparation of this chapter was supported in part by the MACC Fund (Midwest Athletes Against Childhood Cancer), Milwaukee, Wisconsin.

who were mismatched for one or more antigens, have proved to be successful. Most notable has been the Seattle experience. Studies from this center have shown that in patients with leukemia a bone marrow transplant from a family member who was either phenotypically identical or who showed a one locus mismatch (A, B or DR), produced results that were equal to those of patients who received marrow from an HLA phenotypic and genotypic matched sibling (5). However, in cases with more than a single antigen mismatch, there was a significant increase in graft-vs.-host disease, and the infectious complications that are associated with graft-vs.-host disease, along with a decrease in rate of prolonged survival (5). This poor outcome especially occurred if the mismatch was in both the B and D regions.

Other transplant teams have also been successful in utilizing partially matched related donors (11-13). The success of this procedure is related to some extent to the disease being treated. Severe aplastic anemia has been the least rewarding disease to treat by mismatched transplantation, associated with a significant rate of graft rejection (40 to 50%) (9-10). Nearly all of these patients have been heavily transfused and rejection may be secondary to sensitization to major histocompatibility complex (MHC) antigens. Also, the early attempts at partially mismatched transplants did not always include a more intense conditioning regimen. The addition of total body irradiation (TBI) to the standard 4-day cyclophosphamide regimen has decreased the rejection rate in aplastic anemia.

The use of haplo-identical parents as donors for their offspring with severe combined immunodeficiency has met with the most success (11-13). Here the ability to reject is almost nonexistent and the problems of graft-vs.-host disease have been dramatically lessened after soybean lectin T cell depletion of the harvested marrow inoculum (11). Removal of 2–3 logs of T cells by this technique has significantly decreased the incidence of graft-vs.-host disease.

The role of unrelated donors for marrow transplantation is only now coming into sharper focus. The initial attempts at bone marrow transplantation using unrelated donors is depicted in Table 1. (14–21). The disease categories were primarily aplastic anemia and severe combined immune deficiency syndrome (SCIDS). Pre-transplant conditioning was none or minimal for SCIDS patients and the standard regimen of 4 days of cyclophosphamide was given to patients with aplastic anemia. There was successful engraftment in 6 of the 9 patients, but moderate to severe graft-vs.-host disease was detected in 5 out of 6 evaluable patients. Only 2 of these patients are known to be alive.

The role of major histocompatibility complex identity in determining a successful outcome is unclear in these early transplants. While all patients were mixed lymphocyte culture (MLC) compatible with their donors, 6 of 9 were mismatched for one antigen as determined by serological criteria. It must be remembered that our knowledge of the antigenic determinants has increased markedly in the past 10 years. The number of different HLA antigenic determinants (A, B, and DR) essentially doubled during this time pe-

TABLE 1. *The early results for pediatric bone marrow transplantation using unrelated donors.*

Patient	Age	Sex	Disease	Conditioning	HLA	MLC	Engraftment	GVHD	Current status	Reference
1	18 yrs	M	SAA	ALG	=	=	–	NE	Dead day 60; graft failure	19
2	5 mos	M	SCID	None	≠	=	+/–	+/–	Unknown	20
3	7 mos	M	SCID	None	≠	=	+	+	Dead day 31; CMV pneumonia	21
4	5 mos	M	SCID	Cyt	≠	=	+	+	Unknown; chronic GVHD	22
5	Unknown	M	SCID	None	≠	=	+/–	+/–	Dead day 15; pseudomonas	23
6	12 yrs	F	ALL	Cyt	=	=	+	–	Dead day 720; recurrent ALL	24
7	18 yrs	F	SAA	Cyt	≠	=	+	+	Dead day 1535; chronic GVHD	25
8	22 yrs	M	SAA	Cyt	≠	=	+	+	Alive day 1466+	25
9	5 yrs	M	SAA	Cyt	=	=	+	+	Alive day 2500+; chronic GVHD	26

SAA = severe aplastic anemia
SCID = severe combined immunodeficiency syndrome
ALL = acute lymphoblastic leukemia
ALG = antilymphocyte globulin
CYT = cyclophosphamide
TBI = total body irradiation

riod (22). We now also appreciate the significant linkage dysequilibrium between certain B and DR combinations (i.e., B8/DR3).

Over the past few years increasing numbers of marrow transplants using unrelated donors have been performed, and the results appear to be improving at this time. One must remember that when the initial transplants using HLA matched siblings were performed in the early 1970s, the selection of patients was such that almost all were high risk and a number of them had end-stage disease. Similarly, the vast majority of patients given unrelated marrow transplants were either heavily transfused aplastic anemia patients or patients with leukemia, and the patients with leukemia, even if they were not in the end stage of their disease, certainly exhibited resistant leukemia as evidenced by the number of recurrences.

In August 1987, the Congressional Office of Technology Assessment convened a meeting to discuss the current information regarding unrelated donor marrow transplants (23). The major participants in this meeting were from Milwaukee, Minneapolis, Seattle, London, Iowa City and New Orleans. Data were presented covering approximately 160 unrelated marrow transplants of whom about 40% are surviving 5–2500+ days.

The fact that many of the patients were at the end stage of their disease and received marrow from mismatched unrelated donors were reasons cited for the high morbidity and mortality. The major problems encountered were infection, nonengraftment and graft-vs.-host disease. These rates of morbidity and mortality are certainly no worse than those observed in the early days of transplantation when HLA-matched siblings were used. It is hoped these results will improve if fully matched donors can be located more quickly and if patients selected will be in better condition.

This chapter will review the donor selection process, disease categories, supportive measures, conditioning regimens, and quality of survival for the children who have had marrow transplants using unrelated donors. This information is difficult to glean from the literature since there are few reports dealing strictly with marrow transplants in children and utilizing unrelated donors. Therefore, the data cited here should not be construed to be inclusive of every transplant done in a child in whom the donor was unrelated. Rather, it is hoped that the reader will have a sense of where we are at the present time and what our goals should be for the future.

DONOR SELECTION

Obviously, the major impediment to performing unrelated bone marrow transplants lies in the recruitment of donors. The Anthony Nolan Bone Marrow Appeal, the first donor registry, was established in England in 1975 (24). The Laura Graves National Bone Marrow Transplant Foundation was established in 1981 to further the identification and recruitment of unrelated marrow donors in the United States (25). In 1986, the Caitlin Raymond International Donor Registry was set up.

More recently in this country bone marrow donor registries have been established through regional blood centers. Regional blood collection centers have access to large numbers of motivated donors. Also, these centers are already involved in public education, record keeping, inventory control, distribution and billing systems, and communication systems. Most important, these centers are able to provide HLA typing and computer-based donor registries (25,26). As an example, prospective donors have been identified among HLA-typed individuals who have volunteered to be on-call donors for HLA matched platelets. The Blood Center of Southeastern Wisconsin (BCSW) initiated a program to recruit bone marrow donors from its file on 11,000 HLA-typed on-call blood donors. Potential problems of a logistical, ethical, philosophical, medical and technical nature were addressed by this group (26).

As many as 88% of donors solicited by the Blood Center of Southeastern Wisconsin responded favorably, and none of the 763 donors contacted disapproved of being asked to donate bone marrow for a nonrelated individual (27). Marrow donors were individuals who donated whole blood regularly and had agreed to consider donating when blood of their particular type was needed by the blood program. These persons comprised a group motivated toward altruistic behavior, and are not necessarily typical of the population at large. These figures may not reflect the attitudes of individuals currently included on non-blood donor-derived registry lists.

In 1986, a National Bone Marrow Donor Registry was established under a contract from the United States Office of Naval Research given to a consortium of three blood service organizations. These organizations included the American Association of Blood Banks, the American Red Cross, and the Council of Community Blood Centers (23). While this registry is in its infancy (currently 15,000 registered donors as of December 1987), it certainly offers the potential for identifying numerous donors. Although the potential donor pool could increase markedly, since about 5,000,000 different individuals donate blood per year, the initial success encountered by the Blood Center of Southeastern Wisconsin in recruiting donors may not be attained. The BCSW recently reported that when donors were contacted regarding bone marrow donation for a specific patient, 70% (or 2155 out of 3065 contacted) agreed to donate their marrow. However, if blood donors were contacted in terms of signing up for the bone marrow donor registry, only about 25% agreed (1737 out of 6384) (28).

The issue of necessary donor pool size is continually evolving (29,30). Most transplant physicians agree that a donor base of 100,000 donors could result in the identification of "compatible" donors for approximately 10 to 50% of the patients (29). If one is willing to accept serological DR identity and a single A or B antigen mismatch in the direction of graft-vs.-host disease, this availability of compatible donors could be increased another 15 to 20% (29). This wide range is due to the different interpretations of the term "compatible" among the transplant centers.

Additional HLA-A, B, DR and DQ specificities have been identified as a result of new antisera which have "split" antigen determinants. For example, what would have been defined as HLA-A9 a few years ago has now been split into A23 and A24 (31). While these HLA types may be cross-reactive, they are nonetheless, two specific antigens. Obviously, this finding has increased the complexity of the matching and may cause problems if the various transplant centers are using different typing sera. Most centers will strongly prefer a donor who is at least matched in the D region with an A or B locus difference.

When cellular typing is added [specifically, primed lymphocyte testing for D region antigens, and mixed lymphocyte culture (MLC) reactivity], the complexities of selecting a donor are increased exponentially. A given donor-recipient combination may express a certain serologically defined pattern indicating compatibility. However, T cell recognition of the antigenic specificities may signal incompatibility. As an example, individuals who type as DR4 can be further divided into 5 Dw subtypes (Dw4, Dw10, and so on) that are recognized differently by T cells (32).

Furthermore, results of mixed lymphocyte culture studies are sometimes very difficult to interpret in light of the patient's underlying disease. Most notably, patients with chronic myelogenous leukemia frequently have very high background lymphocyte counts, making interpretation of the data extremely difficult if not impossible. Patients with severe aplastic anemia and severe combined immune deficiency do not respond well, or do not respond at all, when challenged by various donor or control lymphocytes.

The transplant physician can usually be relatively assured that if siblings are HLA-A, -B, and -DR serologically identical, they most likely are genotypically identical. However, when working with the unrelated donor, the phenotype cannot always be precisely determined. Even the assignment of haplotypes can only be assumed unless family typing of the prospective donor is available. Consequently, there are transplant centers which will insist upon a serological 6 of 6 antigen match (A, B, and DR) and MLC relative response index of less than 10 to 25% before they will accept the donor as "compatible." On the other hand, there are other institutions which will accept an unrelated donor with one or more A, B or DR incompatibilities (whether they are cross-reactive antigens or not), and also with relative response indices of > 25% in mixed lymphocyte culture.

Currently our program at the Medical College of Wisconsin relies on serological typing which includes A, B, C, DR, DQ and the MLC assays. A major problem has been obtaining sufficient cells expressing DR/DQ in patients with leukemia who are receiving chemotherapy. Culturing cells in phyto-hemagglutinin/interleukin-2 for 7 to 14 days has been helpful in activating and expanding T cells which express D-region antigens (33). MLC assays may be uninterpretable because: (1) of lack of sufficient host cells for stimulation (as in patients with marrow aplasia), (2) of presence of leukemia cells giving high background counts (as in patients with chronic myelogenous leukemia or those with relapsed leukemia), and (3) the MLC assay may be uninterpretable due to other technical problems. Therefore, one may be left dependent on the serological typing for identifying the best donor.

For pediatric patients we will accept a 5 of 6 antigen serological match with relative responses of up to 30% in the donor to recipient direction. In our small group of transplanted patients, graft-vs.-host disease has been tolerable (classified as grades I or II), and the severity of graft-vs.-host disease has not correlated with the degree of mismatching. The degree of major histocompatibility complex identity that is needed for a successful transplant has certainly not been defined at this time. The reasons for this difficulty will become more clear in the section dealing with conditioning regimens and methods of preventing graft-vs.-host disease.

Other techniques for defining the degree of identity at the major histocompatibility complex include: (1) restriction-fragment length polymorphisms (RFLP), (2) complotyping, and (3) HLA-DQ and -DP testing (34–36). These techniques may enhance our ability to identify the *best match,* and a donor pool based on these molecular probes may be very beneficial. There is no question that bone marrow transplantation using unrelated donors can be successfully achieved. However, the total impact of an unrelated donor program is not known at this time.

INDICATIONS

While there have been hundreds of matched related transplants performed using HLA-matched, MLC nonreactive siblings as donors, there have been fewer than 50 unrelated transplants reported in children under 16 years old (1–3,37–40). Children with leukemia account for about 60% of the cases in whom the procedure has been done. Patients with aplastic anemia make up 25% and the remaining 15% of transplants have been performed for treatment of immune deficiencies and for hematological or metabolic disorders (46). Patients who must depend on the availability of an unrelated donor have usually been heavily treated (such as patients with leukemia) or those who have no other viable alternative form of therapy (such as patients with aplastic anemia or SCIDS) and in poor clinical condition.

However, newly diagnosed adult patients with chronic myelogenous leukemia have been most suitable for an unrelated marrow transplant because of the usually slow progression of their disease, allowing the transplant center to have adequate time to identify the best potential donor (42,43). Also, these patients with CML are on minimal therapy or no therapy, and therefore they are not subject to the toxicity of aggressive chemotherapy.

Currently, a child with high-risk acute lymphocytic leukemia (ALL) in first remission would not likely be transplanted if only an unrelated donor were available. In fact, there is no clear consensus among the major pediatric cancer centers on the question of whether any child with acute leukemia should be transplanted in first remission (44). However, recent findings suggest that children who have Philadelphia chromosome positive ALL have a particularly poor prognosis (45). This may be the first type of childhood leukemia in which an unrelated donor, if available, would be utilized for transplantation in a first remission.

Most recently bone marrow transplantation has been advocated for patients with the myelodysplastic syndromes or preleukemia (46,47). We have transplanted 4 patients with myelodysplastic syndrome, and in two instances unrelated donors were used (48).

Severe aplastic anemia has been very successfully treated in minimally transfused patients who have an HLA-identical sibling as donor (39). However, if such a donor is not available, these patients are currently being treated with antithymocyte (or antilymphocyte) globulin. While the success of this therapy approaches 50%, fewer patients than this show full hematopoietic reconstitution (49). Consequently, it is our policy to do matched unrelated marrow transplants in patients with severe aplastic anemia who have not recovered 2 to 3 months after receiving antithymocyte globulin or antilymphocyte globulins. Currently the search for an unrelated donor takes an average of 6 to 12 weeks. Rather than wait this long we feel it is best to start the antithymocyte globulin and evaluate the patient's response while the search for a donor is in progress. Our experience in marrow transplantation using a haplo-identical parent has been poor and we would not consider this option.

According to Gluckman, treatment of Fanconi's anemia when a matched sibling is available, includes a conditioning regimen of low-dose cyclophosphamide and low-dose total lymphoid irradiation. This regimen has proven to be very successful (50). Whether patients with Fanconi's anemia can routinely be successfully transplanted using unrelated donors is not clear at the present time. However, Sokal and colleagues have reported successful engraftment of a patient with Fanconi's anemia following a matched unrelated transplant. Significant graft-vs.-host disease occurred, however, and an autoimmune hemolytic anemia persists (51).

Patients with immune deficiency diseases are particularly amenable to therapy with mismatched donors. First, the problem of graft rejection is less severe than that seen in patients with aplastic anemia. Second, since most patients with immune deficiency diseases are diagnosed at a very young age, graft-vs.-host disease is milder and occurs less frequently (2). Consequently, a number of marrow transplants have been done in those patients using family members as donors, usually only haplo-identical matches, often with excellent results (11). However, these transplants in immunodeficient patients may be a very important situation in which to look for unrelated donors who are more fully matched, especially as a means of promoting immune reconstitution because of concern that SCIDS patients receiving haplo-identical marrows do not always show reconstitution of the humoral (B cell) immune system (52).

Any disease in which bone marrow transplantation using an HLA-matched sibling as a rational choice can be considered a potential setting for use of an unrelated donor. It is very important, however, to balance the risks of the disease itself against the potential increased risk of nonengraftment and graft-vs.-host disease following use of marrow from an unrelated donor.

SUPPORTIVE MEASURES

Unrelated bone marrow transplants have become feasible mainly because of marked improvements in supportive therapies now available. The most important advances in supportive care in our center include: (1) Central venous (Hickman) catheters, (2) trimethoprim-sulfamethoxazole, (3) acyclovir, (4) DHPG (9 [1,3 dihydroxy-2-propoxymethyl] quanine), (5) CMV seronegative blood products, (6) chlorhexidine and, (7) intravenous gamma-globulin preparations.

Central venous catheters (double or triple lumen) enable optimal nutrition, antibiotics and blood products to be more easily administered.

Trimethoprim-sulfamethoxazole has significantly lowered the incidence and improved the results of treatment of *Pneumocystis carinii* pneumonia (53,54). We give 150 mg/m^2 trimethaprim and 750 mg/mm^2 sulfamethoxazole per day in two divided doses daily until the transplant, discontinue the drugs until the absolute neutrophil count is over 500 mg/m^3 post-transplant, and then reinstitute the drug on a Monday, Tuesday, Wednesday schedule (55).

Acyclovir is given at a dose of 5 mg/kg every 8 hours intravenously as prophylaxis for herpes virus infections (56). There are also a few reports suggesting that acyclovir may be of benefit in the prevention of Epstein-Barr virus-induced lymphomas that can arise in the post-transplant period (57). Chlorhexidine and myostatin are given to try to decrease the severity and duration of the discomfort of mucositis and the risk of fungal infections (58).

CMV seronegative patients receive only CMV seronegative, irradiated blood products, a policy which appears to be extremely beneficial in preventing significant cytomegalovirus infection (59,60). The recent introduction of ganciclovir (9 [1,3 dihydroxy-2-propoxymethyl] quanine) appears effective in preventing significant sequelae and mortality caused by infections with this virus (61,62). Foscarnet is another agent which has been reported to be beneficial in the treatment of cytomegalovirus infections (64).

We give immunoglobulin at a dose of 500 mg/kg/wk intravenously in all patients until at least day 120 post-transplant (65).

All patients are cared for in private rooms equipped with HEPA filtration systems, and febrile episodes are treated with broad spectrum antibiotics after appropriate cultures are obtained. Because our patients are transplanted with T cell depleted marrow and there is a risk of contamination (especially with *Staphylococcus epidermidis*), patients routinely are given 12 doses of vancomycin post-transplant.

CONDITIONING REGIMEN

Initially, unrelated donor transplants relied on the same pre-transplant conditioning regimens that were successful in transplants using HLA-matched sibling donors such as cyclophosphamide, 60 mg/kg/day, for 2 days followed by 1000–12000 cGy of total body irradiation or 1320 cGy of total body irradiation given in 11 doses of 120 cGy each, followed by cyclophosphamide, 60 mg/kg/day, for 2 days (66,67).

As more transplants have been performed in the mismatched, unrelated setting, and the HLA disparity between donor and recipient has increased, however, a significant incidence of graft rejection has been observed using these conditioning regimens (68). This was especially true if the marrow inoculum was depleted of T cells (69). Residual host lymphocytes bearing the CD3+, CD8+ phenotype cells thought to play a role in the graft rejection have been detected after such conditioning (70). Some investigators feel that the population of cells present in a nonmanipulated marrow contain T cells which are responsible for eliminating resistant host T cells, and thus increase the likelihood of engraftment (71).

Our regimen now includes cytosine arabinoside 3 gm/m^2 every 12 hours for 6 doses (on days -8 to -5), cyclophosphamide 45 mg/kg/day for 2 days (on days -7 and -6), and methylprednisolone 1 g/m^2 every 12 hours for 3 days (on days -3 to 0) (72). Patients with resistant leukemia and the myelodyspasias are also given busulfan 4 mg/kg/day for 2 days (on days -10 and -9). Irradiation is also more intense. Patients receive 1400 cGy of total body irradiation in 9 fractions over 3 days, in a schedule similar to that used at Memorial-Sloan Kettering Cancer Center (67). The lungs are shielded so that the absorbed dose of irradiation is approximately 1000 cGy. The dose rate is between 10 to 25 cGy/min. This more intense therapy results in fewer problems with graft rejection with no apparent increase in acute toxicity.

Patients with aplastic anemia transplanted with mismatched and/or unrelated donors present more of a challenge. They most often have failed a course of antithymocyte globulin and have been heavily transfused. They may also have cytotoxic antibody to the donor's lymphocytes. A major problem in any heavily transfused patient with severe aplastic anemia is graft failure (73). The standard conditioning regimen of cyclophosphamide 50 mg/kg/day for 4 days does not produce sufficient immunosuppression and currently our patients receive similar conditioning for leukemia without busulfan (74).

Patients who have various types of immune deficiencies also present special problems when unrelated or family mismatched donors are used. Moderate immunosuppression of the recipient is necessary because of the possibility that there may be circulating cytoxic cells derived from the mother (75,76). Most centers utilize either cyclophosphamide alone or in combination with busulfan, depending on the degree of HLA disparity (77).

We have noticed significant renal abnormalities in the form of glomerulosclerosis in a few of our patients, which may be related to the need for intense conditioning regimen in unrelated transplants (76). These patients have also been treated with a number of other nephrotoxic drugs (such as vancomycin, amphotericin and cyclosporine).

GRAFT-VS.-HOST DISEASE

The intensity of the conditioning regimen and its relationship to engraftment goes hand in hand with the steps used to prevent graft-vs.-host disease.

The standard regimen for the prevention of graft-vs.-host disease has consisted of methotrexate 15 mg/m^2 day 1 and 10 mg/m^2 on days 3, 6 and 11 post-transplant, and then weekly for the first 100 days post-transplant (79). This regimen has been modified in recent years in adult patients with the addition of cyclosporine, so that patients now receive a combination of short-term methotrexate (given on days 1, 3, 6 and 11) along with daily cyclosporine (80). In the HLA-matched sibling transplant setting this regimen has been very effective (81).

It is clear from limiting dilution analysis that the harvested bone marrow contains a significant number of proliferating T cells which may be responsible for the graft-vs.-host reaction. Many centers employ purging techniques to remove these T lymphocytes from the marrow inoculum. Such techniques include: (1) monoclonal or polyclonal antibodies, (2) counterflow centrifugation, (3) ricin labelled antibodies, and (4) lectin separation (11,82–88). All methods can successfully remove 2 to 3 logs of T cells. T cell purging has decreased the incidence of significant graft-vs.-host disease but has also resulted in an increased incidence of nonengraftment in transplantation settings that previously had not been associated with graft rejection (89).

The more intense the purging of T lymphocytes, the greater the efficiency in removing proliferating T cells (Figure 1). An untreated bone marrow inoculum contains approximately 1 in 15 proliferating T lymphocytes as determined by limiting dilution analysis (87). If antibody (Ab) T$_{10}$B$_9$ (CD3) is utilized for purging, approximately 1 in 900 cells is shown to be a proliferating T cell. Treatment with antibody T$_{12}$A$_{10}$ (CD12) is even more efficient for purging of T lymphocytes, with only 1 T cell/3000 marrow cells remaining. If a combination of these two antibodies is used, only about 1 in 5000 marrow cells

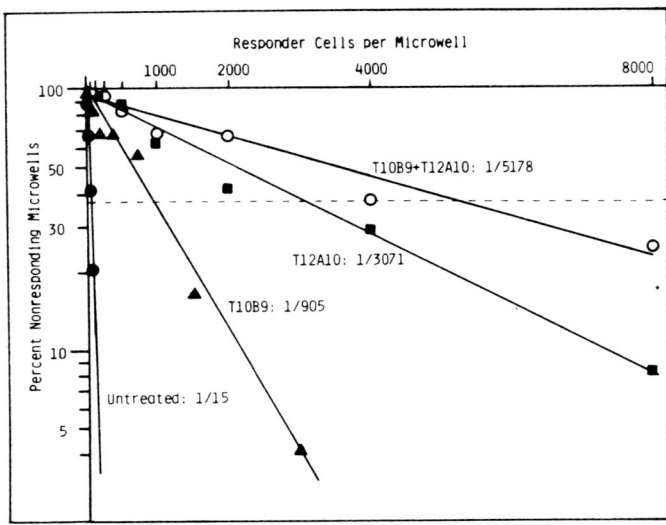

FIG. 1. Representative linear regression curves showing relationship between the number of responder cells per microwell and the percent nonresponding microwells set up at each of the indicated doses of untreated bone marrow (●) or marrow treated with T10B9 (▲), T12A10 (■), or T10B9+T12A10 (○) MoAb+C'. The calculated PTL frequencies are shown. Reprinted from *Cellular Immunotherapy of Cancer* (Truitt, Gale and Bortin, eds.) Alan Liss, 1987.

in the marrow inoculum is a proliferating T cell. Currently we use a single CD3 antibody ($T_{10}B_9$) to purge the bone marrow inoculum (72).

The $T_{10}B_9$ antibody has significant activity against human T cells and was derived from fusion of SP2 myeloma cells with Balb C splenocytes after immunization with human T cells (90). This antibody has the following characteristics: (1) it has the IgM isotype, (2) it is lytic for T lymphocytes in the presence of fresh autologous human serum, and (3) it does not affect human pluripotential (CFU-GEMM) and committed (GFU-GM, BFU-E, CFU-E and CFU-MK) hemopoietic progenitors (91).

The harvested marrow inoculum is initially diluted with RPMI medium and separated on Ficoll-Hypaque to obtain a mononuclear cell population. After washing, the monoclonal antibody (MoAb) is added to a final concentration of 10 μg/ml. Marrow cells and monoclonal antibody are incubated with complement for 90 to 120 minutes at 37°C in the presence of DNAse. The final product is washed and resuspended in HBSS with 4% human albumin for infusion. The number of infused nucleated cells usually range from 1 to 3.7 × 10^8/kg following T cell depletion.

The procedure results in approximately a 97–98% depletion of T cells. The addition of several antibodies can increase the efficiency of T cell removal to greater than 99% (87). A similar efficiency of T cell depletion can be obtained by using a combination of soybean lectin agglutination and E rosette depletion (92). However, with this greater efficiency, problems with nonengraftment are magnified (69,93).

It has been postulated that T lymphocytes present in the marrow inoculum are necessary for engraftment (71). Whether these T lymphocytes are needed to eradicate any remaining host cells responsible for rejection is still unknown (94). It has been shown that host T cells remain after certain intense conditioning regimens and increasing the intensity of the conditioning regimen may allow the effects of various depletion techniques to be studied (70).

Cyclosporine A is employed as an adjunct to prevent graft-vs.-host disease in transplants of T lymphocyte depleted unrelated marrow in a dose of approximately 3 mg/kg/day intravenously. Once the medication can be taken orally the dosage is increased to 9 mg/kg/day and then tapered starting at day 40 if there are no signs of graft-vs.-host disease. Methylprednisolone (2–6 mg/kg/day) is added when there are signs of graft-vs.-host disease. We do not use methotrexate because of the intensity of our conditioning regimen and because this drug often produces mucositis.

From recent studies, it appears that infusion of a CD5 antibody labelled with immunotoxin (ricin A chain), used for the treatment of severe graft-vs.-host disease, may be of benefit in patients given unrelated marrow transplants (95). Among the first 25 patients treated, 86% showed improvement, with 41% being complete responders. Use of this technique for treating graft-vs.-host disease may allow one to be less aggressive in depleting the marrow of T cells, thereby decreasing the problem of nonengraftment.

Another problem also related to T cell depletion is the reported increased incidence of recurrent leukemia, with leukemia almost always being of host origin (96). A graft-vs.-leukemia effect has been observed in mice after allogeneic marrow transplantation together with identification of the cell(s) responsible (97,98). A similar clinical finding has been reported in man but the mechanism of this phenomenon has not been elucidated (99,100). As with nonengraftment, the nature of the T lymphocyte depletion is most likely a critical factor. Thus, not all methods of T lymphocyte depletion are likely to result in an increased rate of leukemic recurrence. However, T cell depletion is another variable which must be taken into consideration.

The occurrence of B cell lymphoproliferation due to infection with Epstein-Barr virus has also been observed following mismatched marrow transplantation. The majority of these tumors are of donor origin (101). Patients who receive bone marrow that is T cell depleted are at highest risk for this complication. While we have not seen B cell tumors in our first 10 T depleted unrelated transplants, we noted this complication in 2 cases out of 14 T depleted mismatched related transplants.

A fine balance will have to be struck between the intensity of the conditioning regimen and the manipulation of the marrow inoculum to prevent significant graft-vs.-host disease and recurrence of leukemia.

IMMUNE RECONSTITUTION

Patients who have undergone bone marrow transplantation for any of a variety of disorders routinely develop a combined cellular and humoral immune deficiency (102). Three factors may contribute to this deficiency. These are: (1) pre-transplant conditioning, (2) histocompatibility differences between donor and recipient and, (3) abnormalities of processing of donor lymphocytes in the thymus of the recipient (103).

In patients transplanted with marrow that was not T cell depleted, donor derived T and B cells repopulate the peripheral blood within the first 3 months (104). The new population of T cell subsets does not reach normal numbers during the first year postgrafting in the setting of graft-vs.-host disease and intercurrent infection (105). Diminished T cell function has been attributed to the presence of suppressor cells, inadequate helper activity, the effects of graft-vs.-host disease, or to a combination of these factors (106). However, patients with SCIDS transplanted with T cell depleted mismatched marrow are able to reconstitute their T cell immunity. This observation suggests that stem cells present in the donor marrow can give rise to a complete set of mature T cells in the recipient (107). While depleted T cells are repopulated relatively quickly, mitogenic and allogeneic responses of these cells often remain significantly reduced for 9 to 12 months post-transplant (108).

B cell reconstitution is far slower. Even when there is T cell repletion following transplant of marrow from a matched sibling the ability of the recipient to produce antibody to specific antigen can be impaired for years (109,110). Children receiving T depleted haplo-identical marrow from their parents for treatment of severe combined immunodeficiency syndrome in several instances did not develop normal B cell function (52).

Once again information on immune reconstitution in children receiving marrow from unrelated individuals is limited. Our own experience indicates that development of the phenotypic T lymphocyte subpopulations is very similar to that which occurs in the allogeneic transplant using matched donor marrow. The limited data regarding mitogenic response is depicted in Figure 2. Patients were tested at various times following transplant. The study included 9 unrelated recipients, 7 who were mismatched related, and 12 who were matched related recipients. Marrows from the unrelated and mismatched related donors were T cell depleted.

In all instances the response compared to normal controls was best for the matched related transplants, followed by the unrelated and then the mismatched related transplants. The mismatched related donors were, in many instances, haplo-identical parents and the unrelated donors showed, at most, a single serological antigenic disparity with the patient. These early data indicate that marrow transplants from unrelated donors are able to repopulate T cell subsets and early T cell function. Whether normal B cell reconstitution

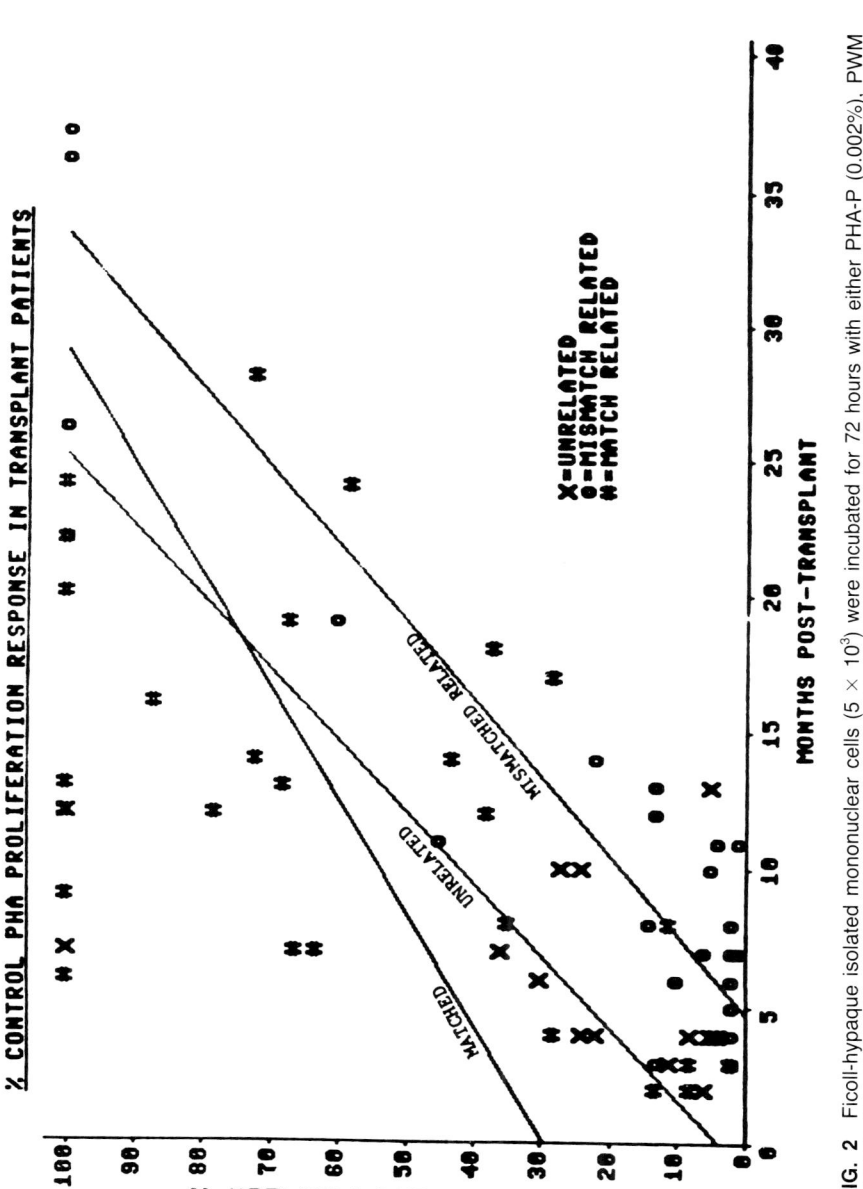

FIG. 2 Ficoll-hypaque isolated mononuclear cells (5×10^3) were incubated for 72 hours with either PHA-P (0.002%), PWM (0.02%), Con-A (0.01%) or media alone. After addition of 0.75 Ci of ^{3}H-thymidine, cells were incubated another 24 hours, harvested with an automated cell harvester and counted using liquid scintillation techniques. The results are expressed as the percent stimulation index of the patient compared to a simultaneously run normal control.

FIG. 2 (Continued)

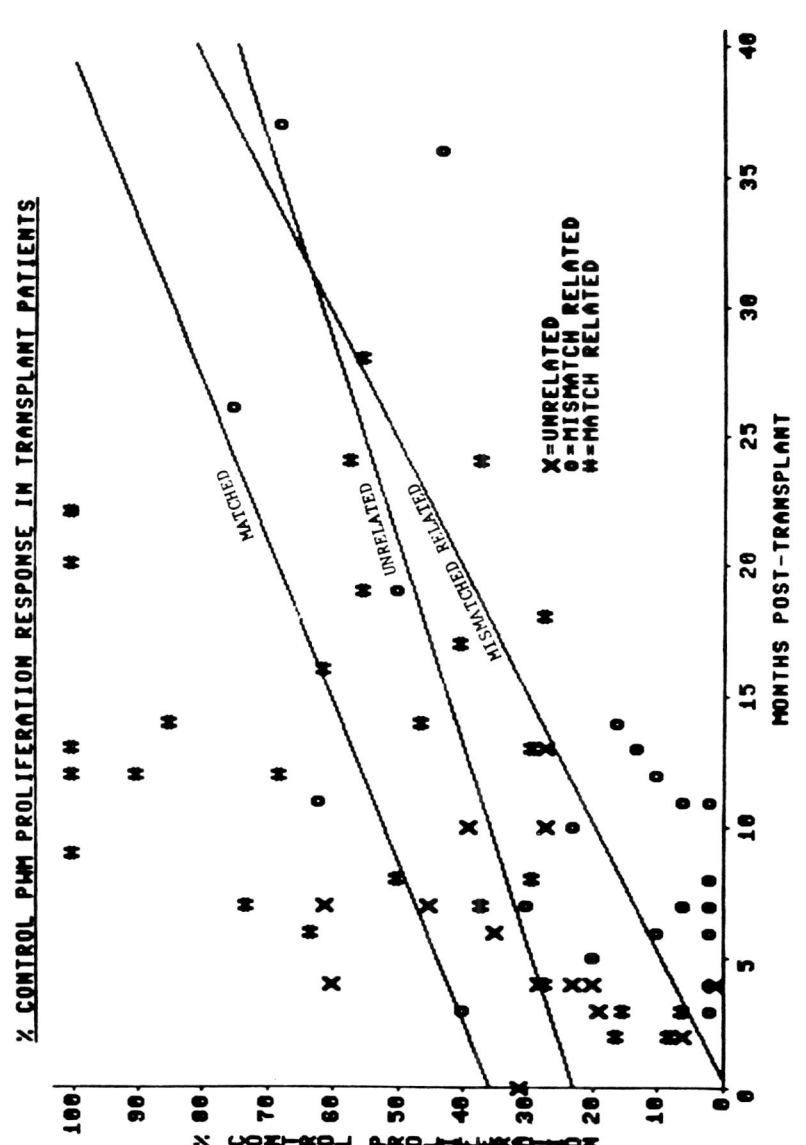

FIG. 2 (Continued)

also occurs following transplant of marrow from unrelated donors remains unknown.

CURRENT SURVIVAL

The true long-term survival and sequelae following transplantation of marrow from unrelated donors in children cannot be accurately assessed at this time, given the few published reports. Through personal communication and literature search, we found that at most 50 such transplants have been reported (23). Approximately 40% of these patients had documented engraftment and are alive beyond 100 days post-transplant.

Ten children have been treated by unrelated marrow transplantation at the Children's Hospital of Wisconsin and followed at least 100 days (Table 2). The patients ranged in age from 1 to 12 years (median, 5 years). There were 7 boys and 3 girls. The primary diseases treated were severe aplastic anemia, 2; juvenile chronic myelogenous leukemia, 2; severe combined immune deficiency, 1; preleukemia, 3; and acute lymphoblastic leukemia, 2. The degree of mismatching varied: 3 patients were serologically identical, 3 an A locus mismatch, 2 a B locus mismatch, and 2 patients a D region mismatch with their donor. Relative responses were greater than 10% in 5 of the 9 evaluable mixed lymphocyte culture assays. All of the donor marrows were T cell depleted using monoclonal antibody $T_{10}B_9$ (CD3) and normal rabbit serum.

In all 10 patients grafted, the absolute neutrophil counts reached 500/mm^3 at a median of 18 days and the platelet counts spontaneously reached 25,000/mm^3 at a median of 12 days following transplantation. Graft-vs.-host disease of severity greater than grade II was not seen in any of these patients. Eight patients are alive and disease-free from 111 to 458 days post-transplant (median, 260 days). One patient died of cytomegalovirus infection on day 76. A second patient, who had anaphylactic reactions to trimethoprim-sulfamethoxazole, died of *Pneumocystis carinii* pneumonia on day 127.

This is not a large group of patients, but with very short follow-up, the results to date compare favorably with the matched and mismatched related transplants that we have performed. Data from other centers indicate that the proportion of patients surviving is about 40%, but the conditioning regimens used and the T cell depletion techniques employed vary.

Many questions still need to be answered. What is the most effective (not necessarily the most efficient) means to deplete the marrow of T cells? Is it possible to decrease the toxicity related to conditioning without sacrificing an antileukemic effect and engraftment? An important question which will be very difficult to answer lies in the selection of a donor. Is a 2 antigen B/D incompatible sibling a better donor than an A or B single antigen mismatched unrelated donor? Our small numbers would favor using the single antigen mismatched unrelated individual as the best donor. The next few years, hopefully, will see answers forthcoming to the perplexing questions raised.

TABLE 2. *Patient characteristics and outcome in 10 patients receiving marrow transplants from unrelated donors.*

Unique patient number	Histocompatibility								GVHD	Age	Disease	Status	Clinical problems
	R→D				D→R								
	A	B	DR	MLC	A	B	DR	MLC					
086	=	=	≠	NE	=	=	≠	NE	2	5	JCML-Accel	Dead (76)	CMV
092	=	=	=	0	=	=	=	0	1	3	AA-Heavy transfusion	Dead (127)	P. carinii
121	≠	=	=	0	≠	=	=	0	1	12	Pre-Leuk	Alive (458+)	Nephritis
124	=	=	=	NE	=	=	=	0	0	7/12	SCID	Alive (413+)	None
134	=	≠	=	NE	=	≠	=	45	1	2	JCML	Alive (384+)	None
157	≠	=	=	17	≠	=	=	65	1	9	Pre-Leuk	Alive (269+)	None
158	=	=	=	32	=	=	=	51	2	3	ALL-2nd PR	Alive (260+)	None
170	=	≠	=	14	=	≠	=	0	1	5	AA-Heavy transfusion	Alive (160+)	None
171	≠	=	=	0	≠	=	=	0	1	6	ALL-2nd remission	Alive (155+)	VOD-resolved
177	=	=	=	36	=	=	≠	57	1	6	Pre-Leuk	Alive (111+)	Adenovirus resolved

= : match
≠ : mismatch
R = recipient
D = donor
VOD = hepatic veno-occlusive disease
JCML = juvenile chronic myeloid leukemia
NE = nonevaluable
AA = aplastic anemia

SUMMARY

Although the first successful unrelated bone marrow transplants were performed in the mid-1970s, progress in this area has remained stagnant. However, advances in three major areas have rekindled interest making the procedure more readily available and successful. They are: (1) an increased understanding of the major histocompatibility complex in man; (2) improved techniques for the prevention of graft-vs.-host disease (i.e., T cell depletion, cyclosporine); and (3) the establishment of bone marrow donor banks. Approximately 160 unrelated transplants have been performed worldwide with about 40–50 of these in pediatric patients. The initial success has been low due to the end-stage nature of the diseases being treated. However, our early experience with 10 patients (8 alive) is encouraging and certainly indicates the feasibility of using even mismatched unrelated donors for transplanting children with otherwise incurable disease.

Acknowledgments

The authors are grateful to the bone marrow transplant team at the Medical College of Wisconsin and the dedication of the nursing staff of the Bone Marrow Transplant Unit at Children's Hospital of Wisconsin. We thank Bettie Lyles for secretarial help in the preparation of this manuscript.

REFERENCES

1. Sanders JE, Whitehead J, Storb R, et al.: Bone marrow transplantation experience for children with aplastic anemia. *Pediatr* 1986;77:179–186.
2. Fischer A, Friedrich W, Levinsky R, et al.: Bone marrow transplantation for immunodeficiencies and osteopetrosis: European Survey. *Lancet* 1986;2:1080–1084.
3. Thomas ED, Clift RA, Fefer A, et al.: Marrow transplantation for the treatment of chronic myelogenous leukemia. *Ann Int Med* 1986;104:155–163.
4. Hows JM, Yin JL, Marsh J, et al.: Histocompatible unrelated volunteer donors compared with HLA nonidentical family donors in marrow transplantation for aplastic anemia and leukemia. *Blood* 1986;68:1322–1328.
5. Beatty PG, Clift RA, Mickleson EM, et al.: Marrow transplantation from related donors other than HLA identical siblings. *N Engl J Med* 1985;313:765–770.
6. Powles RL, Kay HEM, Clink HM, et al.: Mismatched family donors for bone marrow transplantation as treatment for acute leukæmia. *Lancet* 1983;1:612–615.
7. Trigg ME, Sondel PM, Billing R, et al.: Mismatched bone marrow transplantation in children with hematologic malignancy using T lymphocyte depleted bone marrow. *J Biol Response Med* 1985;4:602–612.
8. Powles RL, Morgenstern GR, Leigh M et al.: Cyclosporin A following matched and mismatched family allogeneic bone marrow transplants. *Hematol Bluttransfus* 1983;28:87–89.
9. Clift RA, Hansen JA, Thomas ED, et al.: The role of HLA in marrow transplantation. *Transplant Proc* 1981;13:234–236.
10. Storb R, Thomas ED, Appelbaum FR, et al.: Marrow transplantation for severe aplastic anemia: The Seattle experience. In: Young NS, Levine AS, Humphries RK, eds.; *Aplastic Anemia: Stem Cell Biology and Advances in Treatment;* New York, Alan R. Liss, Inc., 1984;pp. 297.
11. O'Reilly RJ, Kapoor N, Kirkpatrick D, et al.: Transplantation for severe combined

immunodeficiency using histoincompatible parental marrow fractionates by soybean agglutinin and sheep red blood cells. *Transplant Proc* 1983;15:1431–1435.

12. O'Reilly RJ, Kapoor N, Kirkpatrick D: Transplantation of hematopoietic cells for lethal congenital immunodeficiencies. In, Wedgwood RJ, Rosen FS, Paul NW, eds.; *Primary Immunodeficiency Diseases;* New York, Alan R Liss, Inc., 1983;129–137.

13. Cowan MJ, Wara DW, Weintrub PS, et al.: Haploidentical bone marrow transplantation for severe combined immunodeficiency disease using soybean agglutinin-negative, T-depleted marrow cells. *J Clin Immunol* 1985;5:370–376.

14. Speck B, Zwaan FE, van Rood JJ, et al.: Allogeneic bone marrow transplantation in a patient with aplastic anemia using phenotypically HLA-identical unrelated donor. *Transplantation* 1973;16:24–28.

15. L'Esperance P, Hansen JA, Jersild C, et al.: Bone marrow donor selection among unrelated four locus-identical individuals. *Transplantation Proceedings* 1975;7:823–831.

16. Horowitz SD, Bach FH, Groshong T, et al.: Treatment of severe combined immunodeficiency with bone marrow from an unrelated, mixed-leucocyte-culture nonreactive donor. *Lancet* 1975;2:431–433.

17. O'Reilly RJ, Dupont B, Pahwa S, et al.: Reconstitution in severe combined immunodeficiency by transplantation of marrow from an unrelated donor. *N Engl J Med* 1977;297:1311–1318.

17a. Thomas ED, Storb R, Clift RA, et al.: Bone marrow transplantation. *N Engl J Med* 1975;292:832–843, 895–902.

18. Jeannet M, Speck B, Sartorius J: Donor selection for bone marrow transplantation. Predictive value of DR typing for mixed lymphocyte culture compatibility between unrelated individuals. *Transplantation* 1978;26:448–449.

19. Hansen JA, Clift RA, Thomas ED: Transplantation of marrow from an unrelated donor to a patient with acute leukemia. *N Engl J Med* 1980;303:565–567.

20. Gordon-Smith EC, Fairhead SM, Chipping PM, et al.: Bone marrow transplantation for severe aplastic anæmia using histocompatible unrelated volunteer donors. *Brit Med J* 1982;285:835–837.

21. Duquesnoy RJ, Zeevi A, Marrari M, et al.: Bone marrow transplantation for severe aplastic anemia using a phenotypically HLA-identical, SB-compatible unrelated donor. *Transplantation* 1983;35:566–571.

22. Nomenclature for Factors of the HLA System 1984. In: Albert ED et al., eds.; *Histocompatibility Testing* 1984; Berlin, Springer-Verlag, 1984.

23. Council of Community Blood Centers Newsletter: Current events and trends relevant to blood services. December 1987.

24. James DCO: Addition of 100,000 bone marrow donors to the Anthony Nolan register—a report (Abstr). *Bone Marrow Transplantation* 1987; Suppl 1, 2:80.

25. McCullough J, Bach FH, Coccia P, et al.: Bone marrow transplantation from unrelated volunteer donors: Summary of a conference on scientific, ethical, legal, financial, and other practical issues. *Transfusion* 1982;22:78–81.

26. Proceedings of the Symposium: "Ethics and Blood Transfusion" XVII Congress of the International Society of Hematology and XV Congress of the International Society of Blood Transfusion, Paris, 1978.

27. McElligott MC, Menitove JE, Aster RH: Recruitment of unrelated persons as bone marrow donors. A preliminary experience. *Transfusion* 1986;26:309–314.

28. Bass GM, Menitove JE: Assessment of methods for recruiting unrelated bone marrow donors (Abstr). *Transfusion* 1987;27:524.

29. Bradley BA, Gilks WR, Gore SM, et al.: How many HLA typed volunteer donors for bone marrow transplantation (BMT) are needed to provide an effective service? (Abstr) *Bone Marrow Transplantation* 1987; Suppl 1, 2:79.

30. Hows JM: Histocompatible unrelated donors for bone marrow transplantation. *Bone Marrow Transplantation* 1987;1:259–263.

31. Dausset J: The genetics of transplantation antigens. *Transplant Proc* 1971;3:8–14.

32. Bach FH, Sachs DH: Current concepts: Immunology. Transplantation immunology. *N Engl J Med* 1987;317:489–492.

33. Adams PW, Ferguson RM, Vaidya S, et al.: Clinical utility of serologic HLA-DR antigen identification using activated T-lymphocytes. *Human Immunology* 1986;16:295–303.

34. Carlsson B, Wallin J, Bohme J, et al.: HLA-DR-DQ haplotypes defined by restriction fragment analysis. *Human Immunol* 1987;20:95–113.
35. Alper CA, Raum D, Karp S, et al.: Serum complement supergenes of the major histocompatibility complex in man (complotypes). *Vox Sang* 1983;45:62–67.
36. Awdeh ZL, Eynon E, Stein R, et al.: Unrelated individuals matched for MHC extended haplotypes and HLA-identical siblings show comparable responses in mixed lymphocyte culture. *Lancet* 1985;2:853–855.
37. Clift RA, Buckner CD, Thomas ED, et al.: The treatment of acute nonlymphoblastic leukemia by allogeneic marrow transplantation. *Bone Marrow Transplantation* 1987;2:243–258.
38. Sanders JE, Flournoy N, Thomas ED, et al.: Marrow transplant experience in children with acute lymphoblastic leukemia: An analysis of factors associated with survival, relapse, and graft-vs.-host disease. *Med Pediatr Oncol* 1985;13:165–172.
39. McGlave PB, Haake R, Miller W, et al.: Therapy of severe aplastic anemia in young adults and children with allogeneic bone marrow transplantation. *Blood* 1987;70:1325–1330.
40. Lucarelli G, Galimberti M, Polchi P, et al.: Marrow transplantation in patients with advanced thalassemia. *N Engl J Med* 1987;316:1050–1055.
41. Storb R: Critical issues in bone marrow transplantation. *Transplantation Proc* 1987;19:2774–2781.
42. Goldman JM: Management of chronic myeloid leukaemia. *Scand J Hæmatol* 1986;37:269–279.
43. McGlave P, Scott E, Ramsay N, et al.: Unrelated bone marrow transplantation therapy for chronic myelogenous leukemia. *Blood* 1987;70:877–881.
44. Champlin RE, Ho WG, Gale RP, et al.: Treatment of acute myelogenous leukemia: A prospective controlled trial of bone marrow transplantation versus consolidation chemotherapy. *Ann Intern Med* 1985;102:285–291.
45. Williams DL, Harber J, Murphy SB, et al.: Chromosomal translocations play a unique role in influencing prognosis in childhood acute lymphoblastic leukemia. *Blood* 1986;68:205–212.
46. O'Donnell MR, Nademanee AP, Snyder DS, et al.: Bone marrow transplantation for myelodysplastic and myeloproliferative syndromes. *J Clin Oncol* 1987;5:1822–1826.
47. Guinan E, Tarbell N, Rappeport J, et al.: Bone marrow transplantation (BMT) for children with *de novo* or secondary myelodysplastic syndromes (Abstr). *Blood* 1987;70:294a.
48. Bunin NJ, Casper JT, Chitambar C, et al.: Partially matched bone marrow transplantation (BMT) using T-cell depletion in patients with myelodysplastic syndromes (MDS) (Abstr). *J Clin Oncol* 1988; 6:1851–1855.
49. Doney K, Storb R, Buckner CD, et al.: Treatment of aplastic anemia with antithymocyte globulin, high-dose corticosteroids, and androgens. *Exp Hematol* 1987;15:239–242.
50. Gluckman E, Berger R, Dutreix J: Bone marrow transplantation for Fanconi's anemia. *Semin Hematol* 1984;21:20–26.
51. Sokal E, Michel M, Ninane J, et al.: Bone marrow transplantation from an unrelated donor for Fanconi's anæmia: Two unusual complications. *Bone Marrow Transplantation* 1987;2:99–102.
52. Friedrich W, Goldmann SF, Vetter U, et al.: Immunoreconstitution in severe combined immunodeficiency after transplantation of HLA-haploidentical, T-cell-deleted bone marrow. *Lancet* 1984;1:761–764.
53. Meyers JD: Infection in bone marrow transplant recipients. *Am J Med* 1986;81:27–38.
54. Engelhard D, Marks MI, Good RA: Infections in bone marrow transplant recipients. *J Pediatr* 1986;108:335–346.
55. Hughes WT, Rivera GK, Schell MJ, et al.: Successful intermittent chemoprophylaxis for pneumocystis carinii pneumonitis. *N Engl J Med* 1987;316:1627–1632.
56. Gluckman E, Lotsberg J, Devergie A, et al.: Prophylaxis of herpes infections after bone marrow transplantation by oral acyclovir. *Lancet* 1983:2:706.
57. Trigg ME, Finlay JL, Sondel PM: Prophylactic acyclovir in patients receiving bone marrow transplants. *N Engl J Med* 1985;312:1708–1709.
58. Ferretti G, Lillich T, Rayboult T, et al.: Effect of chlorhexidine on the oral complications of patients receiving intensive chemotherapy (Abstr). *Proceed Am Soc Clin Oncol* 1987;6:268.
59. Ash RC, Bratanow NC, Raybould T, et al.: Prevention of primary cytomegalovirus infection in allogeneic bone marrow transplant patients by cytomegalovirus-negative blood products and anticytomegalovirus intravenous immunoglobulin. *Blood* 1986;68:279A.
60. Bowden RA, Sayers M, Gleaves CA, et al.: Cytomegalovirus-seronegative blood compo-

nents for the prevention of primary cytomegalovirus infection after marrow transplantation. *Transfusion* 1987;27:478–481.

61. Bratanow N, Ash RC, Turner P, et al.: The use of 9(1,3-dihydroxy-2-propoxymethyl)guanine (ganciclovir, DHPG) and intravenous immunoglobulin (IVIG) in the treatment of serious cytomegalovirus (CMV) infections in thirty-one allogeneic bone marrow transplant (BMT) patients. *Blood* 1987;70:302A.

62. Erice A, Jordan MC, Chace BA, et al.: Ganciclovir treatment of cytomegalovirus disease in transplant recipients and other immunocompromised hosts. *JAMA* 1987;257:3082–3087.

63. Laskin OL, Cederberg DM, Mills J, et al.: Ganciclovir for the treatment and suppression of serious infections caused by cytomegalovirus. *Am J Med* 1987;83:201–207.

64. Akesson-Johansson A, Lernestedt JO, Ringden O, et al.: Sensitivity of cytomegalovirus to intravenous foscarnet treatment. *Bone Marrow Transplantation* 1986;1:215–220.

65. Sullivan KM: Immunoglobulin therapy in bone marrow transplantation. *Am J Med* 1987;83:34–45.

66. Thomas ED, Sanders JE, Flournoy N, et al.: Marrow transplantation for patients with acute lymphoblastic leukemia in remission. *Blood* 1979;54:468–476.

67. Brochstein JA, Kernan NA, Groshen S, et al.: Allogeneic bone marrow transplantation after hyperfractionated total body irradiation and cyclophosphamide in children with acute leukemia. *N Engl J Med* 1987;317:1618–1624.

68. Trigg ME, Billing R, Sondel PM, et al.: Clinical trial depleting T lymphocytes from donor marrow for matched and mismatched allogeneic bone marrow transplants. *Cancer Treat Reports* 1985;69:377–386.

69. Martin PJ, Hansen JA, Buckner D, et al.: Effects of *in vitro* depletion of T cells in HLA-identical allogeneic marrow grafts. *Blood* 1985;66:664–672.

70. Bordignon C, Kernan NA, Keever CA, et al.: Graft failures following T-cell depleted grafts for leukemia: Emergence of host T-lymphocytes (CD3+ CD8+) with donor-specific reactivity. *Blood* 1987;5:303a.

71. Storb R: The role of T cells in engraftment: Experimental models, clinical trials. In: Gale RP, Champlin R, eds.; *Progress in Bone Marrow Transplantation;* New York, Alan R. Liss Inc, 1987;23–25.

72. Ash RC, Casper J, Serwint MS, et al.: Extending the application of allogeneic marrow transplantation for leukemic patients who lack matched sibling donors, utilizing partially matched donors in concert with T-cell depletion for GVHD prophylaxis. In: Gale RP and Champlin R, eds; *Progress in Bone Marrow Transplantation;* New York, Alan R. Liss Inc, 1987;365–379.

73. Storb R, Prentice RL, Thomas ED, et al.: Factors associated with graft rejection after HLA-identical marrow transplantation for aplastic anemia. *Brit J Hæmatol* 1983;55:573–585.

74. Casper J, Bunin N, Hunter J, et al.: Unrelated bone marrow transplantation in children (Abstr). *Bone Marrow Transplantation: Current Concepts;* UCLA Symposium, in press.

75. Friedrich W, Goldmann SF, Ebell W, et al.: Severe combined immunodeficiency: Treatment by bone marrow transplantation in 15 infants using HLA-haploidentical donors. *Eur J Pediatr* 1985;144:125–130.

76. Pollack MS, Kirkpatrick D, Kapoor N, et al.: Identification by HLA typing of intrauterine-derived maternal T cells in four patients with severe combined immunodeficiency. *N Engl J Med* 1982;307:662–666.

77. Fischer A, Durandy A, de Villartay JP, et al.: HLA-haploidentical bone marrow transplantation for severe combined immunodeficiency using E rosette fractionation and cyclosporine. *Blood* 1986;67:444–449.

78. Sheth KJ, Segura AD, Bunin NJ, et al.: Renal involvement in partially matched bone marrow transplantation (BMT) (Abstr). The Society of Pediatric Research 1988; in press.

79. Thomas ED, Storb R, Clift RA, et al.: Bone marrow transplantation. *N Engl J Med* 1975;292:832–895.

80. Storb R, Deeg HJ, Whitehead J, et al.: Methotrexate and cyclosporine compared with cyclosporine alone for prophylaxis of acute graft-vs.-host disease after marrow transplantation for leukemia. *N Engl J Med* 1986;314:729–735.

81. Storb R, Deeg HJ, Farewell V, et al.: Marrow transplantation for severe aplastic anemia: Methotrexate alone compared with a combination of methotrexate and cyclosporine for prevention of acute graft-vs.-host disease. *Blood* 1986;68:119–125.

82. Herve P, Cahn JY, Flesch M, et al.: Successful graft-vs.-host disease prevention without graft failure in 32 HLA-identical allogeneic bone marrow transplantations with marrow depleted of T cells by monoclonal antibodies and complement. *Blood* 1987;69:388–393.

83. Mitsuyasu RT, Champlin RE, Gale RP, et al.: Treatment of donor bone marrow with monoclonal anti-T-cell antibody and complement for the prevention of graft-vs.-host disease. *Ann Int Med* 1986;105:20–26.

84. Filipovich AH, Youle RJ, Neville DM, et al.: *Ex vivo* treatment of donor bone marrow with anti-T-cell immunotoxins for prevention of graft-vs.-host disease. *Lancet* 1984;1:469.

85. Storb R, Thomas ED: Graft-vs.-host disease in dog and man: The Seattle experience. *Immunol Rev* 1985; 8:215–238.

86. Atkinson K, Farrelly H, Cooley M, et al.: Human marrow T cell dose correlates with severity of subsequent acute graft-vs.-host disease. *Bone Marrow Transplantation* 1987; 2:51–57.

87. Truitt RL, Ash RC: Manipulation of T-cell content in transplanted human bone marrow: Effect on GVH and GVL reactions. In, *Cellular Immunotherapy of Cancer;* New York, Alan R. Liss, Inc, 1987;409–421.

88. Takaue Y, Roome AJ, Turpin JA, et al.: Depletion of T lymphocytes from human bone marrow by the use of counterflow elutriation centrifugation. *Am J Hematol* 1986;23:247–262.

89. Blazar BR, Filipovich AH, Kersey JH, et al.: T-cell depletion of donor marrow grafts: Effects on graft-vs.-host disease and engraftment. In: Gale RP, Champlin R, eds; *Progress in Bone Marrow Transplantation;* New York, Alan R. Liss Inc, 1987;381–397.

90. Ash RC, Marshall ME, Rhoades J, et al.: Development of monoclonal antibody "cocktail" for *in vitro* T cell removal for graft-vs.-host disease (GVHD) prophylaxis in human bone marrow transplantation. *Blood* 1983;62:217A.

91. Ash RC, Fitzpatrick L, Kersey J, et al.: Effect of depletion of marrow T lymphocytes by monoclonal antibody OKT3 on human pluripotential (CFU-GEMM) and committed hematopoietic progenitors (CFU-C, BFU-E, CFU-E). *Clin Res* 1981;29:761A.

92. Reisner Y, Kapoor N, Kirkpatrick D, et al.: Transplantation for severe combined immunodeficiency with HLA-A,B,D,DR imcompatible parental marrow cells fractionated by soybean agglutinin and sheep red cells. *Blood* 1983;61:341–348.

93. O'Reilly RJ, Keever C, Kernan NA, et al.: HLA nonidentical T cell depleted marrow transplants: A comparison of results in patients treated for leukemia and severe combined immunodeficiency disease. *Transplantation Proceedings* 1987;19:55–60.

94. Deeg HJ, Storb R, Weiden PL, et al.: Abrogation of resistance to and enhancement of DLA-nonidentical unrelated marrow grafts in lethally irradiated dogs by thoracic duct lymphocytes. *Blood* 1979;53:552–559.

95. Vitetta ES, Fulton RJ, May RD, et al.: Redesigning nature's poisons to create antitumor reagents. *Science* 1987;238:1098–1104

96. Apperley JF, Jones L, Hale G, et al: Bone marrow transplantation for patients with chronic myeloid leukæmia: T-cell depletion with Campath-1 reduces the incidence of graft-vs.-host disease but may increase the risk of leukæmic relapse. *Bone Marrow Transplantation* 1986;1:53–66.

97. Truitt RL, Shih C C-Y, LeFever AV: Manipulation of graft-vs.-host disease for a graft-vs.-leukemia effect after allogeneic bone marrow transplantation in AKR mice with spontaneous leukemia/lymphoma. *Transplantation* 1986;41:301–310.

98. Shih C C-Y, Truitt RL: Downregulation of L3T4+ cytotoxic T lymphocytes by interleukin-2. *Science* 1987;283:344–347.

99. Weiden PL, Sullivan KM, Flournoy N, et al.: Antileukemic effect of chronic graft-vs.-host disease. *N Engl J Med* 1981;304:1529–1533.

100. Weisdorf DJ, Nesbit ME, Ramsay NKC, et al.: Allogeneic bone marrow transplantation for acute lymphoblastic leukemia in remission: Prolonged survival associated with acute graft-vs.-host disease. *J Clin Oncol* 1987;5:1348–1355.

101. Martin PJ, Shulman HM, Schulaach WH, et al.: Fatal Epstein-Barr virus-associated proliferation of donor B cells after treatment of acute graft-vs.-host disease with a murine anti-T-cell antibody. *Ann Intern Med* 1984;101:310–315.

102. Gale RP, Opelz G, Mickey MR, et al.: Immunodeficiency following allogeneic bone marrow transplantation. *Transplant Proc* 1978;10:223–227.

103. Franceschini F, Gale RP: Immune reconstitution following bone marrow transplantation in man. In: Gale RP, Champlin R, eds; *Progress in Bone Marrow Transplantation;* New York, Alan R. Liss, Inc, 1987;607–622.
104. Lum LG: The kinetics of immune reconstitution after human marrow transplantation. *Blood* 1987;69:369–380.
105. Gratama JW, Naipal A. Oljans P, et al.: T lymphocyte repopulation and differentiation after bone marrow transplantation. Early shifts in the ratio between T4+ and T8+ T lymphocytes correlate with the occurrence of acute graft-vs.-host disease. *Blood* 1984;63:1416–1423.
106. Rozans MK, Smith BR, Burakoff SJ, et al.: Long-lasting deficit of functional T cell precursors in human bone marrow transplant recipients revealed by limiting dilution methods. *J Immunol* 1986;136:4040–4048.
107. Voltarelli JC, Stites DP: Immunological monitoring of bone marrow transplantation. *Diagnostic Immunol* 1986;4:171–193.
108. Odum N, Hofmann B, Platz P, et al.: The immunodeficiency of bone marrow-transplanted patients. *Scand J Immunol* 1985;22:259–266.
109. Lum LG, Munn NA, Schanfield MS, et al.: The detection of specific antibody formation to recall antigens after human bone marrow transplantation. *Blood* 1986;67:582–587.
110. Aucouturier P, Barra A, Intrator L, et al.: Long-lasting IgG subclass and antibacterial polysaccharide antibody deficiency after allogeneic bone marrow transplantation. *Blood* 1987;70:779–785.

Bone Marrow Transplantation in Children, edited by F. Leonard Johnson and Carl Pochedly. Raven Press, Ltd., New York © 1990.

Bone Marrow Transplantation Using Partially Matched Family Donors

Michael E. Trigg

Department of Pediatrics, University of Iowa School of Medicine, and Pediatric Bone Marrow Transplantation Program, University of Iowa Hospitals and Clinics, Iowa City, Iowa 52240

Introduction
A. Historical perspective
B. Problems and methodology
C. Eligibility of patients for transplant with marrow from partially matched family donors
D. Immune reconstitution following transplant of histoincompatible marrow
E. Future prospects
Summary

INTRODUCTION

More than half of all children with acute leukemias or lymphomas remain in long-term remission following conventional chemotherapy (1). Unfortunately, many children still relapse and ultimately succumb to their disease (2,3). Bone marrow transplantation has become widely accepted as a curative treatment for children with acute leukemias and non-Hodgkin's lymphomas who relapse following initial therapy (4–7).

No curative therapy, other than bone marrow transplantation, has been found for patients with chronic myelogenous leukemia (CML) (8,9). In addition, for those with severe aplastic anemia, marrow transplantation has become the accepted modality of therapy, if there is a matched bone marrow donor in the family.

Limitations to use of bone marrow transplantation are imposed by the lack of available histocompatible related donors and the high incidence of graft-vs.-host disease which occurs when using donor marrow from other than a related immunologically matched donor (10–15). Many chemotherapeutic and immunomodulating agents have been used to try to diminish or prevent acute graft-vs.-host disease in those undergoing marrow transplantation with alternative-type donors (16). Despite use of these measures, the incidence of severe graft-vs.-host disease is very high when using other than a matched related donor (17).

Experiments in animals have shown that histoincompatible donor marrow can be used for transplantation without producing the expected severe graft-vs.-host disease if the T lymphocytes, which are responsible for this complication, are removed from the bone marrow (18). In another chapter in this volume, issues related to the use of T lymphocyte depletion for prevention of graft-vs.-host disease are discussed in detail. (See Chapter 4 on treatment and prevention of graft-vs.-host disease.) This chapter discusses the rationale for using histoincompatible family donors, and the relationship of these transplants to the use of unrelated donors (as reviewed in the preceding chapter by Casper et al.).

HISTORICAL PERSPECTIVE

Only 30% of children who might benefit from bone marrow transplantation for treatment of aplastic anemia, malignancies that have relapsed or that are resistant to other therapy, and immune deficiencies, have a matched histocompatible related bone marrow donor available (19–23). Three avenues of approach have been tried to resolve this dilemma.

For those children with leukemias and lymphomas, transplantation of autologous bone marrow has been used. Unfortunately, the autologous marrow in these patients is contaminated with leukemic cells. Thus, methods have to be developed to purge the leukemic cells from the donated marrow. In addition, in those situations where autologous marrow is used for hematopoietic reconstitution and there is no graft-vs.-host disease, presumably there is no graft-vs.-leukemia effect either. As a result, the recurrence rate of the malignancy following such transplants is predictably high.

The second type of alternative donor for transplantation is the use of marrow from a closely matched unrelated donor (24). In some situations, such as in the University of Iowa program, individuals have been recruited specifically to serve as bone marrow donors. In other situations, donors who previously agreed to be part of pheresis programs at various blood centers have indicated a willingness to also donate bone marrow. These individuals usually have had incomplete tissue typing. On the basis of these computerized registries of individuals, it is possible to locate a donor for 10 to 50% of children who might need a donor. The main difficulty in using such unrelated donors is the period of time required to find such a donor.

Most donors who have been identified on computer searches have had incomplete tissue typing. Thus, once an individual is identified as a close match at the HLA A and B loci, additional typing is usually necessary. This further testing requires the donor to return to the medical center to give additional blood for Dr typing by serologic methods, for testing in mixed lymphocyte culture (MLC) with the potential recipient, or both. In addition, at the present time there is lack of experience using incompletely matched unrelated donors, as well as with the use of MLC-reactive unrelated donors. Thus, most centers performing transplants with use of such unrelated donors are demanding that donors must match serologically at 5 out of 6 of the HLA A, B and Dr loci and that the MLC reactivity must be low (less than 25%). The author and his colleagues believe that these restrictions on donor use are too extreme. In addition, in our program we have completely typed all the possible donors. As a result of this prior testing, it is possible in only 1 hour to complete a search through the donor pool to identify histocompatible individuals, but this is not the usual routine. In some cases the search for an unrelated donor may take up to 3 months at a minimum in order for such a donor to be identified.

Then we deal with the logistical problem of deciding where the transplant will be done. For example, if the individual requiring a transplant using a particular unrelated donor is in Boston and the donor lives in Seattle, then either the patient needing the transplant must go to Seattle or the donor from Seattle must go to Boston. The alternative would be to have the marrow harvested in Seattle and then sent to Boston for use in the transplant. In the situation where the recipient has to travel, this becomes very inconvenient for a family and creates other social and emotional problems. When the donor has to travel, this adds additional expense not covered by the center doing the search nor is this cost covered by the recipient's insurance. Thus, the donor's travel expenses would have to be paid by the recipient, which most families would find difficult to do. Finally, the donor's marrow could conceivably be harvested at the institution where the donor was identified. This requires the physicians and technical staff to be available to perform the procedure and coordination of the harvest with the recipient's transplant center may be difficult.

For these reasons, one would like to be very certain that the results following use of marrow from histoincompatible family members are significantly worse than when unrelated donors are used before embarking on the establishment of a national program.

Histoincompatible family donors have been used for some time as bone marrow donors (25). However, it is critical in evaluating the results of marrow transplantation using histoincompatible donors to define the level of histoincompatibility. The Seattle group has reported extensive studies on this issue. These studies indicate that the use of phenotypically identical related (sibling) donors produces results similar to those observed following use of genotypically identical (unrelated) donors. Transplant results using donors who differ at one of the HLA A or B loci, with a negative MLC, are similar to those using fully matched related donors. The results are much worse when the degree of histoincompatibility increases to two or more of the HLA loci and, in particular, when the donor and recipient pair differ at one of the two HLA Dr loci producing a positive MLC reaction (26). In fact, in most centers reporting such data, rejection rates have been extremely high and graft-vs.-host disease has been quite severe (27,28). So, it was not until the development of methods to decrease the likelihood of graft-vs.-host disease that such transplants were attempted in large enough numbers to demonstrate the curative potential of bone marrow transplantation in children (29,30,31).

PROBLEMS AND METHODOLOGY

The identification of family donors is far easier than the identification of an unrelated donor—clear advantage for a child requiring such a transplant. Donors can be identified relatively quickly. Family members can be tissue typed weeks or months before the time when the transplant might be needed, and these tissue typing data would be available on hand if acutely needed (31,32).

The use of histoincompatible donors would predictably result in two potential problems (Table 1). The first is severe graft-vs.-host disease. Both the Seattle group and the Royal Marsden group in London utilized unmanipulated marrow from the histoincompatible donors with methotrexate or cyclosporine for prevention of graft-vs.-host disease (17,25). Both groups documented severe graft-vs.-host disease in 75 to 90% of patients, and this complication limited survival. In these studies, the majority of the histoincompatible donors who were haplo-identical at the HLA A, B and DR loci showed reactivity in mixed lymphocyte culture with the recipients' cells.

TABLE 1. *Major problems following bone marrow transplantation with histoincompatible donors*

1. Problems with engraftment
    a. graft rejection
    b. graft-vs.-host disease
2. Problems with infections—causes
    a. immune responsiveness and HLA restriction
    b. T lymphocyte depletion
    c. delayed hematopoietic recovery (neutropenia)
    d. continued immunosuppression to prevent graft-vs.-host disease
3. Problems with recurrent malignancy
    a. no graft-vs.-malignancy effect
    b. malignant disease resistant to treatment

The second anticipated problem would be graft rejection. Rates of graft rejection in these two studies appeared to be low, although evaluation of rejection was difficult as many patients died of severe graft-vs.-host disease before they achieved full hematopoietic reconstitution (Figure 1).

In order to achieve stable hematopoietic engraftment when using histoincompatible marrow from related donors, an immunosuppressive regimen of increased intensity was necessary to completely ablate the bone marrow of the recipient animal (19,32,33). These observations have since been confirmed in studies done in humans as well (32).

In the initial experience at the University of Wisconsin, 3 patients of the first 10 receiving histoincompatible related donor marrow engrafted (32). These were the only patients who had been given significantly increased pretransplant immunosuppression. This finding documented the need for giving increased immunosuppression to permit marrow engraftment. As a result of that study, marrow rejection is believed to be the result of persistence of host lymphocytes, those remaining after completion of the standard ablative chemotherapy and radiotherapy given to prepare the patient for marrow transplant (35). Subsequent to that discovery, other centers have also published findings showing that persistence of cells of the host immune system is a possible mechanism to explain the rejection of histoincompatible marrow (28).

One of the methods to prevent graft-vs.-host disease is by depleting T lymphocytes from the donor marrow, and such an approach in matched transplants has been associated with a decreased incidence of severe graft-vs.-host

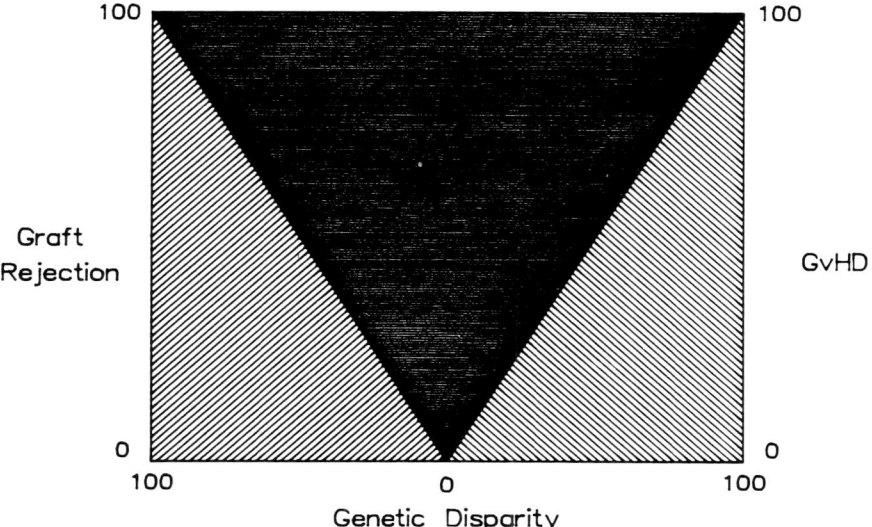

FIG. 1. Diagram showing the relationship of genetic disparity between donors and the occurrence of graft rejection and graft-vs.-host disease. In each case, there is an inverse relationship.

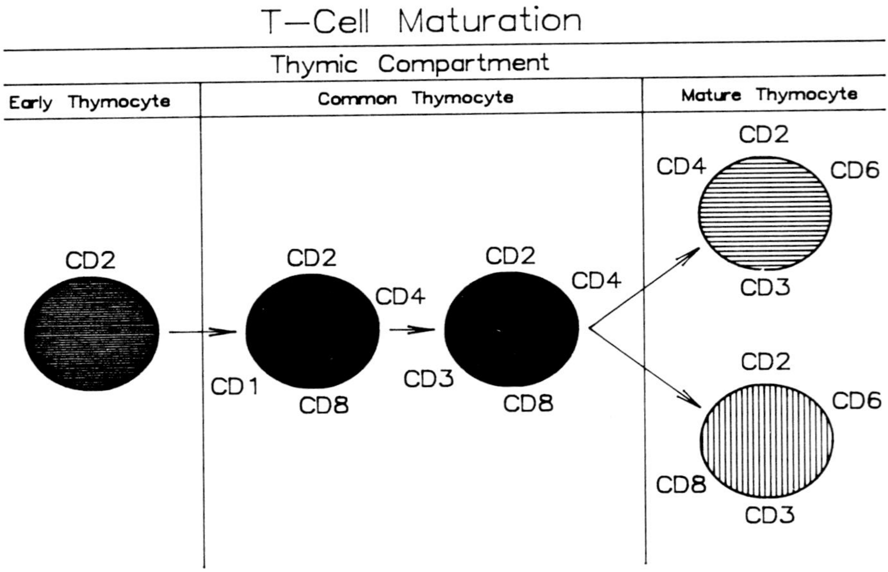

T—Cell Maturation

FIG. 2. T lymphocyte maturation by division of the thymic compartment into various components. T lymphocyte depletion has been accomplished with a variety of methodologies and reagents. As demonstrated here, an anti-CD2 antibody (CT2) reacts with cells in each of the thymic compartments.

disease (Figures 2 and 3) (36–43). However, the incidence of graft rejection was found to be very high when the donor marrow had been depleted of mature T lymphocytes (28). It was assumed that the lack of donor T lymphocytes in the marrow inoculum accounted, to some extent, for this high rate of graft rejection. This problem of rejection has been successfully overcome by more completely suppressing the recipient's immune system (32,35). We observed a rejection rate of 5% in children who received histoincompatible marrow from family donors.

It is well known that many children transplanted for treatment of leukemia have leukemic recurrence following the transplant. This finding suggests that in selected situations, leukemic cells remain resistant to the ablative preparative regimen of chemotherapy and radiation (44). It is not difficult to accept the concept that some mature lymphocytes of the recipient may also survive the ablative therapy. Furthermore, in some situations hematopoietic and immunologic chimerism may not be possible, and the donor marrow is then rejected once host lymphocytes regrow. Thus, it may never be possible to lower the rejection rate to less than 5%, the currently achievable level, without massively increasing the ablative chemotherapy and radiotherapy given prior to transplant.

Other studies have now shown the importance of giving pre-transplant

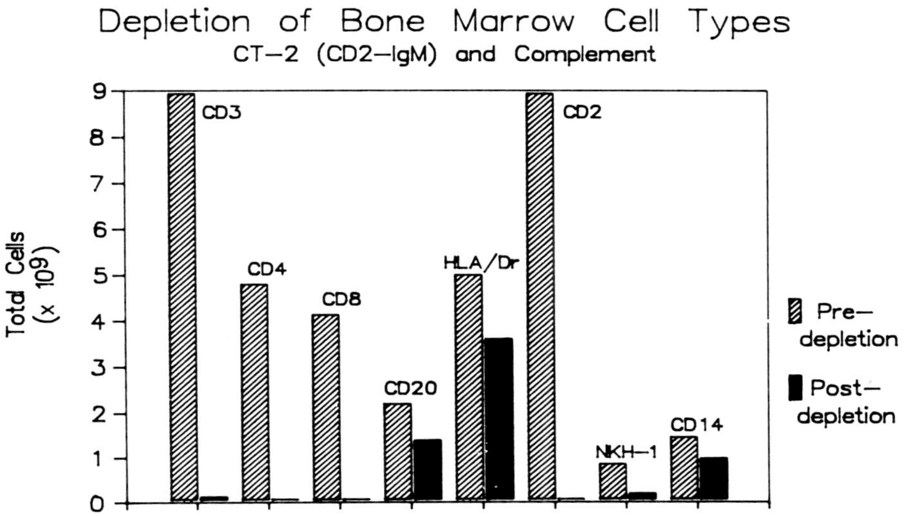

Depletion of Bone Marrow Cell Types
CT—2 (CD2—IgM) and Complement

FIG. 3. Depletion of bone marrow cell types using an IgM anti-CD2 antibody in complement. The extent of T lymphocyte depletion is complete at a level of 99%. Normal hematopoietic stem cells are not harmed with this method and engraftment is quite adequate.

marrow-ablation therapy to permit engraftment of bone marrow from histo-incompatible related donors (45).

Some have speculated that a specific number of T lymphocytes must remain in the marrow graft in order for engraftment to occur. It has even been suggested that, if all of the donor T lymphocytes have been removed for the marrow graft, a certain number should then be added back to facilitate engraftment (45). However, the function of T lymphocytes in the donor marrow and their relationship to marrow growth has not been adequately explained by laboratory studies intended to show the importance of these cells in marrow engraftment (46,47).

ELIGIBILITY OF PATIENTS FOR TRANSPLANT WITH MARROW FROM PARTIALLY MATCHED FAMILY DONORS

Children with acute lymphoblastic leukemia (ALL) in second remission, children with acute nonlymphocytic leukemia (ANLL) in second remission and those with chronic myelogenous leukemia, as well as patients with severe aplastic anemia unresponsive to conventional treatment with androgens, steroids and/or antilymphocyte or antithymocyte globulin qualify for trials of marrow transplants from partially matched family donors.

Initial results with use of transplants of marrow from partially matched family donors in children with leukemias indicate 2-year event-free survivals of approximately 40%. These results are superior to those reported following use of conventional chemotherapy for children with relapsed acute lymphoblastic leukemia or acute nonlymphocytic leukemia. If these data are confirmed by other transplant centers, this would suggest that use of histoincompatible bone marrow transplantation will have application for these children.

For the child with severe aplastic anemia who does not have a histocompatible related donor, most investigators would prescribe a trial of antithymocyte globulin, steroids and/or cyclosporine before recommending a marrow transplant using a histoincompatible donor.

Another difficulty encountered when using marrow from an unrelated donor or marrow from a histoincompatible donor for the treatment of aplastic anemia is a high rejection rate if the recipient's immune system is incompletely ablated prior to the transplant (32). Thus, in order to achieve stable engraftment, the child with severe aplastic anemia who is to be given marrow from an unrelated donor or from a histoincompatible related donor must be as completely immunosuppressed as a child with leukemia being prepared for transplant. Two such patients were transplanted by the author. One child, who lived for almost 4 months after the transplant, had excellent hematopoietic engraftment, as shown by aspirated bone marrow smears which looked completely normal, but died of a disseminated adenovirus infection.

IMMUNE RECONSTITUTION FOLLOWING TRANSPLANT OF HISTOINCOMPATIBLE MARROW

In vitro experiments and studies of immune responsiveness in animals suggest that immune response is HLA restricted. This means that for cells to present antigen properly and to respond to the appropriate antigenic signal, there must be some similarity in HLA phenotype. Thus, when using a histoincompatible donor, it was expected that more significant problems with infections would occur.

In addition, the depletion of T lymphocytes from marrow prior to transplant has also predisposed to an increased number of infections. Several studies have shown delayed recovery of T lymphocytes in patients receiving T lymphocyte-depleted histoincompatible bone marrow, as compared to those receiving unmanipulated bone marrow from histocompatible related donors. It is not known whether this situation is secondary to the use of prolonged immunosuppression in the recipient of the T lymphocyte-depleted graft, or whether it is due to the significantly faster hematopoietic engraftment in those receiving marrow from a histocompatible donor. These studies have also documented an increased incidence of infections and the occurrence of different types of infections in patients who received T lymphocyte-depleted bone marrow (48). Several patients have developed Epstein-Barr virus-related lymphoproliferative disorders, which were previously rarely seen in marrow transplant patients. Similarly, a variety of other viral infections that have occurred in these patients is thought to be related to the use of T lymphocyte-depleted bone marrow, but again these infections may be related only to the use of histoincompatible marrow.

More than 20 long-term survivors of histoincompatible marrow transplants have now been studied. Eventually, all showed normal immunologic reconstitution in both the T lymphocyte and B lymphocyte compartments. Many of these children have not required readmission to the hospital following transplantation and have not suffered any significant infections. This suggests that in time a tolerance develops between the host and the histoincompatible hematologic and immunologic graft, allowing for a normal immune response to occur. Whether this situation is restricted only to certain HLA phenotypes, and whether there are differences between disease types and the age of the recipient, is unknown. It is hoped that future analyses will help to resolve these questions.

Several studies of immunologic reconstitution in children with a variety of immune deficiencies have shown the occurrence of only partial immune reconstitution following marrow transplant. In almost every situation where partial immune reconstitution was observed, the children had not been immunosuppressed pre-transplant. These were primarily children with severe immune deficiencies, in whom the donor marrow was simply infused intravenously. In these selected situations, it is quite probable that there was some immune responsiveness to the donor marrow and that portions of the donor marrow were rejected or were incompletely grafted. As a result, these children have remained partially immune deficient. Of interest is the fact that the major cellular components failing to engraft were the B lymphocytes.

In one study, children with immune deficiencies who failed to engraft following infusion of bone marrow were then immunosuppressed with a preparative regimen similar to that used before transplant for leukemia (49). Complete immunologic reconstitution followed. These findings suggest that the lack of a response *in vitro* to foreign cells may not in itself determine whether complete marrow engraftment will take place. Thus, if marrow engraftment fails to occur promptly and completely, then further immunosuppression followed by a second transplant is warranted. Also, indirect findings suggest that a bone marrow transplant from a histoincompatible donor can reconstitute thymic epithelium in children with severe combined immune deficiency disease (50).

FUTURE PROSPECTS

Marrow engraftment using histoincompatible related donors has been clearly demonstrated. In order to produce stable hematopoietic engraftment and immunologic reconstitution, more immunosuppressive therapy is necessary pre-transplant and adequate methods are needed to prevent or control graft-vs.-host disease. In addition, adequate control over infections is needed during the period preceding normal immune reconstitution. Newer drugs and immunomodulating agents such as gamma globulin can be given to enhance other measures taken to prevent infections. On the other hand, while attempts are made to prevent infections and graft-vs.-host disease until the patient achieves full immunologic recovery, further studies are needed to understand the mechanisms of immunologic recovery following transplantation of histoincompatible marrow. Clearly, tolerance to the new marrow graft develops in some children without occurrence of severe graft-vs.-host disease and normal immunologic and hematopoietic reconstitution occurs. How this reconstitution occurs, and why this happens in some individuals and not in others, is still unclear.

Currently, controlled trials are under way comparing the use of unrelated marrow donors to histoincompatible family donors. It is anticipated that these trials will demonstrate any differences in the results of transplantation using the 2 types of donor marrow. In a study being conducted by the author, only those children who match with an available unrelated donor are eligible for randomization, which is stratified by disease type. Preliminary data indicate that there will be no difference in long-term outcome, regardless of the donor type used. Such a finding would significantly increase the usefulness of bone marrow transplantation in children. All children who would benefit from transplant-type therapy could undergo transplantation using a histoincompatible family donor, except adopted children who might require an unrelated donor.

SUMMARY

When a suitably matched family donor cannot be found, children may undergo transplantation using a partially matched family member or an unrelated donor. Graft rejection and infectious complications are the main problems which occur when using partially matched family donors. However, major progress has been made in overcoming the rejection phenomena by increasing pre-transplant immunosuppression. In addition, with improvements in engraftment and improvements in the prophylactic medications which are used to prevent infections, more patients are surviving free of major infectious problems. How these children develop tolerance to their new grafts is unknown, but certainly normal immune function has been well documented to occur within 1 year post-bone marrow transplantation. It is anticipated that survival rates will reach the same level as those seen using suitably matched family donors.

REFERENCES

1. Steinhorn SC: Improved survival among children with acute leukemia diagnosed in the 1970s. *Cancer Treat Rep* 1984;68:953–958.
2. Johnson FL, Thomas RD: Treatment of relapsed acute lymphoblastic leukemia in childhood. *N Engl J Med* 1983;310:263.
3. Amato KR, Sallen SE, Lipton JM: Combination chemotherapy in relapsed childhood acute lymphoblastic leukemia. *Cancer Treat Rep* 1984;68:411–412.
4. Preisler HD, Brecher M, Browman G, et al.: The treatment of acute myelocytic leukemia in patients 30 years of age and younger. *Am J Hematol* 1982;13:189–198.
5. O'Leary M, Ramsay NKC, Nesbit ME, et al.: Bone marrow transplantation for non-Hodgkin's lymphoma in children and young adults. *Am J Med* 1983;74:497–501.
6. Weinstein HJ, Mayer RJ, Rosenthal DS, et al.: Chemotherapy for acute myelogenous leukemia in children and adults; VAPA update. *Blood* 1983;62:315–319.
7. Kadoat RP, Smithson WA: Bone marrow transplantation for diseases of childhood. *Mayo Clin Proc* 1984;59:171–184.
8. Preisler HD, Raza A: Chronic myelocytic leukemia; comments on new approaches to therapy. *Cancer Treat Rep* 1982;66:1073–1076.
9. Speck B, Bortin MM, Champlin R, et al.: Allogeneic bone marrow transplantation for chronic myelogenous leukemia. *Lancet* 1984;1:665–668.
10. Johnson FL, Thomas ED, Clark BS, et al.: A comparison of marrow transplantation with chemotherapy for children with acute lymphoblastic leukemia in second or subsequent remission. *N Engl J Med* 1981;305:846–851.
11. Beutler E, McMillan R, Spruce W: The role of bone marrow transplantation in the treatment of acute leukemia in remission. *Blood* 1982;59:1115–1117.
12. Gale RP, Kay HEM, Rimm AA, Borten MM: Bone marrow transplantation for acute leukemia in first remission. *Lancet* 1982;2:1006–1009.
13. Thomas ED, Sanders JE, Flournoy N, et al.: Marrow transplantation for patients with acute lymphoblastic leukemia; a long-term follow-up. *Blood* 1983;62:1139–1141.
14. Buckner CD, Clift RA, Thomas ED, et al.: Allogeneic marrow transplantation for patients with acute nonlymphoblastic leukemia in second remission. *Leuk Res* 1982;6:395–399.
15. Dinsmore R, Kirkpatrick D, Flomenberg N, et al.: Allogeneic bone marrow transplantation for patients with acute nonlymphocytic leukemia. *Blood* 1984;63:649–656.
16. Kanojia MD, Angnoustou AA, Zander AR, et al.: High-dose methylprednisolone treatment for acute graft-vs.-host disease after bone marrow transplantation in adults. *Transplantation* 1984;37:246–249.
17. Powles RL, Kay HEM, Clink HM, et al.: Mismatched family donors for bone marrow transplantation as treatment for acute leukemia. *Lancet* 1983;1:612–615.
18. O'Reilly RJ: Allogeneic bone marrow transplantation; current status and future directions. *Blood* 1983;62:941–964.
19. Vallera DA, Youle RJ, Neville DM, et al.: Monoclonal antibody toxin conjugates for experimental graft-vs.-host disease prophylaxis. *Transplantation* 1983;36:73–80.
20. Johnson FL: Marrow transplantation in the treatment of acute childhood leukemia. *Am J Pediatr Hematol/Oncol* 1981;3:389–395.
21. Barrett AJ, Kendra JR, Lucas CF, et al.: Bone marrow transplantation for acute lymphoblastic leukemia. *Br J Hæmatol* 1982;52:181–188.
22. Thomas ED: Marrow transplantation for malignant diseases. *J Clin Oncol* 1983; 1:517–531.
23. Storb R, Thomas ED: Allogeneic bone marrow transplantation. *Immunol Rev* 1983;71:77–102.
24. Gingrich RD, Howe CWS, Goeken NE, et al.: The use of partially matched, unrelated donors in clinical bone marrow transplantation. *Transplantation* 1985;39:526–532.
25. Beatty PG, Clift RA, Mickelson EM, et al.: Marrow transplantation from related donors other than HLA identical siblings. *N Engl J Med* 1985;313:765–771.
26. Clift RA, Beatty PG, Thomas ED, et al.: Marrow transplantation from mismatched donors for the treatment of malignancy. *Transplant Proc* 1985;17:445–446.
27. Filipovich AH, Ramsay NKC, Arthur DC, et al.: Allogeneic bone marrow transplantation with related donors other than HLA, MLC matched siblings and the use of antithymocyte

globulin, prednisone and methotrexate for prophylaxis of graft-vs.-host disease. *Transplant Proc* 1985;39:282–285.

28. Kernan MA, Flomenberg N, DuPont B, O'Reilly RJ: Graft rejection in recipients of T-cell depleted HLA nonidentical marrow transplants for leukemia. *Transplantation* 1987;43:842–847.

29. Trigg ME, Billing R, Sondel P, et al.: *In vitro* treatment of donor bone marrow with anti-E rosette antibody and complement prior to bone marrow transplantation. *J Cell Biochem* 1983; [Suppl] 7A:57.

30. Prentice HG, Janossy G, Price-Jones et al.: Depletion of T lymphocytes in donor marrow prevents significant graft-vs.-host disease in matched allogeneic leukæmic marrow transplant recipients. *Lancet* 1984;1:472–476.

31. Trigg ME, Billing R, Sondel PM, et al.: Depletion of T cells from human bone marrow with monoclonal antibody CT-2 and complement. *J Biol Resp Modif* 1984;3:406–412.

32. Trigg ME, Billing R, Sondel PM, et al.: Clinical trial depleting T lymphocytes from donor marrow for matched and mismatched allogeneic bone marrow transplants. *Cancer Treat Rep* 1985;69:377–386.

33. Vallera DA, Ash RC, Zanjani ED, et al.: Anti-T-cell reagents for human bone marrow transplantation; ricin linked to three monoclonal antibodies. *Science* 1983;333:512–513.

34. Trigg ME, Peterson A, Erickson C, et al.: Depletion of T-cells from bone marrow for allogeneic transplantation; method for treatment of bone marrow in bulk. *Exp Hematol* 1986;14:21–26.

35. Sondel PM, Hank JA, Trigg ME, et al.: Transplantation of HLA mismatched T-cell depleted bone marrow for leukemia. Autologous marrow recovery with specific immune sensitization to donor antigens. *Exp Hematol* 1986;14:278–286.

36. Martin A, Ebell W, Friedrich W, et al.: Transient hemopoietic stem cell engraftment after transplantation of HLA haploidentical T cell depleted bone marrow. *Transplantation* 1987;43:165.

37. Filipovich AH, Ramsay NKC, Warkentin PI, et al.: Pretreatment of donor marrow with monoclonal antibody OKT3 for prevention of acute graft-vs.-host disease in allogeneic histocompatible bone marrow transplantation. *Lancet* 1982;1:1266–1269.

38. Granger S, Janossy G, Francis G, et al.: Elimination of T lymphocytes from human bone marrow with monoclonal T-antibodies and cytolytic complement. *Br J Hæmatol* 1982;50:367–374.

39. Prentice HG, Janossy G, Skeggs D, et al.: Use of anti-T-cell monoclonal antibody OKT3 to prevent acute graft-vs.-host disease in allogeneic bone marrow transplantation for acute leukemia. *Lancet* 1982;1:700–703.

40. Reinherz EL, Geha R, Rappeport JM, et al.: Reconstitution after transplantation with T lymphocyte-depleted HLA haplotype-mismatched bone marrow for severe combined immunodeficiency. *Proc Natl Acad Sci USA* 1982;79:604–651.

41. Hale G, Bright S, Chumbley G, et al.: Removal of T cells from bone marrow for transplantation; a monoclonal antilymphocyte antibody that fixes human complement. *Blood* 1983;62:873–882.

42. Ozer H, Han T, Early A, et al.: An improved method for T cell depletion of allogeneic histoincompatible donor bone marrow. *Cancer Drug Delivery* 1983;1:79–86.

43. Sharp TG, Sachs DH, Fauci AS, et al.: T cell depletion of human bone marrow using monoclonal antibody and complement-mediated lysis. *Transplantation* 1983;35:112–120.

44. Dinsmore R, Kirkpatrick D, Flomenberg N, et al.: Allogeneic bone marrow transplantation for patients with acute lymphoblastic leukemia. *Blood* 1983;62:381–388.

45. Pietryga DW, Blazar BR, Soderling CCV, Vallera DA: The effect of T-subset depletion on the incidence of lethal graft-vs.-host disease in a murine major histocompatibility complex mismatched transplantation system. *Transplantation* 1987;43:442–445.

46. deWitte T, Raymakers R, Plas A, et al.: Bone marrow repopulation capacity after transplantation of lymphocyte depleted allogeneic bone marrow using counterflow centrifugation. *Transplantation* 1984;37:151–155.

47. Filipovich AH, Youle RJ, Neville DM, et al.: *Ex vivo* treatment of donor bone marrow with anti-T-cell immunotoxins for prevention of graft-vs.-host disease. *Lancet* 1984;1:469–472.

48. Skinner J, Finlay JF, Sondel PM, Trigg ME: Infectious complications in pediatric patients

undergoing transplantation with T lymphocyte depleted bone marrow. *Pediatr Infect Dis* 1986;5:319–324.

49. Moen RC, Horowitz SD, Sondel PM, et al.: Immunologic reconstitution after haploidentical bone marrow transplantation for immune deficiency disorders; treatment of bone marrow cells with monoclonal antibody CT-2 and complement. *Blood* 1987;70:664–669.

50. Hong R, Horowitz S, Moen R, et al.: Thymus and B cell reconstitution in severe combined immunodeficiency after transplantation of monoclonal antibody depleted parental mismatched bone marrow. *Bone Marrow Transplantation* 1987;1:405–409.

Graft Rejection

Terry E. Pick

Bone Marrow Transplant Services, Cook-Fort Worth Children's Medical Center, Fort Worth, Texas 76102

Introduction
A. Animal studies
B. Human studies
Summary

INTRODUCTION

Graft failure is a complication of bone marrow transplantation that has been recognized for many years. In early studies of bone marrow transplantation, this was a common occurrence. Graft rejection was first noted in 1939 by Osgood and associates when they injected marrow in an attempt to treat a patient with aplastic anemia (1). There was no evidence of a take of bone marrow in this case or in other cases treated during the next decade.

This failure of engraftment is not surprising since these patients were treated before we had a clear knowledge of the pathophysiology of graft rejection. No conditioning regimen was used before transplant in these early cases. Knowledge of the requirement of host immune suppression by giving high-dose chemotherapy, radiation, or both, to prevent graft rejection only came after animal studies were performed by the pioneers of bone marrow transplantation. When the need was recognized for this host immune suppression by high doses of chemotherapy and radiation, the incidence of graft rejection markedly decreased.

Recently, there has been an increased incidence of graft failure as methods of T cell depletion have been used in clinical transplant trials, in efforts to prevent graft-vs.-host disease. This complication has sparked another look into the treatment and prevention of failure of engraftment.

341

ANIMAL STUDIES

In 1949, Jacobson initiated studies using radiation in mice to doses that produced marrow ablation (3). The spleen was protected by shielding it from the radiation. This was accomplished by exteriorizing the spleen surgically, which allowed for complete shielding. Even when the spleen seemed to become infarcted, this procedure still protected the animal from marrow failure. Jacobson reasoned that these infarcted spleens were equivalent to splenic autografts and thus his findings showed that splenic autografts protected the animals from irradiation (4). In the same year, Jacobson and colleagues also showed that intraperitoneal injection of syngeneic marrow protected the mice from death due to bone marrow failure.

These and subsequent studies demonstrated that marrow could be infused and produce bone marrow engraftment. Ford in 1956 introduced *radiation chimera* to designate an animal which carries a foreign hematopoietic system following marrow ablation by radiation and then subsequent transplantation of foreign hematopoietic cells (5). It was later shown that chemotherapy alone could produce similar chimeras and the word *radiation* was dropped. From these and subsequent studies (6–10), the observed engraftment in bone marrow chimeras led to the concept of graft tolerance. These experiments also produced animals that developed acute graft-vs.-host disease and regained their health and developed tolerance to host antigens.

It was initially believed that a serum factor was responsible for this tolerance (11). Field and colleagues showed that refractoriness to graft-vs.-host disease could be transferred in rats by serum from rats who had recovered from graft-vs.-host disease (11). This factor has subsequently been shown to be a suppressor T cell, probably a T_8 (CD-8) cell (12).

How the animal was prepared for transplant appeared to be an important factor in engraftment. The most widely used conditioning regimen in dogs has been total body radiation (TBI). Engraftment only occurred when the dose of radiation was above 1200 cGy (13,14). Dogs that engraft at this dose are complete chimeras.

In other studies performed in dogs and rodents, cyclophosphamide was substituted for total body irradiation (15). In contrast to the complete radiation chimeras produced by TBI, animals treated with cyclophosphamide alone are usually mixed chimeras, that is, an animal with a combination of host and donor hematopoietic cells.

An adequate number of bone marrow cells harvested for marrow transplantation is very important to insure full engraftment and to prevent marrow failure in both allogeneic and autologous bone marrow transplantation. The dose of cells appears to be particularly important in transplantation in dogs when compatibility at the major histocompatibility complex (MHC) locus, called DL-A, is taken into account. A dose of $2 - 4 \times 10^8$ marrow cells/kg consistently insures engraftment of donors who are identical at the DL-A locus but higher doses of donor marrow cells, on the order of 10^9 cells/kg, are necessary for engraftment in animals nonidentical at the MHC locus (18–20). Consistent engraftment could also be produced even across histocompatible barriers when buffy coat, a source of stem cells and immunologically active cells, was added to the marrow inoculum. (21).

Compatibility at the MHC, then, is also of value in predicting engraftment. Eleven of 12 dogs transplanted with DL-A identical marrow following TBI demonstrated sustained engraftment in contrast to 1 of 10 dogs given DL-A mismatched marrow (30). Attempts to overcome this graft rejection by increasing the dose of TBI treatment with silica particles, ATS, procarbazine and ATS, and high doses of methotrexate failed to prevent graft rejection.

The only treatment that was effective in overcoming this histocompatible barrier was transfusion of viable donor leukocytes. Nine out of 11 dogs achieved a sustained engraftment when donor leukocytes were added to the marrow infusion (33).

The mechanism for prevention of graft rejection by leukocyte transfusions is not completely understood, but three possibilities are: (1) potentiation of graft tolerance by a large amount of donor antigen provided by the infused white blood cells, (2) administration of increased numbers of stem cells, and (3) depression of the host's residual immune reactivity by immunocompetent cells present in large numbers in infused leukocytes. The first explanation is unlikely because irradiated lymphocytes cannot produce marrow engraftment. The third explanation is most likely.

Blood transfusions before bone marrow transplantation is also associated with a higher rate of graft rejection (23). In a study by Weiden and colleagues it was observed that in 41 transplants between MHC matched nontransfused canine littermates, recipient dogs rejected their graft (25).

In the same experiment, 12 littermates were treated with TBI, marrow infusion from mismatched littermates and leukocyte transfusions. None of these 12 rejected their marrow graft (25). In contrast, 6 out of 9 dogs transfused with blood from random donors prior to their transplantation rejected their grafts after an identical transplant protocol. This sensitization could have been due to exposure to either major or minor histocompatibility antigens. Graft rejection was associated with reappearance of peripheral blood lymphocytes with host karyotype suggesting that the graft rejection was related to a cellular immune response of the host (26).

Transplants between unrelated, mismatched dogs also are associated with a high rate of graft failure. Eleven of 72 dogs treated with 1200 cGy of TBI, and given unrelated mismatched marrow and leukocytes, rejected or failed to sustain their grafts (27). If the dogs were previously exposed to donor blood from 24 hours to 3 months prior to transplantation, there was an increased incidence of marrow rejection. Transfusion of leukocyte-poor or platelet-poor blood also produced this increased rate of graft rejection (28).

This sensitization by blood transfusions could be blocked by immunosuppressive agents. Dogs were given 2 donor blood transfusions at 20 and 13 days before bone marrow transplantation. Seven out of 10 dogs developed graft rejection in spite of being conditioned with and being infused with peripheral blood leukocytes as well as marrow (29). When procarbazine (2.5 mg/kg) was given on days −8, −6, and −4, together with rabbit anti-dog antithymocyte serum (0.6 ml/kg) on days −7, −5, and −3, 9 out of 10 dogs so treated sustained successful engraftment. Neither of these agents were able to prevent graft failure when given alone.

In a subsequent study, pairs of dogs were given 6 weekly transfusions of either donor platelet concentrates (22 dogs) or whole blood (8 dogs) before transplantation (29). One dog of each pair was conditioned with TBI only. The other dog received procarbazine and antithymocyte serum in addition to the TBI. Eleven of 15 dogs treated with TBI alone rejected their grafts, in contrast to 3 of 15 dogs conditioned with procarbazine and ATS, confirming the usefulness of more intensive immunosuppression in preventing graft rejection in dogs.

Storb and colleagues showed that graft rejection could be produced with both blood products and skin epithelial cells (33). They transfused 19 dogs with whole blood before transplantation and all 19 dogs rejected their grafts. Graft rejection was believed to be caused by sensitization of the recipient to non-DL-A antigens expressed on leukocytes in the transfused blood from the marrow donor. Tripling the dose of TBI did not prevent graft rejection. This 100% rejection rate also suggested that more than one minor multiallelic antigenic histocompatibility system outside the DL-A may be involved in the sensitization process that leads to graft rejection, an observation consistent with the observed increased incidence of rejection in heavily transfused patients with aplastic anemia. Subcutaneous injections of epithelial cells also led to graft rejection in dogs (33), indicating that antigens involved in the mediation of graft rejection are not found only on hematopoietic cells. All 6 dogs sensitized by injections of epithelial cells rejected their grafts.

Antigens involved in graft rejection are contained in concentrated leukocyte preparations. As many as 50% of transplanted dogs sustained an engraftment when they were transfused with leukocyte-poor products, such as buffy coat-free platelets or red cells, a higher rate of engraftment than earlier studies (34). It was believed that this difference was due to the fact that red cells and platelets express only some of the antigens involved in graft rejection and that the cell separation techniques available during initial studies still allowed contamination by leukocytes. This information may be clinically relevant in aplastic anemia, where leukocyte-poor transfusions might decrease the incidence of graft rejection.

HUMAN STUDIES

Graft failure in transplants for aplastic anemia is a common problem. Up to 30% of patients multiply transfused pre-transplant, prepared with cyclophosphamide alone and transplanted from an HLA-matched donor will reject their grafts (35). This rejection is believed to be due to sensitization by the prior transfusions of blood products and both major and minor antigens are involved in this sensitization. Antigens other than those of the MHC locus may also be involved in this process.

The relative response index (RRI) has been used to predict whether a patient will reject a graft (36). In a study of 34 patients with severe aplastic anemia, the relative response index in the mixed lymphocyte culture was studied as a predictor of graft failure (36). A RRI value greater than 1.6 was defined as positive and a value less than 1.6 was considered negative. Nine out of 12 patients with a positive RRI rejected their grafts. Each of these 9 patients had received more than 10 transfusions of red blood cells or platelets from random donors before transplantation. Twenty-three patients had a negative RRI and only 3 of these patients rejected their grafts.

An analysis of 139 patients transplanted for the treatment of severe aplastic anemia demonstrated that besides a positive RRI, the number of marrow cells infused also correlated with rejection (37). Donor infusions with less than 3×10^8 marrow cells/kg had a higher incidence of graft rejection.

These factors have been used in devising strategies for treating patients who may be expected to have a high likelihood of graft rejection. Nonsensitized patients with RRI values of less than 1.6 were conditioned with cyclophosphamide alone in one study: the rejection rate was 14% and survival was 77% (37). Of the 38 nonsensitized patients, 15 had never received a blood transfusion, and none of these 15 patients rejected their grafts. Patients who had a positive RRI were treated with a more intensive conditioning regimen and buffy coat from the donor was given in addition to the marrow cells. This was done in an attempt to increase the number of stem cells. Eleven sensitized patients were treated in this way. The rejection rate decreased to less than 10% but survival was not improved, due to deaths from graft-vs.-host disease and interstitial pneumonia.

Various other forms of immunosuppression have been studied including total body irradiation, procarbazine, cyclophosphamide, and antithymocyte antiserum (ATS). Of these four agents, only ATS has been shown to be effective when used alone in the treatment and prevention of graft failure (38). All 15 sensitized patients successfully engrafted following ATS in one study (38). Most centers now employ a combination of immunosuppressive agents including cyclophosphamide with cyclosporine A or total nodal irradiation to overcome rejection in sensitized patients. (See Chapter 10.)

In an effort to transplant across major barriers and prevent graft-vs.-host disease, T cell depletion of the marrow has been investigated following the observation in animal models that depleting mature T cells from marrow lessens the severity of graft-vs.-host disease. A major complication of the use of T cell depleted marrow, however, has been an increase in the risk of graft failure and rejection. Failure to graft has been observed in 10 to 35% of HLA identical bone marrow recipients, and in up to 50% of HLA nonidentical matches (39–41). Affected patients either fail to graft or, following initial engraftment and hematopoietic recovery, slowly lose hematopoiesis during the next 6 months. The exact mechanism is uncertain but it is probably due to immunological rejection of the grafted bone marrow. T cells in the donor marrow are probably necessary to destroy immunologically active cells that remain in the host after conditioning regimens have been used.

SUMMARY

Graft rejection was noted in early marrow transplant studies. Animal studies increased our understanding of the mechanisms of graft rejection. Use of much more intensive conditioning regimens have markedly decreased the incidence of graft rejection in patients with malignancies. In aplastic anemia, recognition of the importance of blood transfusions in sensitizing a recipient to produce graft rejection has been noted. The use of a response index (RRI) is a predictive value. Finally, use of the new T cell purging techniques have produced an increased incidence of graft rejection. This problem will need to be overcome in order for marrow transplantation to have an expanding therapeutic role.

REFERENCES

1. Osgood EE, Riddle MC, Mathews TJ: Aplastic anemia treated with daily transfusions and intravenous marrow. *Ann Intern Med* 1939;13:357–367.
2. Santos GW, Sensenbrenner LL: A sensitive and quantitative assay for non-H-2 histocompatibility antigens. *Exper Hematol* 1971;21:19–20.
3. Jacobson LO, Simmons EL, Marks EK, Elredge JH: Effect of spleen protection on mortality following X-irradiation. *J Lab Clin Med* 1949;34:538–543.
4. Jacobson LO, Simmons EL, Marks EK, Elredge JH: Recovery from radiation injury. *Science* 1951;113:510–511.
5. Ford CE, Hamerton JL, Barnes DWH, Loutit JF: Cytological identification of radiation chimeras. *Nature* 1956;177:452–454.
6. Santos GW, Owens AH: Syngeneic and allogeneic marrow transplants in the cyclophosphamide pretreated rat. In, Doussett J, et al. (eds): *Advances in Transplantation* 1968, pp. 431–436.
7. Santos GW, Haghshenass M: Cloning of syngeneic hematopoietic cells in the spleens of mice and rats pretreated with cytotoxic drugs. *Blood* 1968;32:629–637.
8. Van Bekkum DW: Determination of specific immunological tolerance in radiation chimeras. *Transplantation* 1973;1:39–57.
9. Van Bekkum DW, de Vries JJ: *Radiation Chimeras* London, Logos, 1967, p. 277.
10. Branch DR, Gallagher MT, et al.: Endogenous stem cell repopulation resulting in mixed hematopoietic chimerism following total body irradiation and marrow transplantation for acute leukemia. *Transplantation* 1982;34:226–228.
11. Field EO, Cauchi MN, Gibbs JE: The transfer of refractoriness to graft-vs.-host disease in F1 hybrid rats. *Transplantation* 1967;5:241–247.
12. Tutschka PJ, Schwerdtfeger R, Slavin RE, Santos GW. Mechanism of tolerance in long-term rat bone marrow chimeras. *Exper Hematol* 1976;4:170.

13. Thomas ED, Ashley CA, Lochte HL, et al.: Homografts of bone marrow in dogs after lethal total body radiation. *Blood* 1959;14:720.
14. Storb R, Thomas ED: In, Schwarz MR (ed): *Proceedings of the Sixth Leukocyte Conference.* New York, Academic Press, 1972, p. 805.
15. Storb R, Epstein RB, Rudolph RH, et al.: Allogeneic canine bone marrow transplantation following cyclophosphamide. *Transplantation* 1969;7:378.
16. Thomas ED, Buckner CD, Storb R, et al.: Aplastic anemia treated by marrow transplantation. *Lancet* 1972;1:284–289.
17. Storb R, Thomas ED, Buckner CD, et al.: Allogeneic marrow grafting for treatment of aplastic anemia. *Blood* 1974;43:157–180.
18. Storb R, Rudolph RH, Kolb HJ, et al.: Marrow grafts between DL-A-matched canine littermates. *Transplantation* 1973;15:92.
19. Thomas ED, Collins JA, Herman EC, et al.: Marrow transplants in lethally irradiated dogs given methotrexate. *Blood* 1962;19:217.
20. Epstein RB, Storb R, Ragde H, et al.: Cytotoxic typing antisera for marrow grafting in littermate dogs. *Transplantation* 1968;6:45.
21. Storb R, Epstein RB, Bryant J, et al.: Marrow grafts by combined marrow and leucocyte infusions in unrelated dogs selected by histocompatibility typing. *Transplantation* 1968;6:587.
22. Storb R, Rudolph RH, Thomas ED. Marrow grafts between canine siblings matched by serotyping and mixed lymphocyte culture. *J Clin Invest* 1971;50:1272.
23. Storb R, Epstein RB, Rudolph RH: The effect of prior transfusions on marrow grafts between histocompatible canine siblings. *J Immunol* 1970;105:627.
24. Storb R, Floersheim GL, Weiden Pl, et al.: Effect of prior blood transfusions on marrow grafts; abrogation of sensitization by procarbazine and antithymocyte serum. *J Immunol* 1974;112:1508.
25. Epstein RB, Bryant J, Thomas ED. Cytogenetic demonstration of permanent tolerance in adult outbred dogs. *Transplantation* 1967;5:267.
26. Storb R, Thomas ED: In, Schwarz MR (ed): *Proceedings of the Sixth Leukocyte Culture Conference,* New York, Academic Press, 1972, p. 805.
27. Ochs HD, Storb R, Thomas ED, et al.: Immunologic reactivity in canine marrow graft recipients. *J Immunol* 1974;113:1039.
28. Weiden PL, Storb R, Thomas ED, et al.: Preceding transfusions and marrow graft rejection in dogs and man. *Transplant Proc* 1976;3(4):551.
29. Weiden PL, Storb R, Slichter S, et al.: Effects of six weekly transfusions on canine marrow grafts: tests for sensitization and abrogation of procarbazine and antithymocyte serum. *J Immunol* 1976;117:143.
30. Storb R, Weiden PL, Graham TC, Thomas ED: Failure of engraftment and graft-vs.-host disease after canine marrow transplantation. *Transplant Proc* 1978;10(1):113–118.
31. Vriesdendorp HM, Lowenberg B, Visser TP, et al.: Influence of genetic resistance and silica particles on survival after bone marrow transplantation. *Transplant Proc* 1976;8:483.
32. Bull MI, Herzig GP, Graw RG, et al.: Canine allogeneic bone marrow transplantation. *Transplantation* 1976;22:150.
33. Storb R, Deeg HJ, Weiden TC, et al.: Marrow graft rejection in DLA-identical canine littermates; antigens involved are expressed on leucocytes and skin epithelial cells but probably not on platelets and red blood cells. *Transplant Proc* 1979;11(1):504–506.
34. Gottlieb M, Strober S, Hoppe R, et al.: Engraftment of allogeneic bone marrow without graft-vs.-host disease in mongrel dogs using total lymphoid irradiation. *Transplantation* 1980;29(6)487–491.
35. Warren R, Storb R, Weiden P, et al.: Direct and antibody dependent cell mediated cytotoxicity against HLA identical sibling lymphocytes. *Transplantation* 1976;22(6):631–635.
36. Mickelson EM, Feffer A, Storb R, et al.: Correlation of the relative response index with marrow graft rejection in patients with aplastic anemia. *Transplantation* 1976;22:294–300.
37. Storb R: Decrease in the graft rejection rate and improvement in survival after marrow transplantation for severe aplastic anemia. *Transplant Proc* 1979;11(1):196–197.
38. Levey RH, Parkman R, Rappeport J. et al.: Successful bone marrow transplantation in sensitized recipients. *Transplant Proc* 1979;11:199–203.
39. Mitsuyasu R, Champlin RE, Gale RP, et al.: Treatment of donor bone marrow with

     monoclonal anti-T-cell antibody and complement for the prevention of graft-vs.-host disease. *Ann Intern Med* 1986;105:20.

40. Martin PJ, Hansen JA, Buckner D, et al.: Effects of *in vitro* depletion of T-cells in HLA identical allogeneic marrow grafts. *Blood* 1985;66:664.

41. Bozdech MJ, Sondel PM, Trigg ME, et al.: Transplantation of HLA-haploidentical T-cell depleted marrow for leukemia: addition of cytosine arabinoside to the pretransplant conditioning prevents rejection. *Exper Hematol* 1985;13:1201.

Bone Marrow Transplantation in
Children, edited by F. Leonard Johnson
and Carl Pochedly. Raven Press, Ltd.,
New York © 1990.

Etiology and Pathogenesis of Graft-vs.-Host Disease. I. Studies in Animal Models*

Jeffrey Sosman, Richard Hong, and Paul M. Sondel

Center for Health Sciences, University of Wisconsin–Madison, Madison, Wisconsin 53792

Introduction
A. Background
B. Graft-vs.-host disease across major histocompatibility complex (MHC) barriers in an irradiated (immunosuppressed) host
C. Graft-vs.-host disease resulting from minor histocompatibility differences in an irradiated (immunosuppressed) host
D. Parental into F_1 hybrid graft-vs.-host disease in nonimmunosuppressed recipients
E. Syngeneic graft-vs.-host disease in animals treated with cyclosporine A
F. Resolution of graft-vs.-host disease: the development of tolerance and a stable chimera
G. Other factors potentially involved in manifestations of graft-vs.-host disease
Summary

INTRODUCTION

Acute and chronic graft-vs.-host disease is a major complication of human allogeneic bone marrow transplantation (1–4). Acute graft-vs.-host disease occurs in approximately 50% of patients who are given an allogeneic marrow transplant from a major histocompatibility complex (MHC) matched sibling. Those with moderate to severe acute graft-vs.-host disease may have a mortal-

*This research was supported by grants CA-32685 and RR03186 from the National Institutes of Health, and American Cancer Society Grant CH--237C.

ity rate of nearly 60%, while those with no graft-vs.-host disease or only mild involvement have a 20% mortality (2,5). Furthermore, chronic graft-vs.-host disease occurs in 15 to 50% of long-term survivors of marrow transplantation, that is, those surviving over 100 days. Thus, chronic graft-vs.-host disease is the cause of significant mortality and morbidity (4,6). These manifestations of disease and their associated mortality are becoming more important clinically because of the increasing utilization of allogeneic bone marrow transplantation in the treatment of a multitude of diseases, including immunodeficiency, hematologic malignancies, and certain inherited metabolic disorders (1,7–11).

Simonsen (12) and Billingham (13) first identified the basic requirements for the development of the graft-vs.-host reaction. These requirements are (1) the graft must contain immunocompetent cells, (2) the host must possess transplantation antigens which are lacking on the cells of the graft, thereby the host cells induce immunologic stimulation of the graft, and (3) the host must be incapable of mounting an effective immunologic rejection reaction directed against the graft. Since these conditions for graft-vs.-host disease were first proposed, many *in vivo* and *in vitro* studies with experimental animals and bone marrow transplant patients suggest that the factors inducing and controlling this reaction are far more complex than was previously thought (14–16).

This chapter summarizes several of the most thoroughly investigated and best understood animal models of graft-vs.-host disease. Each animal model sheds light on some aspect of human graft-vs.-host disease. These studies have clarified some of the clinical manifestations, cellular requirements of the donor, genetic requirements of the donor and host, the target cells and their antigens, the mechanisms underlying graft-vs.-host disease, and finally, the resolution of this condition. In the next chapter, we will review *in vivo* and *in vitro* studies of bone marrow transplantation which explore the mechanisms underlying the induction, the effector phase, and the resolution of acute and chronic graft-vs.-host disease in the clinical setting (17–22).

A better understanding of the etiology and pathogenesis of graft-vs.-host disease will not only improve our ability to prevent and treat this complication of bone marrow transplantation, but may also lead to a better understanding of a variety of other disease states associated with abnormal immune regulation.

For the remainder of this chapter, we will review the experimental animal studies used to study graft-vs.-host disease.

BACKGROUND

"Runt disease," as first described by Simonsen (12), is a form of graft-vs.-host disease which occurs when an immunologically immature animal is exposed to alloreactive lymphoid cells from an adult donor (Figure 1A). This can occur *in utero*, thus affecting the neonatal animal. It has been demonstrated in mice, rats, rabbits, guinea pigs, and humans (23,24). This is one of

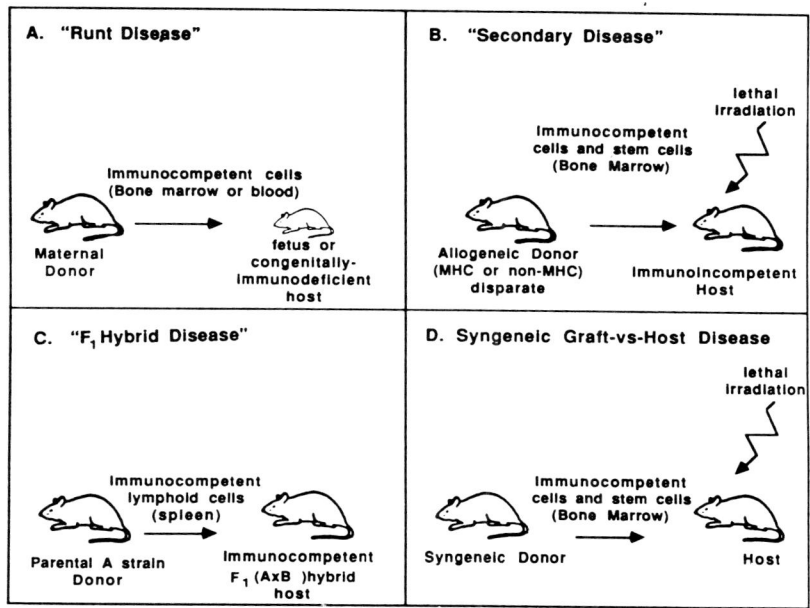

FIG. 1. Various experimental models of graft-vs.-host disease.

the first models of graft-vs.-host disease studied. Human runt disease was observed in infants with thymic immunologic deficiencies or severe combined immune deficiency (SCID) who were given blood transfusions or bone marrow or blood from the mother (25,26). Survival of these infants was brief and was accompanied by multiple organ failure due to graft-vs.-host disease.

"Secondary disease" occurs when a recipient animal has been rescued from the lethal effects of ionizing irradiation by the engraftment of hematopoietic stem cells from an allogeneic donor (Figure 1B) (27,28). This situation is somewhat more analogous to the clinical setting of bone marrow transplantation. Secondary disease can be seen when the donor cells contain immunocompetent lymphoid cells, and the donor and host differ significantly for antigens controlled by either the MHC or other non-MHC (minor histocompatibility) loci (28,29).

A third animal model for graft-vs.-host disease is the "F_1 hybrid disease." This condition occurs when parental lymphoid cells from an inbred homozygous mouse strain are infused into an F_1 hybrid animal, which is derived from a cross between the donor parent and a parent from a separate histoincompatible inbred strain (Figure 1C) (30). In this setting, lymphoid cells from one homozygous parent (strain A) can recognize the F_1 (A × B) hybrid tissues as foreign due to their codominant expression of antigens inherited from the other parent strain (strain B). Because the grafted parental cells do not express any antigens that are foreign to the F_1 host, the host will not eliminate donor cells. For this reason, graft-vs.-host disease can occur even if the host is immunocompetent. Thus, unlike other models of graft-vs.-host disease, in F_1 hybrid disease, the host animal does not need to be immunosuppressed due to congenital abnormalities or secondary to lethal irradiation.

Finally, a fourth animal model is syngeneic (autologous) graft-vs.-host disease. According to this model, a disease with similar manifestations to graft-vs.-host disease occurs in animals which have been irradiated and then rescued with genetically identical hematopoietic stem cells plus lymphoid cells (Figure 1D) (31). The occurrence of syngeneic graft-vs.-host disease emphasizes that the infusion of mature T cells can result in a clinical picture of graft-vs.-host disease, with skin lesions and characteristic organ damage, even when the target is not a major or minor foreign histocompatibility antigen. Whether in a strict sense these phenomena, that is, the skin lesions and damage to other organs, can be considered examples of true graft-vs.-host disease is debatable; but their role in producing the clinical picture seen in bone marrow transplantation must be considered.

The histologic and clinical changes of graft-vs.-host disease which occurs in each of these animal models can be quite dissimilar (27,28,32,33). In general, the animals suffer acutely from wasting and hunched posture and have a high mortality rate. Several organs and tissues appear to be selectively and severely affected by these reactions, including the skin, gastrointestinal tract, liver, the hematopoietic system, and lymphoid organs. Under certain conditions (as described below), a more chronic, indolent reaction can occur, with signs of lymphoid stimulation and autoimmune phenomena, such as, antinuclear antibody, rheumatoid factor, and elevated gamma globulin levels. This process may involve the lungs, muscles, and serosal surfaces as well as the skin, liver, and gastrointestinal tract (32).

Each of these distinct animal models is summarized in the following sections. Taken together, these descriptions may help formulate an overall animal model for the mechanism of graft-vs.-host disease.

GRAFT-VS.-HOST DISEASE ACROSS MAJOR HISTOCOMPATIBILITY COMPLEX (MHC) BARRIERS IN AN IRRADIATED (IMMUNOSUPPRESSED) HOST

The MHC is a localized complex of genes which code for the major cell surface histocompatibility antigens. These antigens play a vital role in graft rejection responses and in the presentation of soluble or viral antigens to host immune T cells (34). The MHC of the mouse (designated H-2) is located on chromosome 17 (34), and in humans it is designated HLA and is situated on chromosome 6 (35). On the basis of tissue distribution, structure of the expressed antigen, and function, 3 separate classes of molecules encoded by the MHC have been defined. Class I molecules (encoded by K, D, and L loci in the mouse, and by A, B, and C loci in humans) are present on all nucleated cells. The molecules consist of a 45 kilodalton (Kd) heavy chain noncovalently associated with a 12-Kd beta-2-microglobulin. These class I surface molecules are the primary targets for most cytotoxic T lymphocytes (34).

Class II molecules are encoded by the I-A and I-E loci in the mouse and by the DR, DQ, and DP loci in humans. They have limited distribution, being found only on monocytes, Langerhans cells, dendritic cells, B lymphocytes, activated T lymphocytes, and occasionally on other types of tissue cells. These molecules are heterodimers consisting of a 29–34 Kd alpha chain non-covalently bound to a 25–28 Kd beta chain. Class II MHC molecules are the primary antigenic stimulus for most T helper/inducer cells and are capable of inducing the *in vitro* mixed lymphocyte proliferative response (MLR) (36). Class III molecules control complement products.

Graft-vs.-host disease occurs when a host is lethally irradiated and then reconstituted, or rescued, with a lympho-hematopoietic graft from an MHC-incompatible (mismatched) allogeneic donor (29). In mice differing for both class I and class II MHC antigens, rapidly lethal graft-vs.-host disease occurs. This condition is characterized by wasting, hunched posture, hair loss, diar-rhea, lympho-hematopoietic atrophy and thymic epithelial dysplasia (37). However, exceptions to this rule exist. Between certain mouse strains, no manifestations of GVH disease occur even when donor and host are MHC incompatible (29). Elimination of Thy1+ cells from the donor graft, using antibody and complement treatment *ex vivo*, prevents the occurrence of clini-cal signs of graft-vs.-host disease and the mice survive (38). Therefore, in this model, presence of a sufficient number of Thy1+ cells or mature T cells in the donor inoculum is required, but may not be sufficient to allow lethal graft-vs.-host disease to develop (29,38,39).

Lyt2+ cells are T cells that recognize class I MHC antigens; they are pre-dominantly cytolytic T lymphocytes (CTL) and T suppressor cells. Further analysis of the donor cellular requirement revealed that depletion of these Lyt2+ cells from donor inoculum had no significant effect on mortality from graft-vs.-host disease. In contrast, depletion of donor L3T4+ cells (T cells recognizing class II MHC antigen, predominantly T helper or inducer cells) from the inoculum significantly reduced mortality (37,40). Furthermore, by depleting both Lyt2+ and L3T4+ T cell subsets, mortality related to graft-vs.-host disease was even further decreased without influencing engraftment of the donor marrow (37,40). Depletion of natural killer cells from the donor inoculum with antibody to Asialo GM-1 had no effect on graft-vs.-host dis-ease (37).

These experiments support the concept that donor L3T4+ T helper cells play a significant role in the initiation phase, in the effector phase or in both phases of graft-vs.-host disease. Others have found no absolute correlation between lethal graft-vs.-host disease and the presence of cytotoxic T lympho-cytes in some donor-recipient matches (41,42). Lethal graft-vs.-host disease can occur in the absence of detectable donor antihost cytotoxic T lymphocytes (41). Intradermal injection of noncytotoxic, class II MHC-reactive, T helper L3T4$^+$ clones led to graft-vs.-host disease limited to the skin (43). Noncytotoxic helper T cell clones or cell lines are able to induce lethal graft-vs.-host disease in allogeneic irradiated recipients in the absence of donor Lyt2$^+$ cytotoxic cells (41).

In contrast to these findings, others observed that elimination of either the L3T4$^+$ or Lyt2$^+$ T cell subset did not prevent lethal graft-vs.-host disease induced by B/6 bone marrow when transplanted into MHC incompatible Balb/c recipients (44). These findings suggest that both Lyt2$^+$ T cells and L3T4$^+$ can play a role in producing graft-vs.-host disease. Piquet studied the role played by MHC class I and class II products of the host in the induction of lethal graft-vs.-host disease (33). The donor inoculum needed to contain 10^6 T cells in order to kill 50% of recipient mice following transplants mismatched for class I antigenic differences. In contrast, as few as 10^5 cells could kill 50% of hosts that were mismatched for class II MHC antigens alone. Enteropathy associated with graft-vs.-host disease was observed only when there were differences of class II loci, and not with class I loci differences between the donor and recipient. Lymphoproliferation in host spleen and lymph nodes was evident soon after injection of T cells different at class II loci, but not after injection of T cells different at class I loci. Limiting dilution analyses revealed that the frequency of donor T cells reactive to class II antigens was 10 to 100 times greater than the frequency of class I reactive T cells. Clonal analysis showed that some donor T cells reactive to host class II MHC antigens were Lyt2$^-$, noncytolytic T cells which proliferated and produced interleukin-2 (IL-2) in response to antigen; other donor T cells were Lyt2$^+$ cytolytic cells. On the other hand, donor T cell clones reactive to host class I MHC antigenic differences were virtually all Lyt2$^+$ and cytolytic.

These findings support the contention that MHC class II antigens are a more potent stimulus of lethal graft-vs.-host disease than are class I antigens. In addition, the mechanism of graft-vs.-host disease in the presence of class II antigenic disparities may involve both cytolytic and helper cells, while class I differences induce more mild graft-vs.-host disease due to more selective activation of cytolytic cells alone. Similarly, it was shown that class I MHC loci can elicit lethal graft-vs.-host disease that is dependent upon Lyt2$^+$, L3T4$^-$ cells in the donor inoculum. However, complete MHC differences or class II differences alone were more dependent upon donor L3T4$^+$ cells for production of lethal graft-vs.-host disease.

Thus, when graft-vs.-host disease develops in irradiated mice inoculated with MHC-mismatched donor lymphocytes, it is the mature T cells in the donor inoculum that are crucial to development of this disease. The role played by Lyt2$^+$ cytolytic T cells may be important in the setting of isolated class I MHC antigenic differences between donor and host. (37) T helper cells that are MHC class II reactive and L3T4$^+$ comprise the major population of T cells involved in most forms of graft-vs.-host disease (37,40). MHC class I and class II antigens of the host can induce this disease; however, class II antigens appear to be the more potent stimuli in pathogenesis (33,37).

GRAFT-VS.-HOST DISEASE RESULTING FROM MINOR HISTOCOMPATIBILITY DIFFERENCES IN AN IRRADIATED (IMMUNOSUPPRESSED) HOST

Several animal models have shown that lethal graft-vs.-host disease can develop in certain irradiated hosts (recipients) after transplantation with immuno-competent cells from MHC-compatible donors differing for non-MHC (minor locus) histocompatibility antigens (30,45,46). This process is demonstrated by the occurrence of graft-vs.-host disease in dogs given marrow from MHC identical littermates (47). This phenomenon was studied extensively in irradiated H-2^k CBA/J mice that received transplants of bone marrow and lymphoid cells from H-2^k compatible B.10BR mice. These two strains of mice differ for at least 6 separate minor histocompatibility loci. Most recipients died within 30 to 80 days with weight loss, hunched posture, lymphoid and hematopoietic atrophy, and infections. Treatment of the donor marrow with anti-Thy1 antibody to remove T cells prevented the occurrence of graft-vs.-host disease. Mortality from graft-vs.-host disease in the recipients was directly proportional to the number of mature T cells contained in the donor marrow (45).

These findings demonstrate that mature T cells are involved in graft-vs.-host disease induced by major as well as minor histocompatibility determinants. Furthermore, it appears that the cells which are induced by minor histocompatibility antigens to mediate graft-vs.-host disease recognize the minor antigen as being restricted by MHC class I (H-2, K, D, and L) antigens. Treatment of donor cells with antibody to Lyt2$^+$ and complement eliminated graft-vs.-host disease. Therefore, an Lyt2$^+$ cell within the donor inoculum appears to recognize minor histocompatibility antigens in the context of an H-2 class I antigen. Among the manifestations of graft-vs.-host disease in this model, skin involvement was minimal. This finding is different from the degree of skin involvement in graft-vs.-host disease observed when donor and recipient are MHC incompatible. In addition, graft-vs.-host disease induced by minor histocompatibility antigenic differences between donor and recipient appears to involve Lyt2$^+$ T cells, while MHC-induced graft-vs.-host disease was more dependent upon the role of Lyt2$^-$, L3T4$^+$ cells (37,40).

Among LP (H-2^b) mice that were lethally irradiated and then transplanted with spleen cells and bone marrow from MHC-compatible C57BL/6 (H-2^b) mice, two forms of graft-vs.-host disease occurred (46). In some mice death occurred early (after 4 to 9 weeks) with disease characterized by wasting, hunched posture, hair loss, skin erythema and ulceration, diarrhea and thymic epithelial dysplasia. This condition was designated as acute graft-vs.-host disease. Other mice died after 6 to 15 weeks with the appearance of wasting, hunched posture, skin and dermal fibrosis, and marked edema. This was designated chronic graft-vs.-host disease. The skin histology was markedly different in the two disease states. There was single cell necrosis of the epidermis in acute graft-vs.-host disease, and dermal fibrosis in the chronic form of the disease.

It was found that the dose of spleen cells is the major determinant of the type of graft-vs.-host disease which occurs (46). When large numbers (5×10^7) of spleen cells were infused, all of the animals died of acute graft-vs.-host disease. Alternatively, if smaller numbers (5×10^6) of spleen cells were infused, some animals showed no evidence of graft-vs.-host disease while others had either the acute or chronic form of the disease. By elimination of Thy1 + cells from the donor inoculum, neither acute nor chronic graft-vs.-host disease occurred, regardless of whether high or low numbers of spleen cells were infused. These same authors demonstrated that in mice with acute graft-vs.-host disease due to minor histocompatibility antigenic differences, the spleen contained donor cytotoxic T lymphocytes with specific antihost reactivity (48). In contrast, those recipients of donor spleen cells which were depleted of mature T cells became stable chimeras. These mice did not develop graft-vs.-host disease and had no antihost cytotoxic T lymphocytes detectable in their spleens.

T cell clones were isolated from some of these engrafted B6 mice at 10 to 14 days post-transplant, while they were exhibiting signs of acute graft-vs.-host disease. T cell clones were isolated from others at day 50 in the presence of signs and symptoms of chronic graft-vs.-host disease (49). Mice with chronic graft-vs.-host disease had T cell clones which were noncytotoxic. These T cells proliferated in response to class II autologous MHC antigens and frequently released lymphokines which could induce collagen production from fibroblasts (49). The phenotype of these T cells was L3T4+, Lyt2−. Clonal analyses of T cells isolated from mice with acute graft-vs.-host disease showed that these T cells were more heterogeneous. Both cytotoxic antihost specific Lyt2+, L3T4− cells and proliferative L3T4+ Lyt2− class II MHC specific cells were isolated. The authors hypothesize that antihost cytotoxic T lymphocytes are instrumental in producing acute graft-vs.-host disease, and that chronic graft-vs.-host disease is characterized by the presence of autoreactive T helper cells. These autoreactive T cells probably develop secondary to early immunologic events post-transplant.

These findings suggest that there is a relationship between the antihost cytotoxic T lymphocytes and the mediation of acute graft-vs.-host disease. However, this relationship does not always hold true. Six separate combinations of H-2 identical strains of mice were observed for presence of graft-vs.-host disease after transplantation; mice of 5 strains developed lethal graft-vs.-host disease, while one developed no signs of this disease (42). Nevertheless, for all 6 combinations of strains, cytotoxic T lymphocytes specific for host antigens could be detected in the spleens 10 to 20 days after the transplant. Therefore, the presence of antihost cytotoxic T lymphocytes detected *in vitro* did not absolutely correlate with lethal graft-vs.-host disease. This finding led the authors to speculate that cytotoxic T lymphocytes may not be the primary effector for graft-vs.-host disease.

However, cytotoxic T lymphocytes could still be the primary effectors of graft-vs.-host disease, if there were also suppressor cells inhibiting functions of cytotoxic T lymphocytes *in vivo* in the strain combination which did not develop graft-vs.-host disease. Another possible explanation for the apparent lack of an active role of cytotoxic T cell in mediation of graft-vs.-host disease was that the *in vitro* target cells (lymphocytes) used to detect activity of cytotoxic T lymphocytes may not be appropriate to correlate with *in vivo* graft-vs.-host disease. Thus, an *in vitro* target which was more involved in graft-vs.-host disease *in vivo* (such as the skin, GI tract, or liver) may have correlated better with the clinical manifestations of this syndrome.

The role of interleukin-2 (IL-2) receptors in the pathogenesis of lethal graft-vs.-host disease induced by differences at minor histocompatibility loci was studied in mice (50). In this study, B10.BR donor bone marrow was infused into CBA host mice. Interleukin-2 is critical for T cell proliferation (51). An antibody to the IL-2 receptor was administered *in vivo* to the CBA host mice for 5 consecutive days after lethal irradiation and transplant of bone marrow and spleen cells from B10.BR mice. The antibody reduced the severity of clinical graft-vs.-host disease. There was a decrease in mortality and weight loss, as well as a reduction in the extent of histologic changes associated with graft-vs.-host disease. These experiments suggest a vital role for interleukin-2 and its cell surface receptor in the pathogenesis of graft-vs.-host disease.

In these models of graft-vs.-host disease, where donor and recipient were MHC matched, several important observations have been made. First, mature T cells in the donor inoculum are vital in the development of this disease state (45). These T cells seem to recognize minor histocompatibility antigens by using receptors that require simultaneous recognition of class I MHC antigens on recipient cells, a process designated "MHC *restriction*" (30). It appears that for at least some minor locus incompatible strains, Lyt2[+] donor cells, and not L3T4[+] T cells, are essential in mediating the graft-vs.-host disease.

Although Lyt2[+] cells are mostly cytotoxic T cells, there is no absolute correlation between the presence of donor cytotoxic cells reactive against the host and the development of graft-vs.-host disease (46). These cytotoxic T lymphocytes can be present in situations where no graft-vs.-host disease occurs, suggesting that other factors are involved. In chronic graft-vs.-host disease, autoreactive helper T cells can be isolated which induce collagen production by fibroblasts (49). Lastly, IL-2 and its receptor probably mediate stimulation and subsequent expansion of the donor T cells which respond to host tissues (50). This model most closely simulates the genetic conditions which occur in human bone marrow transplantation performed with HLA-matched siblings (3). The degree to which conclusions drawn from these animal experiments may be applicable to humans requires further analysis of clinical data.

PARENTAL INTO F_1 HYBRID GRAFT-VS.-HOST DISEASE IN NONIMMUNOSUPPRESSED RECIPIENTS

Results of a series of experiments depicted the manifestations of graft-vs.-host disease which develops when B10 spleen cells are infused into nonirradiated (B10 × DBA/2)F_1 hybrids (31,52,53). The recipients do not recognize the donor cells as being foreign, while the DBA/2 antigens on the host tissues stimulate the donor's T cells. Two forms of graft-vs.-host disease have been observed under these conditions. A severe *suppressive* form is characterized by lympho-hematopoietic atrophy, aplastic anemia, intestinal epithelial lesions, and severe immunosuppression. There is early death preceded by severe wasting and signs of infection. A second form of graft-vs.-host disease is *stimulatory* characterized by clinical findings of lymphoid hyperplasia, hypergammaglobulinemia, autoantibodies, antibodies to double-stranded DNA, and immune complex glomerulonephritis, as well as skin, liver, and salivary gland changes.

Early experiments failed to confirm a significant role for cytotoxic T lymphocytes in the *suppressive* form of graft-vs.-host disease (52). Later experiments utilizing parental donor marrow infused into F_1 hybrid recipients, differing for only class I or class II MHC loci, showed that donor Lyt2$^+$ T cells and L3T4$^+$ cells reacted against class I and class II MHC antigens, respectively, on host cells. (31,53) The authors proposed that T helper L3T4$^+$ cells activate Lyt2$^+$ suppressor cells which are the ultimate effectors of the *suppressive* form of graft-vs.-host disease. On the other hand, the *stimulatory* form of graft-vs.-host disease occurs when only class II MHC differences are present, inducing an L3T4$^+$ donor T cell to stimulate the polyclonal activation of recipient B cells via multiple lymphokines (53). This abnormal T cell-B cell cooperation leads to the lymphoid hyperplasia, abnormal immunoglobulin production, and autoimmune manifestations.

Via noted that while transplanting B/6 bone marrow into (B/6 × DBA/2)F_1 hosts produced a *suppressive* form of graft-vs.-host disease, injection of bone marrow from the other parental strain (DBA/2) into the same (B/6 × DBA/2)F_1 host led to a *stimulatory* graft-vs.-host disease (54). This observation appeared inconsistent with the model proposed by Gleichman (32). Via showed that the DBA/2 inoculum contained one-half the number of Lyt2$^+$ cells and one-ninth the number of cytotoxic T lymphocyte precursors reactive to F_1 tissue compared to the B6 inoculum. Furthermore, following injection of DBA/2 bone marrow cells into F_1 chimera spleen, only L3T4$^+$ T cells of donor origin could be found. No parental anti-F_1 cytotoxic T lymphocytes were present in the chimeric spleen. Therefore, it is likely that the L3T4$^+$ cells from the DBA/2 donor induced recipient B cells to mediate the *stimulatory* features of graft-vs.-host disease.

On the other hand, following injection of B6 bone marrow into F$_1$ chimera spleens, the host animals contained both L3T4$^+$ and Lyt2$^+$ T cells of donor origin. These spleens were reduced by 70% in cellularity, were deficient in "third party" alloantigen responsiveness, and the cytotoxic T lymphocytes showed restricted responsiveness to MHC antigens. At the same time, these spleen cells demonstrated potent activity of cytotoxic T lymphocytes directed against the foreign DBA/2 antigens of the F$_1$ host. These authors suggest that the L3T4$^+$ T cells mediate the *stimulatory* form of graft-vs.-host disease, and the Lyt2$^+$ antihost cytotoxic T cells mediate the *suppressive* form of this disease. Recently, it was confirmed that in the DBA/2 into F$_1$ *stimulatory* model of graft-vs.-host disease, L3T4$^+$ donor T cells are important. But it was also shown that recipient Lyt2$^+$ T cells are required for graft-vs.-host disease (55). When Lyt2$^+$ host cells are eliminated *in vivo* by anti-Lyt2$^+$ antibody and thymectomy, no *stimulatory* or *suppressive* graft-vs.-host disease occurred (55). Furthermore, donor engraftment of both Lyt2$^+$ and L3T4$^+$ cells was increased after elimination of recipient Lyt2$^+$ cells.

Whether increased engraftment suppresses the autoimmunity, or the recipient Lyt2$^+$ T cells play an effector role in autoimmunity is subject to question. Clearly, the immunoregulation of these reactions involves multiple interactions between distinct subsets of host and donor immune cells.

In a slightly different model, Moser studied the graft-vs.-host disease which occurred when parental lymphoid cells were introduced into F$_1$ offspring who differed only by a class II MHC antigenic mutation in the other parental strain (56). These mice developed profound immunodeficiency, probably due to graft-vs.-host disease. They failed to generate effective MHC-restricted cytotoxic responses to self + X, where X may be virus, soluble antigen, or hapten. However, the mice were able to develop cytotoxicity to allogenic targets. These mice are deficient in L3T4$^+$ T helper cells, which may be more essential for responses of cytotoxic T lymphocytes to self + X than they are for alloreactive responses of cytotoxic T lymphocytes. Alternatively, these immunosuppressed mice may have a population of suppressor cells which preferentially suppress responses of cytotoxic T lymphocytes of self + X; these suppressor cells do not suppress responses of alloreactive cytotoxic T lymphocytes.

This model of graft-vs.-host disease has offered some insight into the vast spectrum of manifestations of acute and chronic graft-vs.-host disease observed clinically. The *stimulatory* form of graft-vs.-host disease has many clinical parallels to human chronic graft-vs.-host disease as well as to a variety of other autoimmune disorders. This *stimulatory* form of graft-vs.-host disease appears to be mediated by donor L3T4$^+$ T helper cells. It is probably induced by class II MHC antigenic differences and mediated by lymphokines which stimulate polyclonal proliferation of host B cells. The *suppressive* form of graft-vs.-host disease is more complicated and may involve both helper and cytotoxic/suppressor T cell subsets. Furthermore, the murine effector cells which carry out the suppressive activity are likely to be Lyt2[+]. Whether these are primarily cytolytic or suppressor cells, or a combination of the two, is not obvious from experimental evidence (31,54). Lastly, in this model, where the host is not immunosuppressed before transplant, Lyt2[+] host cells are required in order for the *stimulatory* form of graft-vs.-host disease to manifest itself (55).

SYNGENEIC GRAFT-VS.-HOST DISEASE IN ANIMALS TREATED WITH CYCLOSPORINE A

There have been several case reports describing the development of graft-vs.-host disease in human recipients of bone marrow from identical twin siblings (18,57,58). These observations appear to disregard the requirement for foreign host transplantation antigens, which are recognized by donor cells. Alternatively, since graft-vs.-host disease may be a manifestation of altered immune regulation, it is possible that "self" antigens may be recognized inappropriately as being foreign. Another explanation centers on the role of external influences inducing alteration in self antigens that are not encoded by histocompatibility genes (57,58).

A model for syngeneic graft-vs.-host disease was developed in rats by Santos and his coworkers (31,59). In this model, Lewis rats are lethally irradiated and transplanted with marrow from genetically identical (syngeneic) rats, or from allogeneic rat strains, and then given cyclosporine A subcutaneously for 40 days (31). Cyclosporine A, a potent immunosuppressive agent whose effects are reversible, suppresses allograft rejection and prevents the development of allogeneic graft-vs.-host disease (60). The drug appears to mediate this effect by impairing production of interleukin-2 by stimulated T cells. Upon discontinuation of cyclosporine A in rats given syngeneic bone marrow transplants, the classic manifestations of acute graft-vs.-host disease developed. This is characterized by weight loss, hunched appearance, diarrhea, dermatitis, and red ears, with typical histologic changes of graft-vs.-host disease on skin biopsy (31,59). Furthermore, this graft-vs.-host disease could be transferred through spleen cells from affected animals into irradiated syngeneic recipients that were not given cyclosporine A. This transfer was dependent upon mature T cells from the donor affected by graft-vs.-host disease.

Efforts were made to clarify the mechanism of this form of graft-vs.-host disease. It was later shown that, with discontinuation of cyclosporine A, the manifestations of graft-vs.-host disease were associated with the appearance of polyclonal cytotoxic T lymphocytes reactive to autologous class II MHC antigens (59). These autocytotoxic T cells showed surface markers of the cytotoxic phenotype rather than the helper T cell phenotype. Neither graft-vs.-host disease nor autocytotoxic cells were generated if the thymus was shielded during radiation therapy. This finding demonstrated a role for intact endogenous thymic function in preventing or regulating this syngeneic graft-vs.-host disease. It is possible that this experimentally induced syngeneic graft-vs.-host disease is a manifestation of altered self-recognition. The altered self-recognition is due to the various external manipulations of the thymus resulting in abnormal T cell development and function. Certain features of this process are somewhat analogous to aspects of immunoregulatory disorders seen in rheumatoid arthritis and other autoimmune diseases.

RESOLUTION OF GRAFT-VS.-HOST DISEASE: THE DEVELOPMENT OF TOLERANCE AND A STABLE CHIMERA

Even more remarkable than the development of graft-vs.-host disease may be its resolution and the development of tolerance, as shown by lack of antihost or antidonor responsiveness. This state of tolerance results in the formation of a stable chimera. Several theories have been proposed to account for the establishment of a stable chimera, including: (1) deletion of donor cells responsive to recipient histocompatibility antigens (clonal deletion), (2) induction of specific or nonspecific suppressor cells (T cells or macrophages) which regulate the reaction of donor antihost T cells (active suppression), and (3) decreased expression of alloantigen on host cells so that the allogeneic stimulus is lacking (16).

In a series of experiments in stable rat chimeras, suppressor T cells were identified which specifically inhibited donor antihost reactivity in mixed lymphocyte culture. Upon adoptive transfer these T cells could suppress ongoing graft-vs.-host disease in a secondary host. These suppressor cells, which are adherent to nylon wool, did not suppress other allogeneic responses; they specifically suppressed only donor antihost reactivity. Nonspecific suppressor cells (suppressing all immune responses) are present early during graft-vs.-host disease and are replaced by these specific suppressor cells during resolution of the disease (61). Recently, a T cell clone was isolated from a stable mouse bone marrow chimera, which specifically suppressed the generation of donor antihost responses of cytotoxic T lymphocytes both *in vitro* and *in vivo*. (64) This L3T4+ T cell clone, which was reactive to class II MHC antigens, blocked the *in vitro* donor antihost response in mixed lymphocyte culture. *In vivo*, these T cells specifically suppressed antihost cytotoxic T lymphocytes in the spleen. Most remarkable is the fact that this T cell clone was able to suppress clinical graft-vs.-host disease. This effect produced prolonged survival in lethally irradiated AKR (H-2^k) mice transplanted with SJL (H-2^s) bone marrow and lymphoid cells.

A role for clonal deletion in the development of tolerance and resolution of graft-vs.-host disease has not been substantiated by *in vitro* studies (62,63). It is possible, however, that specific suppressor cells may carry out their function by clonal deletion of donor antihost responding cells. Thus, the "suppression" versus "clonal deletion" mechanisms for development of graft-vs.-host disease are not mutually exclusive.

Another possible mechanism for the resolution or resistance to graft-vs.-host disease has been proposed (65). Previously, it was shown that resistance to lethal graft-vs.-host disease can be induced in the lethally irradiated F_1 hybrid recipients of parental marrow by immunization of the host with small numbers of parental spleen cells prior to irradiation and transplantation (66,67). This resistance to graft-vs.-host disease was mediated by Lyt2$^+$ T cells of the host (F_1 hybrid) origin which were cytotoxic for donor T cells reactive to host tissues (65). One mechanism for this resistance to graft-vs.-host disease could be host T cells which specifically recognize the alloreactive T cell receptor of the donor T cells which recognize host MHC antigens. These cells were induced by previous immunization with donor spleen cells of either L3T4$^+$ or Lyt2$^+$ phenotype.

OTHER FACTORS POTENTIALLY INVOLVED IN MANIFESTATIONS OF GRAFT-VS.-HOST DISEASE

Following lethal irradiation, conventional mice that receive an H-2 histoincompatible marrow graft (containing sufficient T cells) will develop lethal graft-vs.-host disease manifested by emaciation, dermatitis, pneumonia, enteritis, and involution of the lymphoid and hematopoietic systems (29,30). In contrast, mice that are raised in a germ-free environment, or that are decontaminated and maintained with antibiotics in sterile isolation, with sterile diet, food, water, and bedding, do not develop signs of graft-vs.-host disease (68). Their appearance is normal and they show no abnormal morphological changes on biopsy, although they are profoundly immunodeficient. These mice are free of infections due to viruses, parasites, bacteria and mycoplasma. This observation strongly implicates infection as a prime factor in the clinical manifestations of graft-vs.-host disease. Whether a virus or other organism triggers the immune system to induce the lesions of graft-vs.-host disease, or the manifestations are secondary to infection in an immunosuppressed host, is not known (69).

Another important observation is that class II MHC antigens which are normally expressed on B cells, monocytes and activated T cells can be found on keratinocytes of the epidermis and gut epithelial cells of rats with graft-vs.-host disease (70,71). This may be especially important since these tissues are preferential targets of graft-vs.-host disease. The mechanisms of this MHC antigen expression appear to be related to the local release of gamma-interferon (γIFN) by activated T cells. Immune interferon (γIFN) induces transcription of class II MHC genes in endothelial cells and fibroblasts (72). It is possible that release of gamma-interferon by T cells is stimulated by either the alloantigen of the host tissue or by recognition of a viral infection in the host. These two observations further emphasize the multifactorial nature of graft-vs.-host disease. These issues are even more complex in the evaluation of laboratory findings regarding graft-vs.-host disease in humans.

SUMMARY

These experimental animal models of graft-vs.-host disease demonstrate the complexity of the pathophysiology leading to this disease state. As depicted in Figure 1 of the following chapter, a number of host, donor, and environmental factors must interact for the clinical manifestations of graft-vs.-host disease to occur. Mature thymus-derived (T) lymphocytes in the donor inoculum are required to recognize and react to either host MHC, minor histocompatibility antigens or even altered syngeneic antigens. Both host class I and class II MHC antigens play a significant role in stimulating donor T cell responses. The exact importance of cytolytic, suppressor, or proliferative (lymphokine release) functions in mediating this disease is variable and differs considerably between the separate experimental systems studied. Other factors including viral infections or *in vivo* gamma interferon release affect the host milieu and host expression of MHC antigens. These may be essential for full expression of the clinical manifestations of graft-vs.-host disease. The different manifestations of acute and chronic graft-vs.-host disease is a result of quantitative and qualitative differences in both the donor T cells (which induce the disease) as well as the host tissues (which are the target for immune therapy). Finally, resolution of graft-vs.-host disease or establishment of tolerance, can require the induction of specific suppressor cells. The next chapter will extend these results to the review of human graft-vs.-host disease. Both *in vivo* and *in vitro* findings which further elucidate the etiology and pathophysiology of clinical graft-vs.-host disease are summarized.

REFERENCES

See complete list of references at the end of the following chapter.

Bone Marrow Transplantation in
Children, edited by F. Leonard Johnson
and Carl Pochedly. Raven Press, Ltd.,
New York © 1990.

Etiology and Pathogenesis of Graft-vs.-Host Disease. II. Human Studies

Jeffrey Sosman, Richard Hong, Paul M. Sondel

Center for Health Sciences, University of Wisconsin–Madison, Madison, Wisconsin 53792

A. Clinical manifestations
B. Risk factors for graft-vs.-host disease
C. Human *in vitro* and *in vivo* studies of graft-vs.-host disease in bone marrow transplant recipients
Summary

Following preconditioning with total body irradiation and cyclophosphamide, human recipients of HLA-matched sibling bone marrow develop a variety of clinical manifestations believed to result from graft-vs.-host disease (3).

This chapter will review the clinical manifestations of this entity, assess factors that increase the risk of developing graft-vs.-host disease, and discuss *in vitro* and *in vivo* studies of human graft-vs.-host disease in recipients of bone marrow transplants.

CLINICAL MANIFESTATIONS

As in mouse models, three main organ systems (the skin, gastrointestinal tract, and liver) are most frequently involved. A minority of patients have disease limited to the skin, ranging from a mild maculopapular rash to generalized erythema with or without bullous formation and desquamation. Histopathologic changes include focal or diffuse vacuolar degeneration of epidermal basal cells, spongiosis, dyskeratosis (consisting of eosinophilic necrotic degeneration), epidermal-dermal junctional separation, or even frank loss of epidermis.

Gastrointestinal and liver manifestations are considered secondary to graft-vs.-host disease only if accompanied by the above skin changes. Gastrointestinal involvement by graft-vs.-host disease is characterized by diarrhea, nausea, vomiting, abdominal pain and even hemorrhage or paralytic ileus. Intestinal biopsy may reveal only focal dilatation and degeneration of mucosal glands, or there may be severe changes, including focal or diffuse denudation of the mucosa. Finally, liver manifestations include marked increases in serum bilirubin, serum glutamic oxaloacetic acid transaminase (SGOT), and alkaline phosphatase. Histologically, the liver reveals degeneration and eosinophilic necrosis of hepatocytes and degeneration and necrosis of small bile ducts. Patients with these manifestations suffer from fever, wasting, and a decline in performance status.

The disease state described above has been called acute graft-vs.-host disease, occurring within the first 100 days after marrow transplant. The disease usually appears within the first 2 to 10 weeks. Diagnostic biopsy of involved organ systems is considered essential to prove the presence of graft-vs.-host disease, since many of the clinical manifestations could result from the toxicities of drugs, radiation therapy, or infection. Mortality from graft-vs.-host disease is frequently related to concomitant infections. The close interrelationship between acute graft-vs.-host disease and infectious complications is suggested by the following associations: (1) graft-vs.-host disease leads to breakdown of mucosal and skin barriers allowing a portal of entry for pathogens, (2) graft-vs.-host disease allows for latent virus reactivation, (3) graft-vs.-host disease aggravates a state of immunodeficiency, and (4) treatment of this disease is immunosuppressive itself, since treatment includes use of prednisone, anti-T cell globulin, etc (69,73). The mortality due to graft-vs.-host disease is closely related to its severity. In some reports there is a 10% mortality rate if there is only grade I graft-vs.-host disease, while there can be an 80 to 100% mortality rate with grade IV graft-vs.-host disease (5,73).

A very different syndrome has been described in recipients of bone marrow transplants who have survived more than 100 days, and is designated chronic graft-vs.-host disease (4). This pleotropic syndrome has many manifestations similar to a variety of collagen vascular diseases. There is frequent involvement of skin, liver, eyes, mouth, esophagus, upper respiratory tract and less often, serosa, lower gastrointestinal tract, and skeletal muscles. Morbidity can occur secondary to the sclerodermatous skin changes, and the presence of dry eyes and dry mouth similar to the condition seen in Sjögren's syndrome. There may be pulmonary insufficiency due to diffuse interstitial pneumonitis and liver changes similar to those in chronic active hepatitis.

Chronic graft-vs.-host disease has many serologic manifestations indicating immune dysregulation. There are elevated gamma globulin levels, and presence of circulating autoantibodies, such as rheumatoid factors, antinuclear antibodies, antismooth muscle antibodies, and Coombs positive autoantibodies. Eosinophilia and thrombocytopenia may also be present. Frequently, the disease is complicated by serious bacterial infections. Patients who develop chronic graft-vs.-host disease have three patterns of disease evolution: (1) a progressive course of acute graft-vs.-host disease with continuous evolution into the chronic form, (2) a temporally limited course of acute graft-vs.-host disease with resolution followed by a period of no symptoms and then later onset of the chronic form of the disease, or (3) *de novo* late onset chronic graft-vs.-host disease with no preceding evidence of the acute form (4,69,73).

Graft-vs.-host disease is not unique to bone marrow transplantation for treatment of leukemia or aplastic anemia. It has also been observed among children with primary immunodeficiencies who have received transplants of immunocompetent cells (such as cells from bone marrow, fetal liver, or fetal thymus) for the purpose of reconstituting their immune response (74–77). These children with underlying immunodeficiencies frequently do not require immunosuppressive (or ablative) chemotherapy or radiotherapy before their transplant (74,76,77). The graft-vs.-host disease developed is clinically quite similar to the disease previously described for immune-ablated patients with leukemia and aplastic anemia. These patients with immunodeficiencies following transplant have prominent skin, gastrointestinal, and liver involvement as well as showing features of the acute and chronic forms of graft-vs.-host disease (74). The fact that these manifestations occur in immune deficient patients without prior irradiation or chemotherapy suggests that these features of graft-vs.-host disease are independent of any external insults.

Successful marrow transplantations have been performed on children with severe combined immunodeficiency (SCID) using donor marrow from HLA-identical siblings, HLA-matched parents, or even from unrelated donors whose marrow is nonreactive in mixed lymphocyte culture (74,76). Although graft-vs.-host disease has occurred frequently, a number of successful engraftments have been reported without the occurrence of severe graft-vs.-host disease. One may postulate that the underlying host immune deficiency may allow for less graft-vs.-host disease to develop under these circumstances than is expected for patients with leukemia or aplastic anemia.

The spectrum of clinical phenomena associated with acute and chronic graft-vs.-host disease have been analyzed for clues as to the clinical etiology of this complication. Such studies have identified a number of elements that influence the risk of developing graft-vs.-host disease.

RISK FACTORS FOR GRAFT-VS.-HOST DISEASE

In the experience of The International Bone Marrow Transplant Registry, 2036 patients received bone marrow from HLA-matched siblings to treat leukemia or aplastic anemia. This experience was analyzed to identify risk factors for the development of acute graft-vs.-host disease (2). Forty-six percent of the patients developed moderate to severe graft-vs.-host disease, and this complication was the primary cause of death in 22% of the transplanted patients. Thirty-three potential prognostic variables were studied, of which 3 were found to be highly associated with the development of acute graft-vs.-host disease. These were: (1) donor-recipient sex mismatch, with female alloimmunized donors (previously pregnant or transfused) for male recipients having the greatest risk, (2) prophylaxis against graft-vs.-host disease, with patients who received no immunosuppressive prophylaxis at greater risk than patients receiving prophylaxis with cyclosporine A or methotrexate, and (3) age of patients, with older recipients having increased risk for graft-vs.-host disease. Of borderline significance as risk factors for developing graft-vs.-host disease were: (1) Trimethoprim-sulfamethoxazole prophylaxis, (2) poor pre-transplant performance status, and (3) a large number of post-transplant transfusions.

Depending on the presence or absence of these risk factors, a recipient would have a predicted risk of graft-vs.-host disease ranging from 16% to over 85%. The risk of developing acute graft-vs.-host disease in this study was not significantly associated with the dose of bone marrow cells, the number of donor T cells in the inoculum, the dosage and fractionation of irradiation given in the preparative regimen, prior splenectomy, pre-transplant decontamination of the gastrointestinal tract, use of a laminar airflow environment, or underlying diagnosis (such as type of leukemia).

A number of smaller studies from single institutions have identified a variety of different risk factors associated with acute graft-vs.-host disease (5,78–82). Risk factors were analyzed for mortality secondary to graft-vs.-host disease for 65 HLA-matched recipients of bone marrow transplants (71). It was found that increased age, smaller bone marrow doses (less than 3×10^8 cells/kg), and prior splenectomy all increased the risk of death from graft-vs.-host disease.

The Johns Hopkins experience with 136 HLA-identical bone marrow transplant recipients revealed that presence of an increased risk of developing moderate to severe graft-vs.-host disease was associated with the following factors: acute lymphoblastic leukemia, sex mismatched donor-recipient pairs, recipient age older than 24 years, and presence of certain HLA alleles (Cw4, Bw21, B49, and B50) (79). The HLA allele Aw19 was associated with a decreased risk of developing this complication. The association of increased incidence of graft-vs.-host disease with certain HLA alleles is especially intriguing. It suggests that minor histocompatibility antigens associate with certain HLA alleles in a way to affect the clinical manifestations of graft-vs.-host disease. Also, transplant tolerance may be associated with other alleles. This may be similar to the resistance to lethal graft-vs.-host disease exhibited by certain strains of inbred mice (29,42).

Use of female donors with increased age and parity greatly increased the risk of acute graft-vs.-host disease among 40 HLA-identical marrow transplant recipients (80). The number of T cells, T cells of various subsets, NK cells or monocytes in the donor inoculum did not influence the development of this complication. These findings imply that female donors were presensitized to their respective recipients by earlier pregnancies.

The role of immunity to herpes viruses in the development of acute graft-vs.-host disease was studied in 126 bone marrow transplant recipients from HLA-identical siblings. It was found that donor seronegativity for herpes simplex virus (HSV) and recipient seronegativity for Epstein-Barr virus (EBV) were significantly associated with a low incidence of graft-vs.-host disease. Since the likelihood of detecting herpes viral antibodies increases with age, it is possible that effects of recipient age on graft-vs.-host disease may be partly due to the increased viral exposure among these donors. These studies again implicate viral reactivation in the pathogenesis of acute graft-vs.-host disease, either directly or by its affect on the induction of lymphokines such as gamma interferon or interleukin-2 (50–72). In another study, the association of cytomegalovirus (CMV) infection with acute graft-vs.-host disease was assessed in recipients of marrow transplants. It was found that serological evidence of previous CMV infection in the recipient, rather than the donor, correlated best with post-transplant development of CMV infection (82). Furthermore, cytomegalovirus infection was strongly associated with the occurrence of acute graft-vs.-host disease. Acute graft-vs.-host disease frequently preceded clinical evidence of CMV infection.

A univariate analysis of 130 patients with aplastic anemia who received HLA-matched bone marrow transplants showed that use of a protective environment with laminar airflow rooms significantly decreased mortality (5). This beneficial effect was primarily due to a delay in onset and decrease in the incidence of acute graft-vs.-host disease. This association has never been demonstrated for marrow transplant recipients with hematologic malignancies. The authors also found that increasing age of the recipient was associated with increased mortality (5).

Data were reviewed from 105 patients who received bone marrow transplants from HLA-nonidentical relatives (21). Acute graft-vs.-host disease occurred earlier with increased severity and frequency among these patients than for the 728 patients studied concurrently who had received bone marrow transplants from HLA-identical siblings. Interestingly, the risk of graft-vs.-host disease did not differ whether there was disparity for class I (HLA-A or -B) or class II (HLA-D region) MHC loci. These recipients of HLA-nonidentical marrow were also more likely to experience delayed engraftment, granulocytopenia and graft rejection than did the HLA-matched recipients. In a different study, among recipients who received bone marrow which had been depleted of T cells, the presence of graft-vs.-host disease correlated closely with the number of clonable T cells in the donor marrow inoculum (83). Graft-vs.-host disease occurred only in recipients who were given more than 10^5 clonable T cells/kg in the bone marrow inoculum. These results appear in conflict with the numerous studies which have failed to find a correlation between T cell number in the bone marrow inoculum and the occurrence of graft-vs.-host disease (78–80). However, it is possible that among the recipients of non-T cell depleted bone marrow, the number of T cells is in such great excess that it does not represent a limiting factor.

Lastly, *in vitro* assays have been developed to predict the development of graft-vs.-host disease in HLA-identical marrow transplant patients (84,85). In one assay, marrow transplant donor lymphocytes are sensitized for 8 days *in vitro* to recipient lymphocytes and then co-cultured with recipient skin explants. A positive test is characterized by histologic changes of graft-vs.-host disease in the *in vitro* skin explant. This test appeared to predict the occurrence of graft-vs.-host disease at a level of at least clinical stage 2, with a sensitivity of 84% and specificity of 85% (84). *In vitro* proliferative responses of donor lymphocytes to recipient epidermal cells were quantitated (85). A stimulation index of over 1.5 was found in 10 out of 11 patients who developed acute graft-vs.-host disease, but was seen in only 3 out of 10 with no acute graft-vs.-host disease. These same donor-recipient pairs were unresponsive in the classic mixed lymphocyte culture performed with lymphocytes rather than epidermal stimulatory cells from the host. It has been postulated that skin may express specific minor histocompatibility antigens not present on other tissues, such as the Ep-1 antigen identified on murine skin. This epidermal antigen may stimulate better primary *in vitro* lymphocyte proliferative responses (86).

Overall, evaluation of risk factors for acute graft-vs.-host disease among recipients of bone marrow transplants has failed to confirm a role played by total donor T cell number or bone marrow dose, an association which was observed in mouse studies. However, these human studies have tested a narrower dose range than was evaluated in the animal models (2,78–80). In T cell depleted bone marrow recipients, the number of clonable T cells may correlate with occurrence of graft-vs.-host disease (83). Nevertheless, sex mismatch between donor and recipient, allogeneic sensitization of the donor, and increased age of the recipient clearly increase the likelihood of acute graft-vs.-host disease (2).

HUMAN *IN VITRO* AND *IN VIVO* STUDIES OF GRAFT-VS.-HOST DISEASE IN BONE MARROW TRANSPLANT RECIPIENTS

Several authors have described a syndrome with the skin manifestations of acute graft-vs.-host disease occurring in recipients of either autologous or syngeneic (identical twin) bone marrow (18,57,58,87). These observations have raised questions concerning abnormalities of immune regulation and suppressor cell activity which may allow autoreactive cells to attack self-antigen. Alternatively, the toxicity due to radiation, drugs or viral infection may have altered recipient self-antigens so that they are recognized as foreign by the donor lymphocytes.

To further investigate the mechanism behind these observations, the phenotypes of peripheral blood T cells were studied during and after acute and chronic graft-vs.-host disease on marrow transplant recipients. Peripheral

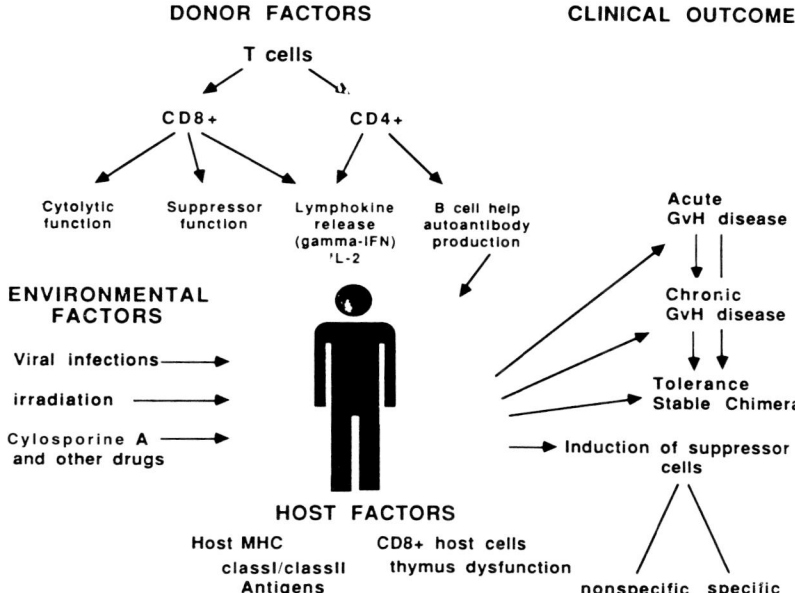

FIG. 1. Some of the complex interactions of host, donor, and environmental factors in the pathophysiology of graft-vs.-host disease.

blood lymphocytes were obtained from marrow transplant patients, who have evidence of graft-vs.-host disease or in whom graft-vs.-host disease had resolved, and lymphocytes were also obtained from control donors. Twenty percent of these lymphocytes were cytotoxic-suppressor phenotype as determined by cell surface marker analysis. This surface marker detected presence of the TH_2+ determinant, which is similar to the CD8 determinant. The 3 patients with acute graft-vs.-host disease, of which one was a twin-donor recipient, had no detectable cytotoxic-suppressor cells in their peripheral blood lymphocytes by this analysis. The circulating T cells in these patients expressed the Ia (HLA-DR) antigen, an indicator of T cell activation. These abnormalities all resolved with resolution of graft-vs.-host disease. Of 6 patients with chronic graft-vs.-host disease, 2 were lacking lymphocytes with the TH_2+ (cytotoxic-suppressor) marker, as were those with acute graft-vs.-host disease. The other 4 patients had increased numbers of TH_2+ Ia^+ T cells which could suppress *in vitro* T cell proliferation to alloantigens and Herpes simplex virus. These findings were consistent with abnormal immune regulation as an underlying mechanism in producing graft-vs.-host disease (18).

Other investigators have also examined the phenotype of peripheral blood T cells in marrow transplant recipients (88,89). T cell phenotypes of these lymphocytes were studied utilizing two monoclonal antibodies: anti-CD4 and anti-CD8. The CD4 (T4) antibody defines a T cell surface molecule which interacts with class II MHC antigens (HLA-DR, -DQ, -DP) and is predominantly found on helper cells. The CD8 (T8) antibody defines a T cell surface molecule which interacts with class I MHC antigens (HLA-A, -B, and -C) and is predominantly found on cytotoxic-suppressor cells (90). During recovery from lethal irradiation and rescue with either allogeneic or autologous bone marrow, peripheral T4$^+$ T cells recover first followed by T8$^+$ T cells 4 to 7 days later. This recovery was faster with autologous than with allogeneic donor cells. In contrast, in patients who developed moderate to severe graft-vs.-host disease, T8$^+$ cells recovered earlier, subsequently leading to lower T4/T8 ratios; the ratios being less than 2.5. Nine out of 11 patients with acute graft-vs.-host disease had a T4/T8 ratio of under 2.5 when symptoms occurred, while only 1 out of 13 patients without significant graft-vs.-host disease had a T4/T8 ratio under 2.5 (88). These findings derived from larger numbers of patients seem to be in conflict with those of other studies (18).

In another study, recipients of HLA-identical sibling marrow all showed evidence of activation markers (T10$^+$ and HLA-DR$^+$), but not interleukin-2 receptors, on both T4$^+$ and T8$^+$ cells. It was found that the numbers of T4$^+$ cells were decreased for prolonged periods relative to the numbers of T8$^+$ cells, independent of the degree of graft-vs.-host disease.

The functional capabilities of T cells and T cell subsets were studied from normal donors, and from marrow transplant recipients with and without chronic graft-vs.-host disease (91). Patients with chronic graft-vs.-host disease had T4$^+$ cells which were defective in their ability to promote pokeweed mitogen induced B cell responses. Several of these same patients had T4$^+$ cells which could suppress normal T cell induced immunoglobulin responses to control B cells. T4$^+$ cells from all 20 normal individuals expressed helper activity, while none suppressed immunoglobulin production. It is clear that underlying mechanisms of chronic graft-vs.-host disease are more complicated than can be inferred from mere differences in ratios of helper to cytotoxic-suppressor T cells. The mechanisms underlying chronic graft-vs.-host disease must involve defective and aberrant functional capacities within these populations, including both T4$^+$ as well as T8$^+$ cells.

Patients with or without acute graft-vs.-host disease were found to have defective *in vitro* production of interleukin-2 when assayed between 30 and 100 days after bone marrow transplantation. On the other hand, long-term survivors of marrow transplant without chronic graft-vs.-host disease have normal *in vitro* production of interleukin-2 while those with chronic graft-vs.-host disease were deficient in their ability to produce interleukin-2 following *in vitro* stimulation. Production of interleukin-1 by monocytes was normal in all of the various populations of patients undergoing bone marrow transplantation.

Others have been able to detect cytotoxic T lymphocyte responses directed toward host minor histocompatibility antigens during chronic graft-vs.-host disease in HLA-matched marrow transplant recipients (19). For some patients, these cytotoxic T lymphocyte responses appeared restricted by HLA-A2 (class

I) MHC antigens. Further analysis could not determine which chromosome contained the gene(s) coding for these minor histocompatibility antigens. Cytotoxic responses directed against H-Y antigens (encoded on the male Y chromosome) have been detected *in vitro* in bone marrow transplant patients. This finding suggests an explanation for the increased incidence of graft-vs.-host disease in sex disparate bone marrow transplants; that is, female donor to male recipient (93,94).

The presence of nonspecific suppressor cells has been observed in patients with chronic graft-vs.-host disease. These cells, which are not present in healthy long-term survivors of bone marrow transplants, are able to suppress donor *in vitro* proliferation induced by allogeneic antigens and concanavalin-A. Similar suppressor cells have been noted frequently in patients shortly (less than 7 days) after bone marrow transplantation, regardless of the presence of acute graft-vs.-host disease (96). However, when these nonspecific suppressor cells were found in long-term survivors, they were frequently associated with clinical manifestations of chronic graft-vs.-host disease.

Among long-term bone marrow transplant recipients who did not show clinical evidence of graft-vs.-host disease, there was the presence of specific radiosensitive suppressor cells which inhibit the ability of donor cells to respond to trinitrophenyl-altered host cells. These suppressor cells were not able to suppress "third-party" alloantigen induced proliferation. Furthermore, it was observed that patients with chronic graft-vs.-host disease have specific cytotoxic cells activated *in vitro* by host tissues, which specifically destroy host fibroblasts (97). This response is absent in patients without chronic graft-vs.-host disease, again suggesting the presence of specific suppressor cells for donor antihost responses. These clinical findings correlate closely with experiments in Lewis rats (61–63). Both authors proposed that nonspecific suppressor cells accompany chronic graft-vs.-host disease, while specific suppressor cells mediate tolerance and the stable chimeric state (95–97).

Recently, a number of groups have published their experience with *in vitro* elimination of T cells from donor bone marrow prior to transplantation (98–100). In most of these studies, the prevalence and severity of acute graft-vs.-host disease was significantly reduced, and has been borne out in randomized trials (98). Several complications have been noted among T cell depleted marrow transplant recipients, including slower engraftment and a higher incidence of graft failure (98,99,101). In several patients studied, graft failure was associated with the emergence of host T lymphocytes which demonstrated *in vitro* antidonor immune specificity (102,103). Further experience in both animals and humans demonstrate that more potent pre-transplant conditioning, either by irradiation or chemotherapy, decreases the incidence of graft failure (101,104).

Taken together, the various studies reviewed above suggest that T cells in the graft help to prevent host mediated graft rejection. A second complication of T cell depletion (in addition to more frequent graft failure) is an increase in leukemic relapse among leukemic recipients (98,105). Acute and chronic graft-vs.-host disease have been noted to be associated with decreased leukemic relapse and prolonged survival (106–110). This effect has been designated the "graft-vs.-leukemia" effect. It has been postulated that mature donor T cells which are required for graft-vs.-host disease are also essential in the graft-vs.-leukemia response. In studies done so far, T cell depletion from the bone marrow inoculum has not led to a significant increase in survival among recipients of HLA-identical marrow transplants. This lack of improved survival in these patients is due to the increase in graft failure and leukemic relapse, even in the absence of graft-vs.-host disease (98).

SUMMARY

Experimental animal studies and human clinical and *in vitro* studies all demonstrate that graft-vs.-host disease represents a complex interaction of many factors. These include immunocompetent cells of the donor, host antigens, infectious agents, lymphokines, and specific and nonspecific regulatory cells. It is likely that mature T lymphocytes within the donor inoculum recognize either MHC or minor histocompatibility antigens within the host as being foreign. The frequency of sensitization of donors and the number of precursor donor cells reactive against the host may effect the likelihood of graft-vs.-host disease. This sensitization may relate to specific MHC haplotypes of host and donor. Recognition of minor histocompatibility antigens appears restricted by MHC antigens, frequently as class I antigens.

The identity of the subset of T cells which mediates graft-vs.-host disease is not clear. Cytotoxic T lymphocytes are definitely not the only mediator of graft-vs.-host disease. There is ample evidence documenting that both cytotoxic-suppressor (CD8+) cells and helper (CD4+) cells can act to mediate graft-vs.-host disease. Simultaneously, latent viral infections may alter host antigens or lead to release of gamma interferon which induces class II MHC antigens on epithelial cells of the skin and the gastrointestinal tract, which are targets of graft-vs.-host disease. Finally, lesions induced by graft-vs.-host disease are sites of entry for microbial agents which give rise to the fulminant infectious complications of graft-vs.-host disease.

Graft-vs.-host disease can resolve as a result of inhibition of antihost responses by specific suppressor cells. On the other hand, chronic graft-vs.-host disease is characterized by immunosuppression with nonspecific suppressor cells, and also manifests signs of autoimmunity associated with polyclonal stimulation of host B cells by donor helper T cells.

Great progress has been made in our understanding of graft-vs.-host disease, but there are still many questions which remain and numerous avenues of research to pursue. With the answers to these questions, there may be improved ability to prevent and treat graft-vs.-host disease as well as other immune-mediated diseases.

REFERENCES

1. Thomas ED, Storb R, Clift RA, et al.: Bone marrow transplantation. *N Engl J Med* 1975;292:895–901.
2. Gale RP, Bortin MM, van Bekkum DW, *et al:* Risk factors for acute graft-vs.-host disease. *Br J Hematol.* 1987;67:397–406.
3. Gleicksberg H, Storb R, Fefer A, et al.: Clinical manifestations of graft-vs.-host disease in human recipients of marrow from HLA-matched sibling donors. *Transplantation* 1974; 18:295–304.
4. Shulman HM, Sullivan KM, Weiden PL, et al.: Chronic graft-vs.-host syndrome in man; a long-term clinicopathologic study of 20 Seattle patients. *Am J Med* 1980;69:204–217.
5. Storb R, Prentice RL, Buckner CD, et al.: Graft-vs.-host disease and survival in patients with aplastic anemia treated by marrow grafts from HLA-identical siblings; beneficial effect of protective environment. *N Engl J Med* 1983; 308:302–307.
6. Storb R, Prentice RL, Sullivan KM, et al.: Predictive factors in chronic graft-vs.-host disease in patients with aplastic anemia treated with marrow transplantation from HLA identical siblings. *Ann Intern Med* 1983;98:461–466.
7. Thomas ED, Buckner CD, Clift RA, et al.: Marrow transplantation for acute nonlympho-blastic leukemia in first remission. *N Engl J Med* 1979;301:597–599.
8. Storb R, Thomas ED, Buckner CD, et al.: Marrow transplantation in 30 "untransfused" patients with severe aplastic anemia. *Ann Intern Med* 1980;92:30–36.
9. Speck B, Bortin MM, Champlin R, et al.: Allogeneic bone marrow transplantation for chronic myelogenous leukemia. *Lancet* 1984;1:665–668.
10. O'Reilly RJ: Allogeneic bone marrow transplantation; current status and future directions. *Blood* 1983;62:941–964.
11. O'Reilly RJ, Brochstein J, Dinsmore R, Kirkpatrick D: Marrow transplantation for congenital disorders. *Semin Hematol* 1984;21:188–221.
12. Simonsen M: The impact on the developing embryo and newborn animal of adult homologous cells. *Acta Pathol Microbiol Scand* 1957;40:480–500.
13. Billingham RE: The biology of graft-vs.-host reactions. *Harvey Lectures* 1968; pp. 21–78.
14. Simonsen M: Graft-vs.-host reaction; the history that never was and the way things happened to happen. *Immunol Rev* 1985;88:5–23.
15. deGast GC, Gratama JW, Ringden O, Gleichman E: The multifactorial etiology of graft-vs.-host disease. *Immunol Today* 1987;8:209–211.
16. Tutschka PJ: Graft-vs.-host disease: immunobiological aspects. *Hæmatology and Blood Transfusion* 1983;28:97–101.
17. Tsoi M-S: Immunological mechanisms of graft-vs.-host disease in man. *Transplantation* 1982;33:459–464.
18. Reinherz EL, Parkman R, Rappaport J, et al.: Aberration of suppressor T cells in human graft-vs.-host disease. *N Engl J Med* 1979;300:1061–1068.
19. Goulmy E, Gratama JW, Blokland E, et al.: A minor transplantation antigen detected by MHC-restricted cytotoxic T lymphocytes during graft-vs.-host disease. *Nature* 1983;302:159–161.
20. Tsoi M-S, Storb R, Dobbs S, Thomas ED: Specific suppressor cells in graft-host tolerance of HLA-identical marrow transplantation. *Nature* 1981;292:355–357.
21. Beatty PG, Clift RA, Mickelson EH, et al.: Marrow transplantation from related donors other than HLA-identical siblings. *N Engl J Med* 1985;313:765–771.
22. Bortin MM: Acute graft-vs.-host disease following bone marrow transplantation in humans; prognostic factors. *Transpl Proc* 1987;19:2655–2657.
23. Beer AE, Billingham RE: Maternally acquired runt disease. *Science* 1973;179:240–247.
24. Neithammer D, Goldmann SF, Flad HD, et al.: Nature of reconstitution with histoincompatible maternal marrow in a case of severe combined immunodeficiency with graft-vs.-host disease following maternofetal transfusions. *Clin Immunol Immunopath* 1981;18:387–401.

25. Hathaway WE, Fulginiti V, Peerce CW, et al.: Graft-vs.-host reaction following a single blood transfusion. *JAMA* 1967;201:139–144.
26. Kadowaki J, Zuelzer WW, Brough AJ, et al.: XX/XY lymphoid chimerism in congenital immunologic deficiency syndrome with thymic lymphoplasia. *Lancet* 1965;2:1152–1156.
27. Santos GW, Cole LJ: Effect of donor and host lymphoid and myeloid tissue injections in lethally X-irradiated mice treated with rat bone marrow. *J Natl Cancer Inst* 1958;21:279–287.
28. Van Bekkum DW, de Vries MJ: *Radiation Chimeras,* Logos Press, London, 1967.
29. Grebe SC, Streilein JW: Graft-vs.-host reactions; a review. *Adv Immunol* 1976;22:119–176.
30. Korngold R, Sprent J: Lethal graft-vs.-host disease across minor histocompatibility barriers; nature of effector cells and role of the H-2 complex. *Immunol Rev* 1983;71:5–29.
31. Glazier A, Tutschka PJ, Farmer ER, Santos GW: Graft-vs.-host disease in cyclosporin-A treated rats after syngeneic and autologous bone marrow reconstitution. *J Exp Med* 1983;158:1–8.
32. Gleichmann E, Pals ST, Rolink AG, et al.: Graft-vs.-host reactions; clues to the etiopathology of a spectrum of immunological disease. *Immunol Today* 1984;5:324–332.
33. Piquet PF: Graft-vs.-host reactions elicited by products of class I or class II loci of the MHC; analysis of the response of mouse T lymphocytes to products of class I and class II loci of the MHC in correlation with graft-vs.-host reaction-induced mortality, medullary aplasia and enteropathy. *J Immunol* 1985;135:1637–1643.
34. Bach FH, Sachs DH: Transplantation immunology. *N Engl J Med* 1987;317:489–492.
35. Auffray C, Strominger JL: Molecular genetics of the human major histocompatibility complex. *Adv Human Genet* 1985;15:197–247.
36. Bach FH: The HLA class II genes and products; the HLA-D region. *Immunol Today* 1985;6:89–94.
37. Korngold R, Sprent J: Surface markers of T cells causing lethal graft-vs.-host disease to class I or class II H-2 differences. *J Immunol* 1985;135:3004–3010.
38. Vallera DA, Soderling CB, Carlson GJ, Kersey JH: Bone marrow transplantation across major histocompatibility barriers in mice; effect of elimination of T cells from donor grafts by treatment with monoclonal Thy-1.2 plus complement or antibody alone. *Transplantation* 1981;31:218–222.
39. Vallera DA, Youle RJ, Neville DM, Kersey JH: Bone marrow transplantation across major histocompatibility barriers. V. Protection of mice from lethal graft-vs.-host disease by pretreatment of donor cell with monoclonal anti-Thy-1.2 couple with toxuricin. *J Exp Med* 1982;155:949–954.
40. Pietryga DW, Blazar BR, Soderling CB, Vallera DA: The effect of T subset depletion on the incidence of lethal graft-vs.-host disease in murine major-histocompatibility complex-mismatched transplantation system. *Transplantation* 1987;43:442–445.
41. Judas HR, Peck AB. Lethal murine graft-vs.-host disease in the absence of detectable cytotoxic T lymphocytes. *Transplantation* 1983;36:281–289.
42. Hamilton BL: Absence of correlation between cytolytic T lymphocytes and lethal murine graft-vs.-host disease in response to minor histocompatibility antigens. *Transplantation* 1984;38:375–380.
43. Shiohara T, Narimatsu H, Nagashima M: Induction of cutaneous graft-vs.-host disease by allo- or self-Ia reactive helper T cells in mice. *Transplantation* 1987;43:692–698.
44. Carmody L, Atkinson K, Cooley M, et al.: Both class I and class II responsive T cell subsets can separately initiate lethal graft-vs.-host disease in H-2-incompatible murine radiation chimeras. *Transplant Proc* 1987;19:2876–2878.
45. Korngold R, Sprent J: Lethal graft-vs.-host diseaes after bone marrow transplantation across minor histocompatibility barriers in mice; prevention by removing mature T cells from marrow. *J Exp Med* 1978;148:1687–1698.
46. Hamilton B, Parkman R: Acute and chronic graft-vs.-host disease induced by minor histocompatibility antigens in mice. *Transplantation* 1983;36:150–155.
47. Storb R, Rudolph RH, Kolb HJ, et al.: Marrow grafts between DLA-matched canine littermates. *Transplantation* 1973;15:92–100.
48. Hamilton BL, Beran MJ, Parkman R: Antirecipient cytotoxic T lymphocyte precursors are present in the spleen of mice with acute graft-vs.-host disease due to minor histocompatibility antigens. *J Immunol* 1981;126:621–625.

49. Parkman R: Clonal analysis of murine graft-vs.-host disease. I. Phenotypic and functional analysis of T lymphocyte clones. *J Immunol* 1986;136:3543–3552.
50. Ferrara JLM, Marion A, McIntyre JF, et al.: Amelioration of acute graft-vs.-host disease due to minor histocompatibility antigens by *in vivo* administration of anti-interleukin-2 receptor antibody. *J Immunol* 1986;137:1874–1877.
51. Robb RJ, Munok JA, Smith KA: T cell growth factor receptors; quantitation, specificity and biologic relevance. *J Exp Med* 1981;154:1455–1467.
52. Rolink AG, Radaszkiewicz T, Pals ST, et al.: Allosuppressor and allohelper T cells in acute and chronic graft-vs.-host disease. I. Alloreactive suppressor cells rather than killer T cells appear to be the decisive effector cells in lethal graft-vs.-host disease. *J Exp Med* 1982; 155:1501–1522.
53. Rolink AG, Gleichman E: Allosuppressor and allohelper T cells in acute and chronic graft-vs.-host (GVH) disease. III. Different Lyt subsets of donor T cells induce different pathologic syndromes. *J Exp Med* 1983;158:546–558.
54. Via CS, Sharrow SO, Shearer GM: Role of cytotoxic T lymphocytes in the prevention of Lupus-like disease occurring in a murine model of graft-vs.-host disease. *J Immunol* 1987;138:1840–1849.
55. Harper SE, Roabinian JR, Seaman WE: Regulation of autoimmunity and donor cell engraftment by recipient Lyt2+ cells during the graft-vs.-host reaction. *J Exp Med* 1987; 166:657–667.
56. Moser M, Mizouchi T, Sharrow SO, et al.: Graft-vs.-host reaction limited to a class II MHC difference results in selective deficiency in the L3T4+ but not in Lyt2+ T helper cell function. *J Immunol* 1987;138:1355–1362.
57. Rappaport J, Reinherz E, Mihm M, et al.: Acute graft-vs.-host disease in recipients of bone marrow transplants from identical twin donors. *Lancet* 1979;2:717–720.
58. Gleichman E, Devergie A, Sohier J, Saurai JH: Graft-vs.-host disease in recipients of syngeneic bone marrow. *Lancet* 1980:253–254.
59. Hess AD, Horwitz L, Beschorner WE, Santos GW: Development of graft-vs.-host disease-like syndrome in cyclosporine-treated rats after syngeneic bone marrow transplantation. I. Development of cytotoxic T lymphocytes with anti-Ia-specificity, including autoreactivity. *J Exp Med* 1985;161:718–730.
60. Morris PJ: Cyclosporin A. *Transplantation* 1981;32:349–354.
61. Tutschka PJ, Hess AD, Beschorner WE, Santos GW: Suppressor cells in transplantation tolerance. I. Suppressor cells in the mechanism of tolerance in radiation oncology. *Transplantation* 1981;32:203–209.
62. Tutschka PJ, Ki PF, Beschorner WE, et al.: Suppressor cells in transplantation tolerance. II. Maturation of suppressor cells in the bone marrow chimera. *Transplantation* 1981;32:321–325.
63. Tutschka PJ, Hess AD, Beschorner WE, Santos GW: Suppressor cells in transplantation tolerance. III. The role of antigen in the maintenance of transplantation tolerance. *Transplantation* 1982;33:510–514.
64. Shih CC-Y, Truitt RL: A class II antigen-specific T cell clone can suppress graft-vs.-host reactivity in murine allogeneic bone marrow chimeras. *Transplant Proc* 1987;19:2664–2667.
65. Kosmatopoulos K, Algara DS, Orbach-Arbouijs S: Antireceptor anti-MHC cytotoxic T lymphocytes; their role in the resistance to graft-vs.-host reaction. *J Immunol* 1987;138:1038–1042.
66. Bellgrau DL, Wilson DB: Immunological studies of T cell receptors. I. Specifically induced resistance to graft-vs.-host disease in rats mediated by host T cell immunity to alloreactive parental T cells. *J Exp Med* 1978;149:234–243.
67. Rose RN: Modification of hybrid responsiveness in the local graft-vs.-host reaction by injection of parental lymphocytes. *Transplantation* 1975;20:248–253.
68. Pollard M, Chang CF, Srivastava KK: The role of microflora in development of graft-vs.-host disease. *Transplant Proc* 1976;8:533–536.
69. Storb R, Thomas ED: Graft-vs.-host disease in dog and man; the Seattle experience. *Immunol Rev* 1985;88:214–238.
70. Lampert IA, Suitters AJ, Chishold PM: Expression of Ia antigen on epidermal keratinocytes in graft-vs.-host disease. *Nature* 1981;293:149–150.

71. Mason DW, Dallman M, Barday AN: Graft-vs.-host disease induces expression of Ia antigen in rat epidermal cells and gut epithelium. *Nature* 1981;293:150–151.
72. Collins T, Korman AJ, Wake CT, et al.: Immune interferon activates multiple class II major histocompatibility complex genes and associated invariant chain gene in human endothelial cells and dermal fibroblasts. *Proc Natl Acad Sci USA* 1984;81:4917–4921.
73. Storb R: Graft-vs.-host disease after marrow transplantation. *Progr Clin Biol Res* 1986; 224:139–157.
74. Parkman R: Treatment of immunodeficiency diseases by organ transplantation. *Proc Clin Immunol* 1977;3:85–102.
75. O'Reilly RJ, Dupont B, Pahwa S, et al.: Reconstitution in severe combined immunodeficiency by transplantation of marrow from unrelated donor. *N Engl J Med* 1977;297:1311–1320.
76. Geha RS, Malakiau A, LeFranc G, et al.: Immunologic reconstitution in severe combined immunodeficiency following transplantation with parental bone marrow. *Pediatrics* 1976; 58:451–455.
77. Gatti RA, Allen HD, Meuwissen HJ, et al.: Immunologic reconstruction of sex-linked lymphophenic immunologic deficiency. *Lancet* 1968;2:1366–1369.
78. Ringden O, Nilsson B: Death by graft-vs.-host disease associated with HLA-mismatched high recipient age, low marrow cell dose, and splenectomy. *Transplantation* 1985;40:39–44.
79. Bross DS, Tutschka PJ, Farmer ER, et al.: Predictive factors for acute graft-vs.-host disease in patients transplanted with HLA-identical bone marrow. *Blood* 1984;63:1265–1270.
80. Atkinson K, Farrel C, Chapman T, et al.: Female marrow donors increase the risk of acute graft-vs.-host disease; effect of donor age and parity and analysis of cell subpopulations in the donor marrow inoculum. *Br J Haematol* 1986;63:231–239.
81. Gratama JW, Strijnen T, Weiland HT, et al.: Herpes-virus immunity and acute graft-vs.-host disease. *Lancet* 1987;1:471–474.
82. Miller W, Flynn P, McCullough J, et al.: Cytomegalovirus infection after bone marrow transplantation; an association with acute graft-vs.-host disease. *Blood* 1986;67:1162–1167.
83. Kernan NA, Collins NH, Juliano L, et al.: Clonable T lymphocytes in T cell-depleted bone marrow transplants correlate with the development of graft-vs.-host disease. *Blood* 1986; 68:770–773.
84. Vogelsang GB, Hess AD, Berkman AW, et al.: An *in vitro* predictive test for graft-vs.-host disease in patients with genotypic HLA-identical bone marrow transplants. *N Engl J Med* 1985;313:645–650.
85. Bagot M, Cordonnier C, Tilkin AF, et al.: A possible predictive test for graft-vs.-host disease in bone marrow graft recipients; the mixed epidermal cell-lymphocyte reaction. *Transplantation* 1986;41:316–319.
86. Tyler JD, Steinmuller D: Establishment of cytolytic T lymphocyte clones to epidermal alloantigen Epa-1. *Transplantation* 1982;34:140–147.
87. Thein SL, Goldman JM, Galton DAG: Acute graft-vs.-host disease after autografting for chronic granulocytic leukemia in transformation. *Ann Int Med* 1981;94:210–211.
88. Gratama JW, Naipal A, Oljans P, et al.: T lymphocyte repopulation and differentiation after bone marrow transplantation early shifts in the ratio between T4+ and T8+ T lymphocytes correlate with the occurrence of acute graft-vs.-host disease. *Blood* 1984;63:1416–1423.
89. Britton K, Atkinson K, Chapman G, et al.: Activation antigen expression on the helper-inducer and cytotoxic-suppressor T cell subpopulation after allogeneic human marrow transplantation. *Transplant Proc* 1986;18:302–304.
90. Reinherz EL, Meuer SC, Schlossman SF: The delineation of antigen receptors on human T lymphocytes. *Immunol Today* 1983;4:5–8.
91. Lum LG, Draitt-Thordarson N, Seigneuret MC, Storb R: The regulation of Ig synthesis after marrow transplantation. IV. T4 and T8 subset function in patients with chronic graft-vs.-host disease. *J Immunol* 1982;129:113–119.
92. Brkic S, Tsoi M-S, Mori T, et al.: Cellular interactions in marrow-grafted patients. III. Normal interleukin-1 and defective interleukin-2 production in short-term patients and in those with chronic graft-vs.-host disease. *Transplantation* 1985;39:30–35.
93. Goulmy E, Termijtelen A, Bradley A, van Rood JJ: Y-antigen killing by T cells of women is restricted by HLA. *Nature* 1977;266:544–545.
94. Goulmy E, Bradley BA, Langsbergen Q, van Rood JJ: The importance of H-Y incompatibility in human organ transplantation. *Transplantation* 1978;25:315–319.

95. Tsoi M-S, Storb R, Dobbs S, et al.: Nonspecific suppressor cells in patients with chronic graft-vs.-host disease after marrow grafting. *J Immunol* 1979;123:1970–1976.

96. Hess AD, Tutschka PJ, Saral R, Santos GW: Nonspecific suppressor cells following bone marrow transplantation. *Exp Hematol* 1982;10(Suppl. 11): 64.

97. Tsoi M-S, Storb R, Dobbs S, et al.: Specific suppressor cells and immune response to host antigen in long-term human allogeneic marrow recipients; implications for the mechanism of graft-host tolerance and chronic graft-vs.-host disease. *Transplant Proc* 1981;13:237–240.

98. Mitsuyasu RT, Champlin RE, Gale RP, et al.: Treatment of donor bone marrow with monoclonal anti-T cell antibody and complement for the prevention of graft-vs.-host disease. *Ann Int Med* 1986;105:20–26.

99. Prentice HG, Janossy G, et al.: Depletion of T lymphocytes in donor marrow prevents significant graft-vs.-host disease in matched allogeneic leukemic marrow transplant recipients. *Lancet* 1984;1:472–475.

100. Herve P, Cahn CY, Flesch M, et al.: Successful graft-vs.-host disease prevention without graft failure in 32 HLA-identical allogeneic bone marrow transplantations with marrow depletion of T cells by monoclonal antibody and complement. *Blood* 1987;69:388–393.

101. Bozdech MJ, Sondel PM, Trigg ME, et al.: Transplantation of HLA-haploidentical T cell depleted marrow for leukemia; addition to cytosine arabinoside to the pre-transplant conditioning prevents rejection. *Exp Hematol* 1985;13:1201–1210.

102. Sondel PM, Hank JA, Trigg ME, et al.: Transplantation of HLA-haploidentical T cell-depleted marrow for leukemia; autologous marrow recovery with specific immune sensitization to donor antigens. *Exp Hematol* 1986;14:278–286.

103. Kernan NA, Flomenberg N, Dupont B, O'Reilly RJ: Graft rejection in recipients of T cell depleted HLA-nonidentical marrow transplants for leukemia; identification of host-derived antidonor allocytotoxic lymphocytes. *Transplantation* 1987;43:842–847.

104. Schwartz E, Lapidot T, Gozes D, et al.: Abrogation of bone marrow allograft resistance in mice by increased total body irradiation correlates with eradication of host clonable T cells and alloreactive cytotoxic precursors. *J Immunol* 1987;130:460–465.

105. Henslec PJ, Thompson JS, Romond EH, et al.: T cell depletion of HLA and haploidentical marrow reduces graft-vs.-host disease, but it may impair a graft-vs.-leukemia effect. *Transplant Proc* 1987;19:2701–2706.

106. Weiden PL, Flournoy N, et al.: Antileukemic effect of graft-vs.-host disease in human recipients of allogeneic marrow grafts. *N Engl J Med* 1979;300:1068–1073.

107. Weiden PL, Sullivan KM, et al.: Antileukemic effect of chronic graft-vs.-host disease, contribution to improved survival after allogeneic marrow transplantation. *N Engl J Med* 1981;304:1529–1532.

108. Gale RP, Champlin RE: How does bone marrow transplantation cure leukemia? *Lancet* 1984;2:28–30.

109. Sosman JA, Sondel PM: The graft-vs.-leukemia (GVL) effect following bone transplantation: a review of laboratory and clinical data. *Hematologic Reviews* 1987;2:77–91.

110. Butturini A, Bortin MM, Gale RP: Graft-vs.-leukemia following bone marrow transplantation. *Bone Marrow Transplantation* 1987;2:233–242.

Bone Marrow Transplantation in Children, edited by F. Leonard Johnson and Carl Pochedly. Raven Press, Ltd., New York © 1990.

Graft-vs.-Host Disease: Hepatic, Gastrointestinal, and Dermal Toxicities

Roger A. Vega

Emory University School of Medicine and Henrietta Egleston Hospital for Children, Atlanta, Georgia 30322

Introduction
A. Cutaneous acute graft-vs.-host disease
B. Liver and gastrointestinal manifestations of acute graft-vs.-host disease
C. Chronic graft-vs.-host disease
D Prevention of graft-vs.-host disease
E. Treatment
Summary

INTRODUCTION

Graft-vs.-host disease is an immunological condition initiated by the engraftment of competent donor T-lymphocytes in patients following allogeneic bone marrow transplantation. Three conditions have to be met in order for graft-vs.-host disease to occur: (1) the presence of alloreactive T lymphocytes contained in the donor's bone marrow, (2) cell membrane antigens in the host which are recognized as foreign by the grafted T cells, and (3) incapability by the host of rejecting the engrafted T cells, which by definition would be host-vs.-graft (1).

The skin, liver and gastrointestinal tract are the organs mainly affected by graft-vs.-host disease. Other affected organs are the lungs, kidneys and the lymphatic system, which are discussed in other sections of this book.

There are two distinct clinical expressions of this disease. The acute form occurs within the first 100 days after bone marrow transplantation and affects 30 to 70% of patients who are transplanted with marrow from an HLA-identical donor. The chronic form of graft-vs.-host disease occurs between 100 and 400 days after transplantation and affects 15 to 40% of transplanted individuals (2).

Many signs and symptoms of graft-vs.-host disease are not specific and may resemble other disorders. The skin rash can mimic irradiation toxicity, drug-related rashes or a viral exanthem. The liver involvement may be confused with drug reactions or viral hepatitis. The gut involvement may resemble viral or bacterial gastroenteritis and, in many cases, it is very difficult to differentiate this complication from irradiation toxicity.

This chapter describes the clinical and pathological manifestations of skin, liver, and gastrointestinal graft-vs.-host disease, together with its treatment.

CUTANEOUS ACUTE GRAFT-VS.-HOST DISEASE

The acute form of the disease may develop very early after transplantation, the peak incidence being between 3 and 6 weeks.

The earliest cutaneous manifestation of acute graft-vs.-host disease is a maculopapular rash that affects the palms, soles and the skin in general (Figures 1 and 2). This rash can be patchy or generalized. It may be superficial or deep in the skin, simulating a third degree burn. The extension of the rash and the degree of involvement of the epidermis is used to grade the disease (Table 1). A grading system of graft-vs.-host disease has been devised to relate clinical and histological changes. The severity of clinical graft-vs.-host disease has been classified ranging from grade 0 in the patient without evidence of graft-vs.-host disease to grade IV in the patient who has life-threatening disease.

It is striking that the target organs of graft-vs.-host disease are restricted mainly to the skin, liver, gastrointestinal tract and oral mucosa, and that these organs are directly or indirectly in contact with pathogenic microorganisms. It has long been speculated that these microorganisms after being ingested by the body cells, induce changes that lead them to express Ia antigens which then function as a target for the ongoing graft-vs.-host disease (3,4). Another hypothesis is that graft-vs.-host disease results from blood-derived host targets as the tissues are replaced by donor cells. Recent studies (5,6) have suggested that the blood-derived cells, such as Langerhans cells in the skin, were the principal targets of alloreactive donor cells in graft-vs.-host disease. Studies by Suitters et al., support the hypothesis that mature host Langerhans cells could be the targets of the graft-vs.-host reaction, and therefore, be selectively depleted (7). Perreault reported that patients with moderate to severe acute graft-vs.-host disease have a significantly lower number of Langerhans cells than those with mild or no graft-vs.-host disease (8).

Most patients who experience the acute form of graft-vs.-host disease will develop spontaneous resolution of this process. It has been postulated that

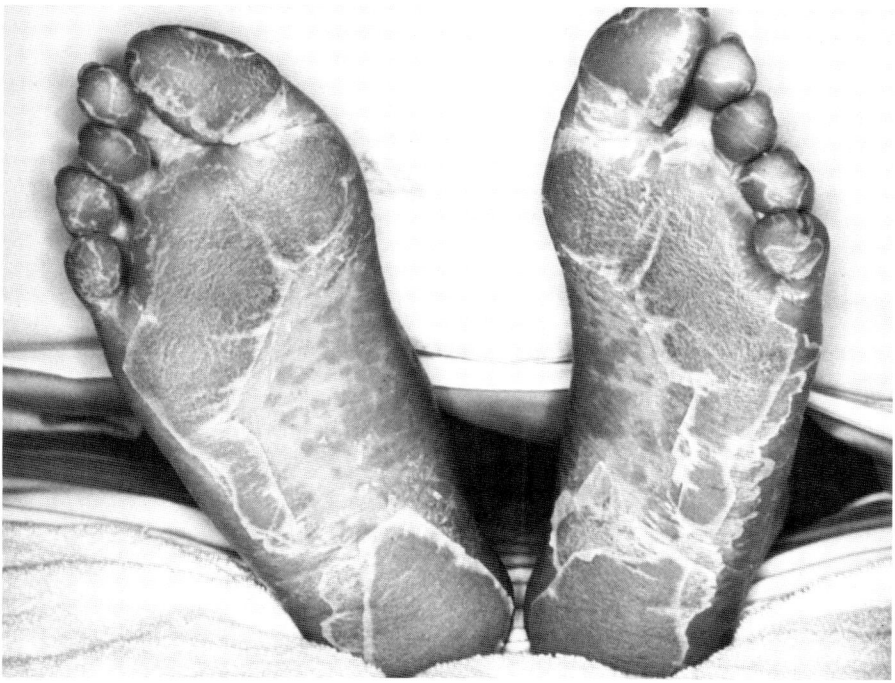

FIG. 1. Maculopapular rash and desquamation compatible with grade IV cutaneous graft-vs.-host disease.

graft-vs.-host tolerance is an active phenomenon that depends upon the development of suppressor cells capable of controlling the graft-vs.-host disease reaction (9).

Pathology of Cutaneous Acute Graft-vs.-Host Disease

In most cases, the skin is the initial target organ of graft-vs.-host disease. The skin lesions are characterized by generalized rash and, in more severe forms, bullae and desquamation occurs.

The conditioning regimen, usually consisting of high-dose chemotherapy, total body irradiation, or both, has a profound effect on these patients. Clinically, the effect of the regimen is manifested by the presence of a skin rash, and the occurrence of nausea and vomiting which may last for days or weeks. At this stage, a persistent mild rash would be clinically and histologically impossible to differentiate from acute graft-vs.-host disease. Lever et al., found that some so-called normal pre-transplant patients had abnormal skin biopsies, and the skin changes were similar to some of the abnormalities

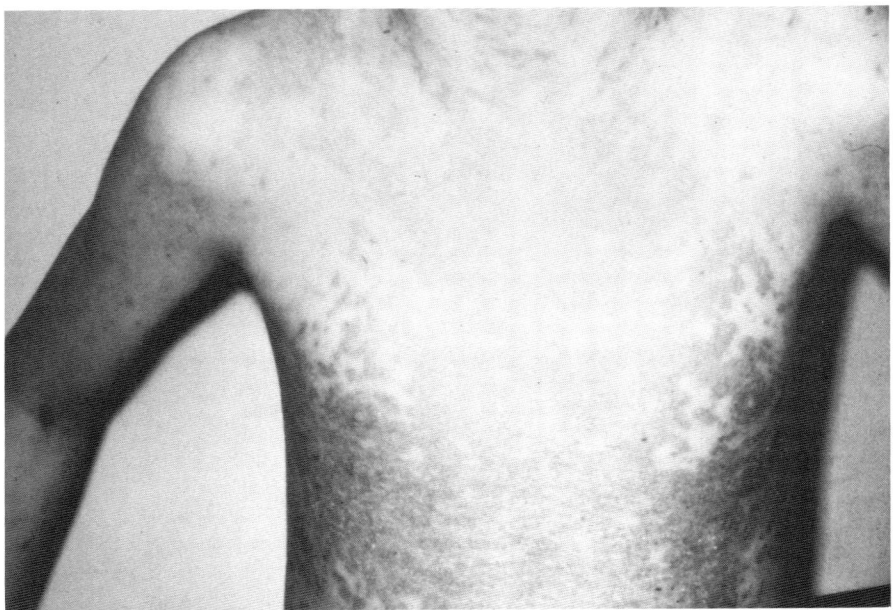

FIG. 2. Generalized maculopapular rash compatible with grade III cutaneous graft-vs.-host disease.

TABLE 1. *Clinical and histopathologic skin stages of graft-vs.-host disease**

Stage	Clinical findings	Histopathology
+	Maculopapular rash (<25% of body surface)	Basal vacuolar degeneration or necrosis (or both)
+ +	Maculopapular rash (25–50% of body surface)	+ plus spongiosis, dyskeratosis and eosinophilic necrosis of epidermal cells
+ + +	Generalized erythroderma	+ + plus focal microscopic epidermal-dermal separation
+ + + +	Generalized erythroderma with bullae formation and desquamation	Frank epidermal loss

*Adopted from Glucksberg H, et al. (14)

found in graft-vs.-host disease (13). These changes can be subtle and nonspecific and can be mistaken by drug and irradiation effects (10).

On histological examination, the mildest change observed in the skin is focal or diffuse vacuolar degeneration of epidermal basal cells and the presence of acanthocytes. In grade II graft-vs.-host disease, focal or diffuse spongiosis (separation and intercellular edema of basal cells and acanthocytes) and dyskeratosis or eosinophilic degeneration of epidermal cells are observed. In grade III graft-vs.-host disease, clefts and spaces (acantholysis and epidermolysis) occurs after necrosis of basal cells and acanthocytes in the basal and more superficial layers of the skin. This results in separation of the dermal-epidermal junction. In grade IV graft-vs.-host disease there is a frank loss of the epidermis (4) (Figure 3). When the epidermal lesions occur, similar changes may be found in the hair-follicle epithelium. The collagen of the papillary dermis displays moderate to severe necrosis in grade III graft-vs.-host disease. Inflammatory changes consist primarily of infiltrates of mononuclear cells in the epidermis and the papillary dermis (11).

The degree of epidermal changes has been used as a criterion in grading graft-vs.-host disease, but great variation may be found within each grade. Hymes et al. (12), retrospectively examined serial biopsies of 54 patients with grade II acute graft-vs.-host disease to try to find a histological factor that could be used to predict progression of the disease. The number of dermal and epidermal mononuclear cells present correlated positively with the probability of developing a more severe form of acute graft-vs.-host disease. In addition, patients who showed cutaneous histological changes early had a more severe form of the disease. None of the other histologic characteristics

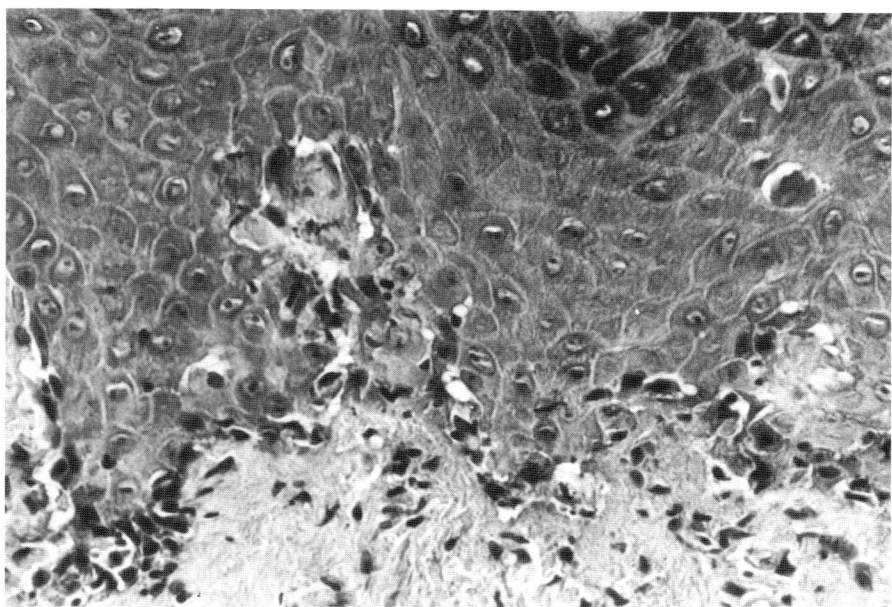

FIG. 3. Skin showing basal spongiosis and chronic inflammation at the dermal-epidermal junction and individual epidermal cell necrosis giving rise to eosinophilic bodies (H and E stain, ×800).

were found to predict progression of graft-vs.-host disease, and they did not predict the subsequent development of chronic graft-vs.-host disease.

LIVER AND GASTROINTESTINAL MANIFESTATIONS OF ACUTE GRAFT-VS.-HOST DISEASE

Hepatic and intestinal manifestations of graft-vs.-host disease can develop concurrently. Also, these findings may precede or follow skin manifestations of graft-vs.-host disease, or they may present without any evidence of skin involvement.

The gastrointestinal tract of individuals suffering from acute graft-vs.-host disease displays lesions in both the small and large intestine. The most severe lesions are found in the distal ileum. Involvement of the gastrointestinal tract is mainly manifested by nausea, vomiting, anorexia and diarrhea. The diarrhea is usually watery or bloody. The volume of diarrhea ranges from a few hundred milliliters to several liters per day. The diarrhea may contain exfoliated epithelium and inflammatory cells that have the appearance of fleshy-like material. The findings of large amounts of cellular debris, occult blood, and leukocytes in green-tinged stool is consistent with acute graft-vs.-host disease. The diarrhea contains a large amount of serum proteins, and this results in a striking decrease in the levels of total serum proteins and albumin (14,15). Other manifestations of severe graft-vs.-host disease of the gastrointestinal tract are abdominal pain and ileus.

Three clinical patterns of acute oral mucosa graft-vs.-host disease have been described: (1) Fine papular presentation. The oral mucosa reveals many small (less than 1 mm) white papules in close proximity to one another, with the resulting impression of generalized mucosal whitening; (2) Reticular or "lichenoid" presentation, in which raised interlacing white striae can be observed. In some cases the reticular presentations appear to be formed as a result of the enlargement coalescence of the papules as described in pattern (1) above; (3) Desquamative presentation. In this condition, exfoliating irregular plaques of whitened mucosa appear following the papular presentation (23).

TABLE 2. *Clinical and histopathologic gastrointestinal stages of graft-vs.-host disease**

Stage	Clinical findings	Histopathology
+	<500 ml diarrhea/day	Dilation of glands, single cell necrosis of epithelial cells
+ +	>1000 ml diarrhea/day	+ plus necrosis plus dropout of entire glands
+ + +	>1500 ml diarrhea/day	+ + plus focal microscopic mucosal denudation
+ + + +	Severe abdominal pain, with or without ileus	Diffuse microscopic mucosal denudation

*Adopted from Glucksberg H, et al. (14)

These clinical manifestations are not pathognomonic of the gastrointestinal form of graft-vs.-host disease. There are 4 possibilities in the differential diagnosis: (1) toxic effect of chemoradiotherapy; (2) intestinal infection; (3) the combination of gastrointestinal graft-vs.-host disease and infection; or (4) all of the above.

The isolation of a pathogen from culture of the diarrhea specimen may suggest an etiology or, more likely, the culture will indicate the presence of a superinfection complicating graft-vs.-host disease. The absence of such microbial pathogens does not exclude their presence in the upper or middle intestine.

X-ray examination of the intestine in patients with acute graft-vs.-host disease show mucosal and submucosal edema, which is most prominent in the distal small bowel. Transit of barium is rapid and often diluted with the intraluminal fluid. Mucosal ulceration and thickened colonic wall may be seen by barium enema (16,17). In patients with abdominal distention, plain abdominal films may show a thickened, edematous small intestine. Pneumatosis cystoides intestinalis may also occur (18). But none of these radiographic findings are pathognomonic of graft-vs.-host disease. The differential diagnosis should include cytomegalovirus enteritis, Henoch-Schonlein purpura, and gastrointestinal toxicity due to irradiation (15,19,20). The X-ray abnormalities of intestinal graft-vs.-host disease may disappear when the abdominal pain and diarrhea ceases, or the abnormalities may progress to segmental involvement of the jejunum and ileum (causing a ribbonlike appearance of the intestine) that may represent an irreversible form of the disease (21)

The pathological manifestations of gastrointestinal graft-vs.-host disease has been reviewed extensively elsewhere (15,22,23). The mild histopathological alterations of gastrointestinal graft-vs.-host disease are described as being focal dilatation and degeneration of the mucosal glands with a concomitant infiltration by hyperbasophilic lymphocytes. Affected crypt cells contain bare nuclei. With progression of the disease, cellular fragmentation develops and eventual disintegration of the entire crypts occurs. With increasing severity, mucosal and submucosal edema, flattening of villi, epithelial cell atypia and necrosis occurs. Mucosal and submucosal mononuclear cell infiltrates, and bacterial and/or fungal infiltrations may be found. In severe cases, diffuse mucosal denudation occurs (4) (Figure 4).

Hepatic involvement with graft-vs.-host disease is manifested as cholestatic jaundice, without a high incidence of hepatocellular failure.

Increased serum alkaline phosphatase follows hyperbilirubinemia, mild hepatomegaly, and clinical jaundice. Usually both skin and gastrointestinal manifestations of graft-vs.-host disease are present by the time jaundice is noted, but liver involvement may be the presenting feature. Alkaline phosphatase values are high and these levels rise in parallel with the total serum bilirubin. Aspartate amino transferase (AST) and other hepatocellular enzymes are elevated as well.

Ascites and liver failure occur primarily in patients with prolonged graft-vs.-

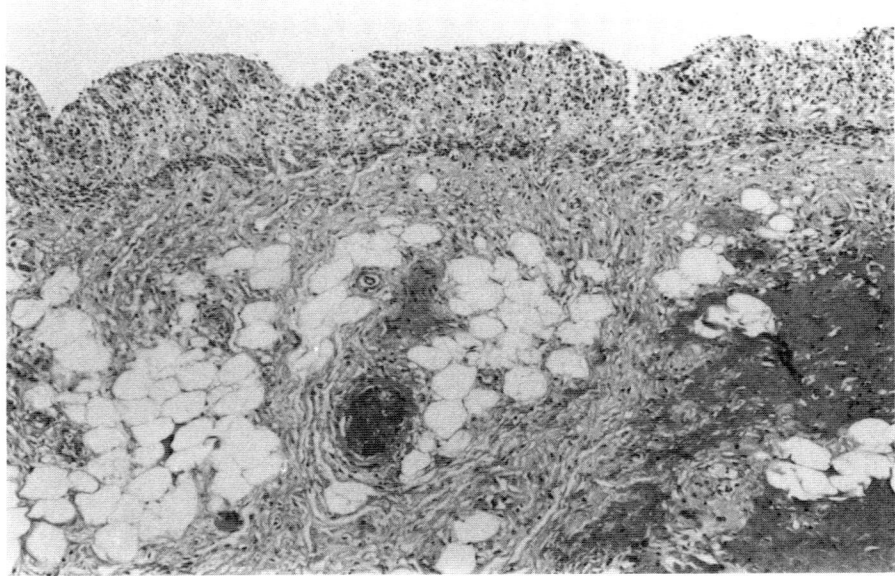

FIG. 4. Colon with complete denudation of the mucosa, chronic inflammation of the lamina propria and prominent edema, congestion and vascular thrombosis in the submucosa (H and E stain, × 400).

host disease and severe multisystem involvement (15,24). Patients with severe graft-vs.-host disease usually die of infection before the natural progression of severe liver involvement leads to liver failure.

Histopathological examination of the liver to establish the diagnosis is not necessary when a patient with proved skin and gastrointestinal graft-vs.-host disease develops liver manifestations typical of this condition. Imaging studies and liver biopsy should be considered when conditions other than graft-vs.-host disease are suspected (25).

TABLE 3. *Clinical and histopathologic liver stages of graft-vs.-host disease**

Stage	Serum bilirubin level	Histopathology of liver
+	Bilirubin (2–3 mg/dl)	<25% abnormal small interobular bile ducts
++	Bilirubin (3–6 mg/dl)	25%–50%
+++	Bilirubin (6–15 mg/dl)	50%–75%
++++	Bilirubin (>15 mg/dl)	>75%

*Adopted from Glucksberg H, et al. (14)

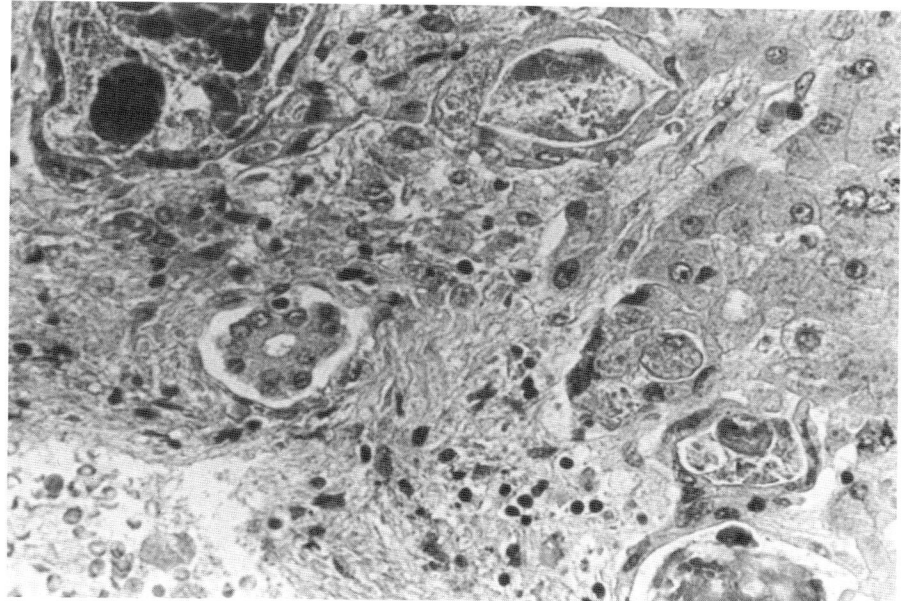

FIG. 5. Liver portal tract with prominent bile duct distension and bile duct plugs. Portal fibrosis and portal chronic inflammation are present with occasional lymphocytes in the bile duct epithelium (H and E stain, × 800).

The histopathology of hepatic graft-vs.-host disease has been discussed elsewhere (15,26,27). The early histopathological findings consist of mild anisonucleosis and anisocytosis throughout the lobules, and infiltration of mononuclear cells and eosinophils in the portal triads. At this early stage, abnormalities of the bile ducts are not usually present. Histological changes in the liver biopsy performed 1 to 2 weeks after the onset of graft-vs.-host disease are more characteristic. At this stage, cholestasis, mild panlobular hepatocellular injury and interlobular bile ducts are found. Abnormalities of the interlobular bile ducts are the most characteristic features of graft-vs.-host disease of the liver. With progression of the disease, destruction of small bile ducts and proliferation of ductules occur.

After weeks of acute graft-vs.-host disease, the liver histopathological change is predominantly characterized by profound cholestasis (Figure 5). In addition, there is ballooning degeneration and heavy pigmentation of the hepatocytes by iron and bile. If the graft-vs.-host disease is not effectively controlled or arrested, hepatocellular dropout, collapse and sclerosis results in portal hypertension and hepatic failure.

CHRONIC GRAFT-VS.-HOST DISEASE

Chronic graft-vs.-host disease is a multiorgan syndrome that resembles many features seen in collagen vascular diseases. The disease usually appears from 3 to 6 months after transplantation.

Chronic graft-vs.-host disease may follow the acute form, or it may appear after a quiescent period following acute graft-vs.-host disease. It also may appear *de novo*. This disease seems to represent a severe intolerance of the repopulation of humoral and cellular immunity, and it is associated with a profound state of immunodeficiency.

Two major types of chronic graft-vs.-host disease have been recognized (28). Approximately 10% of patients will develop a form of the disease with involvement limited to the skin or limited to the skin and liver. In this type of chronic graft-vs.-host disease, the onset of symptoms occurs later and the course is more favorable. Approximately 90% of patients develop a more extensive form of chronic graft-vs.-host disease that involves three or more organs. If this condition is not treated, or if it is not responsive to immunosuppressive therapy, the prognosis is very poor.

Chronic graft-vs.-host disease has been found to be associated with three major independent factors (29,30). These include acute graft-vs.-host disease, increasing age of the patient, and infusion of donor buffy coat cells in addition to the marrow inoculum. The dominant factor is the occurrence of acute graft-vs.-host disease. Its association with chronic graft-vs.-host disease, and the response of chronic graft-vs.-host disease to immunotherapy, suggest that chronic graft-vs.-host disease is the result of a reaction of the immunologically active donor cells to host antigens. The adverse effect of increasing age of the patient may be related to thymic epithelial dysfunction. This thymic dysfunction may result in defective maturation of lymphoid cells generated by the transplanted marrow (29,31). The resulting defective lymphoid cells may result in impaired defenses against infection and inappropriate production of nonspecific suppressor cells. There may also be absence of production of a specific suppressor, which is thought to be involved in the maintenance of graft-host tolerance. The late onset of chronic graft-vs.-host disease in older patients is usually less severe and is less frequently fatal. Also, late onset chronic graft-vs.-host disease responds better to therapy than the chronic graft-vs.-host disease developing after acute graft-vs.-host disease (29).

The third factor associated with increased incidence of chronic graft-vs.-host disease is the infusion of viable donor buffy coat cells in addition to the marrow inoculum. This technique is used to overcome graft rejection in alloimmunized patients with aplastic anemia (32,37). These buffy coat infusions produce a minimal increase in incidence of graft-vs.-host disease; presumably the adverse effect of donor lymphoid cells is prevented so long as the postgrafting immunosuppression is maintained. Once the immunosuppression is discontinued, alloreactive and cytotoxic cells may develop, thus producing the syndrome of graft-vs.-host disease. This observation confirms the concept that chronic graft-vs.-host disease is a cell-mediated disease caused by donor lymphocytes reacting against host tissue antigens. Graft-vs.-host disease which develops in patients receiving buffy coat infusions generally has a better prognosis than that which occurs after acute graft-vs.-host disease (29).

Clinically, chronic graft-vs.-host disease is characterized by an indolent course. It is manifested as malar erythema, scleroderma, oral mucositis, alopecia, sicca syndrome, polyserositis, polymyositis, chronic airway disease, chronic liver disease, involvement of the large intestine, and failure to thrive.

Sclerodermatous changes of the skin, consisting of poikiloderma, thickening and atrophy of the skin and appendages, and telangiectasia, together with hyperpigmentation or hypopigmentation, occur in almost all patients with chronic graft-vs.-host disease. In more severe cases, joint contractures may develop (35). Lichen planuslike lesions in the mouth may lead to pain, dryness of the mouth, and dental decay. Ocular sicca may produce corneal erosions and, in extreme cases, there may be corneal perforation (34). Involvement of the esophagus may produce web and strictures that may cause dysphagia. In untreated patients, worsening of the dysphagia may lead to severe retrosternal pain predisposing the patients to aspirations and insidious weight loss. With the early diagnosis and treatment of chronic graft-vs.-host disease, the scleroderma, contractures and esophageal symptoms are less common. About 90% of patients develop liver involvement characterized by the presence of hepatic enzyme abnormalities. Liver disease rarely leads to cirrhosis, or death, even though a few cases with such outcomes have been reported (35,36). One of the most detrimental effects of chronic graft-vs.-host disease is the development of nonspecific suppressor T cells and partial or total absence of both T cell responsiveness and immunoglobulin synthesis. This immunocompromised condition leads to an increased incidence of bacterial infections in these patients (33,38). In many cases, the final event of chronic graft-vs.-host disease is a lethal infection.

PREVENTION OF GRAFT-VS.-HOST DISEASE

The first approach to the management of graft-vs.-host disease is prevention. Methotrexate has been shown to prolong the survival of experimental animals. For this reason, methotrexate has been used to produce immunosuppression following allogeneic bone marrow transplantation (39,40). However, Lazarus reported no difference in the incidence of acute or chronic graft-vs.-host disease with or without methotrexate prophylaxis in patients given allogeneic bone marrow transplantation (41). In a randomized study comparing methylprednisolone and cyclosporine, the results suggested that cyclosporine is a useful agent in the treatment of acute graft-vs.-host disease, being comparable in efficacy to methylprednisolone (42). Adding antithymocyte globulin (ATG) to the basic methotrexate regimen did not change the incidence of acute graft-vs.-host disease (43). However, Ramsey et al., compared the use of methotrexate to the combination of methotrexate, antithymocyte globulin and prednisone and observed a significant reduction in the incidence of graft-vs.-host disease with use of the 3-drug combination (44).

Two prospective randomized trials were conducted to evaluate the usefulness of the combination of methotrexate and cyclosporine for the prevention of acute graft-vs.-host disease. In the first study, this combination resulted in a significant decrease in the incidence and severity of acute graft-vs.-host disease, with an improvement in survival when compared to use of cyclosporine alone (45). In the second study, the combination of methotrexate and cyclosporine resulted in a significant decrease in the severity of acute graft-vs.-host disease when compared to methotrexate alone (46).

Another approach to the prevention of graft-vs.-host disease involves the depletion of immunocompetent T lymphocytes from the donor's marrow by *in vitro* purging. The severity of acute graft-vs.-host disease is directly proportional to the number of lymphocytes administered, as shown by the inverse relation between survival time and the number of lymphocytes added to mismatched marrow in mice receiving marrow transplants (47).

However, complete depletion of the immunocompetent T lymphocytes introduces the problem of graft rejection, which has been reported to occur in approximately 10% of cases (48). Mature lymphocytes, apart from the adverse effect of causing acute graft-vs.-host disease, may also cause additional immunosuppression that facilitates the beneficial effect of acceptance of the graft.

The various techniques of T cell depletion has been reviewed (50). Some of these techniques include the use of monoclonal antibodies with or without complement (49,56), immunomagnetic beads (50), toxic conjugates (51), counterflow centrifugation (52), and soybean agglutinin with sheep red blood cells (53,54).

TREATMENT

In patients who fail prophylaxis and who develop acute graft-vs.-host disease, treatment with high-dose prednisone, cyclosporine, antithymocyte globulin and monoclonal antibodies directed against the T cell has been attempted. Response to treatment is 30 to 50%, but it is unpredictable, and treatment may be associated with severe toxicity. Even patients who respond to treatment have a high incidence of fatal infections, and 20 to 30% of patients die of graft-vs.-host disease or associated complications.

In patients who develop chronic graft-vs.-host disease, treatment consists of a regimen which includes various drugs, including prednisone, cyclophosphamide, procarbazine, cyclosporine, and azathioprine. The most effective combination appears to be azathioprine and prednisone, which results in arrest of the disease in 30 to 50% of the patients. However, many of these patients are still at high risk of delayed complications, especially fatal infections, even years after transplantation (57).

In a recent report by Bunjes et al., cyclosporine appears to be an effective alternative to cyclophosphamide in the treatment of chronic graft-vs.-host disease (58). The treatment and prevention of graft-vs.-host disease is considered in more detail in Chapter 24.

SUMMARY

Bone marrow transplantation is one of the major advances of modern medicine, but the complications of transplantation presents the clinician with a variety of challenging problems that were unknown until the last decade.

Graft-vs.-host disease is one of the unique complications that the clinicians have to deal with. The early development (7–14 days) of the acute form usually has a poor outcome. High index of suspicion, early diagnosis and treatment of the chronic phase of the disease may help about 50% of the patients to achieve a better life.

Better understanding of the human immune system, the major and minor histocompatibility complex in man, and better immune modulators, will improve the selection of donors and control graft-vs.-host disease if it occurs.

ACKNOWLEDGMENTS

We would like to thank Dr. Kevin Winn from the Department of Pathology of the Henrietta Egleston Hospital for his assistance in supplying the microphotographs.

REFERENCES

1. Simonsen M: Graft-vs.-host reaction; the history that never was and the way things happened to happen. *Immunol Rev* 1985;88:5–23.
2. O'Reilly RJ: Allogeneic bone marrow transplantation; current status and future directions. *Blood* 1983;62,5:941–964.
3. Lampert IA, Suitters AJ, Chisholm PM: Expression of Ia antigen on epidermal keratinocytes in graft-vs.-host disease. *Nature* (London) 1981;293:149–150.
4. Bril H, Benner R: Graft-vs.-host reaction; mechanisms and contemporary theories. *CRC Crit Rev Clin Lab Sci* 1985;22(1):43–95.
5. Elkins WL, Guttman RD: Pathogenesis of a local graft-vs.-host reaction; immunogenicity of circulating host leukocytes. *Science* 1968;159:1250–1254.
6. Streilein WJ, Billingham RE: An analysis of graft-vs.-host disease in Syrian hamsters. *J Exp Med* 1970;132:181–184.

7. Suitters AJ, Lampert IA: The loss of Ia+ Langerhans cells during graft-vs.-host disease in rats. *Transplantation* 1983;36:540–546.
8. Perreault C, Pelletier M, Landry D, et al.: Study of Langerhans cells after bone marrow transplantation. *Blood* 1984;63:807–811.
9. Tutschka PJ, Hess AD, Beschorner WE, et al.: Suppressor cells in transplantation tolerance. I. Suppressor cells in the mechanism of tolerance in radiation chimeras. *Transplantation* 1981;32:203–209.
10. Sale GE, Lerner KG, Barker EA, et al.: The skin biopsy in the diagnosis of acute graft-vs.-host disease in man. *Am J Pathol* 1977;89:621–634.
11. Lerner KG, Kao GF, Storb R, et al.: Histopathology of graft-vs.-host reaction (GVHR) in human recipients of marrow from HLA-matched siblings donors. *Transplant Proc* 1974; 6:367.
12. Hymes SR, Farmer ER, Lewis PG, et al.: Cutaneous graft-vs.-host reaction; prognostic features seen by light microscopy. *J Am Acad Dermatol* 1985;12:468–474.
13. Lever R, Turbitt M, Mackie R, et al.: A prospective study of the histological changes in the skin in patients receiving bone marrow transplants. *Br J Dermatol* 1986;114:161–170.
14. Glucksberg H, Storb R, Feffer A, et al.: Clinical manifestations of graft-vs.-host disease in human recipients of marrow from HLA-matched sibling donors. *Transplantation* 1974; 18:295–304.
15. McDonald GB, Shulman HM, Sullivan KM, et al.: Intestinal and hepatic complications of human bone marrow transplantation. Part I. *Gastroenterology* 1986;90:460–477.
16. Fish JD, Shulman HM, Greening RR, et al.: Gastrointestinal radiographic features of human graft-vs.-host disease. *Am J Roentgenol* 1981;136:329–336.
17. Rosenberg KH, Serota FT, Koch P, et al.: Radiographic features of gastrointestinal graft-vs.-host disease. *Radiology* 1981;138:371–374.
18. Navari RM, Sharma P, Deeg HJ, et al.: Pneumatosis cystoides intestinalis following allogeneic marrow transplantation. *Transplant Proc* 1983;25:1720–1724.
19. Glasier CM, Siegel MU, McAllister WH, et al.: Henoch-Schonlein syndrome in children; gastrointestinal manifestations. *Am J Roentgenol* 1981;136:1081–1085.
20. Rogers LF, Goldstein HM: Roentgen manifestations of radiation injury to the gastrointestinal tract. *Gastrointest Radiol* 1977;2:281–291.
21. McDonald GB, Sale GE: The human gastrointestinal tract after allogeneic bone marrow transplantation. In, Sale GE, Shulman HM (eds.): *The Pathology of Bone Marrow Transplantation.* New York, Masson Publishing, 1984, pp. 77–103.
22. Snover DC, Weisdorf SA, Vercellotti GM, et al.: A histopathologic study of gastric and small intestinal graft-vs.-host disease following allogeneic bone marrow transplantation. *Human Pathol* 1985;16:387–392.
23. Barrett AP, Bilous AM: Oral patterns of acute and chronic graft-vs.-host disease. *Arch Dermatol* 1984;120:1461–1465.
24. Shulman HM, McDonald GB. Liver disease after bone marrow transplantation. In, Sale GE, Shulman HM (eds.): *The Pathology of Bone Marrow Transplantation.* New York, Masson Publishing, 1984; pp. 104–135.
25. Meyers JD, Thomas ED. Infection complicating bone marrow transplantation. In, Rubin RH, Young LS (eds.): *Clinical Approach to Infection in the Compromised Host.* New York, Plenum Publishing, 1981, pp. 507–556.
26. Slavin RE, Woodruff JM: The pathology of bone marrow transplantation. *Pathol Annual* 1974;9:291–344.
27. Sloan JP, Farthing MJ, Powles RL: Histopathological changes in the liver after allogeneic bone marrow transplantation. *J Clin Pathol* 1980;33:344–350.
28. Sullivan KM, Shulman HM, Storb R, et al.: Chronic graft-vs.-host disease in 52 patients; adverse natural course and successful treatment with combination immunosuppression. *Blood* 1981;57:267–276.
29. Storb R, Thomas ED: Graft-vs.-host disease in dog and man; the Seattle experience. *Immunol Rev.* 1985;88:214–238.
30. Deeg HJ, Storb R: Acute and chronic graft-vs.-host disease; clinical manifestations, prophylaxis, and treatment. *JNCI* 1986;76:1325–1328.
31. Santos GW, Vogelsang GB: Graft-vs.-host reaction and disease. *Immunol Rev* 1985;88:169–192.

32. Storb R, Thomas ED, Appelbaum F, et al.: Marrow transplantation with or without donor buffy coat cells for 65 transfused aplastic anemia patients. *Blood* 1982;59:236–246.
33. Gale RP: Graft-vs.-host disease. *Immunol Rev* 1985;88:193–214.
34. Franklin RM, Kenyon KR, Tutschka PJ, et al.: Ocular manifestations of graft-vs.-host disease. *Ophthalmology* 1983;90:4–13.
35. Yau JC, Zander AR, Srigley JR, et al.: Chronic graft-vs.-host disease complicated by micronodular cirrhosis and esophageal varices. *Transplantation* 1986;41:129–130.
36. Knapp AB, Crawford JM, Rappeport JM, et al.: Cirrhosis as a consequence of graft-vs.-host disease. *Gastroenterology* 1987;92:513–519.
37. Deeg HJ, Self S, Storb R, et al.: Decreased incidence of marrow graft rejection in patients with severe aplastic anemia; changing impact of risk factors. *Blood* 1986;68:1363–1368.
38. Lum LG: The kinetics of immune reconstitution after human marrow transplantation. *Blood* 1987;69:369–380.
39. Cheson BD, Curt GA: Bone marrow transplantation; current perspective and future directions. *JNCI* 1986;76:1265–1267.
40. Deeg HJ, Storb R: Graft-vs.-host disease. *Annual Rev Med* 1984;35:11–24.
41. Lazarus HM, Coccia PF, Herzig RH, et al.: Incidence of acute graft-vs.-host disease with or without methotrexate prophylaxis in allogeneic bone marrow transplant patients. *Blood* 1984;64:215–220.
42. Kennedy MS, Deeg HJ, Storb R, et al.: Treatment of acute graft-vs.-host disease after allogeneic bone marrow transplantation; randomized study comparing corticosteroids and cyclosporine. *Am J Med* 1985;78:978–983.
43. Doney KC, Weiden PL, Storb R, et al.: Treatment of graft-vs.-host disease in human allogeneic marrow graft transplants; a randomized trial comparing antithymocyte globuline and corticosteroids. *Am J Hematol* 1981;11:1–8.
44. Ramsay NKC, Kersey JH, Robison LL, et al.: A randomized study of the prevention of acute graft-vs.-host disease. *N Engl J Med* 1982;306:392–397.
45. Storb R, Deeg HJ, Thomas ED, et al.: Bone marrow transplantation for leukemia; a controlled trial of a combination of methotrexate and cyclosporine versus cyclosporine alone for prophylaxis of acute graft-vs.-host disease (Abstract). *Blood* 1985;66(suppl 1):255a.
46. Storb R, Deeg HJ, Thomas ED: Bone marrow transplantation for severe aplastic anemia; methotrexate alone compared with a combination of methotrexate and cyclosporine for the prevention of acute graft-vs.-host disease. *Blood* 1986;68:119–125.
47. Van Bekkum D: The selective elimination of immunologically competent cells from bone marrow and lymphatic cell mixtures. *Transplantation* 1984;2:393–397.
48. Vega RA, Franco CM, Abdel-Mageed AMS, et al.: Bone marrow transplantation in the treatment of children with cancer; current status. *Hematol Oncol Clin N Am* (November) 1987;1(4):777–800.
49. Apperley JF, Jones L, Hale G, et al.: Bone marrow transplantation for patients with chronic myelogenous leukemia; T cell depletion with Campath I reduces the incidence of graft-vs.-host disease but may increase the risk of relapse. *Bone Marrow Transplantation* 1986;1:53–66.
50. Vartdal, Albrechtsen D, Ringden O, et al.: Immunomagnetic treatment of bone marrow allografts. *Bone Marrow Transplantation* 1987;2:(Suppl 2)94–98.
51. Kersey J, LeBieu T, Ramsay N, et al.: Antibodies and immunotoxins for bone marrow purging. *Bone Marrow Transplantation* 1987;2:(Suppl 1)47–49.
52. DeWitte T, Hoogenhout B, dePauw B, et al.: Depletion of donor lymphocytes by counterflow centrifugation successfully prevents acute graft-vs.-host disease in matched allogeneic marrow transplantation. *Blood* 1986;67:1302–1308.
53. Reisner Y, Kapoor N, Kirkpatrick D, et al.: Transplantation for acute leukemia with HLA-A and -B nonidentical parental marrow cells fractionated with soybean agglutinin and sheep red blood cells. *Lancet* 1981;2:327–331.
54. Kernan NA, Collins NH, Cunningham I, et al.: Prevention of GVHD in HLA-identical marrow grafts by removal of T cells with soybean agglutinin and SRBCs. *Bone Marrow Transplantation* 1987;2:(Suppl 2)13–17.
55. Neudorf SML, Filipovich AH, Kersey J: Recent advances in bone marrow transplantation. In, Weiner RS, Hackel E, Schiffer CA (eds.): *Bone Marrow Transplantation*. Arlington, Va, American Association of Blood Banks, 1983;147–160.

56. Martin PJ. T cell purging with antibody—the Seattle experience. *Bone Marrow Transplantation* 1987;2:(Suppl 2)53–57.
57. Winton DJ, Ho WG, Champlin RE, et al.: Infectious complications of bone marrow transplantation. *Exp Hematol* 1984;12:205–215.
58. Bunjes D, Heit W, Arnold R, et al.: Cyclosporine as an alternative to cyclophosphamide in the treatment of chronic graft-vs.-host disease. *Transplantation* 1986;41:170–172.

Bone Marrow Transplantation in
Children, edited by F. Leonard Johnson
and Carl Pochedly. Raven Press, Ltd.,
New York © 1990.

Pulmonary Complications of Bone Marrow Transplantation

*John A. Fort and **John Graham-Pole

*Department of Hematology/Oncology, Children's Hospital National Medical Cancer
Center, Washington, D.C. 20010 and **Department of Pediatrics, College of Medicine,
University of Florida, Gainesville, Florida 32610

INTRODUCTION

Bone marrow transplantation has become a therapeutic modality for the treatment of many diseases which have a poor prognosis for long-term survival. Results of this treatment are improving in terms of both increased efficacy and diminished complications. However, pulmonary problems continue to be a major source of morbidity and mortality for about half of those patients who undergo allogeneic marrow transplants, and in a lesser but significant number of patients given autologous bone marrow (1). Although the course is variable, about half of those patients who develop interstitial lung disease die of its complications (2,3). Lung disease is the most common cause of death in patients receiving bone marrow transplantation, with interstitial pneumonitis accounting for 40% of transplant-related deaths (4).

397

PULMONARY EDEMA

Pulmonary toxicity developing early after bone marrow transplantation is probably due to the individual or collective effects of the conditioning chemotherapy, radiation therapy or marrow infusion (5). Seven to 28 days after transplantation, this lung involvement takes the form of pulmonary edema, presumed to be due primarily to leaky pulmonary vasculature. High-dose cytosine arabinoside, which is used in several conditioning regimens, has been shown to cause capillary leakage of proteinaceous, serous fluid (6). Whole body radiation, which is used to condition many patients, causes similar capillary leakage. Radiation doses of 100 cGy to the lung are associated with increased vascular permeability, alveolar wall edema, alveolar protein leakage, loss of pulmonary surfactant, and alveolar hyaline membrane formation (7). With precise fluid management and judicious use of diuretics, the patient can be assisted through this initial phase of bone marrow transplantation with complete resolution of the process.

Acute hemorrhagic pulmonary edema may also develop early. This is much less common than the edema caused by increased vascular permeability, and seems to affect patients receiving HLA-mismatched transplants (7). The condition is associated with hemorrhage into the alveolar sacs, low central venous pressure, fluid retention, hypotension and renal failure. This complication, once it develops, has a high mortality rate, being about 90%.

In addition to the occurrence of pulmonary edema due to damage to lung parenchyma and vasculature, pulmonary edema may also arise secondary to myocardial damage due to prior chemotherapy, irradiation, or infection. The cardiotoxicity of adriamycin is well documented at doses greater than 450 mg/m^2. The mechanism of damage from adriamycin is by loss of myocardial fibrils, mitochondrial changes and cellular degeneration. Cyclophosphamide, which is frequently used to condition patients for marrow transplantation, is also cardiotoxic when given in very high doses, that is, in doses greater than 150 mg/kg (8). Cardiac failure results from the development of a hemorrhagic myocarditis.

Cardiac irradiation has been associated with the development of pericardial effusions and constrictive pericarditis; both of these conditions predispose the patient to development of pulmonary edema (8,9). Infections in these immunosuppressed patients can also produce myocarditis, which may result in decreased myocardial contractility, diminished cardiac output and secondary pulmonary edema. Among the more commonly implicated infectious agents are adenovirus, *Toxoplasma gondii,* Coxsackie virus, and certain fungi. Myocardial conduction disturbances may also develop from infectious agents invading the cardiac conduction system.

Other less common causes of lung disease associated with bone marrow transplantation are mechanical obstruction or trauma to the pulmonary bed. A syndrome analogous to the adult respiratory distress syndrome has been seen with acute onset following bone marrow transplantation (7). Its mechanism is unclear, since these patients are neutropenic and should not have the normal oxidation products of neutrophil metabolism present to cause damage to the lungs. Pulmonary embolism due to infusing fat particles and bone spicules from unfiltered bone marrow has been seen at autopsy from patients dying from other causes, but their significance is uncertain. Pulmonary veno-occlusive disease has also been documented (7), which is probably an unusual response to high-dose chemotherapy and irradiation.

PULMONARY INFECTIONS

Infections are a major cause of pulmonary pathology after bone marrow transplantation in these immunosuppressed subjects. These infections may take the form either of intra-alveolar lobar consolidation or involve the interalveolar linings to produce interstitial pneumonitis. The symptomatology associated with infectious pulmonary infiltrates consists of dyspnea, tachypnea, cyanosis and cough due to inadequate gas exchange. These symptoms result from abnormal alveolar architecture which produces an alveolar-capillary block. Late effects of pulmonary disease result from inadequate gas exchange secondary to fibrosis and loss of functional pulmonary capacity. Other late effects include obstructive airway problems, recurrent pneumothorax and bronchiectasis (10–13).

Bacterial pneumonia very commonly affects patients within the first 6 months post-bone marrow transplant. Etiologic factors include neutropenia, B cell immune deficiency and chronic graft-vs.-host disease and its treatment. Infections due to both gram-positive organisms (such as *Staphylococcus aureus*, *Staphylococcus epidermidis*, and *Streptococcus pneumoniae*) and gram-negative organisms (such as Klebsiella and Pseudomonas) are common. Resistant strains are being seen more frequently late into treatment, which are sensitive only to vancomycin. Prophylactic use of trimethoprim-sulfamethoxazole may have lowered the frequency of infections due to *Streptococcus pneumoniae* or the frequency of certain gram-negative infections. But the present pneumococcal vaccine seems to provide no protection for the post-marrow transplant patient from contracting pneumococcal infections. (14) The presence of Legionella, Chlamydia, Mycobacteria and Mycoplasma is also being identified more frequently in these patients.

Unlike the consolidation of the alveolar sacs usually seen in lobar pneumonia due to bacterial infections, most other infectious agents cause alveolar wall thickening, producing interstitial pneumonitis. Interstitial pneumonitis usually occurs from day 30 to day 100 following marrow transplantation, and approximately 50% of cases are fatal. There are numerous probable and possible causes of this condition, but about two-thirds of cases have a documented infectious agent causing the pneumonitis (being either viral, fungal,

TABLE 1. *Risk factors for the development of interstitial pneumonitis*

1. Immunosuppressive agents (corticosteroids, methotrexate, cyclosporine-A)
2. High-dose cyclophosphamide prior to bone marrow transplantation
3. Graft-vs.-host disease
4. Blood product transfusions (transmission of CMV infection)
5. High-dose rate of radiotherapy
6. High total lung dose of radiotherapy
7. Single-fraction radiotherapy
8. Total body irradiation
9. Increased age at transplantation

or protozoal), while other cases are attributable to the noxious effects of drugs, radiation, or both.

Table 1 lists some of the most common risk factors associated with the development of interstitial pneumonitis (11,15,16). Viral infections are the most commonly documented cause, with cytomegalovirus (CMV) being the most common pathogen (17). CMV is the etiologic agent in about 50% of all cases of interstitial pneumonitis, and usually presents 6 to 8 weeks after marrow transplantation. It may present either as multifocal, miliary disease suggestive of hematologic dissemination, or it may appear to be strictly localized to the lung and with evidence suggestive of airway dissemination (Figures 1 and 2). Cytomegalovirus infection may arise by any of 3 mechanisms: (1) infection may arise by activation of latent disease in the bone marrow recipient, (2) there may be acquisition of CMV from an infected marrow donor, or (3) CMV infection may be acquired through transfusion with CMV-infected blood products.

Prolonged immunosuppression seems to be the single most important factor in predisposing a patient to development of CMV pneumonitis, with patients who have received antithymocyte globulin for prevention of graft-vs.-host disease and patients with acute graft-vs.-host disease being at particularly increased risk. Resistance to cytomegalovirus infection is mediated by cellular immunity and, although hematologic reconstitution and cytotoxic and phagocytic functions recover within about 100 days post-bone marrow transplantation, cooperative T cell- and B cell-mediated functions are reduced for up to 2 years (18,19).

The most promising current management for cytomegalovirus infection post-marrow transplantation is prevention by use of immune globulin containing a high titer of CMV antibody. Intravenous immunoglobulin administered before and for the first 3 to 4 months after marrow transplantation probably reduces the incidence of CMV pneumonitis, although results of various studies are conflicting. Various antiviral agents, including interferon, probably have no efficacy in preventing or treating CMV pneumonitis (14,20), although

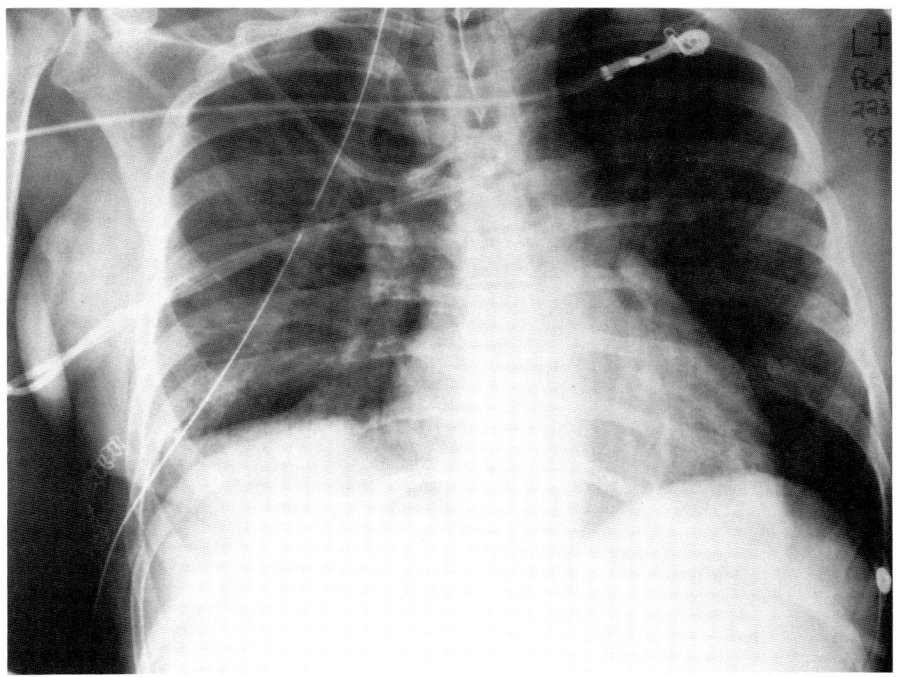

FIG. 1. Chest X-ray showing diffuse interstitial infiltration produced by cytomegalovirus following allogeneic marrow transplantation. Note total lung involvement with an interstitial pattern.

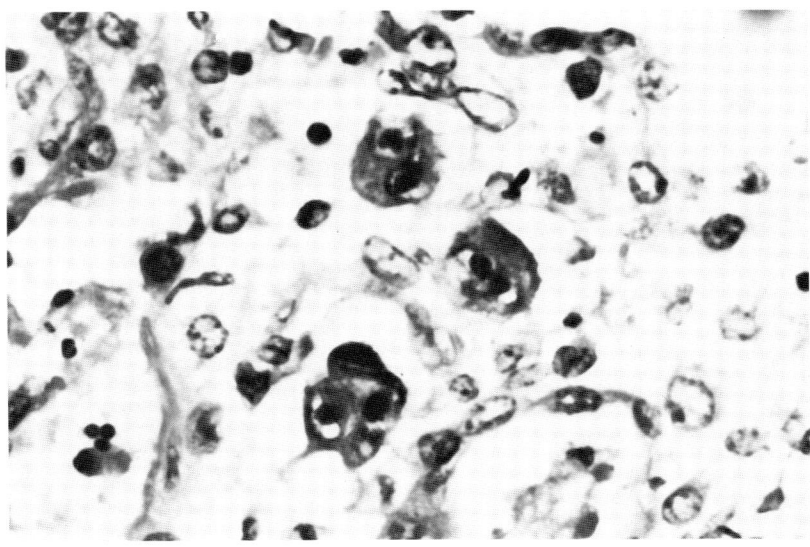

FIG. 2. Histologic section of pulmonary CMV. The infected cells are larger than the surrounding cells with intranuclear inclusions seen (H & E stain, × 200).

early results of studies on use of gancyclovir and acyclovir are promising. Although cytomegalovirus is the most common viral agent linked to the etiology of interstitial pneumonitis, other viruses are occasionally implicated. These include adenovirus, Herpes simplex (HSV) virus, and Varicella zoster (VZ) virus, which account for 7% to 10% of infectious cases of interstitial pneumonitis. Acyclovir given as prophylaxis has decreased the incidence of interstitial pneumonitis due to Herpes virus, and treatment with this drug has reduced the severity of established infections. Epstein-Barr virus (EBV), respiratory syncytial virus, influenza, and parainfluenza infections are rare causes of interstitial pneumonitis in these patients.

Pulmonary fungal infections often present as interstitial lung disease, the most common pathogens being Candida, Aspergillus, the mucormycoses, and *Torulopsis glabrata* (21). Use of protective environments, particularly laminar airflow rooms, seems to decrease the incidence of Aspergillus pneumonitis. This is an important finding in view of the very high mortality rate of Aspergillus infections (Figures 3 and 4).

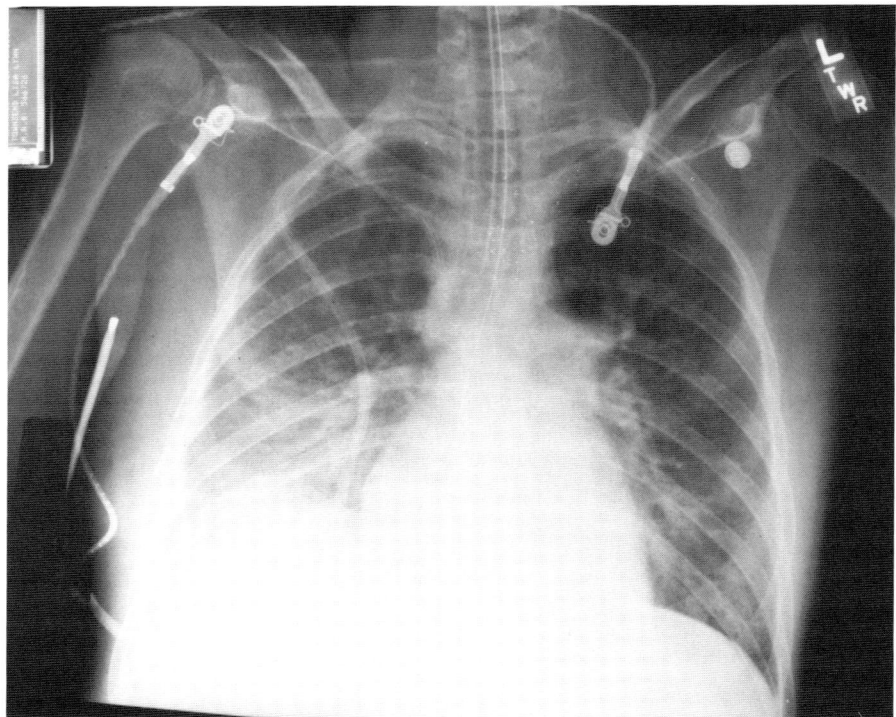

FIG. 3.   Chest X-ray picture of Aspergillus pneumonia following allogeneic marrow transplantation, with bilateral interstitial infiltration, but also with lobar consolidation in the right lung.

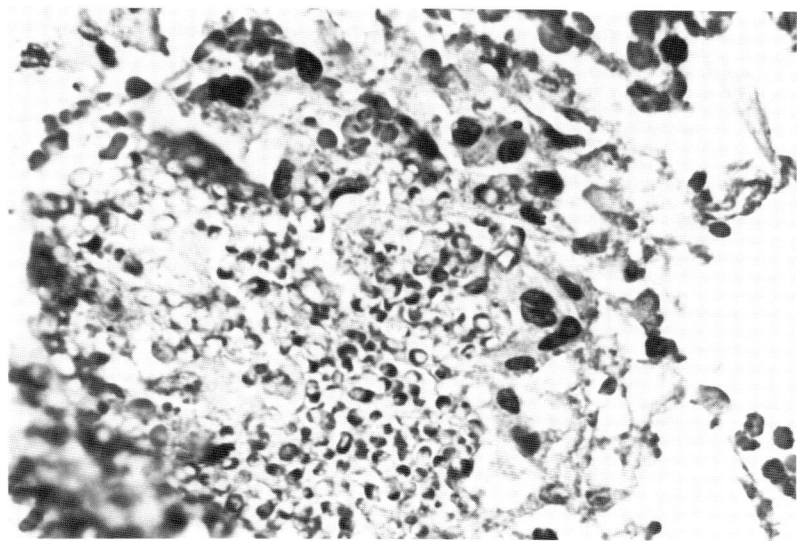

FIG. 4. Histological appearance of the lung in Candida pneumonia. Note the numerous yeast forms of Candida within a necrotic alveolus. This may be present without a corresponding inflammatory response (H & E stain, ×200).

Before the routine use of prophylaxis against *Pneumocystis carinii* with trimethoprim-sulfamethoxazole, this microorganism was a common cause of severe pneumonia in immunocompromised patients. With the institution of trimethoprim-sulfamethoxazole prophylaxis, *Pneumocystis carinii* infections now account for less than 5% of cases of interstitial pneumonitis following bone marrow transplantation. Although interstitial pneumonitis rarely develops in patients who are receiving prophylaxis with trimethoprim-sulfamethoxazole, in such a situation the mortality is high, due presumably to the emergence of resistant strains (Figure 5).

In spite of exhaustive attempts to identify an associated microorganism, the causes of interstitial pneumonitis remain uncertain in about a third of cases. Such idiopathic cases may be due to our inability to identify a causative microorganism, or may be attributable to the combined effects of chemotherapy, immunosuppression, radiation therapy, and other less clearly defined factors.

DRUG-INDUCED DAMAGE TO THE LUNGS

Certain drugs used in the conditioning regimen given prior to bone marrow transplantation are known to be pulmonary toxins. These drugs may be implicated in some cases of idiopathic interstitial pneumonitis. This pulmonary toxicity may be an acute single-dose effect, or the toxicity may be cumulative and additive from a patient being exposed to a combination of different drugs. Such pulmonary toxicity becomes compounded when these drugs are used in

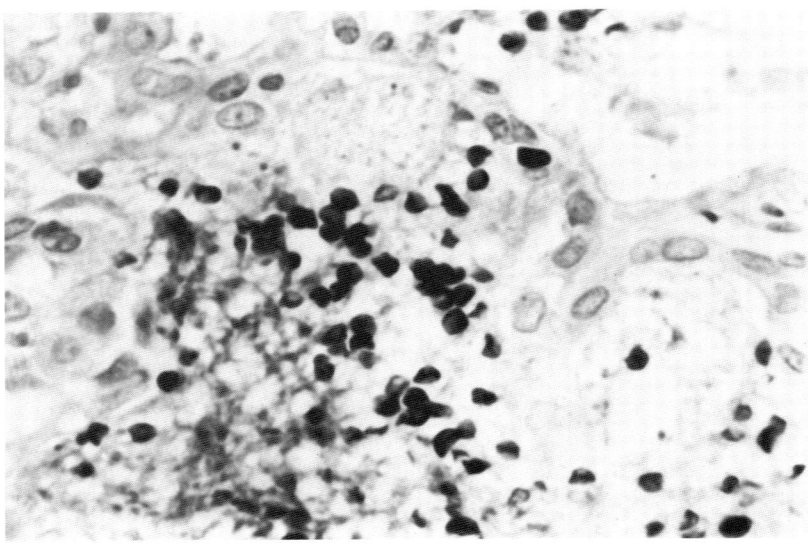

FIG. 5. Histological section showing pulmonary picture in *Pneumocystis carinii* pneumonia. Note the darkly stained cysts of *P. carinii* with surrounding frothy and granular intra-alveolar proteinaceous material (Silver methenamine stain, ×200).

conjunction with radiation therapy and other modalities, such as oxygen therapy and positive pressure ventilation (22,23).

Bleomycin is one of the most pulmonary-toxic chemotherapeutic agents currently in use, since it has preferential distribution in the skin and lungs (23). Pulmonary toxicity due to bleomycin presents with a dry, hacking cough associated with exertional dyspnea that can progress to the occurrence of dyspnea at rest, tachypnea and cyanosis. Abnormal findings on physical exam and abnormal X-ray findings often may be preceded by abnormal pulmonary function tests (PFTs). Bleomycin produces its toxicity by causing pulmonary fibrosis, which appears to be dose-related. Pulmonary fibrosis develops in up to 40% of patients at doses greater than 150 units (22), and is usually irreversible and often fatal. The route of administration of bleomycin may play a role in toxicity, with continuous infusion being possibly less toxic than bolus intravenous or intramuscular therapy. The dose of bleomycin needed to cause pulmonary toxicity is much lower when the drug is combined with other pulmonary toxins, including alkylating agents, radiation therapy, or high oxygen tensions to the lung (22,24).

In one study of patients undergoing operative procedures and receiving elevated oxygen tensions during the procedure, there was 100% mortality in those patients who had received cumulative doses of bleomycin between 200 and 400 units/m^2 (22). All of those patients died of interstitial pneumonitis and progressive pulmonary fibrosis. There is also a synergistic effect when radiation therapy is given in association with bleomycin. The frequency of severe pulmonary toxicity when radiation therapy is given together with bleomycin is 35% to 55%, with 50% of those cases being fatal (24). There is no treatment for the pulmonary fibrosis caused by bleomycin. The occasional hypersensitivity reactions to bleomycin, with fever, eosinophilia and diffuse infiltrates, respond to corticosteroid therapy (24).

The nitrosureas (BCNU, CCNU, semustine and chlorozotocin) are also pulmonary toxins, having a reported incidence of pulmonary toxicity of 20% to 30%. The dose of these drugs at which symptoms develop is unknown, but there is usually a delay of 6 months or longer from drug exposure to the development of symptoms. The symptoms consist of progressive dyspnea, tachypnea and a nonproductive cough. Chest X-rays show a reticulonodular pattern, together with the presence of pulmonary edema and often pleural effusions. Pulmonary function tests reveal a restrictive lung defect, with hypoxemia and a decreased carbon monoxide diffusion capacity (DLCO). In patients examined at autopsy, specimens of lung tissue show interstitial fibrosis, alveolar septal thickening and protein-filled alveoli. Although outcome in cases of pulmonary toxicity due to nitrosureas is variable, and is probably dose-dependent, the mortality rate ranges from 24% to 60%. Corticosteroids are of no benefit for the treatment of pulmonary toxicity from nitrosoureas.

Methotrexate produces a variable degree of pulmonary toxicity which is independent of the dose received. One study reported no changes in pulmonary function tests after a total methotrexate dose of 256 grams/m^2. Pulmonary damage can result from giving methotrexate by any route of administration, and pulmonary function tests usually show hypoxemia, decreased carbon monoxide diffusion capacity and a restrictive defect in the lungs. The observed toxic effects vary, with a reversible drug hypersensitivity being the most common. Leucovorin does not seem to protect against the pulmonary toxicity due to methotrexate, but recovery from lung damage usually occurs after the drug is discontinued, and treatment with corticosteroids appears to have a beneficial effect.

The alkylating agents (cyclophosphamide, busulfan, chlorambucil, and melphalan) probably have additive pulmonary toxicity when combined with bleomycin or BCNU (22,24,25). Cyclophosphamide can cause intra-alveolar inflammation and edema leading to fibrosis, with similar changes in pulmonary function tests to those seen after the nitrosoureas. Intra-alveolar and interstitial infiltration can lead to opacification of the entire lung, but early discontinuation of the drug can lead to complete clinical and radiographic resolution (13). Like methotrexate, route of administration and total dose of cyclophosphamide do not appear to determine toxicity. Symptoms can begin while the patient is being given therapy with cyclophosphamide, or symptoms may appear as early as one month and as late as eight years after stopping therapy. Teenage patients receiving cyclophosphamide during their growth spurt can also show a decrease in relative lung volume (15).

Busulfan can produce similar symptoms referable to hypoxemia with a restrictive ventilatory defect. Toxicity has an insidious onset with dry cough, tachypnea, fever and crepitant rales, usually occurring while on therapy, and often progressing over weeks or months to a fatal outcome. Clinical improvement has been reported after discontinuing the drug and using high-dose steroids. Busulfan is also associated with loss of lung volume during a patient's growth spurt (15).

Melphalan rarely causes pulmonary toxicity. However, this drug occasionally damages the alveolar epithelium, which results in dysplasia that can progress to fibrosis. The histologic appearance consists of proliferation of bronchiolar and alveolar epithelial cells together with infiltration by plasma cells.

Cytosine arabinoside, as mentioned earlier, can increase pulmonary vascular permeability with resulting development of pulmonary edema. The occurrence of this pulmonary edema seems to correlate with the time of drug administration and is not related to the total dose of drug given.

Most drugs that are toxic to the lungs cause toxicity through parenchymal inflammation and fibrosis. However, procarbazine, like methotrexate, causes pneumonitis through a hypersensitivity reaction, with eosinophilia being seen in tissues examined on lung biopsy. Permanent fibrosis of the lung can result from prolonged hypersensitivity and resulting infiltration, following repeated exposure to the drug. But usually the pulmonary infiltration resolves when the drug is stopped.

RADIATION-INDUCED DAMAGE TO THE LUNGS

In addition to pulmonary infections and chemotherapy-induced pulmonary toxicity, radiation therapy is a major cause of lung damage associated with bone marrow transplantation (15). Signs of radiation-induced lung damage usually develop two to three months after exposure (15,23). Shielding the lungs, reducing the total dose exposure of total body irradiation to 600 cGy or less, giving the irradiation as fractionated doses of total body irradiation over several days, and decreasing the rate of delivery of irradiation all seem to decrease the incidence of interstitial pneumonitis. The lung damage usually resolves slowly but may progress to fibrosis.

The clinical signs of radiation pneumonitis are progressive dyspnea, high, spiking fevers, moist cough occasionally associated with hemoptysis, and chest pain secondary to rib fracture or pleural involvement. Late effects are cyanosis, clubbing of the nails, orthopnea and chronic cor pulmonale. Scoliosis, with a shift of alignment of the vertebrae away from the midline, may result from loss of lung volume in the irradiated field. On chest X-ray, the earliest sign of radiation pneumonitis is radiolucency of the irradiated lung. With progressive disease, there is ground-glass opacification associated with hazy pulmonary markings. The radiographic findings are usually sharply demarcated by the margins of the radiation portal. As fibrosis develops, linear streaked consolidation of the lung occurs and occasionally there is shift of midline structures. Bronchiectatic cysts may develop in the fibrosed lung.

On histologic examination, the early changes consist of capillary thrombosis and engorgement, accumulation of lipid-laden macrophages, hyperplasia and desquamation of alveolar spaces, and production of hyaline membranes. The alveolar septae are thickened by deposition of connective tissue, and there is focal necrosis of the bronchial wall mucosa. The time needed for resolution of the pulmonary lesions or for progression of disease is related to the severity of the pulmonary insult (8).

PULMONARY DAMAGE ASSOCIATED WITH
GRAFT-VS.-HOST DISEASE

From 30% to 70% of allogeneic bone marrow transplantation patients develop graft-vs.-host disease as a complication. Such patients are predisposed to lung infections because of the immunosuppression that accompanies graft-vs.-host disease and its treatment. But in addition, graft-vs.-host disease itself appears to have a direct effect on pulmonary epithelium (26,27). The sicca syndrome of chronic graft-vs.-host disease, which is recognized to have other target organs, can also exert its effect on the lungs. Lung involvement in sicca syndrome is associated with decreased production of IgA and reduced local humeral immunity. Because of death of epithelial cells, ciliary function is decreased and bronchial secretions are reduced. The bronchial mucosa is thus exposed, with loss of its normal protective mucociliary action, which predisposes the lung to development of bronchopneumonia (28).

Another complication whose time of occurrence closely follows that of graft-vs.-host disease is lymphocytic bronchitis. However, lymphocytic bronchitis may be caused by ventilator trauma or viral infections (29). The clinical symptoms of lymphocytic bronchitis are dyspnea, tachypnea and a nonproductive cough due to bronchospasm, with occasional development of progressive airway obstruction. There is lymphocytic infiltration of the mucosa, submucosa and muscularis, with necrosis of epithelial cells, loss of cilia and decreased numbers of goblet cells. The decreased ciliary function predisposes to the development of bronchopneumonia.

Bronchiolitis obliterans affects about 10% of patients with chronic graft-vs.-host disease. It is characterized by loss of elastic recoil in lung tissue. On histologic examination, there is infiltration of the walls of the small bronchioles by acute and chronic inflammatory cells, while the upper airways remain normal. Organizing granulomas can plug the alveolar spaces, secondary to the sicca syndrome. Clinically, the patient rapidly develops shortness of breath, inspiratory rales, a nonproductive cough, and airway obstruction. The chest X-ray is usually normal except for presence of mild hyperinflation (Figure 6). The

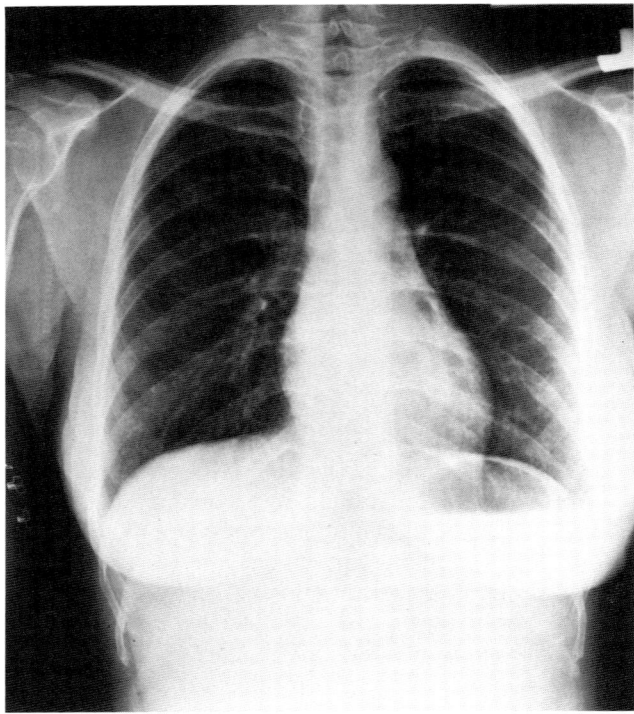

FIG. 6. Chest X-ray showing bronchiolitis obliterans in a patient with chronic graft-vs.-host disease following allogeneic marrow transplantation. Note the marked pulmonary hyperinflation due to the severe obstructive disease.

airway obstruction is irreversible. It is unresponsive to treatment with bronchodilator drugs, mucolytic agents or adrenocorticosteroids. The airway obstruction usually progresses with the development of recurrent pneumothoraces and hypoxia leading to death.

MALIGNANT INFILTRATIONS OF THE LUNGS

There is increasing use of autologous bone marrow transplantation for treatment of malignancies involving the bone marrow. Thus, another possible source of pulmonary disease associated with transplantation is infiltration of the lung with malignant cells (Figures 7 and 8) (30). Although bone marrow purging techniques are frequently used, the procedure may not be adequate to remove all malignant cells from the purged marrow. Although malignant infiltrations of the lungs are infrequent in marrow transplant patients, this possibility must be remembered as part of the differential diagnosis in patients with diffuse pulmonary infiltrates after being given autologous bone marrow.

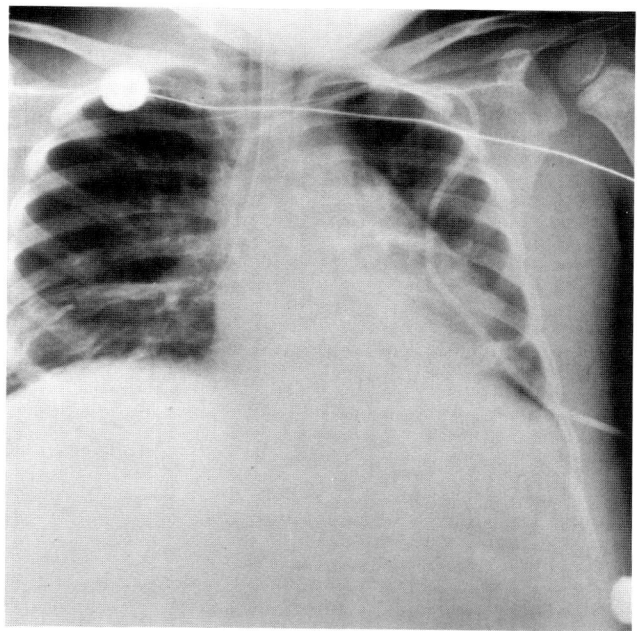

FIG. 7. Chest X-ray showing pulmonary infiltration by neuroblastoma following autologous bone marrow transplantation in a child with metastatic neuroblastoma. Note the diffuse interstitial involvement without lobar consolidation, suggesting metastatic disease occurring at the time of marrow reinfusion.

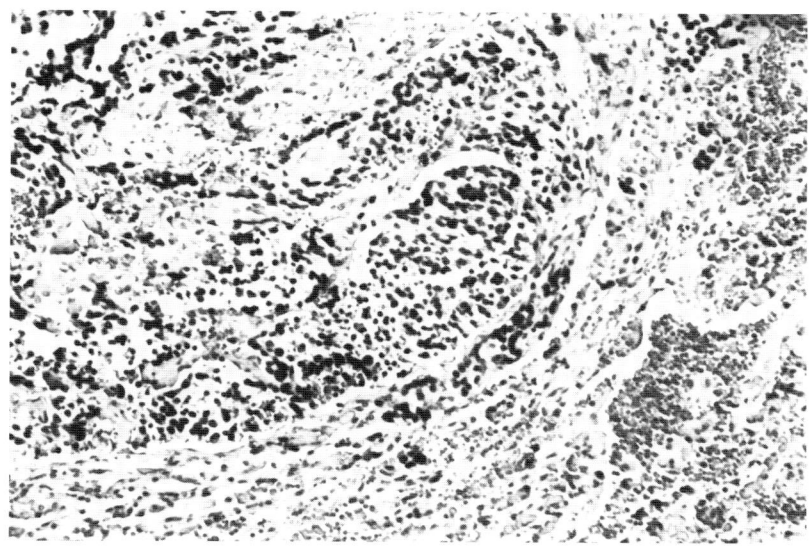

FIG. 8. Histologic section showing infiltration of the lung by metastatic tumor. The neuroblastoma cells are compressing surrounding lung tissue with infiltrates along the alveolar wall (H & E stain, ×80).

SUMMARY

Allogeneic and autologous bone marrow transplantation are promising new modalities for treatment of a wide variety of conditions, both neoplastic and nonneoplastic. At present, however, pulmonary complications following marrow transplants are among the most devastating. There is continuing research to find new ways of diagnosing the causes of idiopathic interstitial pneumonitis, to increase our ability to recognize the risk factors involved, and to develop new treatment options. Various drugs used prior to transplantation and as preparation for transplantation can cause pulmonary damage, some of which is reversible but some of which may be progressive. Graft-vs.-host disease can also play a role in lung disease after allogeneic transplant, and, in autologous bone marrow transplants, infusion of malignant cells must be considered when pulmonary infiltration occurs.

REFERENCES

1. Tutschka PJ: Diminishing morbidity and mortality of bone marrow transplantation. *Vox Sang* 1986;51(Suppl)2:87–94.
2. Link H, et al.: Lung function changes after allogeneic bone marrow transplantation. *Thorax* 1986;41(7):508–512.
3. Cardozo BL, et al.: Lung damage following bone marrow transplantation. I. The contribution of irradiation. *Int J Radiat Oncol Biol Phys* 1985;11(5):907–914.
4. Weiner RS, et al.: Interstitial pneumonitis after bone marrow transplantation; assessment of risk factors. *Ann Int Med* 1986;14:168–175.
5. Glorieux P, et al.: Metastatic interstitial pneumonitis after autologous bone marrow transplantation. A consequence of reinjection of malignant cells. *Cancer* 1986;58(9):2136–2139.
6. Cardozo BL, et al.: Interstitial pneumonitis following bone marrow transplantation; pathogenesis and therapeutic considerations. *Eur J Cancer Clin Oncol: 1985;21:43.*
7. Hamilton, PJ, et al.: Bone marrow transplantation and the lung. *Thorax* 1986;41(7):497–502.
8. Levine AS (ed): *Cancer in the Young,* New York, Masson Publishing USA, 1982, pp. 735–742.
9. Gross NJ: Pulmonary effects of radiation therapy. *Ann Int Med* 1977;86:81–92.
10. Paulin T, et al.: Variables predicting bacterial and fungal infections after allogeneic marrow engraftment. *Transplantation* 1987;43(3):393–398.
11. Weiner RS, et al.: Risk factors for interstitial pneumonitis following allogeneic bone marrow transplantation for severe aplastic anemia; a preliminary report. *Transplant Proc* 1987;19(I, Part 3):2639–2642.
12. Springmeyer SC, et al.: Pulmonary function changes in long-term survivors of allogeneic marrow transplantation. In, Gale RP (ed): *Recent Advances in Bone Marrow Transplantation.* New York, Alan R. Liss, Inc., 1983, pp. 343–353.
13. Meyers JD, et al.: Biology of interstitial pneumonia after marrow transplantation. In, Gale RP (ed): *Recent Advances in Bone Marrow Transplantation.* New York, Alan R. Liss, Inc., 1983, pp. 403–423.
14. Krowka MJ, et al.: Pulmonary complications of bone marrow transplantation. *Chest* 1982;87(2):237–246.
15. Pino y Torres JL, et al.: Risk factors in interstitial pneumonitis following allogeneic bone marrow transplantation. *Int J Radiat Oncol Biol Phys* 1982;8:1301.
16. Neiman PE, et al.: A prospective analysis of interstitial pneumonia and opportunistic viral infection among recipients of allogeneic bone marrow grafts. *J Infect Dis* 1977;136:754.
17. Beschorner WE, et al.: Cytomegalovirus pneumonia in bone marrow transplant recipients; miliary and diffuse pattern. *Am Rev Respir Dis* 1980;122:107–114.

18. Kim TH, et al.: Interstitial pneumonitis following total body irradiation for bone marrow transplantation using two different dose rates. *Int J Radiat Oncol Biol Phys* 1985;11:1285.

19. Lum LG: The kinetics of immune reconstruction after human marrow transplantation. *Blood* 1987;69:369.

20. Winston DJ, et al.: Treatment and prevention of interstitial pneumonia associated with bone marrow transplantation. In, Gale RP (ed.): *Recent Advances in Bone Marrow Transplantation.* New York, Alan R. Liss, Inc., 1983, pp. 425–444.

21. Hackman RC: Lower respiratory tract. In, *The Pathology of Bone Marrow Transplantation.* 1984, pp. 156–170.

22. Weiss BR, et al.: Cytotoxic drug-induced pulmonary disease; update 1980. *Am J Med* 1980;68:259–266.

23. Bortin MM: Pathogenesis of interstitial pneumonitis following allogeneic bone marrow transplantation for acute leukemia. In, Gale RP (ed): *Recent Advances in Bone Marrow Transplantation.* New York, Alan R. Liss, Inc., 1983, pp. 445–460.

24. Ginsberg SJ, et al.: The pulmonary toxicity of antineoplastic agents. *Semin Oncol* 1982; 9(1):34–51.

25. Mark GJ, et al.: Cyclophosphamide pneumonitis. *Thorax* 1978;33:89–93.

26. Ostrow D, et al.: Bronchiolitis obliterans complicates bone marrow transplantation. *Chest* 1985;87(6):828–830.

27. Link H, et al.: Obstructive ventilation disorders as a severe complication of chronic graft-vs.-host disease after bone marrow transplantation. *Exp Hæmatol* 1982;10:92–93.

28. Bortin MM, et al.: Factors associated with interstitial pneumonitis after bone marrow transplantation for acute leukæmia. *Lancet* 1982;1:437.

29. Beschorner WE, et al.: Lymphocytic bronchitis associated with graft-vs.-host disease in recipients of bone marrow transplants. *N Engl J Med* 1978;299:1030–1036.

30. Pecego R, et al.: Interstitial pneumonitis following autologous bone marrow transplantation. *Transplantation* 1986;42(5):515–517.

Bone Marrow Transplantation in
Children, edited by F. Leonard Johnson
and Carl Pochedly. Raven Press, Ltd.,
New York © 1990.

Oral Complications of Bone Marrow Transplantation

*Robert J. Berkowitz, **Joel H. Berg, and †Gerald A. Ferretti

*Department of Pediatric Dentistry, *Children's Hospital National Medical Center,
Washington, D.C. 20010, **University of Texas Dental Branch at Houston, Houston,
Texas 77225; and †School of Dentistry, University of Kentucky, Lexington,
Kentucky 40506*

A. Oral complications during marrow ablative therapy
B. Oral complications during the immediate post-transplant period
C. Oral complications in the postengraftment period
Summary

The oral cavity is a frequent site of complications during bone marrow transplantation (1–8). Morbidity associated with oral involvement may seriously affect the clinical course of these patients. This chapter reviews the clinical manifestations and management of oral complications of the child undergoing marrow transplant.

ORAL COMPLICATIONS DURING MARROW ABLATIVE THERAPY

Oral complications presenting during marrow ablative therapy usually occur in only those patients receiving total body irradiation (TBI) as part of their preparative regimen (1,3,4,7). Patients present with parotitis, xerostomia, and thick, ropy saliva immediately after whole dose TBI or within 24 hours after their second or third dose of fractionated TBI (200 cGy/dose) (1,4,7). The parotitis usually disappears spontaneously within 48 hours. Xerostomia persists for about one week and the xerostomia associated discomfort is effectively relieved by use of synthetic saliva substitutes (1,7).

These adverse reactions to radiation represent inflammation in the salivary glands that gradually resolve. Complete recovery of salivary flow to the rate prior to bone marrow transplantation is gradual, and may take up to 12 months following bone marrow transplantation (9). Also, these clinical effects of TBI have only been reported for adults and adolescents (1,6,7). Prepubertal children do not present with these complications when exposed to fractionated TBI (7).

ORAL COMPLICATIONS DURING THE IMMEDIATE POST-TRANSPLANT PERIOD

Oral complications occurring during this phase of transplantation are a result of the direct effects (stomatotoxicity) of the preparative regimen. In addition, these oral complications may be indirect effects of myelosuppression due to the preparative regimen. Clinically, these effects of stomatotoxicity and myelosuppression present as mucositis, infection, and hemorrhage.

Mucositis

The most common oral complication in the immediate post-transplant period is mucositis (Figure 1) (1–8). Most, if not all, of these patients experience some degree of mucositis. The onset of the mucositis usually occurs 4 to 6 days

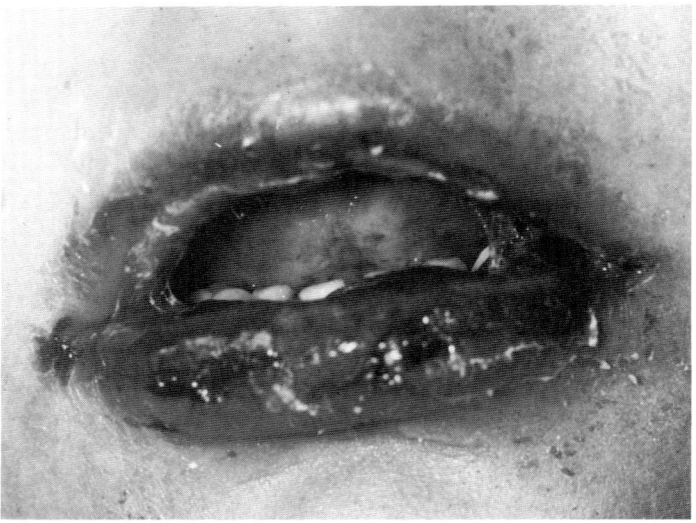

FIG. 1. Mucositis in a 3½-year-old boy undergoing allogeneic bone marrow transplantation for treatment of grade IV neuroblastoma. This photograph was obtained 9 days after bone marrow transplantation. The marrow ablative regimen included melphalan at a dose of 60mg/m^2/day intravenously for 3 doses, followed by fractionated total body irradiation 200 cGy twice a day for 6 doses.

post-transplant when the white blood cell count has fallen to a very low level. The mucositis usually resolves when the absolute neutrophil count exceeds 500/mm^3 (7).

Severity and duration of mucositis varies from patient to patient (3–8), and is dependent on several factors. The relationship between severity and duration of mucositis and several therapeutic variables was studied in 41 pediatric bone marrow transplantation patients (7). Duration of mucositis was statistically correlated with methotrexate administration for prevention of graft-vs.-host disease. The 13 patients receiving methotrexate for graft-vs.-host disease prophylaxis had mucositis for 9 to 23 days, with a mean of 14.33 days; whereas the mucositis persisted for 6 to 18 days, with a mean of 8.46 days, in 28 patients not receiving methotrexate. Stated differently, methotrexate administration was associated with a 6-day increase in the mean duration of episodes, which represents almost a doubling of the duration. None of the other variables (cytosine arabinoside, cyclophosphamide, melphalan, total body irradiation, or type of mouth care) were significantly associated with duration of mucositis.

Severity of mucositis was best predicted by a combination of indicator variables corresponding to melphalan administration and TBI. In particular, patients graded on a severity scale of 0 to 4 according to the criteria of the Eastern Cooperative Oncology Group (Table 1) tended to be at least 1.5 categories worse if melphalan was administered. These patients were also an additional stage or grade worse if they received TBI. None of the other variables (cytosine arabinoside, cyclophosphamide, methotrexate, or type of mouth care) showed a statistically significant association with severity of mucositis. However, the investigators believed that those patients receiving professionally administered mouth care experienced less severe mucositis than those patients receiving unsupervised, self-administered mouth care. Furthermore, there is a direct relationship between decreasing severity and duration of mucositis and improvement in the quality of oral hygiene (6,10–13).

Treatment of mucositis is generally limited to efforts to relieve pain. The discomfort associated with mild to moderate mucositis can usually be relieved by use of topical anesthetic agents. However, anesthetic rinses have the disad-

TABLE 1. *Grading of mucositis: criteria of the Eastern Cooperative Oncology Group*

Degree of stomatitis	Clinical manifestations
0	None
1	Oral soreness, fewer than 3 ulcers
2	Oral soreness, more than 3 ulcers, can eat and swallow
3	Many ulcers, cannot eat
4	Hospitalization and intravenous alimentation required

vantages of poor taste, short duration of action, and the potential for systemic toxicity from mucosal absorption which limits the frequency of their use. Moderate to severe mucositis usually requires the parenteral administration of narcotic drugs for adequate pain control. Commercial mouthwashes which contain alcohol and phenol should not be used. These agents dehydrate the mucosa and intensify the mucositis.

Infections

The risk for oral infection is highest during this phase of marrow transplantation because of leukopenia, immunosuppression, and stripping of mucosal barriers. Consequently, the oral tissues are susceptible to a variety of fungal, bacterial, and viral infections. In addition, the use of high doses of broad-spectrum antibiotics further compromises the oral flora and facilitates colonization of pathogenic microbes as well as opportunistic organisms.

Fungal Infections

Systemic candidiasis is a major cause of morbidity and mortality during bone marrow transplantation (14). DeGregorio and co-workers (15) reported that systemic candidiasis developed almost exclusively in those myelosuppressed patients who had prior oropharyngeal candidiasis. This observation implies that prevention of oropharyngeal candidiasis (Figure 2) would reduce the incidence of systemic candidiasis. In this regard, nystatin has been utilized as a prophylactic agent in the prevention of oropharyngeal candidiasis. However, unsupervised "swishing and swallowing" of this agent has not had a significant effect on prevention of oropharyngeal candidiasis in myelosuppressed patients (15–17).

In contrast, two oral care protocols (8,17) appear to be effective in preventing oropharyngeal candidiasis in bone marrow transplant patients. One of these protocols (17) utilizes a multiagent regimen which consisted of the following: (1) debriding all mucous membrane surfaces within the oropharyngeal cavity with one povidone-iodine swabstick 4 times per day, and (2) swabbing all mucous membrane surfaces within the oropharyngeal cavity with one large cotton pledget saturated with 500,000 units of nystatin 4 times per day.

This multiagent regimen therapy was initiated on the day before marrow ablative therapy commenced and was terminated when the patient's absolute neutrophil count recovered to approximately $500/mm^3$. The povidone-iodine debridement preceded the nystatin application. Most patients were premedicated with intravenous narcotic analgesics in order to permit the procedure to be done thoroughly and quickly. No thyroid dysfunction was noted secondary to the iodine exposure from the povidone-iodine swabsticks. The

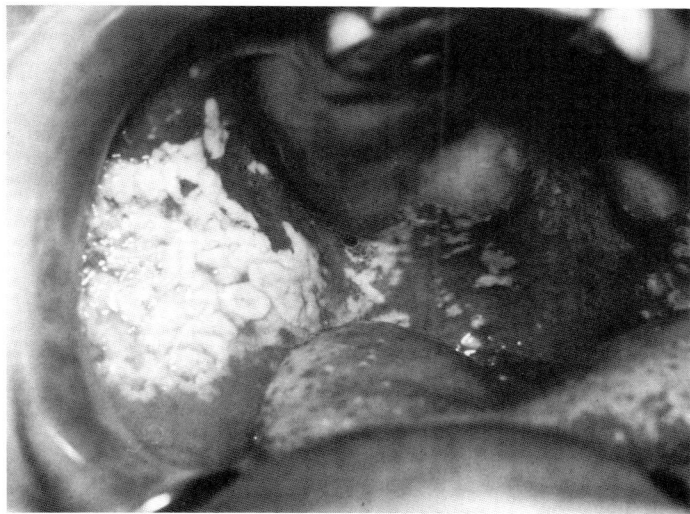

FIG. 2. Oropharyngeal candidiasis in a 9-month-old girl undergoing allogeneic marrow transplantation for treatment of osteopetrosis. This photograph was obtained 13 days after bone marrow transplantation. The marrow ablative regimen included busulfan 2mg/kg/dose by mouth daily for 4 doses followed by cyclophosphamide 50 mg/kg/dose intravenously daily for 4 days.

multiagent regimen appears to be a safe and effective approach for preventing oropharyngeal candidiasis in myelosuppressed patients. In addition, none of the patients who were treated with the multiagent regimen presented with candida sepsis or esophagitis during the immediate post-transplant period.

One other recent approach in preventing oropharyngeal candidiasis is the use of a 0.12% chlorhexidine mouth rinse. A large prospective, double-blind, randomized clinical trial of this agent in marrow transplant patients has recently been reported (8). The agent appears to be safe and extremely effective. In addition to preventing candida infections, use of chlorhexidine was associated with a significant reduction in the frequency and severity of mucositis and gingivitis.

Bacterial Infections

Examinations to detect bacterial infections in the mouth of myelosuppressed patients was formerly limited to the finding of mucosal lesions. However, the importance of periodontal and dental pulp infections have only recently been understood. In particular, necrotic teeth and periodontal infection represent bacterial reservoirs available for bacteremia and may be a source for hematogenous seeding. Therefore, the distinction between mucosal, periodontal, and dental pulp infections is critical for appropriate management of the child undergoing bone marrow transplantation. Infections in these 3 sites will be discussed separately.

In a study of 35 adult bone marrow transplant patients, the incidence of oral mucosa bacterial infections during the immediate post-transplant period was about 23%.[1] Four patients were infected with Pseudomonas, 3 with Staphylococcus, and 1 with Klebsiella. In another study (18) consisting of 1000 adult leukemia patients being treated in the blastic phase, the oral mucosa bacterial infection rate was approximately 11.5%. About 30% of the infecting bacteria were gram-positive cocci and 70% were gram-negative bacilli. On the other hand, among 41 pediatric bone marrow transplant patients none of the children showed evidence of bacterial infections of the oral mucosa during the immediate post-transplant period (7). One likely explanation for this difference between the adult and pediatric groups was that 28 of the 41 children received daily professionally supervised mouth care during the period of bone marrow depletion.

The clinical manifestations of oral mucosal infections may be obscured in myelosuppressed patients. Profound leukopenia may reduce or eliminate abscess formation and pus production. Also, the presence of mucositis induced by a program of intensive multimodal cancer therapy, herpetic stomatitis, or oropharyngeal candidiasis may hamper efforts to make an exact diagnosis of the oral lesions. Symptomatically, oral mucosa bacterial infections are usually characterized by pain, fever, dysphagia, anorexia, and malaise. All sites of suspected infection must be cultured and treated promptly and vigorously.

The periodontium includes the gingiva, alveolar bone, and the periodontal ligament (Figure 3). Failure in providing active oral hygiene results in the accumulation of a dense bacterial mass (dental plaque) around the necks of the teeth at the gingival margin (gum line). If not removed, this dental plaque will give rise to an inflammatory response in the gingiva (gingivitis) (Figure 4). The gingivitis may progress to periodontitis, which causes alveolar bone loss and subgingival accumulation of dental plaque.

Periodontal disease is usually asymptomatic; therefore, many patients are often unaware of its presence or severity. Acute complications associated with periodontal disease may arise during myelosuppression. Thus, in one study acute flares of periodontal infection accounted for 28% of all acute infections in adult patients with acute nonlymphoblastic leukemia during myelosuppression (19). These periodontal lesions may also serve as a portal of entry for septicemia (20). The clinical characteristics of these lesions are variable. Patients usually complain of pain, and the periodontium at the site of the lesion is tender to palpation. Acute periodontal infections that present during myelosuppression usually respond well to local irrigation (such as with betadine) in combination with broad-spectrum antibiotics. However, several studies (7,8,21–23) clearly indicate that dental evaluation and treatment before bone marrow transplantation minimizes the risk for acute flares of periodontal infection during periods of marrow depletion.

Bacterial invasion of the dental pulp (Figure 3) is usually secondary to

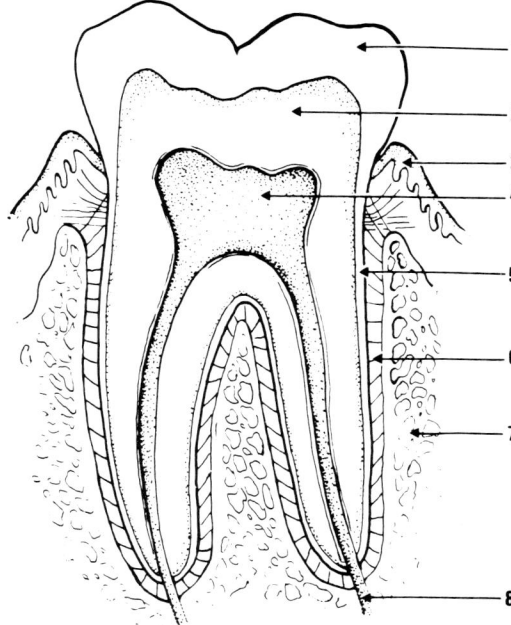

FIG. 3. Diagram showing anatomy of the tooth and adjacent structures. (1) enamel, (2) dentin, (3) gingival margin, (4) pulp, (5) cementum, (6) periodontal ligament, (7) alveolar bone, and (8) neurovascular bundle.

untreated dental caries. Bacterial colonization of the dental pulp initiates an inflammatory response in this tissue. The ensuing pulpitis can elicit significant pain, in the form of toothache. In turn, the pulpal inflammation can progress to necrosis, with subsequent bacterial invasion of the alveolar bone, causing a periapical abcess. This process may be quite painful and is associated with the complications of facial cellulitis, sepsis, and systemic infection. Therefore, dental pulp infections can contribute to the morbidity of the pediatric bone marrow transplant patient.

Prevention of pulp complications is of paramount importance. Technical constraints imposed by patient isolation prevent the safe and efficient performance of endodontic (pulpal) procedures. Likewise, profound neutropenia and thrombocytopenia preclude any extraction of teeth. Dental evaluation and treatment before bone marrow transplantation greatly reduces the risk for dental pulp complications during periods of marrow depletion (7,8).

Viral Infections

Infections due to Herpes simplex virus and Varicella zoster virus usually present with crops of vesicles which quickly rupture, leaving punctate ulcers that may coalesce. It is clinically difficult to differentiate mucosal breakdown secondary to the stomatotoxicity of the preparative regimen from lesions due to viral infections. Involvement of perioral tissues (lips and nose) with vesicu-

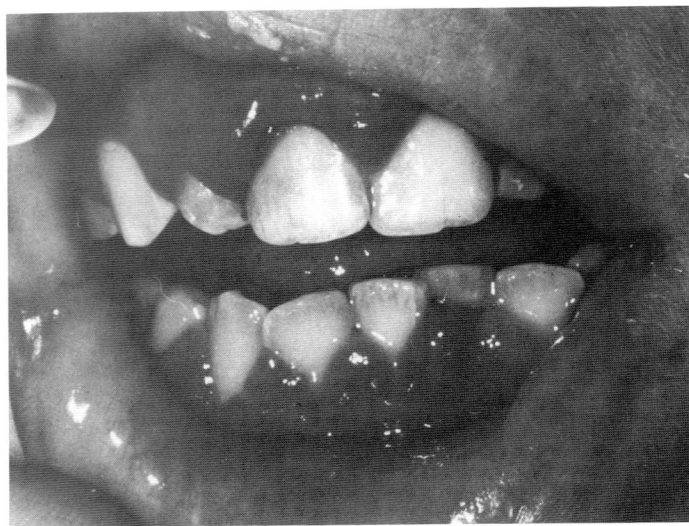

FIG. 4. Acute gingivitis in a 16-year-old girl. Note gingival hypertrophy secondary to inflammatory edema.

lar lesions aids clinical assessment, but definitive diagnosis is established on the results of viral cultures. The more severe the mucositis, the greater the likelihood that the patient is excreting Herpes simplex virus (25). Viral lesions usually do not resolve until the absolute neutrophil count recovers to 500/mm^3. Several reports (25,26) indicate that acyclovir therapy is beneficial.

Hemorrhage

Hemorrhage is a common complication of myelosuppressive therapy and the resultant thrombocytopenia. Oral bleeding is frequent and much variation is noted among patients. Spontaneous gingival bleeding usually occurs with platelet counts of 15,000/mm^3 (27). Patients with periodontal disease are more likely to develop gingival bleeding than children with periodontal health. Hematoma formation may occur at any location on the oral mucosa, but it is more frequent in areas that may be traumatized, such as the lateral border of the tongue. Prior to epithelialization, these areas are a potential nidus of infection and must be carefully observed.

Of particular importance in children are exfoliating primary teeth that are loose. These teeth should be removed prior to initiating marrow ablative therapy. Ten days should be allowed between extraction and the onset of neutropenia to allow adequate time for wound healing. The importance of this delay is that once epithelialization of the extraction wound occurs, the portal of entry for bacteria is reduced. Leaving such a wound open during profound neutropenia can lead to serious infection.

Control of oral bleeding secondary to thrombocytopenia is most effectively achieved by platelet transfusions. However, antiplatelet antibodies may arise following repeated platelet transfusions and, therefore, their use for control of oral bleeding should be kept to a minimum. Local measures include topical thrombin and pressure, topical epsilon aminocaproic acid (Amicar) and pressure, and microfibrillar collagen (Avitene).

ORAL COMPLICATIONS IN THE POSTENGRAFTMENT PERIOD

Oral complications which present in the postengraftment period include: graft-vs.-host disease, dental caries, and infection.

Graft-vs.-Host Disease

Previous studies indicate that oral involvement in the postengraftment period is frequently associated with graft-vs.-host disease (1–8). Oral complications of graft-vs.-host disease include stomatitis, Sjögren's-like xerostomia, and a variety of mucocutaneous lesions that mimic such diseases as lichen planus, scleroderma, and lupus erythematosis. In a recent report (7), acute graft-vs.-host disease developed in 25 out of 36 pediatric patients receiving allogeneic bone marrow transplants, as evidenced by liver dysfunction, generalized dermatitis, diarrhea, enterocolitis, and recurrent stomatitis.

Five of the 25 patients with acute graft-vs.-host disease developed recurrent stomatitis approximately 1 week after their pancytopenia-associated mucositis resolved. Recurrent stomatitis presented as an ulceration of the buccal mucosa, tongue, palate, and chelitis (Figure 5). These ulcerations usually resolved rapidly following therapy with systemic steroids. Eight of the 25 patients with acute graft-vs.-host disease developed chronic graft-vs.-host disease. All of the patients with chronic graft-vs.-host disease showed histopathologic changes in the minor salivary glands and labial mucosa characteristic of graft-vs.-host disease (28). All of the 8 patients with chronic graft-vs.-host disease showed oral findings which included: lichen planus-like lesions (1 out of 8 patients), mucosal erythema (7 out of 8 patients), and xerostomia (4 out of 8 patients). The lichenoid reaction presented as asymptomatic, fine, white, reticular striae on otherwise normal appearing mucosa. This lesion, which was noted 68 days after bone marrow transplantation, completely resolved by 180 days after marrow transplant. The discomfort associated with the mucosal erythema was controlled adequately with anesthetic mouth rinses. The onset of this lesion was associated with premature tapering of corticosteroid therapy. This lesion resolved rapidly by increasing the dose of systemic steroids.

Dryness of the mouth due to xerostomia was palliated with the use of a synthetic saliva substitute. In addition, xerostomia is associated with the development of rampant dental caries (29,30). Thus, the 4 xerostomic patients

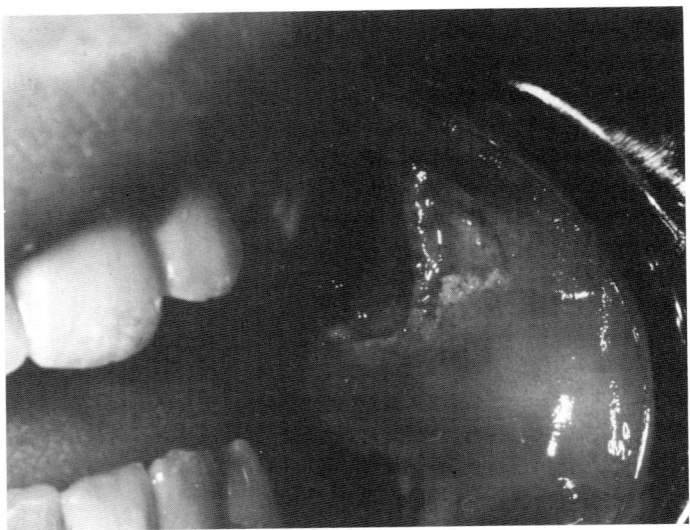

FIG. 5. Large ulceration of the buccal mucosa in a 13-year-old allogeneic bone marrow transplant patient with acute nonlymphocytic leukemia. Lesion was noted 38 days after bone marrow transplantation in association with acute graft-vs.-host disease. The lesion resolved 96 hours after institution of therapy with systemic corticosteroids.

were treated with caries preventive measures which included the daily use of topical fluoride gel (0.4% stannous fluoride), carbohydrate restrictive diets, meticulous oral hygiene, and frequent and regular dental evaluation (at least once every two months). Daily application of a topical fluoride gel was discontinued when the xerostomia disappeared. In this regard, the xerostomia resolved in 2 of the 4 patients within 6 months of onset and persisted in the other 2 patients for 10 and 14 months respectively. None of these 4 patients developed dental caries during their observation periods of 16 to 25 months.

Dental Caries

A recent Swedish study (5) reported that 37% of adult bone marrow transplant patients presented with rampant dental caries during their first year post-transplant. A similar observation was recently observed in a longitudinal study (7) of pediatric bone marrow transplant patients (Figure 6). Neither of these studies could demonstrate an association between the risk for dental caries and several variables, such as carbohydrate intake, presence of xerostomia, chronic graft-vs.-host disease, salivary flow rate and buffer capacity, and cariogenic bacteria counts. However, these observations still suggest that bone marrow transplant patients are at a high risk for developing dental caries, especially during the first year after bone marrow transplant.

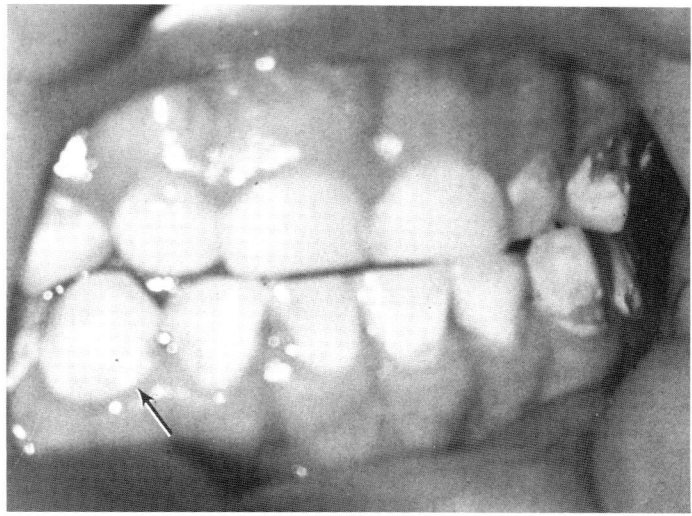

FIG. 6. Rampant dental caries in a 5-year-old allogeneic bone marrow transplantation patient with acute nonlymphocytic leukemia. Lesions were noted approximately 13 months after bone marrow transplantation. Arrow denotes area of enamel decalcification (initial caries lesion).

Infection

Allogeneic bone marrow transplant patients experience delayed immuno-logic recovery during their first year after marrow transplant. Consequently, they are particularly vulnerable to oral fungal and viral infections (13). In addition, patients with active chronic graft-vs.-host disease who are receiving immunosuppressive and prophylactic antibiotic therapy are susceptible to oral infections.

Dental Development

A recent long-term study (31) indicated that pediatric bone marrow trans-plant patients conditioned with TBI exhibited disturbances in dental develop-ment. Multiple dental disturbances were found in most patients and included the following: shortening of roots, agenesis of roots, enamel hypoplasia and microdontia.

SUMMARY

The oral cavity is a frequent site of complications during bone marrow transplantation. Following marrow ablative therapy, patients are susceptible to a variety of problems, including mucositis, infections, and hemorrhage.

These complications are associated with significant morbidity and may be lethal. In addition, oral involvement in the postengraftment period may include: oral complications of graft-vs.-host disease in the form of mucositis, Sjögren's-like xerostomia, and mucocutaneous changes that mimic lichen planus, scleroderma, and lupus erythematosis. There may also be dental caries and infections. Oral care plays an important role in minimizing the morbidity and risk for mortality associated with oral complications.

REFERENCES

1. Dreizen S, McKredie KB, Dicke KA, et al.: Oral complications of bone marrow transplantation in adults with acute leukemia. *Postgrad Med* 1979;66:187–196.
2. Rakocz M, Serota FT, Nelson LP, et al.: Dental management of the child undergoing bone marrow transplantation. *JADA* 1982;104:485–488.
3. Schubert MM, Sullivan KM, Izutsu KT, Truelove EL: Oral complications of bone marrow transplantation. In, Peterson DE, Sonis S (eds.): *Oral Complications of Cancer Chemotherapy.* Boston; Martinus Nijhoff, 1983, pp. 93–112.
4. Berkowitz RJ, Crock J, Strickland R, et al.: Oral complications associated with bone marrow transplantation in a pediatric population. *Am J Pediatr Hematol/Oncol* 1983;5:53–57.
5. Heimdahl A, Johnson G, Danielson KH, et al.: Oral condition of patients with leukemia and severe aplastic anemia. *Oral Surg* 1985; 60:498–504.
6. Seto BG, Kim M, Wolinsky L, et al.: Oral mucositis in patients undergoing bone marrow transplantation. *Oral Surg* 1985;60:493–497.
7. Berkowitz RJ, Strandjord S, Jones P, et al.: Stomatologic complications of bone marrow transplantation in a pediatric population. *Pediatr Dent* 1987;9:105–110.
8. Ferretti GA, Ash RC, Brown AT, et al.: Chlorhexidine for prophylaxis against oral infections and associated complications in patients receiving bone marrow transplants. *JADA* 1987;114:461–467.
9. Izutsu KT, Menard TW, Schubert MM, et al.: Graft-vs.-host disease: related secretory immunoglobulin A deficiency in bone marrow transplant recipients; Finding in labial saliva. *Lab Invest* 1985;52:292–297.
10. Lindquist SF, Hickey AJ, Drake JB: Effect of oral hygiene on stomatitis in patients receiving cancer chemotherapy. *J Prosthet Dent* 1978;40:312–314.
11. Beck S: Impact of a systematic oral care protocol on stomatitis after chemotherapy. *Cancer Nurs* 1979;2:185–199.
12. Hickey AJ, Toth BB, Lindquist SF: Effect of intravenous hyperalimentation and oral care on the development of stomatitis during cancer chemotherapy. *J Prosthet Dent* 1982;47:178–183.
13. Otschega Y: Preventing and treating cancer chemotherapy's oral complications. *Nursing* 1980;10:47–52.
14. Pizzo PA, Robechaud KJ, Gill FA, et al.: Empiric antibiotic and antifungal therapy for cancer patients with prolonged fever and granulocytopenia. *Am J Med* 1982;72:101–111.
15. DeGregorio MW, Lee WF, Ries CA: Candida infections in patients with acute leukemia: Ineffectiveness of nystatin prophylaxis and relationship between oropharyngeal and systemic candidiasis. *Cancer* 1982;50:1780–1783.
16. Carpenterie V, Haggard ME, Lockhart LH, et al.: Clinical experience in prevention of candidiasis by nystatin in children with acute leukemia. *J Pediatr* 1978;92:593–595.
17. Berkowitz RJ, Hughes C, Rudnick M, et al.: Oropharyngeal candida prophylaxis in pediatric bone marrow transplant patients. *Am J Pediatr Hematol/Oncol* 1985;7:82–85.
18. Dreizen S, McKredie KB, Keating MJ, Bodey GP: Chemotherapy-associated oral infection in adults with acute leukemia. *Postgrad Med* 1982;71:133–146.
19. Overholser CD, Peterson DE, Williams LT, Schimpf SC: Periodontal infection in patients with acute nonlymphocytic leukemia; prevalence of acute exacerbations. *Arch Int Med* 1982;142:551–554.
20. Greenberg MS, Cohen SG, McKitrick JC, Cassileth PA: The oral flora as source of septicemia in patients with acute leukemia. *Oral Surg* 1982;53:32–36.

21. Peterson DE, Overholser CD, Williams LT, et al.: Reduced infections in patients with acute nonlymphocytic leukemia following rigorous oral hygiene. *Proc Am Soc Clin Oncol* 1980; 21:438.
22. Peterson DE, Overholser CD, Schimpf SC, et al.: Relationship of intensive oral hygiene to systemic complications in acute leukemia patients. *Proc Am Ped Clin Res* 1981; 29: 440A.
23. Peterson DE: Bacterial infections: periodontal and dental disease, in *Oral Complications of Cancer Chemotherapy*, Peterson DE, Sonis S. (eds.) Boston; Martinus Nijhoff, 1983, pp. 79–91.
24. Meyers JD, Thomas ED: Infection complicating bone marrow transplantation. In *clinical approach to infection in the immunocompromised host*, Young LS, Rubin RH (eds.) New York, Plenum, 1981.
25. Saral R, Burns WH, Laskin DL, et al.: Acyclovir prophylaxis of herpes simplex virus infections: A randomized, double blind, controlled trial in bone marrow transplant recipients. *N Engl J Med* 1981, 305:63–67.
26. Chou SW, Gallagher J, Merigan TC. Controlled clinical trial of intravenous acyclovir in heart-transplant patients with mucocutaneous herpes simplex infections. *Lancet* 1981, 1:1391–1394.
27. Lynch MA, Ship II: Initial oral manifestations of leukemia. *JADA* 1967,75: 932–940.
28. Sale GE, Shulman HM, Schubert MM et al.: Oral and ophthalmic pathology of graft-vs.-host disease in man: predictive value of the lip biopsy. *Hum Path* 1981, 12:1022–1030.
29. Brown, L. Dreizen S, Handler S: Effects of selected caries preventive regimens on microbial changes following irradiation-induced xerostomia in cancer patients. In, Stiles HM, Loesche WJ, O'Brien TC (eds): *Proc Microbial Aspects of Dental Caries*, Vol 1, pp. 275–290, Special Suppl Microbial ABs, Information Retrieval Inc., Washington, D.C., 1976.
30. Dreizen S, Brown L, Daly T, et al.: Prevention of xerostomia-related dental caries in irradiated cancer patients. *J Dent Res* 1977; 56:99–104.
31. Dahllof G, Heimdahl A, Bolme P, et al.: Oral condition of children treated with bone marrow transplantation. *Bone Marrow Trans* 1988; 43–51.

*Bone Marrow Transplantation in
Children*, edited by F. Leonard Johnson
and Carl Pochedly. Raven Press, Ltd.,
New York © 1990.

Infectious Complications

*Wayne L. Furman and **Sandor Feldman†

*St. Jude Children's Research Hospital, Department of Pediatrics, University of
Tennessee College of Medicine, Memphis, Tennessee 38101 and **Department of
Pediatrics, University of Mississippi Medical Center, Jackson, Mississippi 39216*

Introduction
A. Post-transplantation stages of immunologic dysfunction
B. Prevention of infection
C. Bacterial infections
D. Fungal infections
E. Viral infections
F. Interstitial pneumonitis
G. Parasitic infections
Conclusions

INTRODUCTION

Severe, life-threatening infection is a serious obstacle to successful bone
marrow transplantation (BMT). The high risk of infection is a direct consequence of the severe immunologic compromise caused by the pre-transplant
conditioning regimen. Occurrence of immunologic dysfunction also depends
on several other factors. These include the underlying disease for which the
bone marrow transplant was performed, the degree of HLA compatibility, the
time to engraftment, the presence of graft-vs.-host disease (GVHD), the
method of prophylaxis against GVH disease, the treatment of graft-vs.-host
disease (GVHD), and cytomegalovirus status (presence of infection or immunity) before bone marrow transplantation.

The protective mechanisms of an intact immune system include the physical

†The work presented in this chapter was supported by Grant CA-21765 (CORE) and the
American Lebanese Syrian Associated Charities (ALSAC).

barriers of the skin and mucous membranes and the components of the humoral and cellular immune response. Protection afforded by the skin and mucous membranes is enhanced by local factors. Containment of infectious organisms by mucous secretions of the respiratory and gastrointestinal tracts is facilitated by intestinal motility, ciliary action, gastric acidity, and the presence of secretory IgA. The low pH of sebum and sweat and the presence of lysozyme and lactoferrin in tears and saliva also play important roles in protection against infection.

The humoral immune system is composed of nonspecific factors, such as lysozyme, lactoferrin, and complement, as well as specific antibodies to infectious organisms. The cellular immune response includes the phagocytic cells, such as polymorphonuclear cells and macrophages, and the specific cell-mediated immunity provided by the interaction of T lymphocytes and mononuclear phagocytes. Abnormalities of these immunologic components are associated with specific types of infections (1,2,3).

POST-TRANSPLANTATION STAGES OF IMMUNOLOGIC DYSFUNCTION

After transplantation, there are periods during which the various components of the immunologic system are more likely to be affected. By recognizing the stage of the bone marrow transplant and assessing the degree of immunologic dysfunction, one can anticipate the type of infection for which a particular patient is at highest risk. The post-transplantation period can be conveniently divided into three stages (the early, middle, and late periods) that take into account the ablation and recovery of various components of the immune system. Figure 1 and Table 1 list the types of organisms most likely to cause problems during each of these stages.

Early Period

The early period is the time from the day of bone marrow transplant to recovery from neutropenia. Immunologic dysfunction during this period is a consequence of the intensive chemotherapy and radiotherapy that was necessary to prepare a patient for successful transplantation. The resulting neutropenia may last for 3 to 4 weeks. The rate of granulocyte recovery is also influenced by the type of treatment employed to prevent graft-vs.-host disease. For example, recovery of the granulocyte count following cyclosporin prophylaxis is more rapid than following methotrexate (4).

Fever is a universal occurrence during this period, although clinical or microbiological documentation of infection occurs in only 33 to 50% of patients (5). Most documented infections during this period are due to bacteria and fungi. Bacteremia has a peak occurrence 8 to 10 days after bone marrow

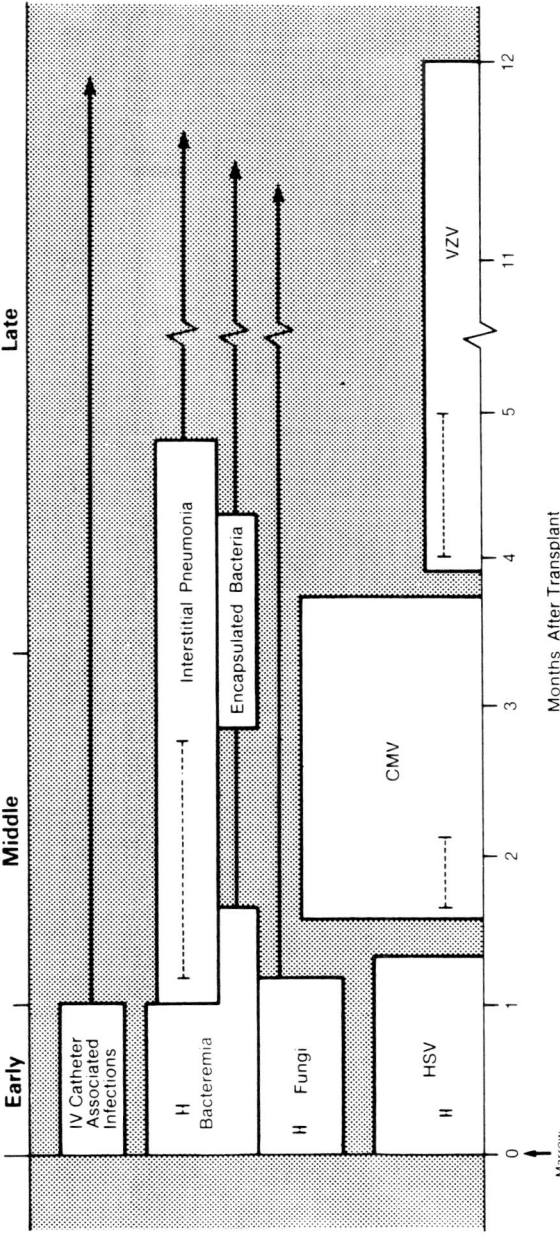

FIG. 1. Infections following bone marrow transplantation. Most infections in bone marrow transplant patients occur during predictable periods. Peak incidence (- - - - -) is indicated for several organisms. HSV, herpes simplex virus; CMV, cytomegalovirus; VZV, varicella zoster virus.

TABLE 1. *Common organisms causing significant infections in bone marrow transplant recipients.*

Organism	Usual time of infection	Clinical syndrome	Specific treatment*
Gram-negative bacteria	early period	septicemia	Ticarcillin, 9.0 g/m^2/day divided every 6 hrs Tobramycin, 240 mg/m^2/day divided every 6 hrs, with or without WBC transfusions
Gram-positive bacteria	early period; some late infections in setting of GVHD	local infections, septicemia	Oxacillin, 3–4.5 g/m^2/day divided every 6 hrs, or Vancomycin, 1.2 g/m^2/day divided every 6 hrs
Staph. epidermidis *Strep. viridans*	early period	local infections, septicemia, endocarditis (rare)	Vancomycin, 1.2 g/m^2/day divided every 6 hrs
Encapsulated Organisms *Strep. pneumonia* *N. meningitidis* *H. influenza*	late period	septicemia, pneumonia, sinusitis, otitis media meningitis, peritonitis	Penicillin G, 100–250,000 U/kg/day divided every 6 hrs Ampicillin, 3–9.0 g/m^2/day divided every 6 hrs, or Cefotaxime, 200 mg/kg/day divided every 6 hrs
Herpes simplex virus	early period	gingivostomatitis, esophagitis, genital infection	Acyclovir, 750 mg/m^2/day divided every 8 hrs
Cytomegalovirus	middle period	pneumonia, anorexia, nausea, vomiting, persistent fever, hepatitis	None available
Varicella zoster virus	late period	localized or disseminated cutaneous infection, pneumonia, gastroenteritis	Acyclovir, 1500 mg/m^2/day divided every 8 hrs
Rotavirus Coxsackie virus Adenovirus	early period	gastroenteritis	None available
Candida	early period	fungemia, pneumonia, thrush	Amphotericin B, 1 mg/kg/day given over 4–6 hrs for 4–6 weeks for disseminated disease
Aspergillus	early period; late period in setting of GVHD	fungemia, pneumonia	

*The particular antibiotics and dosages are those utilized at St. Jude Children's Research Hospital for these infections. Changes may be indicated depending on local antibiotic sensitivities of pathogenic microorganisms.

transplantation (1). The immediate result of the intensive preparative regimen is breakdown of oropharyngeal, gastrointestinal and integumentary barriers to microbial invasion. These defects substantially increase the risk of bacterial and fungal infections during the immediate post-transplant period. Also, reactivation of Herpes simplex virus (HSV) infection occurs in 80% of seropositive patients (6). Patients with oropharyngeal reactivation of herpes virus infection have more severe mucositis and may develop esophagitis, tracheitis, or pneumonia (7).

Middle Period

An arbitrary time, from the recovery from neutropenia to 100 days after bone marrow transplantation, is called the middle period. Patients surviving into this period have two major risks: graft-vs.-host disease and interstitial pneumonitis. Bacterial and fungal infections during this period are a serious threat only to those who develop graft-vs.-host disease, those who reject the graft, or who fail to engraft.

Most infections are viral and are usually associated with the development of interstitial pneumonitis. Cytomegalovirus (CMV) is the most commonly encountered organism, occurring in at least 50% of all patients, with about a third of these developing CMV pneumonia (8). Other viruses, responsible for less than 5% of cases of interstitial pneumonitis during this period, include Herpes simplex virus, varicella zoster virus (VZV), and adenovirus (9). Although nearly 50% of all transplant recipients who survive 6 months or more will develop varicella zoster virus infections, the vast majority of these infections occur after day 100 (10).

Late Period

The late period is arbitrarily defined as 100 or more days after transplantation. A patient who survives this long enters a period of high risk for two types of infections. These infections are caused by: (1) bacteria, due to encapsulated organisms (especially *Streptococcus pneumonia* and *Hemophilus influenzae*) and gram-positive cocci (such as *Staphylococcus aureus* and β-hemolytic streptococci), and (2) viruses, especially due to reactivation of varicella zoster virus (11–13). Infection with encapsulated organisms occurs in 17–27% of transplant recipients who survive 6 months or more (12,13). Approximately 20% of these same patients will develop infection with gram-positive cocci other than the pneumococcus (12), and almost 50% will develop infection with varicella zoster virus (10). The severity of infections seems to be determined by the completeness of immunologic recovery. The major predisposing factors to infection during this period are graft-vs.-host disease, HLA mismatching, and the presence of nonspecific suppressor cells (T lymphocytes) (11).

PREVENTION OF INFECTION

A number of strategies have been employed by investigators to reduce the risk of serious infections in patients during the transplant procedure. In general these approaches have consisted of protecting the patient from exogenous organisms, reducing the patient's burden of potentially pathogenic endogenous microorganisms, and augmenting the patient's defense mechanisms (14).

Some bone marrow transplantation centers use a laminar air flow (LAF) room, oral nonabsorbable antibiotics, skin and mucous membrane decontamination, and a sterile diet. These measures are usually continued until the granulocyte count is above $500/mm^3$. Compared with simple reverse isolation in private rooms, this approach has significantly reduced the incidence of bacterial and fungal infections in the first 50 days after transplantation. A prospective randomized trial compared laminar airflow isolation, skin and mucous membrane decontamination, and a sterile diet with use of simple reverse isolation in private rooms. This trial showed that the incidence of major local infections or documented septicemia was 28% in the laminar airflow group as compared with 70% in the control group (13/46 vs. 31/44; P = 0.008). However, no difference in long-term survival could be demonstrated between the two groups (15).

On the other hand, patients transplanted for severe aplastic anemia who were placed in LAF rooms and were given skin decontamination and a sterile diet, actually had a decreased incidence of graft-vs.-host disease and improved survival when compared with similar patients treated in private rooms (16,17). In 130 aplastic anemia patients transplanted in Seattle, 39 were randomly assigned to LAF rooms, treated with oral nonabsorbable antibiotics, skin decontamination, and a sterile diet. This group had a 20% incidence of graft-vs.-host disease of grade II and greater, compared with a 40% incidence of GVH disease in the 91 patients treated in a conventional manner (P = 0.05). In this same study, estimated long-term survival for the laminar airflow group was 87%, as compared with a survival of 69% in the control group (P = 0.03) (17).

The disadvantages of a total protective environment as a means of preventing infection include cost, poor compliance with oral nonabsorbable antibiotics, and the psychologic effects of the patient's separation from his family (18). The problems of compliance and the anguish due to separation are greatly magnified in pediatric patients.

Daily granulocyte transfusions given during the period of neutropenia, before documented infection develops, have decreased the incidence of early period bacteremia. In a study from Seattle, bone marrow transplant patients were randomized to receive or not receive prophylactic granulocytes for neutrophil counts of under $200/mm^3$. In the first 21 days after transplantation, there were no cases of septicemia in the group of 29 patients that received transfusions of granulocytes, as compared to 10 cases of septicemia out of 40 patients in the control group (P <0.005) (19). However, this method of prophylaxis is associated with significant morbidity including unexplained pneumonitis, occasional occurrence of lethal pulmonary toxicity in association with amphotericin B, and other less severe reactions such as fever, chills, and urticaria (20,21,22).

Granulocyte transfusions have also been implicated in the transmission of cytomegalovirus infections. The incidence of CMV infections was 61% in those given granulocyte transfusions, as compared with 26% in those not receiving granulocytes (P = 0.01) (23). The increased incidence of cytomegalovirus infections is most pronounced in seronegative patients receiving granulocytes from seropositive donors. Thus, in seronegative patients given granulocytes from seropositive donors 75% developed CMV infections as compared to an incidence of CMV infections of only 33% in those patients not given prophylactic granulocytes (P = 0.005) (24). Also, oral nonabsorbable antibiotics given without granulocyte transfusions may be equally effective in preventing serious infections (25). For these reasons, granulocyte transfusions are no longer employed for prevention of infections in BMT patients.

The comparative efficacy of oral nonabsorbable antibiotics in preventing infection outside of isolation in a laminar airflow room is unknown. Studies in adult acute leukemia patients suggest that the antibiotics may be beneficial if the problem of compliance can be overcome (26,27). The optimal combination of antibiotics is not known. However, studies in mice have suggested that drugs that selectively suppress the aerobic flora of the gastrointestinal tract, but do not affect the anaerobes, may prevent colonization with multiple, resistant, hospital-acquired organisms (28). Several trials evaluating oral prophylactic antibiotic combinations in adult leukemic patients suggest that trimethoprim-sulfamethoxazole (TMP-SMZ) (Bactrim or Septra) alone may be the best choice, because it spares the patient's normal anaerobic microbial population (29,30,31). However, a word of caution: TMP-SMZ is ineffective against Pseudomonas. Because bone marrow transplant patients who develop bacteremia are almost always first colonized by an organism infecting the gastrointestinal tract, surveillance cultures are often helpful (3).

The ideal strategy for prevention of infection has not yet been defined, but careful examination of each patient, followed by supportive care that is modified to the individual's needs, can be offered.

BACTERIAL INFECTIONS

Staphylococcus aureus is found in approximately 5–10% of early bacteremias, although it is rarely a cause of mortality. S. *aureus* is a serious problem in patients with graft-vs.-host disease and is a frequent cause of late-period infections (33). Defects in humoral immunity and neutrophil chemotaxis contribute to the increased incidence of late infections with this organism (34–37).

Staphylococcus epidermidis is a component of the normal skin flora. Until recently, it was considered a nonpathogen (38). It is now recognized as a cause of significant disease in severely immunocompromised individuals, in whom it causes extensive soft tissue infections, endocarditis, pneumonia, and infected emboli. Although it may cause a protracted illness, infection is fatal in less than 10% of reported cases (33). At present, *Staphylococcus epidermidis* is the most frequent cause of bacteremias in most bone marrow transplant centers, accounting for about 33% of blood culture isolates (33). The increasing incidence of infections due to this microorganism over the last decade may be related to the more frequent use of indwelling venous catheters in recipients of bone marrow transplants (2,33). This organism is frequently resistant to all antibiotics except vancomycin, which we include in the combination of antimicrobials at the initiation of fever in neutropenic patients.

Streptococcus viridans is second only to *Staphylococcus epidermidis* as a cause of bacteremia and accounts for up to 25% of bacteremias in some centers. Sepsis with this microorganism has been responsible for the sudden onset of shock, pneumonia, and encephalopathy without meningitis (39). Infection develops early after bone marrow transplantation and may be related to placement of indwelling venous catheters, contamination of bone marrow before reinfusion, or oral ulcerations (39,40,41). Vancomycin is the drug of choice for treatment of infections with this organism.

Pneumococcal infections are a particular problem in the late period. The organism may cause sinusitis, pneumonia, otitis media, meningitis, and spontaneous bacterial peritonitis in bone marrow transplant patients (13,42). The risk of late infection with *Streptococcus pneumoniae* does not seem to be confined to those patients with graft-vs.-host disease, and is not correlated with age, underlying disease, type of preparative regimen, or presence of cytomegalovirus infection. There is some evidence that affected patients have decreased specific opsonic activity against the pneumococcus (13). Also, depressed splenic function as a result of total body irradiation or high-dose chemotherapy may contribute to the unusually high incidence of infection with this organism in late survivors of bone marrow transplantation. For these reasons, most patients who are late survivors are given the polyvalent pneumococcal vaccine (Pneumovax), oral prophylactic penicillin, or both.

Diphtheroids (*Corynebacterium* species) are normally present in large numbers on the skin and mucous membranes. In the immunocompetent host, when these organisms are isolated from the blood, they are usually considered contaminants. However, they may cause significant infections in bone marrow transplant recipients. The patients at greatest risk are those who are older than 16 years of age, who have persistent granulocytopenia and have failed to engraft, or have undergone a second bone marrow transplant. Mucosal or epithelial defects of any type (such as rectal fissures, skin or mucosal ulcers or erosions due to indwelling venous catheters) provide this organism with a portal of entry (43). Diphtheroids are frequently resistant to most antibiotics, and vancomycin is the antibiotic of choice.

Anaerobes, such as *Bacteroides* species and *Clostridium difficile*, are an infrequent cause of bacteremia, accounting for less than 5% of the cases (33).

Other reported complications attributed to these organisms are severe gastro-enteritis due to a toxin-producing strain of *C. difficile* (44) and a case of fatal tetanus due to *Clostridium tetani* in an individual who was fully immunized before transplantation (45).

Primary infections of mycobacterial tuberculosis, due to *M. fortuitum* and *M. kansasii*, have occurred in recipients of bone marrow transplantation. Most cases have been treated successfully by use of multiple-drug therapy for pro-longed periods (46). Fatal dissemination of mycobacteria was observed 6 months after a *Bacillus Calmette-Guerin* (BCG) immunization in an infant transplanted for severe combined immunodeficiency (33). This child was immu-nized at birth and had normal healing of the immunization site, suggesting that the transplant procedure was responsible for reactivation of the mycobacteria. Antimicrobial prophylaxis should be considered in patients who previously received BCG immunotherapy, in patients with a history of inadequately treated tuberculosis, in patients with known family contacts, in those with recent skin test conversion, or who had a skin test positivity in the past (46).

Because of their profound immunologic compromise, bone marrow trans-plant recipients may develop significant infection from virtually any organism (42). The traditional signs and symptoms of infection are often absent, and broad-spectrum antibiotics, which are effective against the most likely patho-gens, are initiated at the first hint of infection. The choice of antibiotics is based upon (1) their effectiveness against the major pathogens observed at the particu-lar medical center, (2) the most likely pathogen for the post-transplantation period, and (3) the most synergistic, or least additive, combination (47). In light of the increasing frequency of resistant gram-positive organisms (such as *Staphylococcus epidermidis, Streptococcus viridans,* and *Corynebacterium* spe-cies), initial therapy at our center is vancomycin, amikacin sulfate, and ticarcillin (VAT). Alternate regimens consist of a cephalosporin, with or with-out a semisynthetic penicillin and an aminoglycoside. Antibiotics are usually continued until there is resolution of the neutropenia and fever. For transplant patients who remain febrile and neutropenic, shorter courses of antibiotics result in a slightly higher incidence of bacterial infections and the same inci-dence of systemic fungal infections (48). Therefore, there is no advantage to giving shorter courses of antibiotics in these patients.

FUNGAL INFECTIONS

Fungal infections, both local and systemic, are common in the early period after bone marrow transplantation and account for up to 33% of documented blood isolates. The primary threat of infections with these organisms is dis-semination, for which the mortality rate is almost 90% (49,50). An unsolved problem in the management of these infections is the extreme difficulty in diagnosis. Fungi are ubiquitous in the environment, their growth in cultures is slow, and attempts at serologic diagnosis have been unreliable (51–56). As a consequence, invasive fungal infections remain undiagnosed until autopsy in at least 40% of patients (3,49–51).

The majority of fungal infections occur in the first month after transplantation, with a median onset of 5–6 days (49,50). Infection after the first month is associated with immunosuppression in the treatment of graft-vs.-host disease (49,50). *Candida albicans* is responsible for about 50% of the cases, *Candida tropicalis* for 25%, and *Candida* species and *Aspergillus* species account for the remainder. Occasionally infections occur with various species of Histoplasma (57), Coccidioides, Mucor (58), Blastomyces, Trichosporon (59), Fusarium (60), and with *Pseudallescheria boydii* (61).

Patients transplanted for aplastic anemia are at much higher risk for the development of fungal infections than those transplanted for acute leukemia (46% vs. 20% in one necropsy series) (33). This difference is presumably due to the prolonged neutropenia in aplastic anemia patients before transplantation. Other factors that have been associated with the development of fungal infections are the disruption of mucosal barriers, the prolonged use of broad spectrum antibiotics, and the placement of central venous catheters (62,63).

Candida most commonly causes superficial infections of the skin (especially of the groin and perianal areas) and the oral mucosa. Esophagitis manifested by fever, severe dysphagia, and retrosternal burning is also a common problem (64,65). Other mainfestations of candida invasion include endocarditis, pneumonia, meningitis, peritonitis, osteomyelitis, endophthalmitis, urinary tract infections, renal infections, and infections involving multiple organs (51,62,64).

Aspergillus species most frequently invade the lung, but other sites of disease include the central nervous system, heart, kidneys, gastrointestinal tract and bones. Often the primary infection occurs in the lungs with dissemination to these other sites (62). The hallmark of aspergillus infection is blood vessel invasion with resultant thrombosis, infarction, and hemorrhage (62,66). Infection is fatal in up to 90% of cases (63). Contributing to this high mortality rate is the rarity of premortem diagnosis (33,63,67).

Most transplant recipients are given an oral antifungal agent, such as nystatin, ketoconazole, amphotericin B, or a combination of these agents in an attempt to prevent infection, but the ideal antifungal agent has not yet been identified (68–71). Amphotericin B, a polyene antibiotic, is the drug of choice for treatment of systemic fungal infections. Patients with neutropenia and prolonged fever who are unresponsive to broad spectrum antibiotics may also benefit from empirical use of amphotericin B (72). We administer a test dose of 1 mg, and if tolerated, the remaining dose of 0.25 mg/kg/day is given over 4–6 hours. The dose is increased in increments of 0.25 mg/kg/day until a dose of 0.5–1.0 mg/kg/day is reached. This dose is continued until a total dose of 1.5–2.0 grams is given, which usually takes 4–6 weeks (66,73). In some instances, such as in cases of Candida esophagitis, a shorter course of 10 days to 2 weeks may be effective (74).

The major toxic effects of amphotericin B in children are azotemia, anemia, hypokalemia, thrombocytopenia, and neutropenia. Side effects, such as drug-related fever, chills, and nausea are common but are not a reason to stop administration of the drug (73,75). Acetaminophen may be given to control fever. Meperidine hydrochloride in an intravenously administered dose of 0.5–1.0 mg/kg is frequently used to control chills (66). The release of prostaglandins may be responsible for chills and fever in some patients. A controlled trial evaluating the prostaglandin inhibitor, ibuprofen, to ameliorate these adverse side effects is in progress (76).

The nephrotoxic effects of amphotericin B are a result of damage to the convoluted tubules, which causes renal tubular acidosis and potassium wasting (73). Careful monitoring of electrolytes and potassium supplementation is necessary. If severe azotemia occurs (that is, with a BUN over 35 mg/dl or serum creatinine over 2.0–3.0 mg/dl), the dose of amphotericin B should be adjusted either by lowering the dose or administering the drug on alternate days (73,75). Additive nephrotoxicity is frequently observed with patients who receive amphotericin B, an aminoglycoside, and cyclosporine A simultaneously (2). We have found that substituting a third-generation cephalosporin, such as Cefotaxime, for an aminoglycoside in a febrile, neutropenic patient may be helpful in reducing the additive nephrotoxicity.

Combinations of amphotericin B with other agents, such as 5-fluorocytosine or rifampin, have been advocated for the treatment of systemic fungal disease. There is *in vitro* evidence of synergism in some studies (64,73,77), but controlled trials have not been reported.

VIRAL INFECTIONS

Viral infections, due to primary infection or reactivation of a latent virus, cause morbidity and mortality in recipients of bone marrow transplants (78). The major pathogens are the human herpes viruses: Herpes simplex viruses (types 1 and 2), cytomegalovirus, varicella zoster virus, and Epstein-Barr virus (EBV). Infections with these organisms occur at predictable intervals following bone marrow transplantation. Infections due to papoviruses, enteroviruses, adenoviruses, Coxsackie viruses, and measles viruses have also been reported, and in some instances, fatalities have occurred (2,79–82).

Herpes Simplex Viruses

Nearly 50% of bone marrow transplant recipients will develop Herpes simplex virus infections in the early period before engraftment takes place (79,83). Infections occur in 73–82% of patients seropositive before bone marrow transplant (6,83,84). The median time of onset of infection is 8 days after bone marrow transplant, or approximately 17 days after initiation of the preparative regimen (79,85).

Oral-labial lesions occur in 85% of patients and genital infections occur in the remaining 15% (78,85). Because infection occurs when the severity of mucositis from the conditioning regimen is at its peak, definitive diagnosis can be difficult without a culture or electron microscopic evaluation of vesicular fluid (62,74). Herpes simplex virus is also a frequent cause of esophagitis in these patients (65). Infrequent, but much more serious, are tracheitis and pneumonia due to Herpes simplex virus. Herpes simplex virus accounts for about 5% of nonbacterial pneumonias in bone marrow transplant recipients, and if untreated, these infections are almost always fatal. Mucocutaneous herpes simplex virus infection usually precedes the onset of pneumonia (7), and even if the oral lesions are mild, any patient with oropharyngeal herpes infection who requires intubation should be treated for herpes pneumonia (74).

Acyclovir [9-(2-hydroxyethoxy methyl) guanine], an inhibitor of viral DNA polymerase, is effective in the prophylaxis and treatment of Herpes simplex virus infections (83,84,86–89). To prevent infection, all seropositive patients should be started on acyclovir shortly after bone marrow transplantation (78). The drug is effective when administered orally or intravenously (87,88). In children, the usual dose of acyclovir is 750 mg/m^2/day, in divided doses given every 8 hours.

Although treatment of Herpes simplex virus infections with acyclovir is effective, there is rapid recurrence when the drug is stopped. Thus, there were recurrences in 18 out of 21 cases at a median time of 27 days in one study (90). A possible explanation for some recurrences is that acyclovir given in the first 5–6 weeks after transplantation can delay restoration of specific immunity against Herpes simplex virus (74,90). A potential solution may be to keep these patients on acyclovir for 1–2 months after transplantation. Herpes simplex infections that develop after this time should be less severe, because the patients' immune systems are more mature. Restoration of the specific immune response to Herpes simplex virus would then occur with minimal morbidity (74).

Patients receiving intravenous acyclovir occasionally develop transient neurological symptoms, such as lethargy, agitation, tremor, disorientation, and hemiparesis (81). Other adverse reactions to acyclovir, although rare, include thrombophlebitis, hematuria, hypertension, rash, seizures, and coma (91). A dosage-related impairment of renal function can occur after rapid intravenous bolus administration. This can usually be prevented by slow intravenous infusion (lasting longer than 1 hour), careful attention to hydration, and appropriate dosage reduction in patients with preexisting renal impairment (92).

Cytomegalovirus

Cytomegalovirus (CMV) occurs in 50–60% of all allogeneic marrow recipients, making it the most common viral pathogen in these patients (2,5,93).

TABLE 2. *Factors associated with increased risk for the development of CMV infections in bone marrow transplant recipients**

Caucasian race
Graft-vs.-host disease of over grade II in severity
Increasing age
Lung irradiation at a dose of over 6 Gy
Preceeding recipient seropositivity for CMV
Recipient seronegativity with donor seropositivity for CMV
Granulocyte transfusions
HLA nonidentity between donor and recipient
Risk of CMV infection in hematologic malignancy is greater than in aplastic anemia

*Sources for this information are in references 8, 9, 33, 78, 121.

The median time for the development of infection is 7–9 weeks after transplantation (2,8,74,94). These infections may be derived from a reactivation of the latent virus, either from the donor marrow or from blood products given after transplantation (78,95). CMV infection occurs in approximately 50% of patients who were seronegative before transplantation and in 85% of patients who were seropositive before transplantation (85). About 33% of seronegative patients will develop infection if they receive random donor blood products, and this risk is increased two- to threefold if they receive granulocyte transfusions from a seropositive donor (23,24,74). Additional factors associated with increased risk for the development of cytomegalovirus infection in recipients of bone marrow transplants are listed in Table 2.

The clinical manifestations of CMV infection are highly variable. A significant proportion of infections are asymptomatic, evidenced only by positive cultures with or without seroconversion (74). A symptom complex of persistent anorexia, nausea, and occasional vomiting with or without esophagitis has been described (65). Diffuse gastric and enteric ulcerations with fatal hemorrhage also occurs (74,79,96,97). Other manifestations of CMV infection include fever, a mononucleosis-like syndrome, a transient macular rash, arthralgia and arthritis, hepatitis, and chorioretinitis (62,74,79).

CMV pneumonia occurs in 25–33% of patients who become infected, and is fatal in at least 85% of cases (8,74). The most common symptoms of CMV pneumonia are tachypnea and a nonproductive cough. Fever and rales are usually found on physical examination (98). CMV pneumonia has even been observed after syngeneic bone marrow transplantation. Thus, it has been postulated that the specific immune response, once infection has occurred, is important in determining the severity of the disease (8). Pneumonia due to cytomegalovirus infection can be difficult to distinguish from other causes of interstitial pneumonia.

The diagnosis of cytomegalovirus infection cannot be made solely on the basis of clinical findings. Some of the more frequently used laboratory aids in diagnosis are examination of urine sediment for the presence of large inclusion-bearing cells, a fourfold or greater rise in CMV antibody, and culture of the virus from body fluids. Newer rapid diagnostic techniques are electron microscopic diagnosis by the "pseudoreplica" technique, a method that permits detection of virus particles within 15–30 minutes (100), and DNA hybridization (79,99).

There is no effective therapy for cytomegalovirus infection. CMV-immune globulin or plasma, antiviral agents (such as vidarabine, acyclovir, interferon, cytosine arabinoside, idoxuridine, and transfer factor), and use of combinations of agents (such as acyclovir and interferon or vidarabine and interferon) have all been unsuccessful (8,74,78). Attempts at prophylaxis with several of these agents have failed to reduce the incidence of serious CMV infections. Trifluorothymidine (TFT) and especially 9-(1,3-dihydroxy-2-propoxymethyl)guanine (DHPG, acycloguanosine, or ganciclovir) appear to be effective against CMV (89,101–103).

CMV-immune globulin or plasma may be effective in preventing serious CMV infections in seronegative patients who are not given granulocyte transfusions (104–106). The effectiveness of this approach in seropositive patients has not been demonstrated.

There is increased incidence of CMV infections in seronegative recipients of bone marrow transplants who have received blood products from donors who are seropositive for CMV (23,24). Use of blood products from donors who are seronegative for CMV has reduced the incidence of neonatal CMV infections (107). As a consequence, some authors routinely administer CMV-negative platelets and red blood cells to bone marrow transplant recipients who are seronegative for CMV. This may be an alternative approach to the use of passively administered antibody (78).

Other approaches being considered for the prevention of CMV infections include the use of an attenuated CMV vaccine, use of a CMV subunit vaccine, and supplying cytotoxic T lymphocytes to recipients who fail to generate such cells after bone marrow transplant (78). Clearly, the development of effective prevention or treatment for this organism would have a major impact on the success of bone marrow transplantation.

Varicella Zoster Virus

As many as 90% of varicella zoster virus (VZV) infections occur within the first year after transplantation, with a peak incidence occurring 4 to 5 months following bone marrow transplantation (10). VZV infections develop in 50% of all bone marrow transplant patients, with a 5–8% mortality (10,78,85). In those patients who develop visceral dissemination, the mortality rate is 28% (92). Most infections are due to a reactivation of latent virus. The development of primary varicella infections represents less than 5% of VZV infections that occur after marrow transplantation. The most common presentation of disease is localized dermatome involvement, which occurs in 84% of bone marrow recipients who develop VZV infection (10). Cutaneous dissemination will develop in 30 to 40% of these patients, but only 10% of patients will present with a generalized rash (1,78). Bone marrow transplant recipients who are younger than 10 years of age have a significantly lower incidence of varicella zoster virus infection than older recipients (10). Other risk factors include underlying disease other than chronic myeloid leukemia, graft-vs.-host disease, and the use of antithymocyte globulin (108–109).

The clinical course is characterized by new lesion formation for 3–14 days in some patients. It is during this time that the highest risk of visceral dissemination exists. Severe abdominal pain and back pain, often requiring narcotic analgesia, are associated with visceral dissemination. Other complications of infection are scarring, secondary infection, blindness following herpes zoster infection of the trigeminal nerve area, and postherpetic neuralgia (74).

Intravenous vidarabine and acylcovir are effective in treating varicella zoster virus infections. Use of these drugs has reduced the mortality of VZV infections in patients who are treated within the first few days after the appearance of skin lesions (74,108,109). A recent study demonstrated that acylcovir is more effective than vidarabine in prevention of disseminated infection, in promotion of cutaneous healing, and for the relief of pain (109). The dose of acyclovir is 1500 mg/m^3/day (91). An oral acyclovir preparation is currently being evaluated.

Human leukocyte interferon is also effective in the treatment of established varicella zoster virus infections. But interferon is considerably more toxic than the other agents and, therefore, it is not widely used.

Passive immunization with varicella zoster immunoglobulin (VZIG) is usually effective in ameliorating disease if it is administered within 72 hours of known exposure. The dose is 1 vial (125 U, 1.25 ml)/10kg of body weight, given intramuscularly to a maximum of 5 vials. Fractional doses are not recommended (91). Index cases are contagious at least 24 hours before the appearance of the rash. Failure to consider the fact that cases are contagious at least 24 hours before the rash is seen, may result in administration of varicella zoster immunoglobulin beyond the period of optimal effectiveness (91).

Epstein-Barr Virus

One study showed that over 60% of transplant recipients will develop a reactivation of Epstein-Barr virus (EBV), although no clinical syndromes attributable to the virus have been observed (8,85,111). EB virus may be involved in the development of graft-vs.-host disease, hepatitis, and certain B cell neoplasms, although a clear cause-and-effect relationship has not been established (8,33,111–114).

Other Virus Infections

Rotovirus, Coxsackie virus, and adenovirus have been associated with the occurrence of severe diarrhea and abdominal cramps, occasionally resulting in death. Acute graft-vs.-host disease can mimic the clinical syndrome caused by these enteric pathogens (8,44,55,115). Adenoviruses, especially types 11, 34, and 35, cause pneumonia, hepatitis, hemorrhagic cystitis, and systemic infection with renal impairment (78,80,81,116), occasionally resulting in death.

Papovavirus has been found in the urine of 30 to 80% of recipients of bone marrow transplants. This organism has been associated with mild hepatitis and hemorrhagic cystitis (33,82). No effective therapy for any of these viral pathogens exists.

Interstitial Pneumonitis

Interstitial pneumonitis (IP) occurs in about 40% of recipients of allogeneic bone marrow transplants, and in 15% of recipients of syngeneic marrow transplants. Overall, interstitial pneumonitis accounts for more than 40% of the transplant-related deaths reported in most large series. Patients usually develop interstitial pneumonitis between 5 and 12 weeks after transplantation, with a median time of onset of 8 weeks (2,8). Auscultation of the chest reveals rales or rhonchi. As the disease progresses, patients show tachycardia, dyspnea, cyanosis, and hypoxia, with carbon dioxide retention. Chest X-ray reveals either diffuse bilateral interstitial infiltrates or a patchy alveolar pattern. Less commonly, a nodular or segmental infiltrate is present, which usually progresses to a widespread, bilateral interstitial process (1,5,117).

Table 3 summarizes the significant causes of interstitial pneumonitis. Other, rarely identified etiologic agents include adenovirus, echovirus, respiratory syncytial virus, and chlamydia. Interstitial pneumonitis caused by these viruses or fungi is fatal in at least 80% of cases (118).

The treatment of interstitial pneumonitis depends on the underlying cause. The treatable causes include certain bacteria, a few fungi, *Pneumocystic carinii*, herpes simplex virus and varicella zoster virus (117).

Until recently, the risk factors for the development of interstitial pneumonitis were poorly defined, with different centers reporting disparate results. A recent report from the International Bone Marrow Transplant Registry summarizing data from over 900 allogeneic transplants, identified 6 risk factors associated with interstitial pneumonitis (Table 4). Using these 6 criteria, the risk of developing interstitial pneumonitis ranged from 8% in patients with none of these factors to 94% in patients with all 6 risk factors (118). Another factor, which approached statistical significance in this report, was the increased incidence of interstitial pneumonitis in male patients who received marrow from a female donor (P <0.06) (118). This factor has been previously noted in a smaller series of patients (119).

TABLE 3. *Etiology of interstitial pneumonitis following allogeneic and syngeneic bone marrow transplantation*

Etiologic agent	Allogeneic BMT		Syngeneic BMT	
Cytomegalovirus	239	(39%)*	0*	
Idiopathic	222	(37%)	11	(65%)
Aspergillus and *Candida*	12	(2%)	0	
P. carinii	50	(8%)	1	(6%)
Other viruses, *Torulopsis,* and *Actinomyces*	35	(6%)	1	(6%)
Clinical**	48	(8%)	4	(23%)
	606		17	

*Percentage of pneumonias in 1834 allogeneic transplantations and in 100 syngeneic transplantations.[117,118]
**No histology available.

TABLE 4. *Factors associated with increased risk for the development of interstitial pneumonia**

Incidence with use of methotrexate to prevent graft-vs.-host disease is less than with use of cyclosporine A
Age over 21 years
Severe graft-vs.-host disease
Interval from diagnosis to transplant less than 6 months
Performance rating before transplantation under 100%
Dose rate of total body irradiation over 4.00 Gy/minute in patients given methotrexate for prophylaxis of graft-vs.-host disease

*Source for this material is found in reference 118.

During the first 3 months after transplantation, 40–50% of cases of interstitial pneumonia are idiopathic in origin. Idiopathic interstitial pneumonia is fatal in 47–78% of cases (8,50,117,118). Idiopathic interstitial pneumonia is a diagnosis of exclusion, which can only be made with certainty by an open lung biopsy. Microscopic examination of lung tissue reveals a mononuclear cell infiltrate in the interstitial space between the alveoli (1,2,9). There is no effective treatment for idiopathic interstitial pneumonia, although most centers will give a trial course of steroids, consisting of either 30 mg/m^2 of prednisone by mouth or 2–10 mg/kg/day of methylprednisolone intravenously (1,117).

A report by Graham-Pole et. al. (121) suggests that prevention of interstitial pneumonia as well as other serious infections may be possible through the use of prophylactic intravenous immunoglobulin (IVIG). In a nonrandomized comparative study, 50 children with acute lymphoblastic leukemia had an allogeneic bone marrow transplant for resistant disease. Those that received IVIG (29 patients) were given either 500 mg/kg every week for 12–16 weeks after transplant (21 patients) or 200–300 mg/kg every 2 to 3 weeks, also for 12–16 weeks post-transplantation (8 patients). One of three commercially available IVIG products were used: Gamma-immune®, Cutter in 7 patients; Sandoglobulin®, Sandoz in 18 patients or Gammagard®, Baxter in 4 patients. Only 7 (24.5%) of the IVIG treated group as compared to 14 (66.7%) of the non-IVIG treated patients developed systemic viral, bacterial, or fungal infections and/or interstitial pneumonia (p<0.005). These cases were fatal in 3 out of 7 of the IVIG treated group as compared to 12 out of 14 in the untreated group (p<0.001). These results strongly suggest that prophylactic IVIG infusions may reduce the frequency of all forms of serious infections in children undergoing allogeneic bone marrow transplantation.

In randomized trials the data are less clear. A recent review of more than 300 bone marrow transplant patients treated in 6 controlled trials using either CMV immune plasma or hyperimmune globulin, suggests that the use of IVIG may not necessarily prevent CMV infection, but may modify the severity of infection and prevent CMV interstitial pneumonia in the transplant setting (122). Intravenous immunoglobulin has also been used to treat established CMV infection, but has never been shown to be beneficial (122). Taken together, these data strongly suggest that the use of IVIG in the post-transplantation period (middle period) may play a role in preventing or ameliorating the infectious complications experienced by patients during this period, and this modality has become "standard practice" in a number of transplant centers.

PARASITIC INFECTIONS

Pneumocystis carinii was a cause of interstitial pneumonia in up to 20% of recipients of bone marrow transplants before the advent of prophylaxis with trimethaprim-sulfamethoxazole (TMP-SMZ) (123). Since the institution of prophylaxis in a dose of 5 mg/kg/day of trimethaprim (divided into 2 doses per day) (124), this infection has been virtually eliminated.

Other parasites, such as *Demodex foliculorum,* ancylostoma, Cryptosporidium, Strongyloides, and Giardia, have only rarely been reported (3,74). *Toxoplasma gondii* causes disseminated disease or central nervous system infections in less than 1% of patients. Diffuse encephalopathy, meningoencephalitis, or enlarging mass lesions may be seen in the central nervous system (8,74,125).

CONCLUSIONS

Infectious complications after a marrow transplant are almost a universal occurrence, because the preparative regimen necessary for a successful transplant drastically alters the patient's immune system. As the "new" immune system of the bone marrow recipient matures, specific organisms are likely to cause infections during certain periods. Familiarity with this course of immune recovery assists in anticipating infectious complications before they develop.

Cytomegalovirus infection, interstitial pneumonia, and graft-vs.-host disease continue to limit the success of bone marrow transplantation. Likewise, a significant number of patients who are otherwise cured of their underlying disease by bone marrow transplantation succumb to these complications. However, improvements in the treatment of infections have been achieved with the development of more effective antibiotics, better supportive care, and elimination of *Pneumocystis carinii.*

A recent advance in supportive care has been the development of recombinant human colony stimulating factors for clinical use. These substances are a family of glycoprotein hormones that regulate the proliferation and maturation of hematopoietic progenitor cells. Their use in the marrow transplant setting promises to reduce or eliminate the period of profound myelosuppression post-transplantation. There are several reports which have demonstrated more rapid recovery of hematopoiesis (126) and fewer febrile days and shorter hospital stays (127) in patients receiving autologous bone marrow transplantation. If these studies are confirmed, we may be well on our way to eliminating a majority of the infectious complications after marrow transplant just described.

REFERENCES

1. Blume KG, Petz LD (eds): *Clinical Bone Marrow Transplantation.* Churchill Livingston, New York, Edinburgh, London, Melbourne, 1983; pp. 131–177.
2. Meyer JD, Atkinson K: Infection in bone marrow transplantation. In, Nathan DG (ed): *Clinics in Hematology* 1983;12(3):791–812.
3. Sale GF, Shulman HM (eds): *The Pathology of Bone Marrow Transplantation.* Yearbook Medical Publishers, Chicago, 1984; pp. 199–214.
4. Atkinson K, Biggs JC, Ting A, et al.: Cyclosporin A is associated with faster engraftment and less mucositis than methotrexate after allogeneic bone marrow transplantation. *Br J Hæmatol* 1983;53:265–270.
5. Winston DJ, Winston GH, Champlin RE, Gale RG: Infectious complications of bone marrow transplantation. *Exp Hematol* 1984;12:205–215.
6. Meyers JD, Flournoy N, Thomas ED: Infection with herpes simplex virus and cell-mediated immunity after marrow transplant. *J Infect Dis* 1980;142:338–346.
7. Ramsey PG, Fife KH, Hackman RC, et al.: Herpes simplex virus pneumonia; clinical, virologic and pathologic features in 20 patients. *Ann Intern Med* 1982;97:813–820.
8. Meyers JD, Flournoy JC, Wade JC, et al.: Biology of interstitial pneumonia after marrow transplantation. In, Gale RP (ed): *Recent Advances in Bone Marrow Transplantation.* Proceedings of the UCLA Symposia Conference in Park City, Utah, March 13–18, 1983. Alan R. Liss, Inc., New York, 1983, pp. 405–423.
9. Meyers JD, Flournoy N, Thomas ED: Non-bacterial pneumonia after allogeneic marrow transplantation; review of 10 years' experience. *Rev Infect Dis* 1982;4:1119–1132.
10. Atkinson K, Meyers JD, Storb R, et al.: Varicella zoster virus infection after marrow transplantation for aplastic anemia or leukemia. *Transplantation* 1980;29:47–50.

11. Atkinson K, Farewell V, Storb R, et al.: Analysis of late infections after bone marrow transplantation; role of genotypic nonidentity between marrow donor and recipient and of nonspecific suppressor cells in patients with chronic graft-vs.-host disease. *Blood* 1982; 67;714–720.
12. Atkinson K, Storb R, Prentice RL, et al.: Analysis of late infections in 89 long-term survivors of bone marrow transplantation. *Blood* 1979;53:720–731.
13. Winston DI, Schiffman G, Wang DC, et al.: Pneumococcal infections after human bone marrow transplantation. *Ann Int Med* 1979;91:835–841.
14. Schimpff SC, Green WH, Young VM, et al.: Infection prevention in acute nonlymphocytic leukemia. *Ann Int Med* 1975;82:351–358.
15. Buckner CD, Clift R, Sanders JE, et al.: Protective environment for marrow transplant recipients. *Ann Int Med* 1978;89:893–901.
16. Navari RM, Buckner CD, Clift RA, et al.: Prophylaxis of infection in patients with aplastic anemia receiving allogeneic marrow transplants. *Am J Med* 1984;76:564–572.
17. Storb R, Prentice RL, Buckner D, et al.: Graft-vs.-host disease and survival in patients with aplastic anemia treated by marrow grafts from HLA-identical siblings. *N Engl J Med* 1983;308:302–307.
18. Schimpff SC: Infection prevention during profound granulocytopenia. *Ann Int Med* 1980; 93:358–361.
19. Clift RA, Sanders JE, Thomas ED, et al.: Granulocyte transfusions for the prevention of infection in patients receiving bone marrow transplants. *N Engl J Med* 1978;298:1052–1057.
20. Strauss RG, Connett JE, Gale RP, et al.: A controlled trial of prophylactic granulocyte transfusions during initial induction chemotherapy for acute myelogenous leukemia. *N Engl J Med* 1981;305:597–603.
21. Winston DJ, Ho WG, Gale RP: Prophylactic granulocyte transfusions during chemotherapy of acute nonlymphocytic leukemia. *Ann Int Med* 1981;94:616–622.
22. Wright DG, Robichaud KJ, Pizzo PA, Deisseroth AB: Lethal pulmonary reactions associated wtih the combined use of amphotericin B and leukocyte transfusions. *N Eng J Med* 1981;304:1185–1189.
23. Winston DJ, Winston GH, Howell CL, et al.: Cytomegalovirus infections associated with leukocyte transfusions. *Ann Int Med* 1980;93:671–675.
24. Hersman J, Meyers JD, Thomas ED, et al.: The effect of granulocyte transfusions on the incidence of cytomegalovirus infection after allogeneic marrow transplantation. *Ann Int Med* 1982;96:149–152.
25. Winston DJ, Ho WG, Young LS, Gale RP: Prophylactic granulocyte transfusions during human bone marrow transplantation. *Am J Med* 1980;68:893–897.
26. Storring RA, McElwain TJ, Jameson B, Wiltshaw E: Oral nonabsorbed antibiotics prevent infection in acute nonlymphoblastic leukemia. *Lancet* 1977;2:837–840.
27. Guiot HFL, van der Meer JWM, van Furth R: Selective antimicrobial modulation of human microbial flora; infection prevention in patients with decreased host defense mechanisms by selective elimination of potentially pathogenic bacteria. *J Infect Dis* 1981;143:644–654.
28. Van der Waaij D, Berghuio JM, Lekkerkerk JEC: Colonization resistance of the digestive tract of mice during systemic antibiotic treeatment. *J Hyg Camb* 1972;70:605–610.
29. Starke ID, Catousky D, Johnson SA, et al.: Co-trimoxazole alone for prevention of bacterial infection in patients with acute leukemia. *Lancet* 1982;1:5–6.
30. Watson JG, Powles RL, Lawson DN, et al.: Co-trimoxazole versus nonsorbable antibiotics in acute leukemia. *Lancet* 1982;1:6–9.
31. Wade JC, Schimpff SC, Hargadon MT, et al.: A comparison of trimethoprim-sulfamethoxazole plus nystatin with gentamycin plus nystatin in the prevention of infections in acute leukemia. *N Engl J Med* 1981;304:1057–1062.
32. Cohen ML, Murphy MT, Counts GW, et al.: Prediction by surveillance cultures of bacteremia among neutropenic patients treated in a protective environment. *J Infect Dis* 1983;147:789–793.
33. Watson JG: Problems of infection after bone marrow transplantation. *J Clin Pathol* 1983;36:683–692.
34. Sosa R, Weiden PL, Storb R, et al.: Granulocyte function in human allogeneic marrow graft recipients. *Exp Hematol* 1980;8:1183–1189.
35. Clark RA, Johnson FC, Klebanoff SJ, Thomas ED: Defective neutrophil chemotaxis in bone marrow transplant patients. *J Clin Invest* 1976;58:22–31.

36. Korsmeyer SJ, Elfenbein GJ, Goldman CK, et al.: B cell, helper T cell, and suppressor T cell abnormalities contribute to disordered immunoglobulin synthesis in patients following bone marrow transplantation. *Transplantation* 1982;33:184–190.
37. Atkinson K, Lockhurst E, Penny R, et al.: Immunologic reconstitution after allogeneic marrow transplantation in man. *Transplant Proc* 1983;15:474–479.
38. Bender JW, Hughes WT: Fatal *Staphylococcus epidermitis* sepsis following bone marrow transplantation. *Johns Hopkins Med J* 1980;146:13–15.
39. Henslee J, Bostrom B, Weisdorf D, et al.: Streptococcal sepsis in bone marrow transplant patients. *Lancet* 1984;1:393.
40. Ringdén O, Hermdahl A, Lönquist B, et al.: Decreased incidence of virdans streptococcal septicemia in allogeneic BMT recipients after the introduction of acyclovir. *Lancet* 1984; 1:744.
41. Mascret B, Maraninchi D, Gastant JA, et al.: Risk factors for streptococcal septicæmia after marrow transplantation. *Lancet* 1984;1:1185–1186.
42. Kugler JW, Armitage JO, Helms CM, et al.: Nosocomial Legionnaire's disease; occurrence in recipients of bone marrow transplant. *Am J Med* 1983;74:281–288.
43. Stamm WE, Tompkins LS, Wagner KF, et al.: Infection due to corynebacterium species in marrow transplant patients. *Ann Int Med* 1979;91:167–173.
44. Yolken RH, Bishop CA, Townsend TR, et al.: Infectious gastroenteritis in bone marrow transplant recipients. *N Engl J Med* 1982;306:1009–1012.
45. Kendra JR, Halil O, Barrett AJ: Tetanus after allogeneic bone marrow transplantation. *Br Med J* 1982;285:1393–1394.
46. Navari RM, Sullivan KM, Springmeyer SC, et al.: Mycobacterial infections in marrow transplant patients. *Transplantation* 1983;36:509–513.
47. Pizzo PA: Infectious complications in the child with cancer. I. Pathophysiology of the compromised host and the initial evaluation and management of the febrile cancer patient. *J Pediatr* 19812;98:341–354.
48. Peterson PK, McGlave P, Ramsay NK, et al.: Empirical antibacterial therapy in febrile, granulocytopenic bone marrow transplant patients. *Antimicrob Agents Chemother* 1984; 26:136–138.
49. Winston DJ, Meyer BV, Gale RP, Young LS, UCLA Bone Marrow Transplant team: Further experience with infections in BMT recipients. *Transplant Proc* 1978;10:247–254.
50. Winston DJ, Gale RP, Meyer BV, Young LS, UCLA Bone Marrow Transplant team: Infectious complications of human bone marrow transplantation. *Medicine* 1979;58:1–31.
51. Edwards JE, Lehrer RI, Stiehm ER, et al.: Severe candidal infections; clinical perspective, immune defense mechanisms, and current concepts of therapy. *Ann Int Med* 1978;89:91–106.
52. Miller GG, Witwer MW, Braude AI, Davis CE: Rapid identification of candida albicans septicemia in man by gas-liquid chromatography. *J Clin Invest* 1974;54:1235–1240.
53. Filice G, Yu B, Armstrong D: Immunodiffusion and agglutination tests for candida in patients with neoplastic disease; inconsistent correlation of results with invasive infections. *J Infect Dis* 1977;135:349–357.
54. Segal E, Berg RA, Pizzo PA, Bennett JE: Detection of candida antigen in sera of patients with candidiasis by an enzyme-linked immunosorbent assay-inhibition technique. *J Clin Microbiol* 1979;10:116–118.
55. Kiehn TE, Bernard EM, Gold JWM, Armstrong D: Candidiasis detection by gas-liquid chromatography of D-arabinitol, a fungal metabolite, in human serum. *Science* 1979; 206:577–580.
56. Kerkering TM, Espinel-Ingroff A, Shadom S: Detection of candida antigenemia by counterimmunoelectrophoresis in patients with invasive candidiasis. *J Infect Dis* 1979;140:659–664.
57. Walsh TJ, Catchatourian R, Cohen H: Disseminated histoplasmosis complicating bone marrow transplantation. *Am J Clin Path* 1983;79:509–511.
58. Myskowski PL, Brown AE, Dinsmore R, et al.: Mucomycosis following bone marrow transplantation. *J Am Acad Dermatol* 1983;9:111–115.
59. Gardella S, Nomdedieu B, Bombi JA, et al.: Fatal fungemia with arthritic involvement caused by *Trichosporon beigelii* in a bone marrow transplant recipient. *J Infect Dis* 1985;151:566.
60. Blazar BR, Hurd DD, Snover DC, et al.: Invasive fusarium infections in bone marrow transplant recipients. *Am J Med* 1984;77:645–651.

61. Gumbart CH: *Pseudallescheria boydii* infection after BMT. *Ann Int Med* 1983;99:193–194.
62. Hughes WT, Feldman S, Cox F: Infectious disease in children with cancer. *Pediatr Clin N Am* 1974;21(3):583–615.
63. Peterson PK, McGlave P, Ramsay NKC, et al.: A prospective study of infectious diseases following bone marrow transplant; emergence of aspergillus and CMV as the major causes of mortality. *Infect Control* 1983;4:81–89.
64. Armstrong D: Fungal infections in the compromised host. In, Young LS, Rubin RH (eds): *Clinical Approach to Infection in the Compromised Host.* Plenum Press, New York, 1981;pp.195–228.
65. McDonald GB, Sharma P, Hackman RC, et al.: Esophageal infections in immunosuppressed patients after marrow transplantation. *Gastroenterology* 1985;88:1111–1117.
66. Pizzo PA; Infectious complications in the child with cancer. II. Management of specific infectious organisms. *J Pediatr* 1981;98:513–523.
67. Young RC, Bennett JE, Vogel CL, et al.: Aspergillosis; the spectrum of disease in 98 patients. *Medicine* 1970;49:147–173.
68. Hann IM, Covingham R, Keaney M, et al.: Ketoconazole versus Nystatin plus amphotericin B for fungal prophylaxis in severely immunocompromised patients. *Lancet* 1982;1:826–829.
69. Van Lint MT, Bacigalupo A, Frassoni F, et al.: Ketoconazole vs. mepartricin for the prevention of candida infections in the immunocompromised host. *Exp Hematol* 1980;10(suppl):6–10.
70. Morgenstern GR, Powles R, Robinson B, McElwain TJ: Cyclosporin interaction with ketoconazole and melphalan. *Lancet* 1982;2:1342.
71. Rogers TR: Prevention of infection in neutropenic bone marrow transplant patients. *Antibiot Chemother* 1985;33:90–113.
72. Pizzo PA, Robichaud KJ, Gill FA, et al.: Duration of empiric antibiotic therapy in granulocytopenic patients with cancer. *Am J Med* 1979;67:194–200.
73. Feigin RD, Cherry JD (eds): *Textbook of Pediatric Infectious Disease,* W.B. Saunders Company, Philadelphia, 1981, p. 1495.
74. Bowden RA, Meyers JD: Infectious complications following marrow transplantation. *Plasma Ther Transfus Technol* 1985;6:285–302.
75. Wilson R, Feldman S: Toxicity of amphotericin B in children with cancer. *Am J Dis Child* 1979;133:731–734.
76. Gigliotti F, Shenep JL, Lott L, et al.: Induction of prostaglandin synthesis as the mechanism responsible for the chills and fever produced in fusing Amphotericin B. *J Infect Dis* 1987;156(5):784–789.
77. Kitahara M, Seth VK, Medoff G: Activity of amphotericin B, 5-fluorocytosine and rifampin against 6 clinical isolates of aspergillus. *Antimicrob Agents Chemother* 1976;9:915–919.
78. Saral R: Viral infections in bone marrow transplant recipients. *Plasma Ther Transfus Technol* 1985;6:275–284.
79. Meyers JD: Infections in marrow recipients. In, Mandell GL, Douglass RG, Bennett JE (eds): *Principles and Practice of Infectious Disease,* 2nd ed, John Wiley & Sons, New York, 1985, pp. 960–970 and 1674–1675.
80. Shields AF, Hackman RC, Fife KH, et al.: Adenovirus infections in patients undergoing bone marrow transplantation. *N Engl J Med* 1985;312:529–533.
81. Purtilo DT, White R, Filipovich A, et al.: Fulminant liver failure induced by adenovirus after bone marrow transplantation. *N Engl J Med* 1985;312:1707–1708.
82. O'Reilly RJ, Lee FK, Grossbard E, *et al.:* Papovirus excretion following marrow transplantation; incidence and association with hepatic dysfunction. *Transplant Proc* 1981;13(1):262–266.
83. Saral R, Burns WH, Laskin OL, et al.: Acyclovir prophylaxis of herpes simplex virus infections; a randomized, double-blind controlled trial in bone marrow transplant recipients. *N Engl J Med* 1981;305:63–67.
84. Gluckman E, Devergie A, Melo R, et al.: Prophylaxis of herpes infections after bone marrow transplantation by oral acyclovir. *Lancet* 1983;2:706–708.
85. Saral R, Burns WH, Prentice HG: Herpes virus infections; clinical manifestations and therapeutic strategies in immunocompromised patients. *Clin Hæmatol* 1984;13(3):645–660.
86. Hann IM, Prentice HG, Blacklock HA, et al.: Acyclovir prophylaxis against herpes virus infections in severely immunocompromised patients; randomized double-blind trial. *Br Med J* 1983;287:384–388.

87. Wade JC, Newton B, Flournoy N, Meyers JD: Oral acyclovir for prevention of herpes simplex virus reactivation after marrow transplantation. *Ann Int Med* 1984;100:823–828.
88. Shepp DH, Newton BA, Dandliker PS, et al.: Oral acyclovir therapy for mucocutaneous herpes simplex virus infections in immunocompromised marrow transplant recipients. *Ann Intern Med* 1985;102:783–785.
89. Schaeffer HJ, Beauchamp L, deMiranda P, et al.: 9-(2-hydroxyethoxymethyl)guanine activity against viruses of the herpes group. *Nature* 1978;272:583–585.
90. Wade JC, Day LM, Crowley JJ, Meyers JD: Recurrent infection with herpes simplex virus after marrow transplantation; role of the specific immune response and acyclovir treatment. *J Infect Dis* 1984;149(5):750–756.
91. Feldman S: Varicella zoster virus infection of the fetus, neonate and immunocompromised child. In, Aronoff S, Hughes WT (eds): *Advances in Pediatric Infectious Diseases*, Vol. I, Year Book Publishers, Chicago (in press).
92. Brigden D, Rosling AE, Woos NC: Renal function after acyclovir intravenous injection. *Am J Med* 1982;72(suppl):182–185.
93. Meyers JD, Flournoy N, Thomas ED: Cytomegalovirus infection and specific cell-mediated immunity after marrow transplant. *J Infect Dis* 1980;142(6):816–824.
94. Vilmer E, Mazeron MC, Rabian C, et al.: Clinical significance of cytomegalovirus viremia in bone marrow transplantation. *Transplantation* 1985;40:30–35.
95. Betts RF: Cytomegalovirus infection in transplant patients. *Progr Med Virol* 1982;28:44–64.
96. Diethelm AG, Gore I, Ch'ien LT, et al.: Gastrointestinal hemorrhage secondary to cytomegalovirus after renal transplantation. *Am J Surg* 1976;131:371–374.
97. Campbell DA, Piercey JRA, Shnitka TK, et al.: Cytomegalovirus-associated gastric ulcer. *Gastroenterology* 1977;72:533–535.
98. Meyers JD, Spencer HC, Watts JC, et al.: Cytomegalovirus pneumonia after human marrow transplantation. *Ann Int Med* 1975;82:181–188.
99. Chou S, Merigan TC: Rapid detection and quantitation of human cytomegalovirus in urine through DNA hybridization. *N Engl J Med* 1983;308:921.
100. Lee FK, Nahmias AJ, Stagno S: Rapid diagnosis of CMV infection in infants by electron microscopy. *N Engl J Med* 1978;299:1266.
101. Cheng Y-C, Huang E-S, Lin J-C, et al.: Unique spectrum of activity of 9-(1,3-dihydroxy-2-propoxy-methyl)-guanine against herpes virus *in vitro* and its mode of action against herpes simplex type 1. *Proc Natl Acad Sci USA* 1983;80:2767–2770.
102. Wingard JR, Stuart RK, Saral R, Burns WH: Activity of trifluorothymidine against cytomegalovirus. *Antimicrob Agents Chemother* 1981;20:286–290.
103. Masur H, Lane HC, Palestine A, et al.: Effects of 9-(1,3-dihydroxy-2-propoxymethyl) guanine on serious cytomegalovirus in 8 immunosuppressed homosexual men. *Ann Int Med* 1986;104:41–44.
104. Meyers JD, Leszczynski J, Zaia JA, et al.: Prevention of cytomegalovirus infection by cytomegalovirus immune globulin after marrow transplantation. *Ann Int Med* 1983;98:442–446.
105. Winston DJ, Pollard RB, Ho WG, et al.: Cytomegalovirus immune plasma in bone marrow transplant recipients. *Ann Int Med* 1982;97:11–18.
106. O'Reilly RJ, Reich L, Gold J, et al.: A randomized trial of intravenous hyperimmune globulin for the prevention of CMV infections following marrow transplantation; preliminary results. *Transplant Proc* 1983;15:1405–1411.
107. Yeager AS, Grumet FC, Hafleigh EB, et al.: Prevention of transfusion-acquired cytomegalovirus infections in newborn infants. *J Pediatr* 1981;98:281–287.
108. Whitley RJ, Soong S, Dolin R, et al., for the NAID Collaborative Antiviral Study Group: Early vidarabine therapy to control the complications of herpes zoster in immunosuppressed patients. *N Engl J Med* 1982;307:971–975.
109. Meyers JD, Wade JC, Shepp DH, Newton B: Acyclovir treatment of varicella zoster virus infection in the compromised host. *Transplantation* 1984;37:571–574.
110. Shepp DH, Dandliker PS, Meyers JD: Treatment of the virus infection in severely immunocompromised patients with randomized comparison of acyclovir and vidarabine. *N Engl J Med* 1986;314:208–212.
111. Lange B, Henle W, Meyers JD, et al.: Epstein-Barr virus-related serology in marrow transplant recipients. *Int J Cancer* 1980;26:151–157.

112. Sullivan JL, Wallen WC, Johnson FL: Epstein-Barr virus infection following bone marrow transplantation. *Int J Cancer* 1978;22:132–135.
113. Shearer WT, Ritz J, Finegold MJ, et al.: Epstein-Barr virus-associated B-cell proliferations of diverse clonal origins after bone marrow transplantation in a 12-year-old patient with severe combined immunodeficiency. *N Engl J Med* 1985;312:1151–1159.
114. Martin PJ, Shulman HM, Schubach WH, et al.: Fatal Epstein-Barr virus-associated proliferation of donor B cells after treatment of acute graft-vs.-host disease with a murine anti-T cell antibody. *Ann Int Med* 1984;101:310–315.
115. Townsend TR, Yolken RH, Bishop CA, et al.: Outbreak of Coxsackie A1 gastroenteritis; a complication of bone marrow transplantation. *Lancet* 1982;1:820–822.
116. Zahradnik JM, Spencer MJ, Porter DD: Adenovirus infection in the immunocompromised patient. *Am J Med* 1980;68:725–732.
117. Johnson FL, Schofer O: Pneumonitis in bone marrow transplant recipients. In, Laraya-Cuasay J, Hughes W (eds): *Interstitial Lung Diseases in Children*. CRC Press, Boca Raton, Florida, 1986;(in press).
118. Weiner RS, Bortin MM, Gale RP, et al.: Interstitial pneumonitis after bone marrow transplantation; assessment of risk factors. *Ann Int Med* 1986;104:168–175.
119. Bortin MM, Kay HEM, Gale RP, Rimm AA: Factors associated with interstitial pneumonitis after bone marrow transplantation for acute leukemia. *Lancet* 1982;1:437–439.
120. Meyers JD, Flournoy N, Thomas ED: Risk factors for cytomegalovirus infection after human marrow transplantation. *J Infect Dis* 1986;153:478–488.
121. Graham-Pole J. Camitta B, Casper J, et al.: Intravenous immunoglobulin may lessen all forms of infection in patients receiving allogeneic bone marrow transplantation for acute lymphoblastic leukemia: A Pediatric Oncology Group Study. *Bone Marrow Transplantation* 1988;3:559–566.
122. Stiehm ER, Ashida E, Kim KS, et al.: Intravenous Immunoglobulins as therapeutic Agents, A UCLA Conference. *Ann Int Med* 1987;107:367–382.
123. Neiman PE, Reeves W, Ray G, et al.: A prospective analysis of interstitial pneumonia and opportunistic viral infection among recipients of allogeneic bone marrow grafts. *J Infect Dis* 1977;136:754–767.
124. Hughes WT: Treatment of pneumoncystis carinii pneumonitis. *N Engl J Med* 1976;295:726–727.
125. Hirsch R, Burke BA, Kersey JH: Toxoplasmosis in bone marrow transplant recipients. *J Pediatr* 1984;105:426–428.
126. Brandt SJ, Peters WP, Atwater S: Effect of recombinant granulocyte-macrophage colony-stimulating factor on hematopoietic reconstitution after high-dose chemotherapy and autologous bone marrow transplantation. *N Engl J Med* 1988;318:869–876.
127. Nemunaitis J, Singer JW, Buckner CD, et al: Use of Recombinant human granulocyte-macrophage colony stimulating factor in autologous marrow transplantation for lymphoid malignancies. *Blood* 1988;72:834–836.

Bone Marrow Transplantation in Children, edited by F. Leonard Johnson and Carl Pochedly. Raven Press, Ltd., New York © 1990.

Treatment and Prevention of Graft-vs.-Host Disease

Michael E. Trigg

Pediatric Bone Marrow Transplantation Program, Department of Pediatrics, University of Iowa School of Medicine, and University of Iowa Hospitals and Clinics, Iowa City, Iowa 52242

Introduction
A. What is graft-vs.-host disease and when does it occur?
B. Clinical features
C. Treatment of graft-vs.-host disease
D. Prevention of graft-vs.-host disease
E. Effect of graft-vs.-host disease on duration of survival and rate of recurrence of leukemia
F. Predictors of unfavorable outcome of graft-vs.-host disease
Summary

INTRODUCTION

When viable lymphocytes capable of growth are introduced from one person into another, the environment in that new person may allow these lymphocytes to proliferate. The disorder that results from the reaction of the infused lymphocytes against new tissues is called graft-vs.-host disease. This is not a new disorder. However, it was not recognized until there was a more fundamental understanding of basic immunology in the late 1950s and early 1960s (1).

Along with the increase in number of bone marrow transplant centers, there was increased use of marrow transplantation to treat patients with aplastic anemia, malignancies (such as leukemias resistant to conventional therapy), and genetic diseases. As a result, more pediatric hematologists are now caring for children who have undergone bone marrow transplants and are susceptible to graft-vs.-host disease. Furthermore, more children are now being treated with curative intensive chemotherapy, radiotherapy, or both, for malignancies. As a result of the intensive immunosuppressive effects of this therapy, these children are also susceptible to developing graft-vs.-host disease if they are transfused with blood that contains viable lymphocytes capable of proliferating (2).

During the past few years, there have been a number of clinical trials in search of new ways to treat or prevent graft-vs.-host disease. We now understand more about this complication and its role in bone marrow transplantation. We also see our limitations in understanding how to control this disease and how it may be used for the benefit of the patient undergoing a transplant (3,4). This chapter will present the various modalities for treatment of graft-vs.-host disease and ways to prevent it, as well as the impact of this complication on the outcome of a bone marrow transplant.

WHAT IS GRAFT-VS.-HOST DISEASE AND WHEN DOES IT OCCUR?

Graft-vs.-host disease occurs when viable lymphocytes are transferred from one person to another and those lymphocytes are then allowed to proliferate (1). In the normal course of a blood transfusion, lymphocytes are generally given from one person to another. However, the intact host immune system will recognize those lymphocytes as being foreign and will destroy them. In this way the transfused lymphocytes are prevented from proliferating; they are not able to recognize the new host as foreign and do not react against various tissues in the new host (2). However, when the person receiving lymphocytes, such as through a blood transfusion or through a bone marrow transplant, is immunosuppressed, he is not capable of recognizing the new lymphocytes as being foreign. The lymphocytes are then capable of growing and reacting against tissues of the new host.

A child may be immunosuppressed due to intensive chemotherapy or radiation, due to the preparative regimen given before bone marrow transplantation, or due to high-dose steroid treatment for chronic renal disease. A child may receive viable lymphocytes by transfusion of blood products, or by being given a transplant of a hematopoietic organ, such as a pancreas transplant with part of the spleen attached. Patients in any of these situations are susceptible to graft-vs.-host disease if appropriate measures are not taken to prevent the newly introduced T lymphocytes from proliferating (2).

Graft-vs.-host disease usually does not occur when viable lymphocytes are transferred from one syngeneic twin to another (5). Modern techniques for histocompatibility testing and mixed lymphocyte culture (MLC) are used to determine tissue identity between one individual and another. However, use of these tests will not necessarily predict for or against the occurrence of graft-vs.-host disease in a bone marrow transplant patient (5). For example, approximately 25% of children undergoing a bone marrow transplant who receive marrow from a donor who is HLA compatible and MLC nonreactive, will still develop significant graft-vs.-host disease. This will occur even when appropriate medications are given to try to minimize such an occurrence (6). Thus, modern histocompatibility testing does not reveal or predict the types of immunologic reactions that can occur *in vivo* that result in graft-vs.-host disease. Host immunoincompetence is the ultimate prerequisite for the development of this complication (7).

When a mixed lymphocyte culture test is performed, lymphocytes from one person are mixed with lymphocytes of another to see whether the cells will recognize each other as foreign. In this test, cells from one person are irradiated in a tissue culture flask, thereby rendering them incapable of growing and proliferating. But the cells are still intact so that their surface antigens can be recognized by other cells. The irradiated lymphocytes are then mixed with lymphocytes from another person. The other person's cells are allowed to react against the tested lymphocytes by proliferating and incorporating a radioactive isotope. The extent of incorporation of isotope can be quantitated as a measure of cell growth. If the lymphocytes react in this way, then two individuals are recognized as being not perfectly histocompatible.

It generally takes between 4 and 7 days for lymphocytes that are expected to respond to foreign tissues to display a sufficient degree of response *in vitro* that can be quantitated. Thus the mixed lymphocyte culture test is an *in vitro* laboratory model used to predict whether graft-vs.-host disease will appear following the introduction of lymphocytes that are viable and capable of proliferation in an immunoimcompetent host. Thus, following a bone marrow transplant where the marrow has been infused soon after it was harvested without any *in vitro* manipulation, graft-vs.-host disease generally will appear within about 7 to 10 days after the transplant (5). The delay between marrow transplant and appearance of graft-vs.-host disease is due to the time it takes for those new lymphocytes to respond to the foreign histocompatibility antigens present in the new host.

Graft-vs.-host disease primarily occurs following introduction of hematopoietic tissue. The introduced foreign hematopoietic tissue may be in the form of bone marrow, in bone marrow transplantation, or spleen cells associated with a pancreas transplant. But graft-vs.-host disease has been well recognized to occur following the introduction of any blood product, including concentrates of platelets, granulocytes or red cells, or plasma. These blood products must be irradiated to render any contaminating lymphocytes that may be present incapable of growth and graft-vs.-host reactions (2). Furthermore, autotransfusions from a mother to a congenitally immune deficient infant at the time of birth have also resulted in graft-vs.-host disease in the infant (8). Likewise, premature infants, lacking a competent immune system, may also be susceptible to graft-vs.-host disease even if they are not receiving medications to suppress the immune system and have no underlying congenital immune deficiency (9) (Table 1).

TABLE 1. *When does graft-vs.-host disease occur?*

1. Following bone marrow transplantation
2. Following pancreas transplant with spleen tissue attached
3. Following transfusion of nonirradiated blood products in an immunocompromised host
4. Following autotransfusions from mother to an immune deficient child
5. (?) In premature infants

CLINICAL FEATURES

Acute graft-vs.-host disease usually occurs within the first 100 days following a bone marrow transplant and is generally associated with skin, gastrointestinal and hepatic manifestations (5). The first evidence of graft-vs.-host disease usually recognized is skin involvement. The skin usually takes on a characteristic appearance (Table 2). There is an erythematous maculopapular rash which is usually most prominent on the palms and soles and the upper part of the back and chest. This rash may eventually involve the entire body with a total sunburn-like appearance. During its worst stages the skin rash will resemble toxic epidermal necrolysis, with bullae formation and desquamation.

Such extensive skin involvement not only results in fluid and electrolyte imbalances but also may result in the introduction of organisms into the immunoincompetent host. Areas of previous skin abnormalities, such as radiation burns or areas of severe eczema that a child with Wiskott-Aldrich syndrome may have had pre-transplant are the commonest areas initially involved by the graft-vs.-host reaction.

When the gastrointestinal tract is involved, diarrhea is the most common symptom. The grading system of graft-vs.-host disease as developed by the Seattle group measures the extent of gastrointestinal involvement by the volume of diarrhea produced per day (see Chapter 20) (5). These criteria cannot be used to grade gastrointestinal graft-vs.-host disease in children since the amount of diarrhea it takes to be significant in a child is much less than that in an adult. However, it is clear that the presence of abdominal cramping and bloody stools is a sign of significant gastrointestinal involvement.

Unfortunately, infection by numerous opportunistic microorganisms may result in extensive diarrhea. Also, the chemotherapy-radiotherapy regimens used to ablate the patient's abnormal marrow prior to transplant may also disturb the enteric bacterial flora. The preparative regimen may also prevent growth of gastrointestinal mucosal cells and thus result in massive diarrhea mimicking intestinal graft-vs.-host disease. Because of this possibility, biopsies of rectal mucosal or small bowel mucosa may be necessary in order to differentiate between an infectious diarrhea or a medication-induced

TABLE 2. *Clinical features of acute graft-vs.-host disease*

1. Skin involvement:
    maculopapular rash
    bullae formation
    desquamation
2. GI tract involvement:
    diarrhea
3. Hepatic involvement
    jaundice (cholestatic)
    hepatocellular death
4. Hematopoietic-lymphoid involvement
    lymphopenia
    anemia, leukopenia, thrombocytopenia
5. Widespread infections

diarrhea, as opposed to diarrhea produced by graft-vs.-host disease. Once adequate treatment for graft-vs.-host disease has been started, then the secretory diarrhea usually will resolve.

The liver is the third most commonly involved organ. Liver necrosis and cholestatic jaundice are the acute findings that usually result. The extent of the rise in bilirubin has been established as the most reliable measure of the extent of liver involvement (5). The acute graft-vs.-host reaction also results in lymphocyte depletion. This depletion of lymphocytes is seen particularly in lymph nodes, in the thymus and spleen, as well as in the peripheral blood. This lymphopenia causes a worsening of the immunoincompetent state of the host. Furthermore, the implanted and proliferating new bone marrow may be inhibited both by the severe graft-vs.-host reaction and by infections that result because of the entry of microorganisms through the denuded gastrointestinal tract or skin.

A matrix-supporting cell of the bone marrow, which is derived from the host and not from donor bone marrow, was recently discovered. The normal presence of these cells suggests that one of the target organs of the graft-vs.-host reaction is the bone marrow matrix itself. Loss of these matrix-supporting cells thereby results in a disturbance to the bone marrow matrix and a loss of bone marrow growth. (10) This concept would explain the persistent thrombocytopenia and neutropenia that accompany severe acute graft-vs.-host disease.

In any event, the most common problems in acute graft-vs.-host disease are widespread infections due to opportunistic microorganisms for which there are few if any effective antimicrobial drugs. In some patients, these acute graft-vs.-host reactions resolve with adequate treatment, as if the invading lymphocytes have learned to tolerate the new host. Unfortunately in other patients, periodic exacerbations of these acute graft-vs.-host reactions occur for many years following a transplant. Some of these acute reactions change in severity, or a new end-organ disease may result, thus producing a more chronic form of graft-vs.-

host disease (11). These chronic manifestations frequently do not appear for at least 3 to 4 months following a bone marrow transplant, and they may easily go unrecognized except to the careful observer.

As already mentioned, the skin is the primary target organ and the organ most likely to show evidence of a chronic or persisting graft-vs.-host disease. Cutaneous changes such as dystrophic nails, hyperpigmentation, palmar and planter erythema, vitiligo and partial alopecia may all be signs of graft-vs.-host disease. The skin is frequently thickened and dry and, in more severe cases, the skin may be scleroderma-like in appearance. Fibrosis and tightening of the skin over bony prominences and around joints may result in skeletal contractures.

The gastrointestinal and secretory glands are the next most likely to be affected. Patients with these types of involvement have complaints of dryness in mucous membranes of the nose, mouth, and eyes. Some patients may even complain that they cannot swallow solid food without consuming liquids at the same time (12). Dysphagia, weight loss, anorexia and regurgitation as well as malabsorption are all signs of chronic graft-vs.-host disease.

Synthetic and metabolic functions of liver cells are generally preserved, even with chronic graft-vs.-host disease. But elevations of serum bilirubin and alkaline phosphatase are quite common. Hepatomegaly and reticuloen-dothelial dysfunction may be permanent, resulting in an increased risk to infection from opportunistic microorganisms.

Many of the features of chronic graft-vs.-host disease are similar to the autoimmune phenomena associated with collagen vascular diseases. Likewise, the treatment of chronic graft-vs.-host disease in some circumstances is similar to that used for an autoimmune collagen vascular disease.

Because of the reaction to lymphoid tissues throughout the body, lymphopenia and chronic immunologic deficiencies are a hallmark of severe chronic graft-vs.-host disease (13). Lymphocytic infiltrations into the bronchial tree, as well as disturbances in the action of cilia and impaired mucous production, increase the likelihood of pulmonary infections.

Unfortunately, some of the changes, particularly those in the respiratory tract and the skin that may be ascribed to graft-vs.-host disease, may also be due to the effects of chemotherapy, irradiation, or both, which were given as part of the pre-transplant regimen to ablate the patient's marrow. Thus, in some patients it is difficult to differentiate between the effects of the treatment given and the reaction due to histoincompatibility between the donor and the recipient. For that reason, treatment that would result in improvement of symptoms if the problem were due to graft-vs.-host disease results in no substantial benefit. This failure to improve suggests that the underlying cause of the symptoms present is not due entirely to graft-vs.-host disease.

TREATMENT OF GRAFT-VS.-HOST DISEASE

Experience with the first bone marrow transplants showed that even marrow from HLA-MLC matched donors can cause graft-vs.-host disease. Thus, it is now commonly assumed that efforts for prevention of graft-vs.-host disease are needed for all patients (5). For that reason, most children and adults undergoing a bone marrow transplant will receive medications to prevent graft-vs.-host disease during the first three months post-transplant. The exact types of regimens and medications used will be presented in the next section.

In 1984 the incidence of graft-vs.-host disease in patients not given prophylactic medications was documented (14). This study by the Cleveland group was nonrandomized. The study was simply a retrospective review of the incidence of graft-vs.-host disease in children undergoing marrow transplantation for aplastic anemia or for treatment of resistant malignancies. In the group of 41 patients under 20 years of age, there was no difference in the incidence and severity of acute graft-vs.-host disease in the group receiving prophylactic methotrexate and the group not receiving prophylactic methotrexate. This finding suggests that the incidence of graft-vs.-host disease is low in children undergoing transplantation with marrow from a matched, related donor. When graft-vs.-host disease occurs, selection of drugs for treatment of the condition depends upon the patient's response to drugs given previously.

The majority of children undergoing bone marrow transplantation to this day, despite the findings of the Cleveland group, receive prophylactic medications to prevent graft-vs.-host disease (15). The established regimen at the present time is a combination of methotrexate and cyclosporine, as originally proposed by the Seattle group (16,17). If patients develop significant graft-vs.-host disease while receiving methotrexate and cyclosporine, usually the cyclosporine dose is increased or prednisone is added. Prednisone is given either in an oral form if intestinal absorption is intact or it is given as intravenous methylprednisolone (Table 3).

The vast majority of patients who develop signs of graft-vs.-host disease while receiving methotrexate and cyclosporine will respond to the addition of a corticosteroid. Those patients who have not been on cyclosporine usually will be started on cyclosporine at the time they develop graft-vs.-host disease (18,19). For many years, antilymphocyte globulin (ALG) or antithymocyte globulin (ATG) have been used only for prevention and not as treatment (15,20,21). However, results of certain studies suggest that ALG and ATG are effective for treatment of acute graft-vs.-host disease (21).

If the graft-vs.-host disease fails to respond to the addition of prednisone (in a dose of 2–4 mg/kg/day) or cyclosporine, then usually additional treatment is necessary. This treatment is needed to prevent the debilitating side effects of significant skin involvement or hepatic compromise, or loss of gastrointestinal fluid and electrolytes (22). A commonly used approach to therapy is the use of high-dose methylprednisolone at 2 gm/m^2/day (23). The time it takes for significant skin, gut, and hepatic graft-vs.-host disease to resolve has been documented. It was shown that well-established acute graft-vs.-host disease will not disappear quickly. Although the skin may improve within 7 to 10 days, significant improvement of hepatic and gastrointestinal involvement by graft-vs.-host disease may take longer. In fact, it may take 3 or 4 weeks

TABLE 3. *Drugs and modalities used in treatment of graft-vs.-host disease*

---

1. Prednisone or methylprednisolone
2. Cyclosporine
3. Antilymphocyte globulin
   Antithymocyte globulin
4. Anti-T lymphocyte monoclonal antibodies
5. Topical moisturizers

---

before signs of significant liver necrosis disappears and serum bilirubin levels return to normal. Thus, once significant graft-vs.-host disease has been established, adequate supportive care during a period of waiting is necessary in order for medications to show their beneficial effects.

Although the exact T cell subtype responsible for acute graft-vs.-host disease has not yet been identified, anti-T lymphocyte antibodies have been used in an effort to treat this reaction. Several of these antibodies appear to be very promising and are available in experimental protocols (24). Unfortunately, if a child fails to respond quickly to the antibody preparation, resistance develops. This resistance to antibody therapy is either because of the formation of antimouse antibodies (the monoclonal antibodies being of mouse origin) or somehow a new population of T lymphocytes develops which is resistant to the antibody given.

Most attention has been given to the treatment of the skin involvement by graft-vs.-host disease. This is because skin involvement tends to be the most debilitating feature, and the manifestation that makes patients the most self-conscious about having undergone a bone marrow transplant. Frequent baths and use of drying soaps are avoided. The main goal of treatment is to keep the skin moist, either with a variety of moisturizing creams or by the use of topical steroids. Areas of vitiligo formation secondary to chronic inflammatory changes in the skin may require application of cosmetic creams to cover the skin blemishes (11). Occasionally, some children develop significant scleroderma-like changes requiring treatment with ultrasound and whirlpool to stretch the skin and keep skin contractures from forming, particularly around joints (11).

The use of unrelated donors or donors whose cells are reactive in mixed lymphocyte culture, and who are not completely HLA identical, results in a significant increase in the incidence of acute graft-vs.-host disease (25–29). For that reason, physicians treating such patients have a wide variety of choices as to regimens for treating acute graft-vs.-host disease that occurs in spite of the use of adequate preventive measures. In many situations, there is no rationale for choosing one treatment instead of another. However, individual clinicians will have had more experience with one regimen than another. This individual experience frequently guides the selection of treatment.

The important point to remember is that all of the drugs used to treat well-established acute graft-vs.-host disease are immunosuppressive and will cause lymphopenia. During times of acute exacerbation of symptoms of graft-vs.-host disease and increased immunosuppression, patients are much more susceptible to opportunistic infections, particularly from fungi. These patients need to be observed very closely.

The vast majority of deaths in patients who are more than 30 days from the time of bone marrow transplant, during times when the blood counts are adequate, occurs while the child is often undergoing treatment for an exacerbation of acute graft-vs.-host disease. At this time, the patient was being given increased doses of cyclosporine or prednisone. The beneficial effects of individual infection prophylactic medications, such as acyclovir and high-dose gamma globulin, have now been clearly shown in controlled trials. However, whether the combination of several prophylactic antimicrobials together with the use of high-dose gamma globulin will provide adequate protection during periods of time when the child is receiving increased immunosuppression is not known. This possibility probably will not be adequately studied because of current efforts to try to minimize or to entirely prevent graft-vs.-host disease.

PREVENTION OF GRAFT-VS.-HOST DISEASE

The use of post-transplant immunosuppression to prevent graft-vs.-host disease originated from studies done in dogs (16). Based upon the use of methotrexate in severe graft-vs.-host disease that developed within 2 weeks after marrow transplantation in the dogs, the use of methotrexate became widespread (30). Initially, the regimen consisted of giving methotrexate intravenously 1 to several days prior to the marrow infusion, and continuing to give the drug until at least 3 months post-bone marrow transplant. However since that time, various changes in this regimen have been introduced. Now patients usually receive 1 dose pre-transplant and 4–6 doses post-transplant (31).

Because acute graft-vs.-host disease has continued to be the major impediment to successful outcome following transplantation, new regimens for post-transplant immunosuppression have been studied (32). Most of these studies are flawed from the pediatric viewpoint because they include adults. Also, it was not until publication of the report of the Cleveland group that the true incidence of graft-vs.-host disease in children could be assessed (14). The Cleveland study was a retrospective review of the outcome of children undergoing transplantation with or without methotrexate having been given post-transplant for immunosuppression. The results showed that the incidence and severity of graft-vs.-host disease were essentially the same in the 2 groups of patients (14). The only major difference that was noted between the groups was the delay in hematopoietic recovery in the group of children who received methotrexate. This finding was no surprise considering the fact

TABLE 4. *Drugs and modalities used to prevent graft-vs.-host disease*

1.	Methotrexate
2.	Methotrexate, prednisone, and antithymocyte globulin
3.	Cyclosporine
4.	Methotrexate and cyclosporine
5.	Prednisone
6.	Cyclophosphamide
7.	T lymphocyte depletion of donor marrow
8.	Antilymphocyte globulin and prednisone

that methotrexate had been widely used as a chemotherapeutic agent, and its suppressive effects on hematopoiesis are well known.

A randomized study was done comparing the use of methotrexate to a triple combination of prednisone, methotrexate and antithymocyte globulin. This study showed a significant advantage to use of the triple combination in preventing graft-vs.-host disease (15). However, the advantage was most pronounced in those patients over 19 years of age. In fact, in children under the age of 12, there were essentially no cases of acute graft-vs.-host disease in either treatment group.

The incidence of severe, acute graft-vs.-host disease has been estimated to be as high as 50%, but most authorities consider the incidence of graft-vs.-host disease in children to be about 25%. In marrow recipients under 10 years of age, the actual incidence of graft-vs.-host disease may be no greater than 10%.

Cyclosporine is an effective immunosuppressive agent which has been shown to prevent organ rejection in animals. Initially, cyclosporine was used to treat well-established cases of graft-vs.-host disease. It was found to be ineffective, although more recent findings would suggest otherwise (19,33). Cyclosporine has been used in a variety of prophylactic regimens to prevent acute graft-vs.-host disease and was shown to be very effective. More recently, combinations of methotrexate and cyclosporine have been shown to be far superior in preventing acute graft-vs.-host disease to the use of methotrexate alone (17).

Other studies have shown that the use of prednisone alone, or prednisone in combination with other immunosuppressive agents, to be equally as effective (15). Low-dose cyclophosphamide has been successfully used to prevent acute graft-vs.-host disease, but most of the patients studied were adults (32).

Each of the drugs used in a prophylactic manner to prevent graft-vs.-host disease is associated with unique toxicities. Cyclosporine consistently causes increases in creatinine and blood pressure. These complications may present significant problems in the early post-transplant course, considering the fact that numerous nephrotoxic antibiotics are being used during that same time. Cyclophosphamide and methotrexate are known inhibitors of hematopoiesis and may delay bone marrow recovery following transplantation. Prednisone on the one hand may help stimulate hematopoiesis, but it may be immunosuppressive enough to result in an increased incidence of infections. Preventing severe, acute graft-vs.-host disease still remains a laudable goal. This reaction is associated with an increased incidence of infections due to breakdown in the skin and gastrointestinal mucosa, and there are also significant abnormalities in hepatic functions.

It is well established that T lymphocytes are responsible for acute graft-vs.-host disease. Thus, the question was asked as to whether the removal of T lymphocytes from the donor graft would help prevent graft-vs.-host disease (34,35). This was accomplished using antibodies directed against T lymphocytes and complement to treat the marrow *in vitro* to remove T lymphocytes. A variety of techniques have been used to deplete T lymphocytes from donor bone marrow (36–38).

The most popular method for T lymphocyte depletion of the bone marrow is by the use of an anti-T lymphocyte antibody and complement (26). The antibodies initially used are primarily of murine origin and of IgG_2 class. The most popular antibody now is Campath I, a rat monoclonal antibody of the IgG_2 class (39). Several IgM antibodies have also been developed and were found to be highly effective in removing T lymphocytes from bone marrow (37). One study showed that T lymphocytes are destroyed by treating bone marrow with a nonlytic antibody alone and infusing the antibody coated cells into the transplant recipient where the T lymphocytes presumably were engulfed by cells of the reticuloendothelial system. However, most authorities believe that the reticuloendothelial system cannot remove such antibody-coated cells (39). For that reason, it is important to kill the T lymphocytes *in vitro* before infusing them into the recipient.

Since these early studies were done, a number of other methods have been developed to remove T lymphocytes. These methods include the use of various centrifugation techniques with or without lectins, as well as the use of sheep red cell rosetting. These are the classic ways of identifying human T lymphocytes and removing them from preparations of mononuclear cells. Other methods for using antibodies to remove T lymphocytes from the bone marrow include attaching magnetic particles to the antibody and passing the treated marrow through magnetic fields, thereby physically pulling T lymphocytes from the marrow solution. Another technique involves attaching drugs to the anti-T cell antibodies, thereby poisoning the cells coated with the antibody, and then attaching radioactive isotopes to the antibodies; the isotope delivers a small amount of irradiation to any cell binding to the labeled antibodies. One of the most novel techniques developed was to attach the known plant toxin, ricin, to an anti-T cell antibody. Cells reacting with the antibody eventually ingest both the antibody and ricin and are poisoned. These cells usually die within 24 hours after the ingestion of the ricin (26).

All methods to remove T lymphocytes from marrow are effective *in vitro*.

However, the true test comes when such T lymphocyte depleted bone marrow is used to reconstitute patients whose marrow has been ablated by pre-transplant conditioning. In this regard, trials have produced a wide variety of results in preventing acute graft-vs.-host disease. One trial in children and adults showed that the use of T lymphocyte depleted bone marrow from a matched sibling donor resulted in little to no acute graft-vs.-host disease, even when no prophylactic immunosuppressive drugs were given (28). Others have subsequently confirmed those results, primarily in studies in adults (39). On the other hand, use of these techniques for T lymphocyte depletion have produced a variety of new problems which were not so commonly seen previously (40).

The rate of failure to achieve sustained engraftment of donor marrow is higher than expected in recipients of T lymphocyte depleted bone marrow, even when the donor is a perfect HLA-MLC match with the recipient (41). In select situations, graft rejection has been clearly documented. This finding suggests that the ablative regimen used pre-transplant was not sufficient to result in the total elimination of host T lymphocytes. These lymphocytes then regrew and, when they recognized the new marrow as foreign, they rejected it (40). However, the incidence of graft rejection in a patient undergoing a marrow transplant with a matched, related donor for treatment of acute leukemia had previously been thought to occur with an incidence of less than 1%. Thus, transplanters are left with the difficult task of explaining the high rate of rejection in these clinical situations even with use of T lymphocyte depleted bone marrow (7). The simplest explanation is that there are residual populations of host T lymphocytes remaining in every individual following the ablative therapy given pre-transplant. The donor lymphocytes infused in an unmanipulated marrow graft respond to these host T lymphocytes, and suppress their growth, therefore allowing the new marrow graft to take hold.

In the absence of donor T lymphocytes, the recipient T lymphocytes regrow, thereby rejecting the graft (7). For that reason, some have suggested that a minimum number of T lymphocytes must remain in the donor graft following T lymphocyte depletion. Furthermore, if that minimum number is not present, then additional T lymphocytes should be added in order to allow the graft to take. The latter suggestions may explain why the addition of peripheral buffy coat cells in the initial donor marrow infusion by the Seattle group resulted in fewer graft rejections, better graft takes, and a superior transplant outcome (42).

In addition, some of the methods used to deplete T lymphocytes result in the loss of a significant percentage of normal marrow cells. Graft failure in these situations may be secondary to lack of an adequate dose of infused marrow. This loss of cells has been more commonly associated with the lectin depletion and sheep red blood cell rosetting techniques. With use of these T lymphocyte depletion techniques, only 5–10% of the nucleated marrow cells harvested in the operating room remain after the depletion procedure, and this number of viable bone marrow cells may be insufficient to allow the graft to take (36).

T lymphocyte depletion techniques have also been used in the transplant setting when using a closely matched unrelated donor, or with the use of haplo-identical donors (40). Early experience with these alternative donor types resulted in the expected increased incidence of acute graft-vs.-host disease. The increase in graft-vs.-host disease occurred because of minor histocompatibility differences between donor and recipient or the occurrence of positive MLC reactions between donor and recipient (40,43). Conventional means of preventing graft-vs.-host disease by the use of methotrexate, cyclosporine or steroids have been found by themselves to be inadequate. Thus, T lymphocyte depletion of donor marrow has been used extensively in these clinical situations (28,40).

In order to overcome host resistance to graft take, increased immunosuppression has been found to be necessary by most transplant groups. This increased immunosuppression usually takes the form of increased chemotherapy pre-transplant to further immunosuppress the host and allow the take of new marrow, particularly with use of T lymphocyte depleted marrow (28,44). Only a few investigators have been able to achieve success in getting such marrow grafts to take. Nevertheless, the use of T lymphocyte depletion techniques in this clinical situation and the incidence of graft failure highlight a lack of understanding as to what donor and recipient T lymphocytes actually do. The high incidence of graft failure focuses attention on the interaction between donor and recipient T lymphocytes during the early stages of marrow transplantation (7). Why some investigators have more success than others in getting marrow engraftment may not be solely related to the class of cells removed by the various T lymphocyte depleting techniques or the extent of T lymphocyte depletion. Instead, this difference in rate of marrow engraftment may relate to other factors such as selection of patients and type of immunosuppression used. These marrow transplant techniques are novel enough to deserve further study.

Besides a decreased incidence of acute graft-vs.-host disease, T lymphocyte depletion has also resulted in an increased incidence of unusual opportunistic infections. The most worrisome of these infections is a lymphoproliferative disorder associated with Epstein-Barr virus (40). Although the Epstein-Barr virus has been thought to be associated with a number of infectious problems following transplant, the number of cases of fatal lymphoproliferative disorders after marrow transplants with unmanipulated marrow is nil. However, numerous investigators have reported cases of fatal lymphoproliferative disorders after the use of T lymphocyte depleted marrow. This finding suggests that the lack of T lymphocytes allows infected B cells that either come from the donor, that are infused with blood product transfusions, or that arise due to an acquired infection to develop and grow unchecked. In a few cases, the prophylactic use of acyclovir has been found to result in a decreased incidence of these lymphoproliferative disorders (45).

In continuing trials of bone marrow transplantation in children, a combination of antilymphocyte globulin and prednisone together with T lymphocyte depletion is used. The immunosuppression is used in order to get effective engraftment of marrow from an unrelated donor, or engraftment of marrow from a haplo-identical donor with an extremely low incidence of acute graft-vs.-host disease (less than 5%) within the first several weeks postgrafting. However, once the ALG is discontinued and the graft has taken hold (at least 95% of children will engraft with these techniques), the incidence of acute graft-vs.-host disease rises to about 25 to 50%. The graft-vs.-host disease occurring after engraftment has occurred is usually quite controllable, with very few fatal cases. In adults, controlled trials for study of prevention of graft-vs.-host disease are now going on in patients receiving marrow grafts from closely matched unrelated donors. These studies are comparing use of T lymphocyte depletion in one group to the use of cyclosporine in the other group.

A variety of other techniques and modalities have been used to prevent acute graft-vs.-host disease (46,47). The only one that has been found to be significantly effective in randomized controlled trials was the use of laminar airflow rooms (48). Reduced mortality was particularly evident within the first 4 months after marrow transplantation and was associated with a reduction in the incidence of acute graft-vs.-host disease or delay of onset of this complication. It had been previously well established in animal models that the use of laminar airflow isolation results in a decreased incidence of severe infection, and the occurrence of fewer severe infections is thought to result in a decreased incidence of acute graft-vs.-host disease. Thus, the occurrence of fewer infections and, therefore, the decreased incidence of graft-vs.-host disease produced an improved outcome in patients with aplastic anemia undergoing marrow grafting from HLA-identical siblings.

However, other studies have shown a similar rate and duration of survival in aplastic anemia patients without use of such extensive protective environmental isolation. This finding confirms the fact that the nature of the supportive techniques used at one institution as compared with those used in another have a major impact on transplant outcome. Thus, it is impossible to know for certain whether a technique developed in one transplant center need be applied across the board in all transplant centers if the outcome is reasonably comparable. (49).

EFFECT OF GRAFT-VS.-HOST DISEASE ON DURATION OF SURVIVAL AND RATE OF RECURRENCE OF LEUKEMIA

In patients following marrow transplantation, the incidence and severity of graft-vs.-host disease increases with age (5). This fact has been well demonstrated by a number of studies. The effect of age on survival is most pronounced in patients older than 30 years of age undergoing marrow transplantation for treatment of a malignancy. On the other hand, there appears to be little information regarding the effect of age on occurrence of graft-vs.-host disease in patients less than 20 years old. One study showed a very low incidence of graft-vs.-host disease in children under 12 years of age (15). Also, anecdotal experience suggests that, in the patient with an immune deficiency, acute graft-vs.-host disease almost never occurs when marrow from a matched donor is used (50). However, overall survival in children with aplastic anemia or leukemia has not been shown to be better than those under 10 years of age as compared with patients between 11 and 20 years of age. This suggests that the age effect of graft-vs.-host disease on survival is not present in patients under the age of 20 (14).

A number of studies have shown that the occurrence of graft-vs.-host disease is correlated with leukemic relapse following transplant (51). This finding suggests that graft-vs.-host disease has an antileukemic effect, confirming suspicions obtained from previous studies done in animals (52,53). Thus, occurrence of severe graft-vs.-host disease can impair or reduce survival. However, if one separates into two groups patients with mild-moderate graft-vs.-host disease and those who have none, the leukemic relapse rates are significantly higher in the group having no graft-vs.-host disease (51). In addition, relapse rates have been found to be significantly higher in transplants between identical twins (syngeneic transplant) than when the transplant is from an allogeneic donor. Although the antileukemic effect of graft-vs.-host disease is more pronounced in patients with acute lymphocytic leukemia, this anticancer effect has been seen across the board in all tested malignancies.

These trials showing that graft-vs.-host disease has a beneficial effect in preventing subsequent relapse include mostly adults. The same effect has not been demonstrated with significance in a large number of children undergoing transplantation where the incidence of graft-vs.-host disease tends to be lower anyway (51). In bone marrow transplant trials in children with acute lymphoblastic leukemia, ablative regimens containing cytosine arabinoside show an improved remission duration as compared to children receiving an ablative regimen of cyclophosphamide and total body irradiation (14). This suggests that in children the major impediment to prolonged survival post-transplant is not acute graft-vs.-host disease. Instead, the main stumbling block is adequate control of the underlying malignancy, which may only be achievable by improvements in the pre-transplant ablative therapy.

Soon after the development of T lymphocyte depletion techniques, a well-controlled trial was begun. In this trial, adults undergoing matched marrow transplantation for treatment of acute leukemia were randomized to receive either T lymphocyte depleted marrow or nondepleted marrow (44). Although the survival between the two groups was ultimately the same, those receiving T lymphocyte depleted marrow had a higher incidence of leukemic relapse as compared to those who received unmanipulated marrow. This relapse rate approached that seen in patients receiving marrow from a syngeneic donor. The major cause of death in those receiving unmanipulated marrow was graft-vs.-host disease. No other group has undertaken such a randomized controlled study in adults. However, other investigators have compared the long-term outcome in patients receiving T lymphocyte depleted marrow to historical controls studied in the same institution. These workers found that there is a significant improvement in survival, suggesting that in some hands and when some lymphocyte depletion techniques are used, leukemic relapse is not a major problem (39). Again, the reasons to account for these differences from institution to institution remain unknown.

PREDICTORS OF UNFAVORABLE OUTCOME OF GRAFT-VS.-HOST DISEASE

In children, differences in age have not been shown to affect the occurrence of graft-vs.-host disease. However, there is sufficient anecdotal experience in children with immune deficiencies to suggest that these children have a markedly decreased incidence of graft-vs.-host disease (54). The majority of children with immune deficiencies undergo transplantation either from matched related donors or from mismatched donors, and are under the age of 2 at the time of transplant. On the other hand, the majority of children undergoing transplantation for treatment of aplastic anemia or acute leukemia are over the age of 2 years. Thus, perhaps there may be an age-related effect on the occurrence of graft-vs.-host disease, but this effect has not been demonstrated in controlled studies.

The number of children in various trials of bone marrow transplantation are small compared to the number of adults that have been studied. Also, some of the predictors of graft-vs.-host disease found in adults have not been shown to be present in children. But this difference may simply be related to lack of numbers. Transplanting patients who are in relapse of leukemia or lymphoma is associated with an increased incidence of graft-vs.-host disease in children as well as in adults (51). Patients who are infected and those who are transplanted outside of laminar airflow rooms may have an increased incidence of graft-vs.-host disease. Clearly, the use of marrow which is nonreactive in mixed lymphocyte culture and from donors who are not HLA-matched phenotypically results in a higher incidence of graft-vs.-host disease (28,29). The highest incidence of graft-vs.-host disease seems to result from the use of haplo-identical marrow (mismatched marrow from a family member) or from the use of closely matched marrow from an unrelated donor.

A number of studies have suggested that use of marrow from female donors may increase the risk of acute graft-vs.-host disease (47). It has also been shown that marrow transplantation in patients with acute nonlymphoblastic leukemia is associated with a higher incidence of acute graft-vs.-host disease than transplantation in patients with other types of leukemia (51). Certain donor HLA phenotypes have also been associated with an increased incidence of this complication. As previously mentioned, the occurrence of infections may increase the likelihood of developing acute graft-vs.-host disease (46).

SUMMARY

There are increasing numbers of bone marrow transplant centers and more children are now undergoing marrow transplantation with improved results. Thus, more pediatric hematologists will have under their care children who have undergone transplantation and who may be suffering from the effects of acute or chronic graft-vs.-host disease.

Although there may also be beneficial effects associated with the occurrence of graft-vs.-host disease, uncontrolled graft-vs.-host disease or the requirement for increased immunosuppression to control graft-vs.-host disease may result in an increased incidence of infections. The increase in infections will influence ultimate survival. Furthermore, medications used to prevent graft-vs.-host disease, such as cyclosporine, are associated with major side effects. Thus, it is important for the physician to become familiar with the side effects of medications given in the post-transplant setting in order to either prevent or to appropriately treat graft-vs.-host disease.

The study of graft-vs.-host disease has become a very important area of research. It is suspected that the manipulation of graft-vs.-host disease may help overcome the resistance some malignancies have to the chemotherapy and radiation now used as part of the pre-transplant ablation regimen. It is of vital importance that we discover the identity of the particular T lymphocyte subtype responsible for acute graft-vs.-host disease, and possibly also responsible for the graft-vs.-leukemia effect. Then trials can be done to determine if the removal of only that particular T lymphocyte subtype from donor marrow will result in a decreased incidence of acute graft-vs.-host disease, but still preserve the beneficial graft-vs.-leukemia effect.

REFERENCES

1. Wick MR, Moore SB, Gastineau DA, Hoagland HC: Immunologic, clinical and pathologic aspects of human graft-vs.-host disease. *Mayo Clin Proc* 1983;58:603–612.
2. Fliedner VV, Higby DJ, Kim U: Graft-vs.-host reaction following blood product transfusion. *Am J Med* 1982;72:951–961.
3. Woods WG: Prevention of graft-vs.-host disease. *Am J Pediatr Hematol Oncol* 1984;6:283–286.
4. Gale RP: Graft-vs.-host disease. *Immunol Rev* 1985;88:193–214.
5. Thomas ED, Storb R, Clift RA: Bone marrow transplantation. *N Engl J Med* 1975;292:832–843 and 895–902.

6. Neudorf S, Filipovich A, Ramsay N, Kersey J: Prevention and treatment of acute graft-vs.-host disease. *Semin Hematol* 1984;21:91–100.
7. Gale RP, Reisner Y: Graft rejection and graft-vs.-host disease; mirror images. *Lancet* 1986;1:1468–1470.
8. Bastian JF, Ornelas W, Williams RA, et al.: Maternal isoimmunization resulting in combined immunodeficiency and fatal graft-vs.-host disease in an infant. *Lancet* 1984;1:1435–1437.
9. Perreaul C, Gyger M, Boileau J, et al.: Acute graft-vs.-host disease after allogeneic bone marrow transplantation. *Canad Med Assoc J* 1983;129:969–974.
10. Torok-Strob B: Personal communication to the author, 1987.
11. Shulman HM, Sullivan KM, Weiden PL, et al.: Chronic graft-vs.-host syndrome in man. *Am J Med* 1980;69:204–217.
12. Rodu B, Gockerman JP: Oral manifestations of the chronic graft-vs.-host reaction. *JAMA* 1983;249:504–507.
13. Graze PR, Gale RP: Chronic graft-vs.-host disease; a syndrome of disordered immunity. *Am J Med* 1979;66:611–620.
14. Lazarus HM, Coccia PF, Herzig RH, et al.: Incidence of acute graft-vs.-host disease with and without methotrexate prophylaxis in allogeneic bone marrow transplant patients. *Blood* 1984;64:215–220.
15. Ramsay NKC, Kersey JH, Robison LL, et al.: A randomized study of the prevention of acute graft-vs.-host disease. *N Engl J Med* 1982;306:392–397.
16. Storb R, Epstein RB, Graham TC, Thomas ED: Methotrexate regimens for control of graft-vs.-host disease in dogs with allogeneic marrow grafts. *Transplantation* 1970;9:240–246.
17. Storb R, Deeg HJ, Farewell V, et al.: Marrow transplantation for severe aplastic anemia; methotrexate alone compared with a combination of methotrexate and cyclosporine for prevention of acute graft-vs.-host disease. *Blood* 1986;68:119–125.
18. Powles RL, Clink HM, Spence D, et al.: Cyclosporine A to prevent graft-vs.-host disease in man after allogeneic bone marrow transplantation. *Lancet* 1980;1:327–329.
19. Gluckman E, Devergie A, Poirier O, Lokiec F: Use of cyclosporine as prophylaxis of graft-vs.-host disease after human allogeneic bone marrow transplantation; report of 38 patients. *Transplant Proc* 1983;15:2628–2633.
20. Weiden PL, Doney K, Storb R, Thomas ED: Antihuman thymocyte globulin for prophylaxis of graft-vs.-host disease; a randomized trial in patients with leukemia treated with HLA identical sibling marrow grafts. *Transplantation* 1979;27:227–230.
21. Doney KC, Weiden PL, Storb R, Thomas ED: Failure of early administration of antithymocyte globulin to lessen graft-vs.-host disease in human allogeneic marrow transplant recipients. *Transplantation* 1981;31:141–143.
22. Bacigalupo A, van Lint MT, Frassoni F, et al.: High-dose bolus methylprednisolone for the treatment of acute graft-vs.-host disease. *Blut* 1983;46:125–132.
23. Kanojia MD, Anagostou AA, Zander AR, et al.: High-dose methoprednisolone treatment for acute graft-vs.-host disease after bone marrow transplantation in adults. *Transplantation* 1984;37:246–249.
24. Janossy G, Prentice HG, Hoffbrand AV, et al.: The role of monoclonal antibodies in the prevention of graft-vs.-host disease. *Med Oncol Tumor Pharmacother* 1984;1:279–284.
25. Hansen JA, Clift RA, Beatty PG, et al.: Marrow transplantation from donors other than HLA genotypically identical siblings. In, Gale RP (ed): *Recent Advances in Bone Marrow Transplantation*, New York. Alan R. Liss, Inc., 1983, p. 739.
26. Filipovich AH, Ramsay NKC, McGlave P, et al.: Mismatched bone marrow transplantation at the University of Minnesota: use of related donors other than HLA-MLC identical siblings and T cell depletion. In, Gale RP (ed): *Recent Advances in Bone Marrow Transplantation*, New York. Alan R. Liss, Inc., 1983, p. 769.
27. Powles RL, Morgenstern GR, Crofts M, et al.: Mismatched family bone marrow transplantation. In, Gale RP (ed): *Recent Advances in Bone Marrow Transplantation*, New York. Alan R. Liss, Inc., 1983, p. 757.
28. Trigg ME, Billing R, Sondel PM, et al.: Clinical trial depleting T lymphocytes from donor marrow for matched and mismatched allogeneic bone marrow transplants. *Cancer Treat Rep* 1985;69:377–386.
29. Gingrich RD, Howe CWS, Goeken NE, et al.: The use of partially matched, unrelated donors in clinical bone marrow transplantation. *Transplantation* 1985;39:526–532.

30. Lochte H, Levy A, Guenther D, Thomas ED: Prevention of delayed foreign marrow reaction in lethally irradiated mice by early administration of methotrexate. *Nature* 1982;196:1110.

31. Smith BR, Parkman R, Lipton J, et al.: Efficacy of a short course (four doses) of methotrexate following bone marrow transplantation for prevention of graft-vs.-host disease. *Transplantation* 1985;39:326–329.

32. Santos GW, Tutschka PJ, Brookmeyer R, et al.: Marrow transplantation for acute non-lymphocytic leukemia after treatment with busulfan and cyclophosphamide. *N Engl J Med* 1983;309:1347–1353.

33. Kennedy MS, Deeg HJ, Storb R, et al.: Treatment of acute graft-vs.-host disease after allogeneic marrow transplantation: randomized study comparing corticosteroids and cyclosporine. *Am J Med* 1985;78:978–983.

34. Vallera DA, Soderling CCB, Carlson GJ, Kersey JH: Bone marrow transplantation across major histocompatibility barriers in mice, effect of elimination of T cells from donor grafts by treatment with monoclonal Thy-1.2 plus complement or antibody alone. *Transplantation* 1981;31:218–222.

35. Vallera DA, Youle RJ, Neville DM, et al.: Monoclonal antibody toxin conjugates for experimental graft-vs.-host disease prophylaxis. *Transplantation* 1983;36:73–80.

36. Reisner Y, Kapoor N, Pollack S, et al.: Use of lectins in bone marrow transplantation. In, Gale RP (ed): *Recent Advances in Bone Marrow Transplantation,* New York. Alan R. Liss, Inc., 1983, p. 355.

37. Trigg ME, Billing R, Sondel PM, et al.: Depletion of T cells from human bone marrow with monoclonal antibody CT-2 and complement. *J Biol Response Mod* 1984;3:406–412.

38. Trigg ME, Peterson A, Erickson C, et al.: Depletion of T cells from bone marrow for allogeneic transplantation; method for treatment of bone marrow in bulk. *Exp Hematol* 1986;14:21–26.

39. Prentice HG, Blacklock HA, Janossy G, et al.: Depletion of T lymphocytes in donor marrow prevents significant graft-vs.-host disease in matched allogeneic leukemia marrow transplant recipients. *Lancet* 1984;1:472–476.

40. Trigg ME, Billing R, Sondel PM, et al.: Mismatched bone marrow transplantation in children with hematologic malignancy using T lymphocyte depleted bone marrow. *J Biol Response Mod* 1985;4:602–612.

41. Kernan NA, Flomenberg N, Dupont B, O'Reilly RJ: Graft rejection in recipients of T cell depleted HLA nonidentical marrow transplants for leukemia. *Transplantation* 1987;43:842–847.

42. Storb R, Doney KC, Thomas ED, et al.: Marrow transplantation with or without donor buffy coat cells for 65 transfused aplastic anemia patients. *Blood* 1982;59:236–246.

43. Korngold R, Sprent J: Lethal graft-vs.-host disease after bone marrow transplantation across minor histocompatibility barriers in mice. *J Exp Med* 1978;148:1687–1698.

44. Champlin R, Ho W, Gale RP: Failure of high-dose radiotherapy to abrogate graft rejection following T cell depleted bone marrow transplantation. *Exp Hematol* 1987;15:536.

45. Trigg ME, Finlay JF, Sondel PM: Use of acyclovir in bone marrow transplant patients. *N Engl J Med* 1985;312:1708–1709.

46. Bross DS, Tutschka PJ, Farmer ER, et al.: Predictive factors for acute graft-vs.-host disease in patients transplanted with HLA-identical bone marrow. *Blood* 1984;63:1265–1270.

47. Atkinson K, Farrell C, Chapman G, et al.: Female marrow donors increase the risk of acute graft-vs.-host disease; effect of donor age and parity and analysis of cell subpopulations in the donor marrow inoculum. *Br J Hæmatol* 1986;63:231–239.

48. Storb R, Prentice RL, Buckner CD, et al.: Graft-vs.-host disease and survival in patients with aplastic anemia treated by marrow grafts from HLA identical siblings: beneficial effect of a protective environment. *N Engl J Med* 1983;308:302–307.

49. Anasetti C, Doney KC, Storb R, et al.: Marrow transplantation for severe aplastic anemia. *Ann Int Med* 1986;104:461–466.

50. Good RA: Personal communication to the author, 1987.

51. Weiden PL, Flournoy N, Thomas ED, et al.: Antileukemic effect of graft-vs.-host disease in human recipients of allogeneic marrow grafts. *N Engl J Med* 1979;300:1068–1073.

52. Bortin MM, Truitt RL, Rimm AA, Bach FH: Graft-vs.-host leukemia reactivity induced by alloimmunization without augmentation of graft-vs.-host reactivity. *Nature* 1981;281:490–491.

53. Truitt RL, Shih CY, Kaehler DA, et al.: Alloimmunization of MHC-compatible donor mice. In, Gale RP (ed): *Recent Advances in Bone Marrow Transplantation,* New York. Alan R. Liss, Inc., 1983, p. 243.
54. Hong R, Horowitz S, Moen R, et al.: Thymus and B cell reconstitution in severe combined immunodeficiency after transplantation of monoclonal antibody depleted parental mismatched bone marrow. *Bone Marrow Transplantation* 1987;1:405–410.
55. Sondel PM, Hank JA: Alien driven diversity and alien selected escape; a rationale for allogeneic cancer immunotherapy. *Transplant Proc* 1981;13:1915–1921.

Bone Marrow Transplantation in Children, edited by F. Leonard Johnson and Carl Pochedly. Raven Press, Ltd., New York © 1990.

Late Effects Following Marrow Transplantation*

Jean E. Sanders

Fred Hutchinson Cancer Research Center, Children's Orthopedic Hospital and Medical Center, and University of Washington School of Medicine, Seattle, Washington 98104

Introduction
A. Transplant-related late effects
B. Late effects of chemotherapy and total body irradiation
C. Recurrence of original disease
Summary

INTRODUCTION

Over the past 15 years the success of marrow transplantation for the treatment of malignant and nonmalignant hematologic diseases has steadily increased. This has led to the incorporation of this treatment into the management of an increasing number of patients. The modalities used in the marrow transplant preparative regimens include total body irradiation (TBI), high-dose chemotherapy or both. Since irradiation and chemotherapy affect normal cells as well as abnormal cells, the preparative regimens are associated with toxicities. Some of these toxic effects occur early, while others occur months to years later. Since transplanted children are surviving longer, the late sequelae are becoming more apparent. All physicians who care for long-term survivors following bone marrow transplantation are faced with diagnosing and treating heretofore unknown late effects in this unique patient population.

*This investigation was supported in part by grant numbers CA 30924, CA 18029, CA 15704, CA 18221, CA 31787, and CA 18105 awarded by the National Cancer Institute, Department of Health and Human Services, Bethesda, Maryland.

This chapter will review the late effects described to date. These effects are categorized as (1) effects related to the transplant procedure itself, (2) effects related to the preparative regimen, and (3) those effects arising from the original disease.

TRANSPLANT-RELATED LATE EFFECTS

Engraftment

In general, engraftment in long-term survivors is stable, with all hematopoietic cells being of donor origin. Mixed chimerism, or reappearance of cells of host origin following allogeneic marrow transplantation, has usually been associated with an unstable situation. Thus, reappearance of cells of host origin has often been followed by graft rejection or return of the original disease and has rarely been followed by complete recovery of autologous marrow function. However, at least 5 patients, transplanted for leukemia, have had a stable mixed chimerism for more than 6 years (1,2). A study of 96 patients transplanted for aplastic anemia from HLA-identical sex-mismatched donors has demonstrated that mixed chimerism may persist for up to 395 days before hematopoiesis becomes donor-type (3). Only one patient has been reported to have had long-term stable mixed chimerism after matched allogeneic marrow grafting for aplastic anemia (4).

Patients receiving ABO-incompatible marrow grafts may produce isohemagglutinins of host origin against the ABO group of the donor for up to 330 days after grafting (5). Continuous low-grade hemolysis may result and increased transfusion requirements may be reduced by using blood group O for transfusions (6,7). The marrow may show an absence of mature red cell precursors and reticulocytopenia may be present in the peripheral blood.

Viral infections, especially those due to cytomegalovirus (CMV), may cause a profound drop in a patient's platelet and leukocyte counts when accompanied by positive cultures for cytomegalovirus or a rise in anti-CMV antibody titers (8). If the viral infection is not fatal, then the platelet and leukocyte counts will recover completely. Occasionally the thrombocytopenia is severe enough to require transfusion support.

Infection prophylaxis with trimethoprim-sulfamethoxazole has been associated with temporary depression of granulocyte and platelet counts. Animal studies have shown that treatment with this drug at the usual doses does not interfere with hematopoietic recovery (9). Furthermore, withholding treatment in patients does not regularly lead to prompt recovery of peripheral blood counts. However, if no explanation for granulocytopenia or thrombocytopenia is apparent, trimethoprim-sulfamethoxazole should be stopped. A trial of folinic acid may be helpful.

Varicella Zoster Virus (VZV) Infections

VZV infections are a major cause of morbidity and mortality in marrow graft recipients. Nearly half of the patients who survived for at least 6 months developed infections due to this virus (10,11). The majority of VZV infections occurred during the first year. Patients who received HLA-nonidentical grafts and those with chronic graft-vs.-host disease who had nonspecific suppressor cells had the highest incidence of varicella zoster virus infections, while recipients of syngeneic grafts had the lowest incidence (12). Patients less than 10 years of age had a significantly lower incidence of VZV infections than did patients 11 years of age and older. While most patients initially had localized zoster, nearly one-third of these infections subsequently disseminated and 15% presented with disseminated varicella-like infections. The overall mortality rate was 8%, and all deaths occurred in patients who were less than 9 months post-transplant. Usually, varicella zoster virus infections are self-limited and only occur once after transplantation, suggesting the reacquisition of durable immunity. If dissemination occurs, treatment with adenine arabinoside or acyclovir (given intravenously) has been effective. Recurrent VZV infections have been reported in a few patients (11).

Chronic Graft-vs.-Host Disease

Chronic graft-vs.-host disease occurs in approximately 30% of long-term survivors of allogeneic marrow transplantation (13,14,15). Although most patients have preceding acute graft-vs.-host disease, 20% have late *de novo* onset. Factors associated with the probability of developing chronic graft-vs.-host disease include increasing grade of acute graft-vs.-host disease, increasing recipient age, and transfusion of unirradiated donor buffy coat cells in patients with aplastic anemia (15,16).

Clinical and pathological findings resemble several naturally occurring autoimmune diseases (17). The skin is involved in almost all patients. The abnormalities observed include dryness, dyspigmentation, lichen planus-like lesions, and papular squamous plaques. Additionally, there may be edema, violaceous macules, and erythema with desquamation. Occasionally these lesions are reactivated by sun exposure but they also may be present in nonsun-exposed areas. Abnormalities of the hair, nails, and mucous membranes may occur. After 6 to 18 months, poikiloderma with epidermal atrophy, telangiectasia, progressive sclerosis, and scleroderma with joint contractures may develop in untreated or nonresponding patients. Significant hair loss or frank alopecia may occur.

Oral involvement has been observed in more than 80% of patients with extensive, multiorgan chronic graft-vs.-host disease (18,19). The lichen planus-like lesions of the oral mucosa may be confused with candidiasis. Buccal lesions range from white reticular striae to large plaques in appearance. Also mucosal atrophy, reduced keratinization, and xerostomia may be present. There is increased salivary sodium and decreased or absent secretory IgA (20,21). Extensive dental caries have been observed.

Approximately 80% of patients have ocular involvement (22,23). Keratoconjunctivitis sicca is the most frequent finding. Without artificial tear replacement, corneal wasting and perforation may develop. In addition, uveitis and membranous conjunctivitis have been seen.

Less frequently involved organs include muscles (as polymyositis) and serosal surfaces (in the form of sterile pericardial, synovial, and pleural effusions). Upper esophageal stenosis with desquamation, dysphagia, and retrosternal pain was seen in 17 out of 41 patients with chronic graft-vs.-host disease (24). Vaginal inflammation, sicca, and adhesions were found in 4 of 41 women with chronic graft-vs.-host disease (25).

Evaluation at 80 to 100 days after transplant of the organ systems most frequently involved is helpful in diagnosing early chronic graft-vs.-host disease (Table 1). Biopsy of involved tissues is useful in establishing the diagnosis (26). Dermatopathology of the early phases of chronic graft-vs.-host disease reveals eosinophilic body formation, liquefactive degeneration, and lichenoid reaction along the basal layer. Later dermal fibrosis and epidermal atrophy are present. Oral biopsy findings include squamous cell necrosis and abnormalities similar to Sjögren's syndrome. Thus, chronic graft-vs.-host disease has many clinical and pathologic similarities to scleroderma, lichen planus, Sjögren's syndrome, systemic lupus erythematous, and primary biliary cirrhosis (27,28). Unlike scleroderma, chronic graft-vs.-host disease of the esophagous does not result in myenteric plexus involvement or smooth muscle fibrosis. In addition, the renal lesions often seen in lupus and scleroderma have not been observed with chronic graft-vs.-host disease.

Both humoral and cellular mechanisms may contribute to the pathogenesis of this disease (13). Immunoglobulin and complement are found deposited along the dermal-epidermal junction in 85% of patients with chronic graft-vs.-host disease (29). These deposits serve as a useful clue for the early diagnosis of chronic graft-vs.-host disease, whether or not they represent the true pathologic mechanism. Cell-mediated immunity against host non-HLA antigens has been observed in chronic graft-vs.-host disease patients in the form of undirectional lymphocyte proliferation to stimulation by cryopreserved host cells (30). Patients with chronic graft-vs.-host disease have demonstrated increased suppressor T cell activity (31). One-half of chronic graft-vs.-host disease patients have nonspecific suppression which is rarely found in healthy long-term chimeras (32). Most healthy chimeras have evidence of specific suppressor cell activity which is also absent in chronic graft-vs.-host disease patients (33).

The prognosis is excellent for patients with the limited form of chronic

TABLE 1 *Diagnosis of early chronic graft-vs.-host disease*

Organ system	Study	Abnormality
Skin	Physical examination	Erythema, Dyspigmentation
	Biopsy	Eosinophilic Bodies, Basal Vacuoles
Mouth	Oral Mucous Membrane Examination	Lichen Planus-like Lesions, White Reticular Striae
	Oral Mucous Membrane Biopsy	Mucositis with Squamous Cell Necrosis
Eye	Schirmers Test and Slit Lamp Examination	< 10 mm Wetting, Corneal Stippling
Gastrointestinal	Weight	Weight loss despite adequate caloric intake
	Liver Function Studies	Elevated bilirubin, alkaline phosphatase

graft-vs.-host disease, but it is poor for untreated patients with extensive disease (13). Among the patients with extensive disease, survival is influenced by the type of disease onset. Survival is highest among those who have *de novo* onset (i.e., those without preceding acute graft-vs.-host disease), survival is intermediate among those with *quiescent* onset (i.e., cases of chronic graft-vs.-host disease arising after complete resolution of acute graft-vs.-host disease), and survival is poorest among those with *progressive* onset (i.e., cases of chronic graft-vs.-host disease arising as a direct continuation from acute graft-vs.-host disease). Patients who still have thrombocytopenia 100 days post-transplantation also have a poor prognosis (34).

The administration of corticosteroids for 6 to 18 months after transplant has been reported by one group to be useful in preventing chronic graft-vs.-host disease (35). However, another transplant team found this approach to be of no benefit (36).

Treatment of chronic graft-vs.-host disease with immunosuppressive drugs, prednisone either alone or in combination with procarbazine, cyclophosphamide, or azathioprine given for a year or more, has improved the course of this disease. Prior to 1977, therapy of chronic graft-vs.-host disease was unsatisfactory and less than 20% of patients survived free from disability. Between 1977 and 1980 immunosuppressive therapy with prednisone (at a dose of 1 mg/kg/day and either azathioprine, cyclophosphamide, or procarbazine (all at a dose of 1.5 mg/kg/day) was given to 21 patients with extensive chronic graft-vs.-host disease. Sixteen of these 21 patients had resolution of their chronic graft-vs.-host disease and are disability-free long-term survivors (13). Early treatment prevented disability and joint contractures in most patients. More than half of the patients are surviving with

Karnofsky performance şcores of 100%, and one-fourth have performance scores of 85% to 90%. However, nearly one-fourth died of infectious complications (37).

In 1980 a prospective double-blind randomized trial of early treatment of extensive chronic graft-vs.-host disease was carried out to determine the benefit of azathioprine added to prednisone therapy (34). Supportive care included artificial tear replacement, vigorous oral hygiene, sun-blocking lotions, and daily prophylactic trimethoprim-sulfamethoxazole. Results showed that prednisone, with or without azathioprine, begun 3 to 4 months after transplant, could effectively prevent disability and joint contractures in patients with newly diagnosed extensive chronic graft-vs.-host disease. Treatment with prednisone alone resulted in fewer infections and significantly better survival than prednisone and azathioprine in standard risk patients. Treatment with prednisone alone in high-risk patients with thrombocytopenia was less effective with significantly worse survival. The use of alternating day cyclosporine and prednisone appears to improve survival in these high-risk patients (38).

Immunologic Reconstitution

A number of transplant centers have demonstrated that repopulation of the immune and hematopoietic systems depends on appropriate proliferation, maturation, and differentiation of cells of donor origin (39–47). Time after transplant is the most important factor. Regardless of the type of graft (autologous, syngeneic, or allogeneic), the type of underlying disease, the type of conditioning regimen, the type of postgrafting immunosuppression (use of methotrexate or cyclosporine), or the presence of acute graft-vs.-host disease, all marrow graft recipients have profound impairment of most immune functions during the first 4 to 5 months after transplant. In healthy recipients the immunologic elements return to normal, or to the near normal range, about 1 year postgrafting. Recipients with chronic graft-vs.-host disease have delayed immune reconstitution which leaves them at increased risk for life-threatening infections.

Serum levels of IgG and IgM return to normal 3 to 4 months posttransplant, but serum levels of IgA may remain low for more than a year (41–44,48). The levels of total hemolytic complement (CH_{50}), the third component of complement (C_3), and the fourth component of complement (C_4) are normal in the first 3 months after transplant (43).

Cellular responses (as delayed-type hypersensitivity) and humoral responses (as rises in antibody titers) to recall and neoantigens recover to normal levels by 1 year in healthy recipients, but in those with chronic graft-vs.-host disease the responses remain impaired. Patients with chronic graft-vs.-host disease have defective primary responses to bacteriophage OX174 and fail to switch from IgM to IgG production in secondary responses (45).

The kinetics of T and B cell repopulation in the peripheral blood by 3 to 4 months after grafting has been described by a number of investigators (41–44,48–55). Although the absolute numbers of T and B cells is restored to normal early, subsets of T lymphocytes repopulate at different rates. During the first year the OKT_8 (suppressor-cytotoxic) subset of T lymphocytes recovers to higher than normal levels, but the OKT_4 (helper) subset recovers to lower than normal levels, leading to an abnormal ratio of OKT_4/OKT_8 (helper-suppressor) cells. After 1 year, healthy recipients usually have normal proportions of OKT_4 and OKT_8 cells in their peripheral blood. However, patients with chronic graft-vs.-host disease continue to have high levels of OKT_8 cells, with low levels of OKT_4 cells in peripheral blood beyond 1 year (47,56,57). Proliferative responses to alloantigens and mitogens and cytotoxic functions such as natural killer activity against K562 cells, antibody-dependent and lectin-dependent cellular cytotoxicity, recover early (44,58). Neutrophil chemotaxis, however, is impaired early after grafting (59,60). No significant correlations were found between the results of these *in vitro* tests and infections, graft-vs.-host disease, or relapse.

In order to improve understanding of the combined cellular and humoral immunologic deficiency seen after grafting, studies with cultures of lymphocyte subpopulations *in vitro* with polyclonal activators have been used. When T and B cells from graft recipients in the first 3 months were co-cultured with normal T and B cells in the presence of pokeweed mitogen, a number of defects were discovered. The B cells failed to secrete immunoglobulin, the T cells in nearly half the recipients failed to provide T cell helper activity, and half the patients had T cells which suppressed immunoglobulin production by normal T and B cells (61,62,63).

The long-term healthy survivors have few of the above-mentioned abnormalities, but long-term survivors with chronic graft-vs.-host disease continue to demonstrate these abnormalities in T and B cell function (46,54,57,61,63–65). Among those with chronic graft-vs.-host disease, two-thirds have B cell defects, one-half have failure of T cell helper function, and one-half have T cells with excessive suppressor activity (56,64). The increased proportions of OKT_8 cells may account for the excessive suppressor cell activity, and the low proportions of OKT_4 cells may account for the failure of helper activity. Studies with other polyclonal activators of immunoglobulin synthesis demonstrate functional diversity in the OKT_4 and OKT_8 subsets from long-term survivors with and without chronic graft-vs.-host disease (66). In patients with or without chronic graft-vs.-host disease, monocytes functioned normally with immunoglobulin production after mitogen stimulation (67).

Recent studies have been done using enzyme-linked immunosorbent assays (ELISA) to measure serum antibody titers to tetanus toxoid, diphtheria toxoid, and measles virus. Results show that most healthy long-term survivors have specific antibody titers to these antigens. However, patients with chronic graft-vs.-host disease do not exhibit specific antibody titers to these same antigens (68). None of the transplant recipients were reimmunized to test these antigens. Several donor-recipient pairs clearly exhibited transfer of positive serum antibody titers from donor to recipient, when the recipient previously (before transplant) was negative for measles virus or diphtheria toxoid titers. Additional *in vitro* studies have demonstrated that tetanus toxoid-stimulated mononuclear cells from peripheral blood of recipients surviving more than 1 year after transplant were able to produce specific IgG anti-tetanus toxoid (69,70).

These studies suggest transfer of specific immunity in health marrow graft recipients. The studies also help to explain why more transplant recipients do not develop life-threatening infections with diseases against which their donors had been immunized. Only one case of measles has occurred in over 1500 patients transplanted in Seattle. Also, a recipient developed measles after being exposed to his donor who developed measles following the graft. This donor was probably not immune to measles before the transplant.

Many recipients appear to be protected by specific antibodies to recall antigens produced from donor-derived B cells. The proportion of marrow graft recipients who develop specific antibody titers, or the levels of specific antibody titers, might be increased by booster immunizations given to the donor prior to the transplant. Healthy recipients, or recipients with chronic graft-vs.-host disease who have not developed specific antibody titers by 1 year, should be immunized and evaluated with specific antibody titers. The use of live virus vaccines is attended by risk of morbidity in immunosuppressed hosts, and therefore the use of routine live virus vaccines is not recommended.

LATE EFFECTS OF CHEMOTHERAPY AND TOTAL BODY IRRADIATION

Pulmonary System

After marrow transplantation pulmonary complications are associated with considerable morbidity and mortality. Upper airway obstruction, pulmonary edema syndromes, and nonbacterial pneumonias are problems which usually occur within the first 100 days after transplant and will not be discussed here (71,72). Late interstitial pneumonia has recently been observed in patients with chronic graft-vs.-host disease (73,74). Among 198 patients with extensive chronic graft-vs.-host disease there were 31 episodes of interstitial pneumonia, either of viral or pneumocystis etiology or of idiopathic nature, observed between 3 and 24 months post-transplant (73). Patients who received trimethoprim-sulfamethoxazole had an 8% incidence of interstitial pneumonia, whereas those who did not receive trimethoprim-sulfamethoxazole had a 28% incidence of interstitial pneumonia (p < .001).

In order to determine delayed effects on lung function, sequential pulmonary function tests were performed in all marrow transplant recipients returning for yearly evaluations (75). The testing included spirometry, lung volumes, and a diffusion study (diffusion capacity of lung function for carbon monoxide or DLCO). At 1 year post-transplant, restrictive ventilatory changes occurred with a mean loss in total lung capacity of 0.81 liters, loss in vital capacity of 0.54 liters, and loss in DLCO of 4.4 ml/min. These changes were not significantly associated with prior total body irradiation or with chronic graft-vs.-host disease. Patients with prior interstitial pneumonia had greater restrictive changes than those who had not had interstitial pneumonia. In most patients these restrictive changes normalized or improved within 3 to 4 years after grafting.

Airflow obstruction, which may develop into functionally severe disease, affects increasing proportions of long-term survivors (75–82). Several transplant centers have observed the development of obstructive lung disease in marrow transplant recipients (75–79). This disorder usually became manifested clinically from 6 to 12 months after transplant. Examination of lung tissue has shown bronchiolitis obliterans, a pathologic finding associated with viral pneumonia in children, toxic fume exposure, autoimmune diseases and heart-lung transplantation (80,81). A study of adult marrow transplant patients has identified chronic graft-vs.-host disease and prolonged methotrexate treatment as important risk factors for development of airflow obstruction after marrow transplantation (82).

Central Nervous System

The late effects to the central nervous system of the marrow transplant procedure has received little attention. Leukoencephalopathy has been reported after marrow transplantation (83–86). Frequently the etiology remains obscure, and methotrexate, cranial irradiation, total body irradiation, and virus infections may contribute (87). A retrospective study of 415 patients transplanted for acute leukemia revealed that leukoencephalopathy was seen in 7% of patients who had received central nervous system irradiation, intrathecal chemotherapy, or both prior to marrow transplantation with TBI, and who were given intrathecal methotrexate after the transplant. Furthermore, the risk of developing leukoencephalopathy was not age-related, with 3 out of 7 who developed leukoencephalopathy being more than 20 years of age (83).

Whether there is impairment of cognitive function and occurrence of learning disabilities after transplantation remains to be determined. Casual reports from some parents suggest that children who received cyclophosphamide only in their preparative pre-transplant regimen had no major problems in school, but some of the children who received TBI in the preparative regimen did have difficulties in school. Whether this learning difficulty is related directly to the transplant procedure, to the treatment given before transplant, or is related to the amount of formal schooling missed is unknown.

Patients given mechlorethamine as part of the conditioning regimen have been observed to develop personality changes, seizures, confusion, diplopia, or dementia as late as 8 months after transplant (88). Computerized tomography usually showed ventricular enlargement and electroencephalograms showed diffuse slowing. The prognosis for these patients was poor.

Ophthalmologic Abnormalities

The eye has been recognized as a target organ for chronic graft-vs.-host disease, as mentioned previously, but other abnormalities not related to graft-vs.-host disease have been less well studied. Cataracts are a known late complication of exposure to ionizing irradiation. The incidence of cataracts in 277 patients followed for up to 13 years after transplant has been evaluated (89). All patients had complete ophthalmologic examinations. Of these, 96 patients with aplastic anemia were conditioned with cyclophosphamide only. The 105 patients with leukemia received cyclophosphamide and 10 Gy of total body irradiation, and 76 patients with leukemia received cyclophosphamide and 12 to 15 Gy of total body irradiation in fractions of 2 to 2.25 Gy over 6 to 7 days (Gy = grays, which equals 100 rad). Posterior capsular cataracts began to develop in 86 patients by 1 year after grafting. Among the 105 patients given single-dose TBI, as many as 80% are expected to develop cataracts by 6 years. Only 19% of the 76 patients receiving fractionated TBI are likely to develop cataracts, and only 18% of the patients not receiving TBI (96 patients with aplastic anemia) are expected to develop cataracts (Figure 1).

These data suggest that causes other than total body irradiation, such as adrenocorticosteroids, contribute to the development of cataracts after transplantation. One-half of the patients with cataracts occurring after single-dose TBI required surgical repair at a median of 6 years post-TBI. On the other hand, only 20% of cataract patients given fractionated TBI and none of the patients not given TBI required surgical repair. Cataract treatment for these patients is the same as for cataracts of other etiologies. Use of lens implants should be considered, but in younger children contact lenses may be preferred. Glasses are a less desirable alternative and should be chosen only if sicca syndrome exists concurrently. All patients who are marrow transplant survivors should have a complete ophthalmologic examination annually.

Endocrine Dysfunction

Endocrine abnormalities have been observed in patients given irradiation (90,91); Therefore, the occurrence of hormonal insufficiencies following total

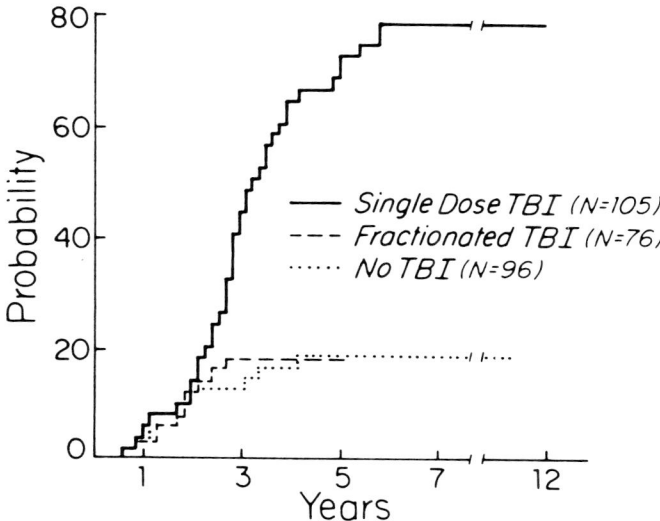

FIG. 1. Kaplan-Meier probability of developing cataracts after transplantation with single dose total body irradiation (TBI), fractionated TBI or no TBI.

body irradiation is not surprising. There may be thyroid dysfunction, gonadal dysfunction, or retarded growth.

The delivery of ionizing irradiation to the thyroid gland has been associated with the development of compensated hypothyroidism, overt hypothyroidism, thyroiditis, and thyroid neoplasms. Among 23 patients who were given TBI and marrow transplantation, 10 developed subclinical hypothyroidism (92). In 8 patients this hypothyroidism was compensated with elevated thyroid stimulating hormone (TSH) and normal thyroxine (T_4) levels. In 116 children prepared with total body irradiation and transplanted for hematologic malignancy, 18% developed compensated hypothyroidism, 11% developed asymptomatic hypothyroidism and 7% developed asymptomatic elevations in TSH and T_4 (93).

Cyclophosphamide and other alkylating agents have been associated with gonadal damage, which is related to patient age, drug dosage, and duration of treatment (94,95). Gonadal function was evaluated in 108 patients transplanted for aplastic anemia following preparation with cyclophosphamide, given at a dose of 200 mg/kg (96,97,98). Fourteen girls who were prepubertal at the time of transplant have developed normally through puberty, as evidenced by normal Tanner developmental scores, normal gonadotropin levels, and the achievement of menarche between 12 and 13 years of age (Figure 2). Similarly, the 19 boys who were prepubertal at the time of transplant have developed normally through puberty and have normal gonadotropin levels (Figure 3).

Among 43 women who were postpubertal at the time of transplant, the 27

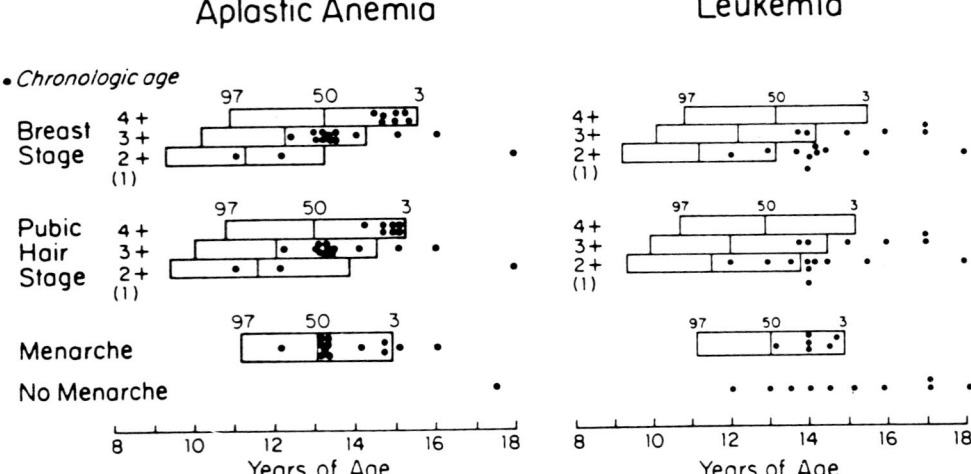

FIG. 2. The Tanner pubertal developmental scores after marrow transplantation for 12 girls transplanted for aplastic anemia following cyclophosphamide preparation and for 16 girls transplanted for leukemia after cyclophosphamide and total body irradiation preparation.

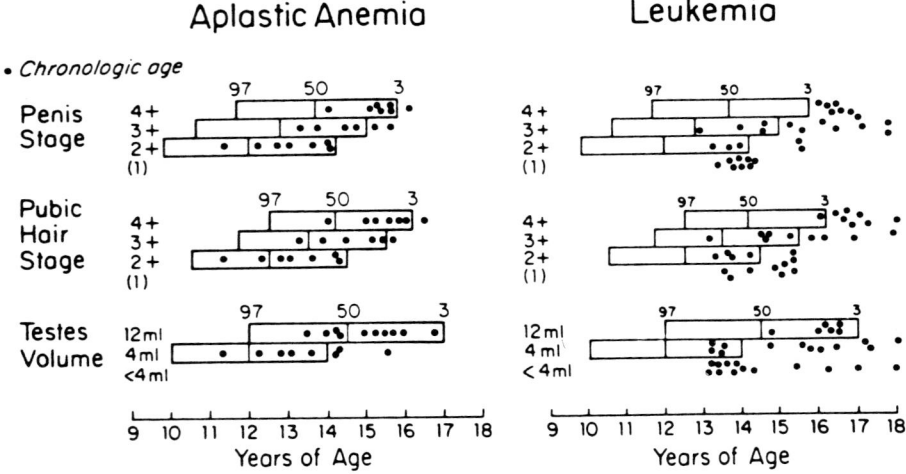

FIG. 3. The Tanner pubertal developmental scores after marrow transplantation for 18 boys transplanted for aplastic anemia following cyclophosphamide preparation and for 31 boys transplanted for leukemia following cyclophosphamide and total body irradiation preparation.

who were under 26 years of age have had return of normal gonadotropin levels and onset of menses at a median of 6 months following transplant (97,98). Thirteen of the 16 women who were over 26 years of age at the time of transplant had early onset of menopause with elevation of gonadotropin levels and amenorrhea. Twenty of 31 postpubertal men have had return of normal gonadotropin levels and two-thirds of the men tested had a normal semen analysis. Twelve normal children have been born to women after transplant for aplastic anemia in which cyclophosphamide was used in preparation (98–103). Also, 7 normal children have been fathered by 8 men transplanted for aplastic anemia with use of the same conditioning regimen (97).

The dose of irradiation needed to produce permanent sterility in females appears to be related to age, number of oocytes remaining at the time of irradiation, and the dose of irradiation. To produce a 50% incidence of sterilization for more than 5 years requires fractionated doses of more than 20 Gy (104). Irradiation experiments have demonstrated that as little as 0.20 Gy can cause germinal epithelial damage resulting in increased follicle stimulating hormone (FSH) levels and a decreased sperm count (105). Gonadal function was evaluated in 142 children followed for 1 to 14 years after treatment with 120 mg/kg cyclophosphamide and total body irradiation before marrow transplantation (93). Delayed development of secondary sexual characteristics was observed in 69% of girls (11 of 16) and boys (21 of 31) who were prepubertal at the time of transplant and were more than 13 years of age at time of analysis (Figures 2 and 3). The majority of these children had elevated gonadotropin levels and low levels of estradiol or testosterone.

All 144 postpubertal females developed amenorrhea after cyclophosphamide and TBI and at the time of transplant for leukemia (97,98). They all developed evidence of primary ovarian failure with elevated lutenizing hormone and FSH levels and low estradiol levels. More than 70% developed symptoms of menopause. Two women had return of ovarian function at 3.5 and 6.0 years after TBI, both became pregnant, and both had abortions (one spontaneous and one elective). Among the 41 males who were postpubertal at the time of transplant and who were prepared with total body irradiation, all developed gonadal failure associated with elevated FSH levels and azoospermia. Most of these males, however, had normal function of Leydig cells with normal luteinizing hormone and testosterone levels. Two men have had return of spermatogenesis approximately 6 years after transplant and one has fathered two normal children (97).

Thus, it appears that prepubertal girls and boys will develop secondary sex characteristics normally, and all younger women and the majority of men can expect recovery of gonadal function following high-dose cyclophosphamide and marrow transplantation for aplastic anemia. Total body irradiation produces gonadal failure in nearly all prepubertal girls and boys and in almost all postpubertal patients. Younger children may need hormone supplementation to promote growth and development of secondary sexual characteristics.

Postpubertal women should receive cyclic hormone therapy to prevent complications of early menopause.

Growth hormone deficiency and abnormal growth velocity have been described in children with leukemia who were given cranial irradiation (106–111). The threshold for impairment of growth hormone production is a radiation dose to the pituitary of greater than 30 Gy (111). Following total body irradiation and marrow transplantation for leukemia, height measurements were determined for a follow-up period of 1 to 14 years (median 4 years) in 142 children (93). The growth velocity curves for these 90 boys and 52 girls demonstrate decreased growth velocity in all patients, but those with chronic GVH disease were the most severely affected (Figure 4). Stimulated growth hormone levels were subnormal in 63% of all patients, and all of the patients with subnormal stimulated levels had received previous cranial irradiation. In contrast, the 57 children transplanted for aplastic anemia following high-dose cyclophosphamide all had normal growth velocity and growth hormone levels (Figure 4) (96). All children, especially those who have received previous cranial irradiation, TBI, or both, need careful long-term follow-up. Further studies are needed to determine if growth hormone supplementation will benefit these children.

Second Malignancy

The development of second tumors following marrow transplantation is most likely caused by more than one contributing factor. Experiments in nonirradiated and irradiated mice given hematopoietic grafts showed that,

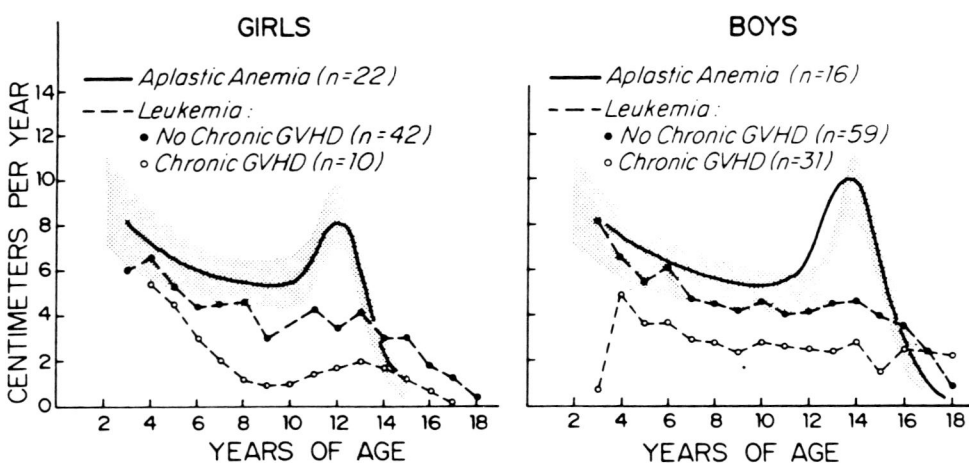

FIG. 4. The mean growth velocity in centimeters growth per year of age for girls and boys transplanted for aplastic anemia following cyclophosphamide or leukemia following cyclophosphamide and total body irradiation preparative regimens.

under specific experimental conditions, the recipient animals developed lymphoid malignancies (112,113). These malignancies, however, were related to graft-vs.-host disease and to virus infections and not necessarily related to irradiation. The question of irradiation-related tumors was studied in 153 dogs given 6.1 to 21.3 Gy of total body irradiation followed by autologous or allogeneic grafts and observed for 6 months to 10 years (114). The incidence of malignant tumors in those dogs was compared to that of 242 untreated dogs observed for 6 months to 16 years. In addition, the outcome of 15 chimeras conditioned with chemotherapy alone was studied. Thirteen nonhematologic malignant tumors were seen in 11 radiation chimeras and 54 malignancies were observed in 44 control dogs. None of the chemotherapy chimeras developed a tumor. Time-dependent regression analysis indicated that the relative risk of developing a malignancy was 5 times higher in irradiated dogs than in controls. Similar results have been reported in rhesus monkeys. Sixteen of 23 monkeys developed solid tumors following treatment with fission neutrons or X-irradiation, whereas no tumors were observed in 21 unirradiated monkeys (115).

In reports of secondary malignancies in man after marrow transplantation, secondary tumors have been recognized in more than 30 patients, but the exact number of patients at risk is not known (116–132). Except for 1 patient transplanted for aplastic anemia, all malignancies occurred in patients transplanted for leukemia. The aplastic anemia recipient and 2 leukemia recipients were prepared with chemotherapy only (118,119,129). These malignancies can be divided into three groups. In the first group, 8 patients had recurrence of leukemia in donor cells 2 months to 6 years after transplant (116–120,126–128). The pathogenesis of these recurrences is not clear. Conceivably, infectious or host environmental factors were responsible. In the second group of secondary malignancies, 7 patients developed lymphopoietic malignancies. These included Hodgkin's disease in 1 (123), diffuse lymphoma in 1 (127), and immunoblastic sarcoma in 5 (121,122,124,130–132). The 12 who developed immunoblastic sarcoma were 2 to 6 months after grafting, and malignancies were of the host type in 4 and were of the donor type in 8 patients. Postgrafting immunosuppression directed at T lymphocytes may have led to uncontrolled proliferation of B cells. In at least 11 instances the Epstein-Barr virus antigen or DNA was present in the malignant cells (121,130,132). In the third group of secondary malignancies following transplant, 5 patients developed solid tumors, which included glioblastoma multiforme in 2, adenocarcinoma of the rectum in 2, and undifferentiated sarcoma in 1 (123,125,126). Both patients who developed glioblastoma had received cranial irradiation 45 to 49 months before transplantation. It is possible that the irradiation was a factor in the etiology of the second tumor in this group of patients.

Further studies are needed in order to assess the true incidence of malignancies following marrow transplantation. It is of interest that in over 250 patients transplanted for nonmalignant diseases, who were prepared with chemotherapy alone and followed for more than 14 years, only 1 patient has developed leukemia and this was of host origin (129). We recommend that any patient who develops a tumor after marrow transplantation be evaluated to determine whether (1) the malignancy is of donor or host origin and (2) whether it is related to the Epstein-Barr virus. Only systematic study can provide data on the incidence of these tumors. Furthermore, studies in animals indicate that much longer follow-up is needed in order to determine the magnitude of this problem.

RECURRENCE OF ORIGINAL DISEASE

Aplastic Anemia

Most patients who are given bone marrow transplants achieve sustained engraftment and are cured of their disease. Only 11 out of more than 150 patients followed from 1 to 13 years after transplantation have demonstrated late loss of the graft and return of host-type hematopoiesis (133,134). In 3 of these 4 patients, hematopoietic function has been normal for 6 to 10 years after transplant, whereas 1 patient developed severe pancytopenia at 2½ years. This patient responded favorably to a course of immunosuppression with antithymocyte globulin and has had normal host-type hematopoietic function for more than 4 years (135). Seven patients were given a second marrow transplant and 5 of these are surviving with full hematopoietic reconstitution of donor type (134). About 10% of patients given cyclosporine after grafting have been reported to develop graft failure after the drug was stopped (4). Several patients have showed recovery of the bone marrow function following administration of cyclosporine and steroids with either recovery of donor-type hematopoiesis or reversion to autologous (host-type) hematopoiesis. However, a few patients have remained aplastic.

Leukemia

Relapse of leukemia continues to be a major problem after marrow transplantation. Except for the small number of cases discussed earlier, in more than 95% of relapses the leukemic cells were of host origin and occurred during the first 2 years after transplant (136). This suggests that the conditioning regimens were not sufficiently intense or cytocidal to eliminate all residual leukemic cells.

For children transplanted for acute nonlymphoblastic leukemia in first remission, the probability of remaining in remission ranges between 50% and 80% (137–141). For children with acute lymphoblastic leukemia who are transplanted in their second or subsequent remission the probability of remaining in remission ranges between 30% and 70% (140,142–144). Once relapse occurs, the management of the patient becomes an important question. Of interest are a small number of patients with Ph¹-positive chronic myelogenous leukemia who were transplanted in the chronic phase, in whom the recurrence of the Ph[1] chromosome did not always herald impending relapse. Careful follow-up of this group of patients revealed that some developed overt leukemia and others showed eventual disappearance of the Ph[1] chromosome. Approximately 25% of boys with acute lymphoblastic leukemia developed isolated testicular relapse without marrow relapse (14). All these boys were treated with orchiectomy and local and para-aortic lymph node irradiation. Maintenance chemotherapy was given to only 1. Three of the 6 who received only local treatment have become long-term survivors, now being 3 to 10 years after testicular relapse. Additional testicular irradiation seems to eliminate this problem (14,140). All patients who sustained an isolated central nervous system relapse eventually died either of complications of treatment to the central nervous system or of subsequent marrow relapse (14,85). The majority of relapses are in the marrow. These patients should be treated with chemotherapy since some will achieve remissions of significant duration (14,136,137).

The question often arises as to whether a second marrow transplant will be of benefit. The experience of second transplants has been disappointing when employed for end-stage patients with persistent leukemia or patients whose post-transplant remission were short (146–149). Recent studies suggest that second marrow transplants are more likely to result in some long-term disease-free survivors if they are performed 1 year or more after the initial transplant (148–150). Since the majority of these patients will have already received maximum tolerated total body irradiation, the design of the preparative regimen may also be an important factor in determining outcome of the second graft.

After an initial transplant containing total body irradiation, the successful second transplants that have been reported after regimens of busulfan and cyclophosphamide, busulfan and etoposide, cyclophosphamide and melphalan are summarized in Table 2 (147–150). It is reasonable to assume that patients who relapse after an initial transplant regimen of chemotherapy only may be successfully prepared for second transplant with a regimen containing total body irradiation (151,152).

Until more effective transplant preparative regimens are designed, recurrent leukemia after transplantation will remain a significant problem. To date 10 of 39 reported patients are surviving from 2 months to 3 years after second marrow transplants. While these results are encouraging and at least 2 patients have sustained remissions after second transplant that is longer than after first transplant, it is too soon to determine how many will be cured.

Graft-vs.-Leukemia Effect

About 30 years ago, Barnes et al., observed in mice that grafted marrow could destroy host leukemia cells which survived irradiation (153). It has been suggested that graft-vs.-host disease might be used against leukemia in the form

TABLE 2. *Second marrow transplants for leukemia*

Diagnosis	No. of patients	Regimen	After second transplants	
			Relapse (months)	Disease free survival (months)
ALL[a]	10[147,149]	BU/CY[d]	3 (2–6)	2 (> 12,23)
	2[148]	CY/L–PAM[e]	1 (16)	—
	3[150]	CY/VP–16[f]	2 (8,17)	1 (> 2)
ANL[b]	7[147,149]	BU/CY[d]	3 (3–38)	2 (> 30–52)
	6[148]	CY/L–PAM[e]	2 (6,8)	1 (> 9)
	1[150]	BU/VP–16[f]	—	1 (> 12)
CML[c]	8[149]	BU/CY[d]	2 (1,15)	2 (> 41–44)
	1[148]	CY/L–PAM[e]	—	1 (> 36)
	1[150]	BU/VP–16[f]	—	—

[a]Acute Lymphoblastic Leukemia
[b]Acute Non-lymphoblastic Leukemia
[c]Chronic Myelogenous Leukemia
[d]Busulfan, 16 mg/kg and Cyclophosphamide, 200 mg/kg
[e]Cyclophosphamide, 300 mg/m^2 and Melphalan, 180 mg/m^2
[f]Busulfan, 16 mg/kg and Etoposide, 60 mg/kg

of adoptive immunotherapy (154). Murine models have been developed in which animals with disseminated tumor are rescued by infusions of donor lymphocytes sensitized to tumor antigens (155). In man, disappearance of leukemia during episodes of acute graft-vs.-host disease has been reported (156). Analysis of clinical data has supported this observation and has suggested an antileukemia effect of both acute and chronic graft-vs.-host disease (14,157–159). The probability of remaining in remission was highest in patients who had acute and chronic graft-vs.-host disease. The probability of being induced into remission was intermediate in those with either acute or chronic graft-vs.-host disease, and the probability was lowest in those who did not have graft-vs.-host disease (157,159). Eighty percent of the recipients who developed *de novo* chronic graft-vs.-host disease were alive at 2 years; 50% of those who had acute graft-vs.-host disease and 25% of those who did not have graft-vs.-host disease were surviving at 2 years. These results suggest that one could possibly manipulate graft-vs.-host disease to augment its antileukemic effect without adversely affecting survival.

SUMMARY

During the past 15 years, marrow transplantation has become a lifesaving procedure for increasing numbers of children and young adults. With continued follow-up, it has become apparent that, as presently used, this procedure is associated with significant chronic and delayed effects. These late effects are related to the chemotherapy and radiotherapy used in the conditioning regimens, to the immunodeficiency after transplantation, to the development of chronic graft-vs.-host disease, and to the immunosuppressive treatment given after transplant.

Attempts need to be made to develop less toxic conditioning regimens, to eliminate chronic graft-vs.-host disease, to accelerate immune reconstitution, and to prevent recurrence of the original disease. In the meantime, careful follow-up with attention to the potential development of these late complications will contribute to the long-term well-being and normal life of these children.

REFERENCES

1. Singer JW, Keating A, Ramberg R, et al.: Long-term stable hematopoietic chimerism following marrow transplantation for acute lymphoblastic leukemia: A case report with *in vitro* marrow culture studies. *Blood* 1983; 62: 869–872.
2. Branch DR, Gallagher MT, Forman SJ, et al.: Endogenous stem cell repopulation resulting in mixed hematopoietic chimerism following total body irradiation and marrow transplantation for acute leukemia. *Transplantation* 1982; 34: 226–228.
3. Hill RS, Petersen FB, Storb R, et al.: Mixed hematologic chimerism after allogeneic marrow transplantation for severe aplastic anemia is associated with a higher risk of graft rejection and a lessened incidence of acute graft-vs.-host disease. *Blood* 1986; 67: 811–816.
4. Hows JM, Palmer S, Gordon-Smith EC: Use of cyclosporine A in allogeneic bone marrow transplantation for severe aplastic anemia. *Transplantation* 1982; 33: 382–386.
5. Witherspoon RP, Storb R, Ochs HD, et al.: Recovery of antibody production in human allogeneic marrow graft recipients: Influence of time post-transplantation, the presence or absence of chronic graft-vs.-host disease, and antithymocyte globulin treatment. *Blood* 1981; 58: 360–368.
6. Bensinger WI, Buckner CD, Thomas ED, et al.: ABO-incompatible marrow transplants. *Transplantation* 1982; 33: 427–429.
7. Hows J, Beddow K, Easton C, et al.: Positive direct antiglobulin tests in BMT recipients. *Br J Hæmatol* 1984; 58: 181–182.
8. Meyers JD, Thomas ED: Infection complicating bone marrow transplantation. In, Rubin RH, Young LS, (eds): *Clinical Approach to Infection in the Immunocompromised Host*, New York, Plenum Press, 1981, pp. 507–551.
9. Deeg JH, Meyers JD, Storb R, et al.: Effect of trimethoprim-sulfamethoxazole on hematological recovery after total body irradiation and autologous marrow infusion in dogs. *Transplantation* 1979; 28: 243–246.
10. Atkinson K, Meyers JD, Storb R, et al.: Varicella zoster virus infection after marrow transplantation for aplastic anemia or leukemia. *Transplantation* 1980; 29: 47–50.
11. Saral R, Burns WH: Viral infections and antiviral chemotherapy. In, Gale RP, (ed): *Recent Advances in Bone Marrow Transplantation*, New York, Alan R. Liss, 1983, pp. 461–469.
12. Atkinson K, Farewell V, Storb R, et al.: Analysis of late infections after human bone marrow transplantation: Role of genotypic nonidentity between marrow donor and recipient and of nonspecific suppressor cells in patients with chronic graft-vs.-host disease. *Blood* 1982; 60: 714–720.
13. Sullivan KM, Shulman HM, Storb R, et al.: Chronic graft-vs.-host disease in 52 patients: Adverse natural course and successful treatment with combination immunosuppression. *Blood* 1981; 57: 267–276.
14. Sanders JE, Flournoy N, Thomas ED, et al.: Marrow transplant experience in children with acute lymphoblastic leukemia: An analysis of factors associated with survival, relapse and graft-vs.-host disease. *Med Pediatr Oncol* 1985; 13: 165–172.

15. Sanders JE, Whitehead J, Storb R, et al.: Marrow transplant experience for children with aplastic anemia. *Pediatrics* 1986; 77: 179–186.
16. Storb R, Prentice RL, Sullivan KM, et al.: Predictive factors in chronic graft-vs.-host disease in patients with aplastic anemia treated by marrow transplantation from HLA-identical siblings. *Ann Intern Med* 1983; 98: 461–466.
17. Sullivan KM, Parkman R: The pathophysiology and treatment of graft-vs.-host disease. *Clin Hæmatol* 1983; 12: 775–789.
18. Schubert M, Sullivan KM, Izutsu KT, et al.: Oral complications of bone marrow transplantation. In, Peterson DE, Sonis ST, (eds): *Oral Complications of Cancer Chemotherapy*, Boston, Martinus Nijhoff, 1985, pp. 93–112.
19. Schubert MM, Sullivan KM, Morton TH, et al.: Oral manifestations of chronic graft-vs.-host disease. *Arch Intern Med* 1984; 144: 1591–1595.
20. Izutsu KT, Sullivan KM, Schubert MM, et al.: Disordered salivary immunoglobulin secretion and sodium transport in human chronic graft-vs.-host disease. *Transplantation* 1983;35:441–446.
21. Izutsu KT, Menard TW, Schubert MM, et al.: Graft-vs.-host disease (GVHD) related secretory IgA deficiency in bone marrow transplant recipients: Findings in labial saliva. *Lab Invest* 1985; 52: 292–297.
22. Jack MK, Jack GM, Sale GE, et al.: Ocular manifestations of graft-vs.-host disease. *Arch Ophthalmol* 1983; 101: 1080–1084.
23. Franklin RM, Kenyon KR, Tutschka PJ, et al.: Ocular manifestations of graft-vs.-host disease. *Ophthalmology* 1983; 90: 4–13.
24. McDonald GB, Sullivan KM, Schuffler MD, et al.: Esophageal abnormalities in chronic graft-vs.-host disease in humans. *Gastroenterology* 1981; 80: 914–921.
25. Corson SL, Sullivan K, Batzer F, et al.: Gynecologic manifestations of chronic graft-vs.-host disease. *Obstet Gynecol* 1982; 60: 488–492.
26. Shulman HM, Sullivan KM, Weiden PL, et al.: Chronic graft-vs.-host syndrome in man: A long-term clinicopathological study of 20 Seattle patients. *Am J Med* 1980; 69: 204–217.
27. Graze PR, Gale RP: Chronic graft-vs.-host disease: A syndrome of disordered immunity. *Am J Med* 1979; 65: 611–619.
28. Gratwohl AA, Moutsopoulos HM, Chused TM, et al.: Sjögren-type syndrome after allogeneic bone-marrow transplantation. *Ann Intern Med* 1977; 87: 703–706.
29. Tsoi M-S, Storb R, Jones E, et al.: Deposition of IgM and complement at the dermo-epidermal junction in acute and chronic cutaneous graft-vs.-host disease in man. *J Immunol* 1978; 120: 1485–1492.
30. Tsoi M-S, Storb R, Dobbs S, et al.: Cell-mediated immunity to non-HLA antigens of the host by donor lymphocytes in patients with chronic graft-vs.-host disease. *J Immunol* 1980, 125: 2258–2262.
31. Reinherz EL, Parkman R, Rappeport J, et al.: Aberrations of suppressor T cells in human graft-vs.-host disease. *N Engl J Med* 1979; 300: 1061–1068.
32. Tsoi M-S, Storb R, Dobbs S, et al.: Nonspecific suppressor cells in patients with chronic graft-vs.-host disease after marrow grafting. *J Immunol* 1979, 123: 1970–1976.
33. Tsoi M-S, Storb R, Dobbs S, et al.: Specific suppressor cells in graft-vs.-host tolerance of HLA-identical marrow transplantation. *Nature* 1981; 292: 355–357.
34. Sullivan KM, Witherspoon RP, Storb R, et al.: Prednisone and azathioprine compared to prednisone and placebo for treatment of chronic graft-vs.-host disease: Prognostic influence of prolonged thrombocytopenia after allogeneic marrow transplantation. *Blood* 1988; 72:546–554.
35. Forman SJ, Farbstein MJ, Scott EP, et al.: Prevention and therapy of graft-vs.-host disease. *N Engl J Med* 1982; 307: 376.
36. Ringden O, Lönnquist B, Lundgren G, et al.: Experience with a cooperative bone marrow transplantation program in Stockholm. *Transplantation* 1982; 33: 500–504.
37. Sullivan KM, Dahlberg S, Storb R, et al.: Infection prophylaxis in patients with chronic graft-vs.-host disease (GVHD). *Exp Hematol* 1983; 11(Suppl 14): 193a (Abstract 346).
38. Sullivan KM, Witherspoon RP, Storb R, et al.: Alternating-day cyclosporine and prednisone for treatment of high-risk chronic graft-vs.-host disease. *Blood* 1988;72:555–561.
39. Stolrb R, Thomas ED: Allogeneic bone-marrow transplantation. *Immunol Rev* 1983;71: 77–102.

40. Witherspoon RP, Kopecky K, Storb RF, et al.: Immunological recovery in 48 patients following syngeneic marrow transplantation for hematological malignancy. *Transplantation* 1982; 33: 143–149.

41. Fass L, Ochs HD, Thomas ED, et al.: Studies of immunological reactivity following syngeneic or allogeneic marrow grafts in man. *Transplantation* 1973; 16: 630–640.

42. Elfenbein GJ, Anderson PN, Humphrey RL, et al.: Immune system reconstitution following allogeneic bone marrow transplantation in man: A multiparameter analysis. *Transplant Proc* 1976; 8: 641–646.

43. Noel DR, Witherspoon RP, Storb R, et al.: Does graft-vs.-host disease influence the tempo of immunologic recovery after allogeneic human marrow transplantation? An observation of 56 long-term survivors. *Blood* 1978; 51: 1087–1105.

44. Gale RP, Opelz G, Mickey MR, el al., for the Bone Marrow Transplant Team: Immunodeficiency following allogeneic bone marrow transplantation. *Transplant Proc* 1978; 10: 223–227.

45. Witherspoon RP, Storb R, Ochs HD, et al.: Recovery of antibody production in human allogeneic marrow graft recipients: Influence of time post-transplantation, the presence or absence of chronic graft-vs.-host disease, and antithymocyte globulin treatment. *Blood* 1981; 58: 360–368.

46. Lum LG, Witherspoon RP, Storb R: The role of T cells and T cells subsets in immune reconstitution after marrow grafting in humans. *J Behring Inst Mitteil* 1982; 70: 188–195.

47. Witherspoon RP, Lum LG, Storb R: Immunologic reconstitution after human marrow grafting. *Semin Hematol* 1984; 21: 2–10.

48. Halterman RH, Graw RG Jr, Fuccillo DA, et al.: Immunocompetence following allogeneic bone marrow transplantation in man. *Transplantation* 1972; 14: 689–697.

49. de Bruin HG, Astaldi A, Leupers T, et al.: T lymphocyte characteristics in bone marrow-transplanted patients. II. Analysis with monoclonal antibodies. *J Immunol* 1981; 127: 244–251.

50. Atkinson K, Hansen JA, Storb R, et al.: T-cell subpopulations identified by monoclonal antibodies after human marrow transplantation. I. Helper-inducer and cytotoxic-suppressor subsets. *Blood* 1982; 59: 1292–1298.

51. Elfenbein GJ, Bellis MM, Ravlin HM, et al.: Phenotypically immature Bu cells in the peripheral blood after bone marrow grafting in man. *Exp Hematol* 1982; 10: 551–559.

52. Forman SJ, Nocker P, Gallagher M, et al.: Pattern of T cell reconstitution following allogeneic bone marrow transplantation for acute hematological malignancy. *Transplantation* 1982; 34: 96–98.

53. Schroff RW, Gale RP, Fahey JL: Regeneration of T cell subpopulations after bone marrow transplantation: Cytomegalovirus infection and lymphoid subset imbalance. *J Immunol* 1982; 129: 1926–1930.

54. Friedrich W, O'Reilly RJ, Koziner B, et al.: T-lymphocyte reconstitution in recipients of bone marrow transplants with and without GVHD: Imbalances of T-cell subpopulations having unique regulatory and cognitive functions. *Blood* 1982; 59: 696–701.

55. Storb R, Ochs HD, Weiden PL, et al.: Immunologic reactivity in marrow graft recipients. *Transplant Proc* 1976; 8: 637–639.

56. Lum LG, Orcutt-Thordarson N, Seigneuret MC, et al.: The regulation of Ig synthesis after marrow transplantation. IV: T4 and T8 subset function in patients with chronic graft-vs.-host disease. *J Immunol* 1982; 129: 113–119.

57. Lum LG, Seigneuret MC, Jin N-R, et al.: Transfer of antigen-specific memory cells from marrow donors to marrow recipients. In Gale RP, Champlin R, (eds): *Progress in Bone Marrow Transplantation*, UCLA Symposia on Molecular and Cellular Biology, New Series, Vol. 53. New York: Alan R. Liss, Inc. 1987, pp. 635–639.

58. Livnat S, Seigneuret M, Storb R, Prentice RL: Analysis of cytotoxic effector cell function in patients with leukemia or aplastic anemia before and after marrow transplantation. *J Immunol* 1980; 124: 481–490.

59. Clark RA, Johnson FL, Klebanoff SJ, Thomas ED: Defective neutrophil chemotaxis in bone marrow transplant patients. *J Clin Invest* 1976; 58: 22–31.

60. Sosa R, Weiden PL, Storb R, et al.: Granulocyte function in human allogeneic marrow graft recipients. *Exp Hematol* 1980; 8: 1183–1189.

61. Ringden O, Witherspoon RP, Storb R, et al.: Increased *in vitro* B-cell IgG secretion during

acute graft-vs.-host disease and infection: Observations in 50 human marrow transplant recipients. *Blood* 1980; 55: 179–186.

62. Witherspoon RP, Lum LG, Storb R: *In vitro* regulation of immunoglobulin synthesis after human marrow transplantation. II. Deficient T and non-T lymphocyte function within 3–4 months of allogeneic, syngeneic, or autologous marrow grafting for hematologic malignancy. *Blood* 1982; 59: 844–850.

63. Bacigalupo A, Mingari MC, Moretta L, et al.: T cell subpopulations after allogeneic bone marrow transplantation. In, Thierfelder S, Rodt H, Kolb HJ, (eds): *Immunobiology of Bone Marrow Transplantation,* Berlin/New York: Springer-Verlag, 1980, pp. 125–140.

64. Lum LG, Seigneuret MC, Storb RF, et al.: *In vitro* regulation of immunoglobulin synthesis after marrow transplantation. I. T-cell and B-cell deficiencies in patients with and without chronic graft-vs.-host disease. *Blood* 1981; 58: 431–439.

65. Korsmeyer SJ, Elfenbein GJ, Goldman CK, et al.: B cell, helper T cell, and suppressor T cell abnormalities contribute to disordered immunoglobulin synthesis in patients following bone marrow transplantation. *Transplantation* 1982; 33: 184–190.

66. Lum LG, Seigneuret MC, Orcutt-Thordarson N, et al.: Functional diversity in OKT4 and OKT8 subsets from long-term survivors after HLA-identical marrow grafting. *Diagnostic Immunol* 1983; 1: 179–187.

67. Shiobara S, Witherspoon RP, Lum LG, et al.: Immunoglobulin synthesis after HLA-identical marrow grafting. V. The role of peripheral blood monocytes in the regulation of *in vitro* immunoglobulin secretion stimulated by pokeweed mitogen. *J Immunol* 1984; 132: 2850–2856.

68. Lum LG, Munn NA, Schanfield MS, et al.: The detection of specific antibody formation to recall antigens after human bone marrow transplantation. *Blood* 1986; 67: 582–587.

69. Lum LG, Shiobara S, Culbertson NJ, et al.: T and B cell collaboration for tetanus toxoid induction of *in vitro* IgG antitetanus toxoid synthesis after human bone marrow grafting. *Exp Hematol* 1984; 12: 390 (abstract).

70. Lum LG: Defects in specific antibody synthesis after human marrow grafting. *Clin Immunol Today* 1985; 12: 1–3.

71. Meyers JD, Flournoy N, Thomas ED: Nonbacterial pneumonia after allogeneic marrow transplantation; a review of ten years' experience. *Rev Infect Dis* 1982; 4: 1119–1132.

72. Buckner CD, Meyers JD, Springmeyer SC, et al.: Pulmonary complications of marrow transplantation: Review of the Seattle experience. *Exp Hematol* 1984; 12(Suppl 15): 1–5.

73. Sullivan KM, Meyers JD, Flournoy N, et al.: Early and late interstitial pneumonia following human bone marrow transplantation. *Int J Cell Cloning* 1986; 4: 107–121.

74. Depledge MH, Barrett A, Powles RL: Lung function after bone marrow grafting. *Int J Radiat Oncol Biol Phys* 1983; 9: 145–151.

75. Springmeyer SC, Flournoy N, Sullivan KM, et al.: Pulmonary function changes in long-term survivors of allogeneic marrow transplantation. In, Gale RP, (ed): *Recent Advances in Bone Marrow Transplantation,* New York, Alan R. Liss, 1983, pp. 343–353.

76. Ralph DD, Springmeyer SC, Sullivan KM, et al.: Rapidly progressive airflow obstruction in marrow transplant recipients: Possible association between obliterative bronchiolitis and chronic graft-vs.-host disease. *Am Rev Respir Dis* 1984; 129: 641–644.

77. Roca J, Granena A, Rodriguez-Roisin R, et al.: Total airway disease in an adult with chronic graft-vs.-host disease. *Thorax* 1982; 37: 77–78.

78. Kurzrock R, Zander A, Kanojia M, et al.: Obstructive lung disease after allogeneic bone marrow transplantation. *Transplantation* 1984; 37: 156–160.

79. Sorenson PG, Ernst P, Panduro J, Moller J: Reduced lung function in leukæmia patients undergoing bone marrow transplantation. *Scand J Hæmatol* 1984; 32: 253–257.

80. Burke CM, Theodore J, Dawkins KD, et al.: Post-transplant obliterative bronchiolitis and other late lung sequelae in human heart-lung transplantation. *Chest* 1984; 86: 824–829.

81. Epler GR, Colby TV, McLoud TC, Carrington CB, Gaensler EA: Bronchiolitis obliterans organizing pneumonia. *N Engl J Med* 1985; 312: 152–158.

82. Clark JG, Schwartz DA, Flournoy N, et al.: Risk factors for airflow obstruction in recipients of bone marrow transplants. *Ann Intern Med* 1987; 107: 648–656.

83. Atkinson K, Clink H, Lawler S, et al.: Encephalopathy following bone marrow transplantation. *Eur J Cancer* 1977; 13: 623–625.

84. Johnson FL, Thomas ED, Clark BS, et al.: A comparison of marrow transplantation with chemotherapy for children with acute lymphoblastic leukemia in second or subsequent remission. *N Engl J Med* 1981; 305: 846–851.
85. Thompson CB, Sanders JE, Flournoy N, et al.: The risks of central nervous system relapse and leukoencephalopathy in patients receiving marrow transplants for acute leukemia. *Blood* 1986; 67: 195–199.
86. Meyers JD, Hansen JA, Anasetti C, et al.: Prophylactic use of human leukocyte interferon after allogeneic marrow transplantation. *Ann Intern Med* 1987; 107: 809–816.
87. Bleyer WA: Neurologic sequelae of methotrexate and ionizing radiation: a new classification. *Cancer Treat Rep* 1981; 65(Suppl 1): 89–98.
88. Sullivan KM, Storb R, Shulman HM, et al.: Immediate and delayed neurotoxicity after mechlorethamine preparation for bone marrow transplantation. *Ann Intern Med* 1982; 97: 182–189.
89. Deeg JH, Flournoy N, Sullivan KM, et al.: Cataracts after total body irradiation and marrow transplantation: A sparing effect of dose fractionation. *Int J Radiat Oncol Biol Phys* 1984; 10: 957–964.
90. Prentice RL, Kato H, Yashimoto K, Mason M: Radiation exposure and thyroid cancer incidence among Hiroshima and Nagasaki residents. *Natl Cancer Inst Monogr* 1982; 62: 207–212.
91. Fleming ID, Black TL, Thompson EI, et al.: Thyroid dysfunction and neoplasia in children receiving neck irradiation for cancer. *Cancer* 1985; 55: 1190–1194.
92. Sklar CA, Kim TH, Ramsay NKC: Thyroid dysfunction among long-term survivors of bone marrow transplant. *Am J Med* 1982; 73: 688–694.
93. Sanders JE, Pritchard S, Mahoney P, et al.: Growth and development following marrow transplantation for leukemia. *Blood* 1986; 68: 1129–1135.
94. Warne GL, Fairley FK, Hobbs JB, et al.: Cyclophosphamide-induced ovarian failure. *N Engl J Med* 1973; 289: 1159–1162.
95. Schilsky PR, Lewis BW, Sherins RJ, et al.: Gonadal dysfunction in patients requiring chemotherapy for cancer. *Ann Intern Med* 1980; 93: 109–114.
96. Sanders J, and the Seattle Marrow Transplant Group: Eleven years of marrow transplantation for children with aplastic anemia. *Blood* 1982; 60(Suppl 5): 1972a (Abstract).
97. Sanders JE, Buckner CD, Leonard JM, et al.: Late effects on gonadal function of cyclophosphamide, total body irradiation, and marrow transplantation. *Transplantation* 1983; 36: 252–255.
98. Sanders JE, Buckner CD, Amos D, et al.: Ovarian function following marrow transplantation for aplastic anemia or leukemia. *J Clin Oncol* 1988;6:813–818.
99. Jacobs P, Dubovsky DW: Bone marrow transplantation followed by normal pregnancy. *Am J Hematol* 1981; 11: 209–212.
100. Card RT, Holmes IH, Sugarman RG, et al.: Successful pregnancy after high-dose chemotherapy and marrow transplantation for treatment of aplastic anemia. *Exp Hematol* 1980; 8: 57–60.
101. Deeg HJ, Kennedy MS, Sanders JE, Thomas ED, Storb R: Successful pregnancy after marrow transplantation for severe aplastic anemia and immunosuppression with cyclosporine. *JAMA* 1983; 250: 647.
102. Hinterberger-Fischer M, Hinterberger W, Kos M, et al.: Three successful pregnancies and deliveries after bone marrow transplantation for severe aplastic anemia (SAA). European Cooperative Group for Bone Marrow Transplantation XIII Annual Meeting of the EBMT and III Annual Meeting EBMT Nurses Group. March 1–5, 1987, 58: 59, (abstr).
103. Schmidt H, Ehninger G, Dopfer R, et al.: Pregnancy after bone marrow transplantation for severe aplastic anemia. *Bone Marrow Transplantation* 1987; 2: 329–332.
104. Lushbaugh CC, Casarett GW: The effects of gonadal irradiation in clinical radiation therapy: A review. *Cancer* 1976; 37: 1111–1125.
105. Rowley MJ, Leach DR, Warner GA, et al.: Effect of graded doses of ionizing radiation on the human testis. *Radiat Res* 1974; 59: 665–678.
106. Richards GE, Wara WM, Grumbach MM, et al.: Delayed onset hypopituitarism: Sequelae of therapeutic irradiation of central nervous system, eye, and middle ear tumors. *J Pediatr* 1976; 89: 553–559.

107. Oliff A, Bode U, Bercu BB, et al.: Hypothalamic-pituitary dysfunction following CNS prophylaxis in acute lymphocytic leukemia: Correlation with CT scan abnormalities. *Med Pediatr Oncol* 1979; 7: 141–151.
108. Romshe CA, Zipf WB, Miser A, et al.: Evaluation of growth hormone release and human growth hormone treatment in children with cranial irradiation-associated short stature. *J Pediatr* 1984; 104: 177.
109. Griffin NK, Wadsworth J: Effect of treatment of malignant disease on growth in children. *Arch Dis Child* 1980; 55: 600–603.
110. Inati A, Sallan SE, Cassady JR, et al.: Efficacy and morbidity of central nervous system "prophylaxis" in childhood acute lymphoblastic leukemia: Eight years' experience with cranial irradiation and intrathecal methotrexate. *Blood* 1983; 61: 297.
111. Shalet SM, Beardwell CG, Pearson D, et al.: The effect of varying doses of cerebral irradiation on growth hormone production in childhood. *Clin Endocrinol* 1976; 5: 287–290.
112. Cole LJ, Nowell PC: Parental-F_1 hybrid bone marrow chimeras: High incidence of donor-type lymphomas. *Proc Soc Exp Biol Med* 1970; 134: 653–657.
113. Gleichmann E, Gleichmann H, Schwartz RS, et al.: Immunologic induction of malignant lymphoma. Identification of donor and host tumors in the graft-vs.-host model. *J Natl Cancer Inst* 1975; 54: 107–116.
114. Deeg HJ, Prentice R, Fritz TE, et al.: Increased incidence of malignant tumors in dogs after total body irradiation and marrow transplantation. *Int J Radiat Oncol Biol Phys* 1983; 9: 1505–1511.
115. Broerse JJ, Hollander CR, Van Zwieten MJ: Tumour induction in rhesus monkeys after total body irradiation with X-rays and fission neutrons. *Int J Radiat Biol* 1981; 40: 671–676.
116. Fialkow PJ, Thomas ED, Bryant JI, et al.: Leukæmic transformation of engrafted human marrow cells *in vivo*. *Lancet* 1971; 1: 251–255.
117. Thomas ED, Bryant JI, Buckner CD, et al.: Leukæmic transformation of engrafted human marrow cells *in vivo*. *Lancet* 1972; 1: 1310–1313.
118. Goh K, Klemperer MR: *In vivo* leukemic transformation: cytogenetic evidence of *in vivo* leukemic transformation of engrafted marrow cells. *Am J Hematol* 1977; 2: 283–290.
119. Elfenbein GJ, Brogaonkar DS, Bias WB, et al.: Cytogenetic evidence for recurrence of acute myelogenous leukemia after allogeneic bone marrow transplantation in donor hematopoietic cells. *Blood* 1978; 52: 627–636.
120. Newburger PE, Latt SA, Pesando JM, et al.: Leukemia relapse in donor cells after allogeneic bone marrow transplantation. *N Engl J Med* 1981; 304: 712–714.
121. Bloom RE, Dinsmore R, O'Reilly RJ, et al.: B-cell lymphoma of host origin in a marrow transplant (BMT) recipient in remission of acute myeloid leukemia. *Blood* 1982; 60(Suppl 1): 165a (Abstract).
122. Gossett TC, Gale RP, Fleischman H, et al.: Immunoblastic sarcoma in donor cells after bone marrow transplantation. *N Engl J Med* 1979; 300: 904–907.
123. Serota FT, Burkey ED, August CS, D'Angio GJ: Total body irradiation: Single vs. fractionated exposure as preparation for bone marrow transplantation in treatment of acute leukemia and aplastic anemia. *Int J Radiat Oncol Biol Phys* 1983; 9: 1941–1949.
124. Schubach WH, Hackman R, Neiman PE, et al.: A monoclonal immunoblastic sarcoma in donor cells bearing Epstein-Barr virus genomes following allogeneic marrow grafting for acute lymphoblastic leukemia. *Blood* 1982; 60: 180–187.
125. Sanders JE, Sale GE, Ramberg R, et al.: Glioblastoma multiforme in a patient with acute lymphoblastic leukemia who received a marrow transplant. *Transplant Proc* 1982; 14: 770–774.
126. Witherspoon RP, Schubach W, Neiman P, et al.: Donor cell leukemia developing six years after marrow grafting for acute leukemia. *Blood* 1985; 65: 1172–1174.
127. Deeg HJ, Sanders J, Martin P, et al.: Secondary malignancies after marrow transplantation. *Exp Hematol* 1984; 12: 660–666.
128. Smith JL, Heerema NA, Provisor A: Leukemic transformation of engrafted bone marrow cells. *Br J Hæmatol* 1985; 60: 415–422.
129. Klingemann H-G, Storb R, Sanders J, et al.: Acute lymphoblastic leukæmia after bone marrow transplantation for aplastic anæmia. *Br J Hæmatol* 1986; 63: 47–50.
130. Martin PJ, Shulman HM, Schubach WH, et al.: Fatal Epstein-Barr virus-associated prolif-

eration of donor B cells after treatment of acute graft-vs.-host disease with a murine monoclonal anti-T-cell antibody. *Ann Intern Med* 1984; 101: 310–315.

131. Zutter MM, Loughran T, Martin PJ, et al.: T-cell lymphoproliferation after bone marrow transplantation. *Blood* 1987; 70(Suppl 1): 1122a (Abstract).

132. Zutter MM, Martin PJ, Sale GE, et al.: Epstein-Barr lymphoproliferation after bone marrow transplantation. *Blood* 1987; 70(Suppl 1): 1123a (Abstract).

133. Tsoi M-S, Warren RP, Storb R, et al.: Autologous marrow recovery and sensitization to non-HLA antigens after HLA-identical marrow transplantation for aplastic anemia. *Exp Hematol* 1983; 11: 73–81.

134. Storb R, Weiden PL, Sullivan KM, et al.: Second marrow transplants in patients with aplastic anemia rejecting the first graft: Use of a conditioning regimen including cyclophosphamide and antithymocyte globulin. *Blood* 1987; 70: 116–121.

135. Doney KC, Torok-Storb B, Dahlberg S, et al.: Immunosuppressive therapy of severe aplastic anemia. In, Young NS, Levine AS, Humphries RK, (eds): *Aplastic Anemia: Stem Cell Biology and Advances in Treatment,* New York, Alan R. Liss, 1984, pp. 259–270.

136. Witherspoon RP, Buckner CD, Thomas ED, et al.: Results of allogeneic marrow transplantation in patients transplanted for acute leukemia: A long-term follow-up. In, Hagenbeek A, Lowenberg B, (eds): *Minimal Residual Disease in Acute Leukemia,* Dordrecht, Martinus Nijhoff, 1986, pp. 318–322.

137. Sanders JE, Thomas ED, Buckner CD, et al.: Marrow transplantation for children in first remission of acute nonlymphoblastic leukemia: An update. *Blood* 1985; 66: 460–462.

138. Sanders JE, Thomas ED, Buckner CD, Doney K: Marrow transplantation for children with acute lymphoblastic leukemia in second remission. (Concise Report) *Blood* 1987; 70: 324–326.

139. Feig SA, Nesbit ME, Buckley J, et al.: Bone marrow transplantation for acute nonlymphocytic leukemia: A report of 67 children transplanted in first remission. *Bone Marrow Transplantation* 1987; 2: 365–374.

140. Brochstein JA, Kernan NA, Groshen S, et al.: Allogeneic bone marrow transplantation after hyperfractionated total body irradiation and cyclophosphamide in children with acute leukemia. *NEJM* 1987; 317: 1618–1624.

141. Woods WW, Nesbit ME, Ramsay NKC, et al.: Intensive therapy followed by bone marrow transplantation for patients with acute lymphoblastic leukemia in second or subsequent remission: Determination of prognostic factors. *Blood* 1983; 61: 1182–1189.

142. Sanders JE, Thomas ED, Buckner CD, et al.: Marrow transplantation for children in first remission of acute nonlymphoblastic leukemia: An update. *Blood* 1985; 66: 460–462.

143. Weisdorf DJ, Nesbit ME, Ramsay NKC, et al.: Allogeneic bone marrow transplantation for acute lymphoblastic leukemia in remission: Prolonged survival associated with acute graft-vs.-host disease. *J Clin Oncol* 1987; 5: 1348–1355.

144. Zwaan FE, Hermans J, Barrett AJ, et al.: Bone marrow transplantation for acute lymphoblastic leukemia: A survey of the European Group for bone marrow transplantation (E.G.B.M.T.). *Br J Hæmatol* 1984; 58: 33–42.

145. Thomas ED, Clift RA, Fefer A, et al.: Marrow transplantation for the treatment of chronic myelogenous leukemia. *Ann Intern Med* 1986; 104: 155–163.

146. Wright SE, Thomas ED, Buckner CD, et al.: Experience with second marrow transplants. *Exp Hematol* 1976; 4: 221–226.

147. Champlin RE, Ho WG, Lenarsky C, et al.: Successful second bone marrow transplants for acute myelogenous leukemia or acute lymphoblastic leukemia. *Transplant Proc* 1985; 17: 496–499.

148. Atkinson K, Biggs J, Concannon A, et al.: Second marrow transplants for recurrence of hematological malignancy. *Bone Marrow Transplantation* 1986; 1: 159–166.

149. Sanders JE, Buckner CD, Clift RA, et al.: Second marrow transplants in patients with leukemia who relapse after allogeneic marrow transplantation. *Bone Marrow Transplantation* 1988; 3: 11–19.

150. Blume KG, Forman SJ: High dose busulfan/etoposide as a preparative regimen for second bone marrow transplants in hematologic malignancies. *Blut* 1987; 55: 49–53.

151. Santos GW, Tutschka PJ, Brookmeyer R, et al.: Marrow transplantation for acute nonlymphocytic leukemia following treatment with busulfan and cyclophosphamide. *N Engl J Med* 1983; 309: 1347–1353.

152. Sullivan KM, Witherspoon RP, Storb R, et al.: Alternating-day cyclosporine and prednisone for treatment of high-risk chronic graft-vs.-host disease. *Blood*, in press.
153. Barnes DWH, Corp MJ, Loutit JF, Neal FE: Treatment of murine leukæmia with X-rays and homologous bone marrow. *Br Med J* 1956; 11: 626–627.
154. Mathé G, Amiel JL, Schwarzenberg L, et al.: Adoptive immunotherapy of acute leukemia: Experimental and clinical results. *Cancer Res* 1965; 25: 1525–1531.
155. Fefer A, Einstein AB, Cheever MA: Adoptive chemimmunotherapy of cancer in animals: A review of results, principles and problems. *Ann New York Acad Sci* 1976; 277: 492–504.
156. Odom LF, August CS, Githens JH, et al.: Remission of relapsed leukæmia during a graft-vs.-host reaction: A graft-vs.-leukæmia reaction in man? *Lancet* 1978; 2: 537–540.
157. Weiden PL, Flournoy N, Thomas ED, et al.: Antileukemic effect of graft-vs.-host disease in human recipients of allogeneic marrow grafts. *N Engl J Med* 1979; 300: 1068–1073.
158. Weiden PL, Sullivan KM, Flournoy N, et al.: Antileukemic effect of chronic graft-vs.-host disease: Contribution to improved survival after allogeneic marrow transplantation. *N Engl J Med* 1981; 304: 1529–1533.
159. Gale RP: Bone marrow transplantation in acute myelogenous leukemia in first remission: Evidence for an antileukemic effect of graft-vs.-host disease. *Exp Hematol* 1982; 10: 20a (abstract).

Bone Marrow Transplantation in
Children, edited by F. Leonard Johnson
and Carl Pochedly. Raven Press, Ltd.,
New York © 1990.

Ethical and Psychosocial Issues in Bone Marrow Transplantation in Children

Thomas E. Williams

Division of Pediatric Hematology/Oncology, Department of Pediatrics, University of Texas Health Science Center at San Antonio, San Antonio, Texas 78284

Bone marrow transplantation has been proved beneficial to children with aplastic anemia (1,2), acute lymphocytic leukemia in second and subsequent remissions (3), acute myeloblastic leukemia in first remission (4), severe combined immunodeficiency disease (5,6), as well as in a few inherited conditions such as thalassemia and osteopetrosis (7,8). The following discussion deals with the ethical dilemmas and psychosocial issues encountered during allogeneic bone marrow transplantation for such conditions.

However, it will be seen that when allogeneic bone marrow transplantation is used in the therapy of diseases where its benefits remain unclear, these ethical issues become more serious or at least amplified in their complexity. Occasionally the ethical concepts have been embodied in the law. Where illustrative, I will refer to court decisions which addressed them. Also, for the purposes of this review, infusions of autologous bone marrow are not considered transplantation per se and will not be discussed.

ETHICAL DILEMMAS INHERENT IN TRANSPLANTATION PROCEDURES IN CHILDREN

In the aftermath of World War II, the world became aware of the importance of a strict code of medical behavior in medicine. Two principles were sanctified: (1) the autonomy of the individual to act in his or her own best interests, and (2) the requirement that the medical procedure be intended only for therapeutic benefit. Some have argued that justice is a third moral principle that must be included in any discussion of medical ethics and that persons must have access to all medical procedures that may be useful in the diagnosis and treatment of their condition (9). Autonomy and beneficence are now embodied in the informed consent procedures that are the backbone of ethical medical practice in the civilized world.

Much has been written about the doctrine of informed consent. Until recently, few laws or quasi-judicial guidelines addressed the issue of the adequacy of medical informed consent; the issue was apparently allowed to be settled in the adversarial climate of the courts. However, the major components of informed consent are codified in regulations adopted by the Department of Health and Human Services (10), for all federally sponsored research. Rules for informed consent were also specified by the Food and Drug Administration for patients given experimental drugs under an investigational new drug application (11). These guidelines derive in large part from the deliberations of the National Commission for the Protection of Human Subjects of Biomedical and Behavioral Research.

In summary, the three essential elements of informed consent include: (1) a description in layman's terms of the research procedures, their purpose and anticipated duration, and the pain, immediate harm and long-term sequelae if known; (2) a discussion of the potential benefits to the patient and/or others, as well as an effort to make a balanced presentation of the risks and benefits ("risk/benefit ratio"); and (3) an explanation of the therapeutic alternatives. Patients are also told that confidentiality will be maintained and that they may withdraw their consent at any time without prejudice to their future care. In case of injury, patients are told whether compensation, medical attention, or both, is available, and where. If they believe their rights have been violated, they may appeal to the institution's committee on the protection of human rights, which is usually a subcommittee of the institutional review board (IRB).

Medical justice, on the other hand, remains elusive, as nations wrestle with their own unique difficulties in the delivery of medical care to their citizenry. Nowhere are the dilemmas raised by these principles more readily apparent than in organ transplantation in children in general and in bone marrow transplantation in particular. While the adequacy of informed consent for any risky medical procedure is a thorny issue for any patient, it is amplified in children where often the decision is made for them by parental proxy. In addition, the rights of a minor donor might appear inherently to be in conflict with ethical principles, because he or she derives no therapeutic benefit from the donation procedure. These concerns are magnified when the benefits of bone marrow transplantation are as yet unproved for the patient's condition. It is unclear whether parents can consent to research for their minor children or if they can give consent on behalf of a minor donor to partake in research from which the child derives no direct benefit. Last, we are confronted with socioeconomic problems which preclude equal access to the therapeutic benefits of bone marrow transplantation or to its potential benefits.

BONE MARROW TRANSPLANTATION FOR DISEASES WHERE THE BENEFITS ARE KNOWN

A close inspection of the diseases amenable to allogeneic bone marrow transplantation reveals that they are all conditions whose prognosis was considered hopeless before the advent of bone marrow transplantation. Most of these diseases have been the subject of randomized and controlled trials which demonstrated the superiority of bone marrow transplantation over other treatment methods (1,3). Nonetheless, as noted in other chapters of this book, allogeneic bone marrow transplantation remains a rigorous procedure with many complications which are not preventable and for which therapy is often ineffective. The explanation to the patient and family of the procedure's attendant risks and the relative merits of alternative therapies is a considerable undertaking. The transplant team must often devote many hours to this task in order to insure adequacy of informed consent.

Some bone marrow transplantation centers have developed a standard procedure for obtaining informed consent. In many hospitals a medical ethics committee acts to consult with physicians and other members of the bone marrow transplant team when complex issues relating to consent are encountered (12–14). The committee is usually composed of doctors, nurses, lawyers, ministers, ethicists and other laypersons from various walks of life. Their recommendations are seldom binding, but are usually highly respected. If substantial disagreement about a particular course of action is encountered between the committee and the parents, or between the committee and the medical staff, the courts, through appointed child advocates or guardians *ad litum,* are asked to resolve the issue.

Some centers argue that the patient's pediatric hematologist/oncologist, if he or she is also a member of the bone marrow transplant team, may be biased in favor of bone marrow transplantation. To counter this bias, another knowledgeable but uninvolved physician, that is, one uninvolved from the point of view of direct care of the patient, is asked to explain the procedures and to be sure that the patient and parents have adequately understood the information. Because it is felt that parents cannot divorce themselves from their desire to find a cure at any price, some centers provide for a guardian *ad litum* to act in the best interest of the patient. For similar reasons, bone marrow transplant centers also provide child advocates for the minor donor, to explain the risk of being a donor. In their desire to find a cure for their afflicted child, it is possible that parents may underestimate the risks to the donor and thus misinform their child-donor.

It is generally agreed that it is appropriate to obtain assent from the minor patient and child-donor. It is accepted that a child may be too young to understand the risks and potential benefits to the same degree as an adult. Nonetheless, efforts should be made to inform the child and to document his or her level of understanding. While there is no uniformity of opinion on this point, the age at which the child has attained a sufficient level of cognitive development that would permit sufficient understanding ranges from 7 to 10 years (15).

Despite the rarity of serious complications following bone marrow donation, no one has ever been compelled to donate their bone marrow. Notable is the case of Robert McFall. This was a patient with aplastic anemia whose histocompatible cousin decided to withdraw implied consent for bone marrow donation. The cousin's refusal to be a bone marrow donor was upheld by the court (16). More recently, a leukemia patient, who accidentally learned that an unrelated person was a potential histocompatible donor, was denied the right to contact that person directly (17).

ETHICAL ISSUES ARISING WHEN BONE MARROW TRANSPLANTATION IS A COMPONENT OF A THERAPEUTIC RESEARCH PROGRAM

All of the foregoing concerns are relevant to the situation in which the bone marrow transplant procedure is part of a research program. However, the issues are further complicated by the unknowns and uncertainties that are attendant on research endeavors (18).

Nearly all bone marrow transplantations are performed at research hospitals or academic medical centers which have federally mandated institutional review boards (IRBs). It might be assumed that these bodies are unbiased peer review groups. In addition to researchers, most institutional review boards have lawyers and laypersons who could be expected to act in the best interest of the child. However, the board seldom reviews the medical history of an individual child before the research is conducted. The instruments of the IRB are the informed consent document and the patient eligibility criteria of the research protocol. It does not act *in loco parentis* (in place of the parents). The informed consent document is executed by 2 parties, the parents and the researcher, who may not be unbiased. The parents, because of their concern for the life of their child, may be driven to accept certain risks that a "disinterested" guardian might find unacceptable. The research physician may be biased because he or she is driven by the desire to serve future generations of sick children and by the need for personal achievement in medical research (19). One might even ask whether institutional review boards can be considered to be truly impartial, since most boards are weighted in their membership with individuals who are members of the research institution or hospital. The notoriety and financial fortunes of these individuals may be dependent upon the successful completion of clinical research.

To avoid these potential conflicts of interests, a number of approaches have been suggested. Ethics committees or ethics review committees have been developed in many hospitals, but few have addressed specific issues regarding research involving bone marrow transplantation or cancer research in children in general (20). Another suggestion is a court-appointed guardian *ad litum* to act in the interest of the child patient, or, in some instances, to act in the interest of the "captive" donor (21). Until recently, the court has not sought to override parental consent, but instead, interposes itself only to be certain that the consent or unwillingness to consent was made under the best circumstances possible. Consent must have been given free from duress, and the child patient or child donor must be adequately informed. Some court-appointed child advocates or guardians have assumed that their role is to make medical judgments; other assume that their role is to assure the court that there is strict adherence to all legal procedures.

On the other hand, other court-appointed child advocates have favored a particular position for or against the research, choosing to base their judgments upon an admixture of medical, legal and ethical considerations. Still others have abstained from giving their opinions as to whether or not the research is in the best interests of the patient. Instead, they maintain the position that their role is to assure the court that all facts pertinent to that judgment are before the court. Moreover, in at least one bone marrow transplantation center the court-appointed child advocate does not necessarily have an extensive medical or legal background. In place of this, the appointee is particularly familiar with child custodial procedures, such as those arising from adoption, divorce and child abuse. Nonetheless, the child advocate has been appointed to judge *inter alia* whether, as the transplant physician maintains, transplantation is preferable to alternate therapy. Also, the medical risks, such as general anesthesia and blood loss, must be deemed acceptable. In addition, the child advocate must rule that the parents and research subject have given their consent after being fully informed of the risks and benefits, and that the consent was not given under duress.

The child advocate is assisted, in large measure, by prior extensive medical and psychosocial evaluations, as well as by peer review of those evaluations. Thus, the court appointee can often attest to the adequacy of informed consent after interviews and a brief review of the documentation.

The view that there is an inherent conflict of interest in the position of those who are parents of the research subject is not evident in *Hart vs. Brown*. The Harts sought to allow a kidney transplantation between their identical twin daughters. In approving their request, the court appeared to be influenced by the fact that a kidney transplantation from a completely histocompatible sibling was more likely to be successful than a graft from a less histocompatible relative. The court was also influenced by the likelihood of an adverse emotional effect on the donor, who in later life might feel guilty if not allowed to donate her kidney (22).

PSYCHOSOCIAL ASPECTS OF BONE MARROW TRANSPLANTATION

The "price" of bone marrow transplantation is high in both psychological (23) and socioeconomic terms. In many transplantation centers the team includes an array of social workers, psychologists, clergymen, patient ombudsmen and financial consultants. Even families burdened by the many arduous experiences encountered during the early part of their child's illness may find it difficult to cope with the rigors of bone marrow transplantation. Frequently, the only alternative to bone marrow transplantation is a course of less aggressive, noncurative therapy that will eventually lead to death. Bone marrow transplantation may be the last remaining hope of a cure for the disease. Nonetheless, patients may be less able to cope with the relative isolation of the transplant unit or the painful diagnostic procedures that they heretofore had been able to tolerate. The use of indwelling venous access devices and hyperalimentation have softened, somewhat, the difficulties associated with frequent blood tests and the occurrence of mucositis, but the patient may balk at the prospect of having more frequent bone marrow biopsies.

Family disruption is often accentuated by the fact that one parent is usually at the bedside. The transplant center may be far from home, sometimes thousands of miles away. Nonetheless, most centers provide for a home-away-from-home, such as a Ronald McDonald House or other suitable lodging, in the vicinity of the hospital. Family disruption may aggravate preexisting sibling rivalries since the time spent away from home by the parents may be 3 months or more. Or the guilt experienced by a sibling may be enhanced by the death of the patient, particularly if the sibling were the donor of the bone marrow that failed to cure the patient.

Bone marrow transplantation is expensive in economic terms as well; medical services alone may often exceed $100,000 (24). The living expenses for donor and parents while away from home usually inflates the costs more. Needless to say, few families can afford a bone marrow transplant from personal savings; they must depend on third-party payers if the procedure is to be available at all. Those patients fortunate enough to have health insurance policies which will cover the cost of bone marrow transplantation are welcome at transplant centers. However, some third-party payers will not approve bone marrow transplantation. Some government medical assistance programs will not approve bone marrow transplantation.

SUMMARY

Bone marrow transplantation is one of many new medical technologies that have raised complex ethical and psychosocial issues. A planned dialogue among members of numerous disciplines will enhance the development of bone marrow transplantation. Public policy concerning bone marrow transplantation must be shaped by the leveling influence that the medical profession can bring to such discussions, and physicians must take the initiative to lay the foundations for such dialogues. It is hoped that these discussions will help enhance, and not impede, the application of bone marrow transplantation to more children.

REFERENCES

1. Camitta BM, Thomas ED, Nathan DG, et al.: A prospective study of androgens and bone marrow transplantation for treatment of severe aplastic anemia. *Blood* 1979;53:504–514.
2. Barrett AJ: Allogeneic bone marrow transplantation for severe aplastic anemia, the London experience. *Clin Lab Hæmatol* 1979;1(2):95–107.
3. Johnson FL, Thomas ED, Clark BS, et al.: A comparison of marrow transplantation with chemotherapy for children with acute lymphoblastic leukemia in second or subsequent remission. *N Engl J Med* 1981;305:846–851.
4. Dinsmore R, et al.: Allogeneic bone marrow transplantation patients with acute nonlymphocytic leukemia. *Blood* 1984;63(3):649–656.
5. Bortin MM, Rimm AA: Severe combined immunodeficiency disease; characterization of the disease and results of transplantation. *JAMA* 1977;238:591–600.
6. O'Reilly RJ, Kapoor N, Pollack M, et al.: Reconstitution of immunologic function in a patient with severe combined immunodeficiency following transplantation of marrow from an HLA-A,B,C nonidentical but MLC-compatible paternal donor. *Transplant Proc* 1978; 11:1934–1937.
7. Coccia PF, Krivit W, Cervenka J, et al.: Successful bone marrow transplantation for infantile malignant osteopetrosis. *N Engl J Med* 1980;302:701–708.
8. Spruce WE: Bone marrow transplantation, II. Use for aplastic anemia, hereditary diseases, and hemoglobinopathies. *AM J Pediatr Hematol/Oncol* 1983;5(3):295–300.
9. Moskop JC: Organ transplantation in children; ethical issues. *J Pediatr* 1987;10(2):175–180.
10. *Federal Register* 46 (January 26):8366(1981).
11. *Federal Register* 43 (August 8):35.186(1978).
12. Robinson RJ: Ethics committees and research in children (editorial). *Br Med J (Clin Res)* May 16, 1987;294(6582):1243–1244.
13. Treatment decisions for infants and children. Bioethics Committee. Canadian Pediatric Society. *Can Med Assoc J* 1986;135(5):447–448.
14. Cross AW, Churchill LR: Pediatric ethics committees; learning from our experience (editorial). *J Pediatr* 1986;108:242–243.
15. Verzemnieks IL, Nash D: Ethical issues related to pediatric care. *Nurs Clin N Am* 1984;19(2):319–328.
16. Culliton BJ: Courts uphold refusal to be medical good samaritan. *Science* 1978;201:596–597.
17. Caplan A, Lidz CW, Meisel A, et al.: Mrs. X and the bone marrow transplant. *Hastings Center Report* 1983;13(3):17–19.
18. Pearn JH: The child and clinical research. *Lancet* (Sep. 1) 1984;2(8401):510–512.

19. Quadggin A: Do doctors consider the risks in research involving children? *Can Med Assoc J* 1987;136(2):189–191.
20. British Pediatrics Association: Guidelines to aid ethical committees considering research involving children. *Arch Dis Child* 1980;55:75–77.
21. Serota FT, August CS, O'Shea AT, et al.: role of a child advocate in the selection of donors for pediatric bone marrow transplantation. *J Pediatr* 1981;98:847–850.
22. *Hart vs. Brown*, 289 A.2d 386 (Connecticut, 1972).
23. Gardner GG, et al.: Psychological issues in bone marrow transplantation. *Pediatrics* 1977;60:625–631.
24. Kay HE, et al.: Cost of bone marrow transplants in acute myeloid leukemia. *Lancet* (May 17) 1980;1(8177):1067–9.

Bone Marrow Transplantation in Children, edited by F. Leonard Johnson and Carl Pochedly. Raven Press, Ltd., New York © 1990.

Bone Marrow Transplantation: Future Prospects

Robert A. Good

Department of Pediatrics, University of South Florida, St. Petersburg, Florida 33701

Introduction
A. Making marrow transplantation safer
B. Broader uses of BMT in treatment of more diseases
C. Marrow transplantation as an outpatient procedure
Summary

INTRODUCTION

In the 20 years that have passed since our first successful marrow transplantation to cure a child with otherwise fatal severe combined immunodeficiency disease (SCID), more than 60 otherwise lethal diseases have been cured using bone marrow transplantation (1,2). These diseases include at least 12 different forms of primary genetically determined immunodeficiency, at least 8 separate forms of aplastic anemia, as many as 15 different forms of high-risk leukemia, several different inborn errors of metabolism, a number of different hematopoietic disorders, and several different forms of cancer. The oldest of the many children we cured of SCID have now passed their twenty-first birthdays. For the first time, such children have been able to grow up and to come of age.

Following these initial successes in treatment of SCID, the greatest impetus to the use of allogenic marrow transplantation has come from the efforts of the group led by E. Donall Thomas. They used marrow transplantation after lethal total body irradiation and cyclophosphamide in the treatment of patients with high-risk leukemias (3). Allogeneic bone marrow transplantation, which is often imbued with an almost ritualistic technology, is being applied to an increasing number of malignant diseases (4). Autologous marrow transplantation, with or without purging of cancer cells from the patient's marrow, represents another somewhat specialized modality of therapy. This technique permits irradiation and chemotherapy to be used in larger and otherwise potentially lethal doses. With such treatment, perhaps more cancers will be cured (5).

MAKING MARROW TRANSPLANTATION SAFER

As bone marrow transplantation has become more widely used, the difficulties that severely limited its application and caused a forbiddingly high mortality rate associated with the procedure are being overcome one by one. Major progress in technique has made bone marrow transplantation, once a most hazardous undertaking, a much less hazardous procedure.

Several practical adaptations have been particularly effective in reducing morbidity and mortality of allogeneic bone marrow transplantation. These include the use of laminar airflow isolation along with gut and skin decontamination; microbial monitoring of transplant patients; and early antimicrobial antibiotic and chemotherapy of bacterial, fungal and certain viral infections when these are suspected (6). We have learned which microorganisms are likely to cause clinical trouble at certain intervals after marrow transplantation. Thus, early and anticipatory treatment is often indicated and effective.

Antibody deficiencies as well as other rather broadly based cellular immunodeficiencies are regularly present in the lethally irradiated bone marrow transplant patients for variable, usually prolonged, intervals following marrow transplantation. In this context, effective prophylaxis against high-grade encapsulated bacterial pathogens and certain viruses can be achieved by intravenous administration in replacement dosages of these immunoglobulin preparations which contain many antibodies.

Large doses of intravenous immunoglobulin (IVIG) preparations, especially large doses of IVIG that contain high titers of antibody against cytomegalovirus (CMV), have been shown to be effective in preventing CMV pneumonitis which often complicates active cytomegalovirus infections in bone marrow transplantation patients (7,8). Ganciclovir has been used with apparent benefit along with intravenous immunoglobulin in large doses to treat complicating infections due to CMV (9). Ganciclovir (DHPG) may have increasing usefulness if given along with high-titered anti-CMV immunoglobulin in patients with CMV infections of the gastrointestinal tract, including those of the liver.

Use of acyclovir in a prophylaxis regimen during those periods following bone marrow transplantation, when Herpes simplex virus infections are likely to be reactivated, has proved helpful in preventing severe Herpes simplex infection in patients who are seropositive for the Herpes simplex viruses (10).

Early and intensive treatment with acyclovir by the intravenous route has been proved to be an effective treatment of otherwise highly lethal complicating varicella zoster infections (11). In this regard, it has been observed that it is sometimes necessary to treat complicating varicella zoster infections in these immunodeficient patients with doses of acyclovir considerably higher than the recommended dosage of 1500 $mg/m^2/day$ intravenously. Dosages as high as 2500 $mg/m^2/day$ may sometimes be indicated (12).

Studies of the use of ganciclovir and intravenous immunoglobulin as prophylaxis in selected bone marrow transplantation patients must still be evaluated in randomized trials. However, clinical observations point to the urgent need for such trials of both IVIG and newer antivirals as they are developed. Oral administration of immunoglobulins given in large doses in patients who have undergone bone marrow transplantation provide antibodies of the IgG class throughout the gastrointestinal tract. Trials are already underway to evaluate the effectiveness of such passive immunoprophylaxis and immunotherapy to reduce complicating viral and bacterial infections (13). IVIG prophylaxis has almost completely eliminated the complicating infections with high-grade intracellular bacterial pathogens such as *Streptococcus pneumoniae, Hemophilus influenzae B, Neisseria meningitidis,* and *Streptococcus pyogenes.* This approach may also have reduced complications due to infections with Pseudomonas. We now rarely see in marrow transplantation units the previously forbidding pulmonary infection with *Pneumocystis carinii.* This is because we employ highly effective prophylaxis with trimethoprim-sulfamethoxazole or pentamidine (14) given by the inhalation route.

When measures such as the latter are used, and when the irradiation dosage to the lungs is reduced by lung shielding and also by fractionation of the irradiation dosage, the incidence of idiopathic interstitial pneumonitis is decreased (15,16). Thus, when a matched sibling donor is available for bone marrow transplantation, this previously life-threatening procedure can be used to cure otherwise lethal diseases while incurring risks of treatment-associated morbidity and mortality that are quite acceptable.

Twenty years have now elapsed since we performed our first successful bone marrow transplant using a matched sibling donor to cure X-linked severe combined immunodeficiency disease and to correct a complicating aplastic anemia. This achievement was followed almost immediately by a partial success in treating a patient with Wiskott-Aldrich syndrome and to cure successfully a patient with an autosomal recessive form of SCID. Since these beginnings, we have witnessed a logarithmic growth of both the indications for use of marrow transplantation and in the numbers of bone marrow transplants, so that more than 10,000 marrow transplants have been performed. In recent years, the most serious limitations to the use of marrow transplantation have been: (1) the slow rate of hematopoietic recovery, and the slowness of immunologic recovery following bone marrow transplantation; (2) the lack of availability of a suitably matched sibling donor for the marrow transplant, a good match being available only 30 to 40% of the time; and (3) inability to eradicate all the cells of widely disseminated cancers and the prevailing threat of graft-vs.-host disease.

Exciting approaches to each of these obstacles are now being pursued. Strategies have been devised to solve the problem of lack of a matched sibling donor. These include the use of bone marrow from an MHC-matched donor located by extended study of family members, marrow from a haplo-identical family member, or marrow from a matched or incompletely matched donor from the general population.

The haplo-identical family donor marrow must have been thoroughly purged of unwanted and hazardous T lymphocytes and T precursors that can mature into cells which cause acute and chronic graft-vs.-host disease (17–22). The approach using a haplo-identical donor has already been employed to permit successful treatment of numerous children with SCID who did not have a matched sibling donor (23,24). This purging of the donor's marrow is dependent upon lectin-based agglutination and removal of T cells and T cell precursors. An alternative approach is the application of monoclonal antibody technology (25). Both techniques are being developed and applied in an effort to make a suitable marrow donor available for all patients who need a marrow transplant.

A related approach, which was among the methods that led us to employ purging of haplo-identical marrow donors, was also successfully applied to cure a few children with SCID. This is the use of fetal liver as a source of hematopoietic stem cells. The fetal liver for use in hematopoietic transplantation must be obtained from fetuses less than 14 weeks of gestational age. In experimental systems, development of isolated stem cell transplants and stem cell cultures are beginning to show promise. This direction may be developed much further in the years ahead so that it ultimately may be applied to humans.

Thus far, the lectin separation method applied to haplo-identical marrow transplantation has not been effective in making available bone marrow donors who will serve well for treatment of patients with leukemias, lymphomas and other diseases (26). Although these approaches can be made to work well in treatment and prevention of disseminated malignancies in animals, the maximally tolerated doses of irradiation and cytotoxic chemotherapy given during cytoreduction have curbed their applicability to man. The purged marrow too often fails to engraft, or even when it does engraft, the cancer or leukemia may return or the marrow may be rejected.

Further extensive research in primates or in other large animals will be necessary to develop appropriate methods to allow successful use of the purged marrow technique in man. The purged marrow technique has been used successfully to overcome all major and minor histocompatibility barriers to marrow transplantation in mice. Thus, supralethal irradiation in rodents requires relatively larger doses of irradiation than is used in human marrow transplantation.

Nonetheless, such doses can be used to establish long-lasting chimeras that are tolerant of donor and tolerant also of recipient strains. At the same time, these chimeras are fully reactive and immunologically responsive to tissues and organs of third parties. Such full chimeras have been shown for prolonged periods to be immunoincompetent to a degree. This immunoincompetence has not proved very limiting in specific pathogen-free environments, or when the donor and recipient have been kept in specific pathogen-free environments before transplantation but in conventional environments after transplantation. After very prolonged periods, such fully allogeneic chimeras seem to develop impressive immunoincompetence and may not be nearly so handicapped as has been predicted by the futile early experiments of Zinkernagel (27).

Design of effective regimens for cytoreduction and T cell elimination, to be used in preparation for mismatched human marrow transplantation, seems a realistic goal. But such techniques are not now available.

BROADER USES OF BMT IN TREATMENT OF MORE DISEASES

Bone marrow transplantation has become a most useful approach to treatment of life-threatening human diseases. Indeed, it is now possible to cure more than 60 otherwise lethal diseases by treatment programs which include bone marrow transplantation. It remains for the future to determine how useful such fully allogeneic transplants will be. However, the immunological limitations should not be a problem with haplo-identical donors or more complete matches between donor and recipient. As the methods and techniques used in bone marrow transplantation are refined and simplified, this powerful modality to therapy promises to become an even more important basis for treatment of an increasing number of human diseases.

Marrow transplantation currently represents the medical application of a most demanding and somewhat uncertain scientific technology. Although it is being progressively improved as the causes of failures are identified and eliminated, it still represents a hazardous undertaking. As such, marrow transplantation is still limited largely to treatment of highly lethal diseases and disorders which generally cannot be treated by any other means. The use of recombinant DNA technology and other techniques of molecular biology has resulted in the identification, isolation, purification and production of increasing quantities of hematopoietic and immunologic growth factors, differentiation factors, cytokines and lymphokines. This achievement promises that some day, perhaps very soon, bone marrow transplantation can become much safer and more generally applicable, because the interval from cytoreduction to full hematopoietic reconstruction will be greatly shortened.

Bone marrow transplantation is now limited in application to diseases and conditions that are uniformly fatal or that have a high mortality rate or that carry extreme morbidity. However, I believe that the technology may soon be developed to the point that marrow transplantation can become an outpatient procedure which can safely be applied to treat or cure many more diseases in many more patients than is currently the case. Indeed, from present-day research with experimental animal models, I visualize that there may be a role for bone marrow transplantation or a variant of this approach using defined stem cells or stem cells and stromal cell precursors in treatment of an extremely wide variety of diseases. This would perhaps include diabetes, vascular diseases and disorders, cardiovascular and renal diseases, systemic autoimmune diseases, mesenchymal diseases, and certain inborn errors of metabolism additional to those for which this procedure has already been shown to be corrective. Indeed, bone marrow transplantation may even ultimately be used as a method for introducing resistance genes against cancers which occur in humans, as we have already done in experimental animals (28). This technique, by facilitating induction of immunological tolerance, might facilitate organ, tissue and cellular transplantation and might serve as an initial basis for somatic cell gene therapy. These possibilities no longer seem the remote vision of a daydreamer but may actually be proximate realities.

When appropriate care is taken to use exactly the right preparative regimen for cytoreduction and immunosuppression, it is now possible in experimental systems in rodents to cure many diseases, in addition to those for which marrow transplantation is now used. Diseases now curable in rodents by BMT include juvenile insulin-dependent diabetes mellitus (28–29), and also every one of the genetically determined autoimmune diseases in which it has been tried (30–31). We have already obtained evidence from our experimental work that even certain stages of advanced renal disease can be corrected by bone marrow transplantation. Recent studies report that in an experimental system (e.g., the twitcher mouse), a disease very similar to Krabbe's disease of humans apparently has been cured or arrested by bone marrow transplantation (33,34). Furthermore, it appears that a variety of metabolic and genetically determined disorders of man may be corrected by this means. Krivit (35–36), following the lead of Hobbs (37), has presented impressive evidence that bone marrow transplantation can be used to delay, if not prevent, progression of certain mucopolysaccharidoses and mucolipidoses (see chapter by Krivit in this book). The most impressive responses among the metabolic diseases thus far treated have been in multifocal leukodystrophy.

In addition, by using bone marrow transplantation we have found that one can produce long-lasting immunological tolerance which permits, by a single procedure, both tissue and organ transplantation without causing signs of rejection. This approach and its derivatives may at long last make organ and tissue transplantation possible without need for concomitantly creating immunodeficiency diseases of varying severity as is now the usual practice.

Thus, when we can apply in the clinic those experimental achievements with bone marrow transplantation already possible in animal models, many presently incurable but not immediately fatal diseases and disorders will be effectively addressed. I firmly believe that the results of trials already carried out show that organ transplantations, in the not too distant future, will be done without need for continuous suppression of the vital immune systems (38,39).

MARROW TRANSPLANTATION AS AN OUTPATIENT PROCEDURE

I have been very impressed by the development of the science that involves the defined growth and differentiation factors, in some instances better viewed as the newer growth and differentiation hormones. This new knowledge makes it likely that, within a decade or so, bone marrow transplantation may actually become an outpatient procedure. With rodents, it has always been possible to see impressive hematopoietic and immunologic restoration within 10 days following supralethal irradiation, and to witness almost full recovery of hematopoiesis and immunocompetence within 30 days. When such rapid recovery of the bodily defenses occurs, one can achieve impressive survival rates from marrow transplantation that approach 100 percent in the animal models. Also, the engrafted bone marrow is tolerated in almost 100 percent of cases. Perhaps such tolerance of bone marrow transplantation can also be accomplished in man if it becomes possible to achieve the same rapid correction of the hematopoietic and immunologic deficits produced by myeloablation and immunosuppression. When this is accomplished, many more diseases that are genetically or developmentally intrinsic to the molecules or cells of the bone marrow derived system will be curable.

I am convinced, from the evidence already in hand, that bone marrow transplantation can thus be further developed into a simple and safe therapeutic modality. This will be a great change from its current high technological requirements and attendant risks. Developed in this way, bone marrow transplantation could provide a major technology that would permit us to address many additional diseases for which our current therapeutic and prophylactic approaches are feeble or ineffective. This would include autoimmune diseases, cardiovascular diseases, diabetes mellitus, and many others.

One can even look further along toward the methodologies which ultimately will use cultured marrow stem cell transplantation (40) to treat disease in lieu of allogeneic whole marrow transplantations. Ultimately, use of cultured marrow stem cells could be a point of departure for accomplishing forms of genetic engineering to harness host stem cells as carriers of genes that can be introduced and made to function in somatic cells to correct a number of genetically based diseases.

Yes, we have already come a long way in the first 20 years since the initial successful marrow transplants were accomplished to treat otherwise lethal human diseases. We still have far to go in the development of the art and science of marrow transplantation. We have seen only the bare beginnings.

SUMMARY

Since the two original successful marrow transplants were done to cure both severe combined immunodeficiency disease and an iatrogenic aplastic anemia in the same patient, bone marrow transplantation has experienced a rapid evolution. Indeed, marrow transplantation has already been employed as an effective means of treating and often curing 60 otherwise fatal diseases. These diseases range from numerous different primary immunodeficiency diseases and different forms of aplastic anemia to a variety of metabolic abnormalities, hematopoietic abnormalities, leukemias, lymphomas and other neoplastic diseases. The diseases and disorders for which bone marrow transplantation has been used are conditions for which other treatments remain woefully inadequate.

For bone marrow transplantation, this great progress appears to be only a beginning. Technical advances, improvements in clinical management and ability to cope with the many clinical complications that may be encountered in bone marrow transplantation have led to timely developments of a prophylactic and therapeutic nature which have improved the safety and efficacy of bone marrow transplantation. Thus, we now treat diseases effectively with bone marrow transplants from identical twins, MHC genotypically matched sibling donors, MHC matched relative donors, and completely matched or even imperfectly matched donors located within or outside the family. Progress in development of local registries has led to efforts to develop a national voluntary bone marrow donor program. The early success of these registries promises that ultimately bone marrow transplantation with a reasonably matched donor may become available to anyone in need of a marrow transplant.

Progress in identifying and, by means of gene cloning, production of growth factors, lymphokines and cytokines promises that in the near future reconstitution of bone marrow following myeloablation may be achieved much more rapidly than has yet been possible. With such progress it may not be too soon to begin to explore the usefulness of bone marrow transplantation to treat diseases which, although not lethal, are associated with high morbidity.

In experimental systems, bone marrow transplantation has already been found to provide a dramatic cure for juvenile diabetes in nonobese diabetic mice and also for numerous autoimmune diseases. With the development of safer, more rapid restoration of hematopoietic function following total body irradiation or other forms of myeloablation, bone marrow transplantation may become a viable strategy for treatment of similar highly morbid diseases of man.

Marrow transplantation that produces permanent immunological tolerance of both donor and recipient may also be the basis of, or may become, one of the components useful for induction of long-lasting immunological tolerance. As such, this technique could contribute greatly to bringing the era of organ and tissue transplantation to full fruition.

Finally, progress is being made in identifying and culturing stem cells and stromal cells which may be useful as a basis for cellular engineering or even somatic cell genetic engineering. Perhaps techniques of cellular engineering will be increasingly applied and ultimately somatic cell genetic engineering may become an approach to treatment of many human diseases.

REFERENCES

1. Good RA: Bone marrow transplantation. In, Lockey RF, Bukantz SC (eds): *Fundamentals of Immunology and Allergy*. Philadelphia, W.B. Saunders Company, 1987, pp. 31–152.
2. Good RA, Kapoor N, Reisner Y: Bone marrow transplantation; an expanding approach to treatment of many diseases. *Cell Immunol* 1983;82:36–54.
3. Thomas ED: Bone marrow transplantation. In, Bach FH, Good RA (eds): *Clinical Immunobiology*. New York, Academic Press, 1974, pp. 2–32.
4. Storb R, Deeg HJ, Whitehead J, et al.: Methotrexate and cyclosporine compared with cyclosporine alone for prophylaxis of acute graft-vs.-host disease after marrow transplantation for leukemia. *N Engl J Med* 1986;814:729–735.
5. Bone Marrow Autotransplantation In Man; Report of an International Cooperative Study. *Lancet* 1986;2:960–962.
6. Good RA: Historic aspects of cellular immunology. In, Gallin JI, Fauci AS (eds): *Advances in Host Defense Mechanisms:Lymphoid Cells*, Vol 2. New York, Raven Press, 1983, pp. 1–42.
7. O'Reilly RJ, Reich L, Gold J, et al.: A randomized trial of intravenous hyperimmune globulin for prevention of cytomegalovirus (CMV) infections following marrow transplantation; preliminary results. *Transplant Proc* 1983;15:1405.
8. Winston DJ, Ho WG, Lin CH, et al.: Intravenous immunoglobulin for modification of cytomegalovirus infection associated with bone marrow transplantation; preliminary results of a controlled trial. *Am J Med* 1984; 76(3A):128–133.
9. Arice E, Jordan C, Chace BA, et al.: Ganciclovir treatment of cytomegalovirus disease in transplant recipients and other immunocompromised hosts. *JAMA* 1987;257:3082–3087.
10. Prentice HG: Use of acyclovir for prophylaxis of herpes infections in severely immunocompromised patients. *J Antimicrob Chemother* (Suppl. B). 1983;12:153–159.
11. Kapoor N, Good RA: Bone marrow transplantation in 1985. In, Aiuti F, Rosen F, Cooper MD (eds): *Recent Advances in Primary and Acquired Immunodeficiencies*. New York, Raven Press, 1986, pp. 327–381.
12. Pahwa R, Good RA: Unpublished observations, 1988.
13. Tutschka PJ: Infections and immunodeficiency in bone marrow transplantation. *Pediatr Infect Dis* 7(Suppl):1988; 22–29.
14. Good RA, Kapoor N: Unpublished observations, 1988.
15. Hughes WT: *Pneumocystis carinii* pneumonitis. *N Engl J Med* 1988;317:1021–1023.
16. Hughes WT: Treatment of *Pneumocystis carinii* pneumonia. *The Medical Letter on Drugs and Therapeutics* 1987;29:103–104.
17. Sprent J, Von Boehmer H, Nabholz M: Association of immunity and tolerance to host H-2 determinants in irradiated F_1 hybrid mice reconstituted with bone marrow cells from one parental strain. *J Exp Med* 1975;141:322.
18. von Boehmer H, Sprent J, Nabholz A: Hematopoietic reconstitution obtained in F_1 hybrids by grafting of parental marrow cells. In Dupont B, Good RA (eds): *Immunobiology of Bone Marrow Transplantation*. Grune & Stratton, New York, 1976, pp. 29–32.
19. Onoe K, Fernandes G, Good RA: Humoral and cell-mediated immune responses in fully allogeneic bone marrow chimera in mice. *J Exp Med* 1980;151:115–132.
20. Reisner Y, Itzicovitch L, Meshorer A, Sharon N: Hemopoietic stem cell transplantation using mouse bone marrow and spleen cells fractionated by lectins. *Proc Natl Acad Sci USA* 1978;75:2933–2936.
21. Reisner Y, Kapoor N, Kirkpatrick D, et al.: Transplantation for acute leukemia with HLA-A

and -B nonidentical parental marrow cells fractionated with soybean agglutinin and sheep red blood cells. *Lancet* 1981;2:327.

22. Reisner Y, Kapoor N, Hodes MZ, et al.: Enrichment for CFU-C from murine and human bone marrow using soybean agglutinin. *Blood* 1982;59:360–363.

23. O'Reilly RJ, Kirkpatrick D, Flomenberg N, et al.: Transplantation of hematopoietic cells for lethal congenital immunodeficiencies. *Birth Defects* 1983;19:173–175.

24. Buckley RH, Schiff SE, Sampson HA, et al.: Development of immunity in human severe primary T cell deficiency following haploidentical bone marrow stem cell transplantation. *J Immunol* 1988;136:2398–2407.

25. Ramsay NK, Kersey JH: Bone marrow purging using monoclonal antibodies. *J Clin Immunol* 1988;8:81–88.

26. Kapoor N, Jung L, Bogardis C, et al.: An immunosuppressive, myeloablative preparative regimen adequate for matched sibling transplant, inadequate in histoincompatible, T cell depleted marrow transplant in leukemia. In, *The Fourth International Symposium on Immunological Monitoring of the Transplant Recipient*, 1983, p. 6.

27. Zinkernagel RM, Althage A, Callahan G, Welsh RM: On the immunoincompetence of H-2 incompatible irradiated bone marrow chimeras. *J Immunol* 1980;124:2356.

28. Naji A, Silvers WK, Kimura H, et al.: *Transplant Proc* 1983;15:1424–1426.

29. Ikehara S, Ohtsuki H, Good RA, et al.: Prevention of type I diabetes in nonobese diabetic mice by allogeneic bone marrow transplantation. *Proc Natl Acad Sci USA*. 1985; 82:7743–7747.

30. Ikehara S, Good RA, Nakamura T, et al.: Rationale for bone marrow transplantation in the treatment of autoimmune diseases. *Proc Natl Acad Sci USA* 1985;82:2483–2487.

31. Oyaizu N, Yasumizu R, Miyama-Inaba M, et al.: (NZW $\times$ BXSB)F_1 mouse; a new animal model of idiopathic thrombocytopenia purpura. *J Exp Med.* 1988;167:2017–2022.

32. Ikehara S, Good RA: Unpublished observations, 1988.

33. Hoogerbrugge PM, Suzuki K, et al.: Donor-derived cells in the central nervous system of twitcher mice after bone marrow transplantation. *Science* 1988;239:1035–1038.

34. Suzuki K, Hoogerbrugge PM, Poorthuis BJHM, et al.: The twitcher mouse; central nervous system pathology after bone marrow transplantation *Lab Invest* 1988;58:302–309.

35. Krivit W, Paul N (eds): *Bone Marrow Transplantation for Lysosomal Storage Diseases*. New York, Alan R. Liss, Inc., 1986.

36. Krivit W, Pierpont ME, Ayaz K, et al.: Bone marrow transplantation in the Maroteaux-Lamy syndrome (mucopolysaccharidosis VI). *N Engl J Med* 1984;311:1606.

37. Hobbs JR: Bone marrow transplantation for genetic diseases. *N Eng J Med* 1985;312:1260

38. Nakamura T, Good RA, Yasumizu R, et al.: Successful liver allografts in mice by combination with allogeneic bone marrow transplantation. *Proc Natl Acad Sci USA* 1986; 83:4529–4532.

39. Yasumizu R, Sugiura K, Iwai H, et al.: Treatment of type I diabetes mellitus in nonobese diabetic mice by transplantation of allogeneic bone marrow and pancreatic tissue. *Proc Nat Acad Sci USA* 1987;84:6555–6557.

40. Sugiura K, Inaba M, Ogata H, et al.: Wheat germ agglutinin-positive cells in stem cell enriched fraction of mouse bone marrow have potent natural suppressor activity. *Proc Natl Acad Sci USA*. In press, 1988.

Subject Index

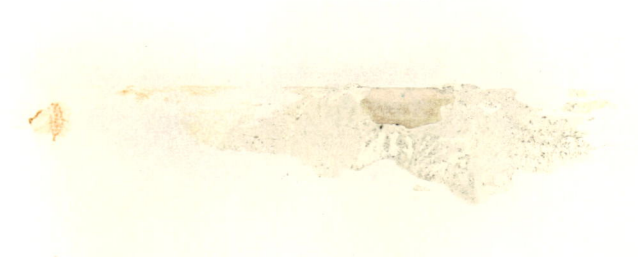